HEALTH
HUMANITIES
READER

HEALTH HUMANITIES
READER

EDITED BY

Therese Jones, Delese Wear, and Lester D. Friedman

ASSISTANT EDITOR

Kathleen Pachucki

RUTGERS UNIVERSITY PRESS
New Brunswick, New Jersey, and London

Fourth paperback printing, 2020

Library of Congress Cataloging-in-Publication Data
Health humanities reader / edited [by] Therese Jones, Delese Wear, and
Lester D. Friedman ; assistant editor Kathleen Pachucki.
    p. ; cm.
Includes bibliographical references and index.
ISBN 978-0-8135-6247-6 (hardcover : alk. paper)
ISBN 978-0-8135-6246-9 (pbk. : alk. paper)
ISBN 978-0-8135-6248-3 (e-book)
I. Jones, Therese, editor of compilation. II. Wear, Delese, editor of
compilation. III. Friedman, Lester D., editor of compilation.
IV. Pachucki, Kathleen, editor of compilation.
[DNLM: 1. Philosophy, Medical. 2. Education, Medical. 3. Health
Personnel—education. 4. Humanities.
W 61]
RA418
362.101—dc23
2013021942

A British Cataloging-in-Publication record for this book is available
from the British Library.

Visit our website: http://rutgerspress.rutgers.edu

Manufactured in the United States of America

CONTENTS

Too Long Too Short

MARK VONNEGUT, MD

As a second-year medical student, I was still trying to do everything perfectly because if I didn't maybe they wouldn't let me be a doctor. I was cutting sutures for a surgeon who was closing after an abdominal procedure.

"Cut."

I tried my best.

"Too long."

"Cut."

I tried again.

"Too short."

And so forth, for the next twenty minutes or so.

"Cut."

"Would you like the next one too short or too long?"

I spent two years as part of the admissions committee at Harvard Medical School. I was surprised by how many applicants had professional-caliber artistic talents. It seemed unfair that these young, gifted applicants could do other things so well. The committee referred to artistic accomplishments as "extras."

The arts are about as extra as breathing. The arts keep you awake and let you make use of your remarkably advantaged point of view.

Well over 90 percent of the time, the diagnosis is in the story—what the patient tells us. The physical exam and imaging and lab tests are mostly done to confirm what we learn from what our patients tell us.

The differential diagnosis is a list of competing narratives.

You need the arts to help you figure out who your patients are. Huck Finn, Lady Chatterley, Willy Loman, and Ophelia, to name just a few, will all come to see you disguised as patients.

There have been many great writers who were also doctors. My favorites are Anton Chekhov and William Carlos Williams.

A writer is not a confectioner, a cosmetic dealer, or an entertainer. He is a man who has signed a contract with his conscience and his sense of duty.
  ANTON CHEKHOV, 1897

The same is true of being a health professional. There's a seriousness about what we do. We're not confectioners, cosmetic dealers, or entertainers, or we're not supposed to be. We're serious observers and students of the human condition, or we're doomed to boredom and falling asleep on the job. We're dedicated to expanding the limits of what medicine can do. We're driven by a conviction that things don't have to be the way they are. We are hopefully useful malcontents who have the power to help, change small things, and be a part of changing bigger things.

A society that gets rid of all its troublemakers goes downhill.
ROBERT A. HEINLEIN, 1973

There's a perception that the arts and sciences are in competition. Sigmund Freud was famous, among other things, for not being able to figure out what women wanted. He was obsessively jealous and worried that his fiancé, Martha, would be—must be—attracted to musicians and artistic types, of which he accused her on a regular basis. How could he, a dogged, 5'7" neurologist compete? Maybe by winning the Nobel Prize for his work on cocaine, a prize that ultimately went to some silly ophthalmologist who noted its anesthetic properties, thus making a long engagement even longer. (The money from the Nobel Prize would have let Freud buy a house and get married.) In spite of the considerable lengths that Martha went to reassure him, he could never believe that the answer to what she wanted was him.

Although he tried always to be a scientist and to bring order to the messy business of what it means to be human, Freud was incapable of leaving the borders of what we know and what we need to know alone. He was eventually awarded a Nobel Prize, but it was for literature because he wrote so beautifully because he had to write to figure out what he thought.

To be a good clinician you have to shut up and let the patient be the most important person in the room. To create the space and opportunity for the patient to tell you what's wrong, you frequently have to refrain from reflexively doing something.

Don't just do something, stand there.
ELVIN SEMRAD, MD, 1954

Nothing in science will teach you how to be quiet, curious, hopeful, or tenacious. Art gives you a way to move forward without knowing exactly where you are going. You have to be open to luck and to what the situation gives you. Without art, you're stuck with yourself the way you are and life as you think it is. If you want to change the world or need to change the world, use art.

I strongly recommend that everyone, but especially health professionals and students, take a shot at making something out of nothing. Whether it's music or painting or writing and regardless of how well it turns out, making art changes the world from one where you can't make art to a world where you can. And maybe it will be beautiful or maybe you can see how to make it better or maybe you can have a conversation with a loved one about it.

And it will make you a better professional and a happier person. Do not believe all that stuff about tortured artists. You should have seen them before they wrote those poems, painted those pictures, wrote those symphonies.

I paint and know other doctors who do as well. Painting has the advantage that you can't possibly make a living at it. I think a lot more about the lines and colors I get wrong than the ones I get right. The principal clinical usefulness of my paintings is that they give nervous patients something to look at and talk about.

"Did you really paint that?"

"Yup."

When I paint I think more clearly. I notice my notes and observations. Things are less repetitive, routine. I connect dots. I write more than "ST TC+ AMOX250TIDX10."

Don't let anyone tell you that it's not about you. It's about you. How honestly you go about the job. How open you are to being taught. How willing you are to be uncomfortable and need more.

The arts grow your soul.

Actively reading good writing is a creative act that can open your world. Writing makes you more genuinely curious and less placated by platitudes. Unless you try to write it out, you don't really know what you think. Freud was amazed to learn what he thought; books' and books' worth that he would never have known about without writing.

If you write, paint, or play music, you change yourself, and you change the world from one where you can't do such a thing to one where you can. It might make you a better health professional, or it might save your life.

How we construct a diagnosis, how we fall short, try again, succeed, and question our successes is exactly how we read or write a story.

History of present illness plucks out salient details from the maelstrom and constructs a story that makes sense—or not. The problem is that you're often expected to write these stories in less time than it takes to wash your face and brush your teeth. Being a health professional means you never have to make stuff up anymore if you don't want to.

A student once asked the French writer, André Gide, if he should try to be writer. "Only if you have to," said Gide.

Study the humanities and the arts as part of your professional training only if you have to. You probably have to.

ACKNOWLEDGMENTS

We deeply appreciate the financial support of the Arnold P. Gold Foundation for this project. We would also like to acknowledge and thank our colleagues/contributors for their outstanding scholarship, brilliant creativity, and unwavering commitment to health humanities education. And finally, we are forever grateful to our cheerful and conscientious assistant editor, Kathy Pachucki.

HEALTH
HUMANITIES
READER

INTRODUCTION

The Why, the What, and the How
of the Medical/Health Humanities

THERESE JONES, DELESE WEAR, AND LESTER D. FRIEDMAN

The delicate balance between biology and culture, as it alters in a continuous flow, is what constitutes the elusive truth of illness.

DAVID MORRIS (1998, 9)

THE WHY

Why introduce and integrate the humanities into science—and clinically based curricula such as medicine, nursing, pharmacy, and allied health programs? Why aren't the scientific basis of knowledge and the apprentice model of training adequate for healthcare practitioners to enter their chosen professions? K. Danner Clouser, the first philosopher to teach ethics at a medical school in the United States, eloquently attempted to answer such questions in a 1980 keynote address at a conference on the role of humanities in health education:

What's missing in a vocational training? . . . It leaves out everything that makes us uniquely human. Where (in a vocational program) do we train for understanding, suffering and joy? Where do we gain ideals and models—for motivations, for patterning our lives, for fashioning our goals, emotions, attitudes, and character? Where do we think about and entertain purposes, goals, and styles of life? Where do we gain perspective on our own life, on others', and the relationships between them? These things don't just happen, however much we like to believe they do.

At the time, Clouser was espousing one of the most commonly advanced political and pedagogical justifications for the still-nascent medical humanities "movement"—the belief that something vital and fundamental was missing in health professions education and that the humanities could fill in those gaps and omissions.

Such ideas and opinions had been simmering since the educational reforms of the 1960s when relatively modest medical schools were dramatically expanding to become vast academic medical centers. In his comprehensive history of American medical education, Kenneth Ludmerer argues that a major consequence of the boom in biomedical research and clinical service across campuses was a diminished focus on student education, what he calls "the forgotten medical student" (1999, 196). With a broad mandate to reform the curriculum, medical educators

1

hurried to incorporate new knowledge and accommodate larger changes affecting clinical practice, such as shifting disease patterns and emerging methods and technologies for diagnosis and treatment (197). However, although biomedical content continued to evolve dramatically, the struggle to encourage student compassion and empathy, to include family and community health needs in addition to those of the individual patient, and to emphasize reasoning and analysis over rote memorization remained remarkably similar in approach to those methods identified throughout the previous century.

With the 1970s came the emergence of seemingly miraculous but morally troubling medical and technological advances such as organ transplantation, standards of death, in vitro fertilization, and complex pharmaceuticals. Educators inserted humanities materials and methodologies into the medical curriculum and clinical practice with the intention of remedying the growing imbalance between the technological aspects of health care and the human aspects of caregiving (Hawkins and McEntyre 2000, 3–4) while, at the same time, radical shifts in the traditional fields of academic study were occurring across the educational landscape. For example, literary criticism, occupied with the intricacies of the reader-writer dyad, excluded social issues, leaving those scholars and educators interested in the cultural or historical context of literature, or in a text's political force, out of step and out of fashion. Described by the literature and medicine scholar Kathryn Montgomery Hunter as the "intellectually underemployed," these disenchanted faculty members, along with a growing cadre of newer scholars interested in interdisciplinary education, were drawn to medical education as fertile ground for their ideas and passions (1991a, 5).

During the inaugural session of the Institute on Human Values in Medicine, physician and ethicist Edmund Pellegrino declared the hope of bringing "some of us in medicine who are concerned with issues involving human values into close discourse with those . . . in the disciplines outside of medicine who have interest in, and perhaps a desire to help us with, the human problems that arise in medicine for the patient and the physicians" (1972, 4). He noted that on almost every medical campus a "subterranean current of interest in exploring potential contributions from the humanities" already existed, a current that has not only remained strong at health sciences centers but has also continued to grow, as the number and quality of programs across the country now demonstrate.

Nothing in the early proceedings and publications of this burgeoning discipline—the medical humanities—suggested a rigid prescription for which areas of academic study should be "invited" into the curriculum, although the usual ones—history, literature, philosophy—were consistently mentioned. In fact, presenters at this first institute session were mindful about casting a wide net to include all humanities disciplines as well as the social sciences, confident and excited about what such a collective and interdisciplinary presence might bring to medical education. Clouser suggested that "each [humanities] discipline should be working to interrelate conceptually with some discipline of the medical world. They should be seeking areas of overlap, where each from its own perspective, methods, and resources can raise questions or shed light to the mutual benefit of both. It is an interdisciplinary enterprise aiming for new insights and understanding" (1972, 50). Yet, then and now, one fundamental question remains: What *particular* knowledge and skills do the humanities disciplines bring to this enterprise of educating healthcare practitioners?

Literature offers a compelling example of how that question can evoke both inventiveness and defensiveness among its practitioners. Over twenty years ago, literature and medicine scholar Anne Hudson Jones (1990) described two major approaches to teaching literature and medicine, each with the same goal of improving patient care. What she calls the *aesthetic* approach focuses on the literary skills of reading, writing, and interpretation for use in medical practice. Joanne Trautmann Banks, the first literature scholar to join the faculty of a medical school in 1972, writes from this orientation in "The Wonders of Literature in Medical Education," the single most important essay in the emerging field. Banks argues that "to teach a student to read *in the fullest sense* is to train him or her medically" (Trautmann [Banks] 1982, 26). She refers to the interpretive skills necessary for the exploration of literary texts that require students to study subtle, ambiguous, and rich detail, to fill in gaps, to understand relationships, to look at "what is being said," and to approach "words in their personal and social contexts and when several things are being said at once" (26). Because medicine is a practice profession that focuses not only on how to do things but also on how to do things better, the imparting and practicing of literary analysis and critical reading has instrumental value by virtue of supplying specific intellectual tools to the multiple dimensions of medicine.

The other approach, also in the service of patient care, has more to do with *moral reflection* rather than with merely introducing medical students to basic literary elements such as point of view, plot, imagery, setting, and narrative stance. This approach engages students with cultural perspectives on health and illness, social justice, and the moral dimensions of patient encounters through literary works that "illuminate a particular set of human experiences and . . . encourage moral reflection in treating patients confronting these experiences" (Hunter et al. 1995, 789). Those favoring this approach often cite the work of philosopher Martha Nussbaum, known for her exploration of literature in developing the moral emotions. In the preface to *Poetic Justice* (1995), she argues that the ability to imagine the concrete ways in which people different from us grapple with their disadvantage can have practical and public value, given the deep prejudice and rampant oppression in the world enacted through sexism, racism, classism, able-ism, homophobia, and ethnic discrimination.

Arising from and enmeshed with Nussbaum's view that attending carefully to the nuances and complexities of literature can sharpen and deepen moral sensibilities is a third approach—the focus on empathy. This approach suggests that studying literature has the potential to enhance a student's ability to understand others' feelings, plights, and values, requiring the reader "to suspend his or her own point of view and enter the reality of another character or another world" (Hunter et al. 1995, 789). However, this approach has become increasingly challenged, particularly when humanities inquiry is tied directly and specifically to the development of humanism and humanistic professionals.

As literary theorist Jonathan Culler (2005) notes, the *human* in *humanities* leads us astray: "The crisis of the humanities might even be linked to the fact that our language proposes a strong link not just between the humanities and the human being but between *humanistic* thinking and even *humane* behavior" (38). Just as medical humanities scholars and educators have become less willing to adapt their research interests and pedagogical practices to the exigencies of clinical practice and medical education over the past forty years, so too have they become less comfortable with the tacit assumption that teaching literature to health professions students is the means of enlightenment *and* empathy. Returning again to Anne Hudson Jones for one of the original articulations of and justifications for the medical humanities in *Literature and Medicine: A Claim for a Discipline* (1984), we see her challenge and caution against any notion that studying the humanities makes one more humane: "This expectation makes me very uncomfortable. This expectation is a burden, not just for literature, for all of the humanities. We all hope that it will [make one more humane], but there have been too many examples to the contrary for me to believe in any guarantee" (32).

Thus, there has been and continues to be a tension between the instrumental justification for the humanities in health professions education, which ostensibly enables and promotes more caring professionals and better caring practices—what physician and bioethicist Jeffrey Bishop (2008) calls the "dose effect" of the humanities (17)—and the intellectual practice of the humanities, which enables and encourages fearless questioning of representations of caregivers and patients in all their varieties, challenges abuses of power and authority, and steadfastly refuses to accept the boundaries that science sets between biology and culture. Increasing numbers of theoretical justifications for humanities in health professions education suggest that the "ethical imperative" of the humanities has been outgrown. As Culler writes, the humanities in any environment, including health care, enable learners to "see situations in another light" (2005, 37)—re-presenting, re-describing, and re-contextualizing—whether it be as humanities scholar or clinical ethicist. Geoffrey Rees calls attention to the "dangerous possibilities organized through collective engagement in the work of the medical humanities" (2010, 277), and medical educator Alan Bleakley predicts that, as a democratizing force, the medical humanities will play a bigger role in health professions education and clinical practice than we might imagine (see chap. 45).

In the next section, we move from questions of rationale—the why—to questions of content—the what: which disciplines or areas of inquiry and what ways of making knowledge constitute the medical humanities or, as it is increasingly known, the *health* humanities.

THE WHAT

The humanities disciplines traditionally represented and integrated in health professions education include history, literature, philosophy, bioethics, and comparative religion as well as those aspects of the social sciences that have humanistic content and employ humanistic methods relevant to medical inquiry and practice, particularly sociology, anthropology, and psychology. The field has been further developed and influenced by such philosophical and pedagogical projects as postmodernism, feminism, disability studies, cultural studies, media studies, and biocultures.

Moreover, the influence of narrative inquiry on the medical/health humanities cannot be overstated, in particular physician and literary scholar Rita Charon's pioneering work in the theoretical development of narrative in medicine. Charon builds on the research of psychiatrist and anthropologist Arthur Kleinman, who writes in *The Illness Narratives: Suffering, Healing, and the Human Condition* (1988) that "the interpretations of narratives of illness ... is a core task in the work of doctoring" (17) as well as on the work of bioethicists such as physician Howard Brody, who introduces the nature, complexities, and rigor of narrative ethics in his book, *Stories of Sickness* (1987).

Arguing that physicians must have the ability to listen to patients' stories, to understand the meanings of such stories, and to be stirred in order to act in support of patients, Charon proposes that narrative competence is what humans use "to absorb, interpret, and respond to stories ... [which] enables the physician to practice medicine with empathy, reflection, professionalism, and trustworthiness. Such a medicine can be called *narrative medicine*" (2001a, 1897). She continues:

Not only medicine but also nursing, law, history, philosophy, anthropology, sociology, religious studies, and government have recently realized the importance of narrative knowledge. Narrative knowledge is what one uses to understand the meaning and significance of stories through cognitive, symbolic, and affective means. This kind of knowledge provides a rich, resonant comprehension of a singular person's situation as it unfolds in time, whether in such texts as novels, newspaper stories, movies, and scripture or in such life settings as courtrooms, battlefields, marriages, and illnesses. (2001a, 1898)

Narrative in the contemporary health professions curriculum is interdisciplinary in both nature and application: its tenets appear in patient interviewing, in making deeper sense of the medical record, in acts of diagnosing, and in psychosocial aspects of patienthood. Moreover, narrative inquiry is also the source of an explosion of reflective writing across the curriculum.

As the field and its practitioners have become less a novelty or an upstart in health professions education (over 60 percent of medical schools currently report both required and elective humanities courses), the benchmarks by which academics chart the successful growth of a discipline have been slowly and steadily met. These include several well-respected peer-reviewed journals; a professional society; annual meetings in the United States and international conferences; active Listservs, blogs, resource databases, and networks; and graduate programs awarding both master's degrees and doctorates. In addition, the development and implementation of undergraduate programs in the medical/health humanities has been nothing short of phenomenal, as many colleges and universities now offer undergraduate minors, concentrations, and/or certificates as a valuable complement to science-based curricula and as independent programs that address current and complex issues in the humanities and social sciences. Such programs simultaneously defy and transcend C. P. Snow's 1959 division of human thought and endeavor into two antagonistic cultures (Snow [1959] 1993). In her contribution to this reader, literary scholar Catherine Belling discusses the long-standing effects of this dualism, especially in education, and identifies the essential role of the humanities as the analysis and critique of both cultural texts—art *and* science (see chap. 39).

Indeed, it is the expansion and variety of humanities inquiry across all educational settings that prompt this book, the *Health Humanities Reader*. While there is still ongoing debate between scholars and educators about the desirability of a core humanities curriculum in health professions education and undergraduate programs that would create standards and establish a common body of knowledge, a consensus exists that both teachers and students need a text—one that is a readily available, fairly representative introduction to and illustration of the field. We believe, as do many of our colleagues and our students, that a central reader such as this will serve

- as a touchstone for both theory and practice among scholars and educators,
- as an accessible and useful text across a variety of settings, and
- as an illustration of how the humanities have identified issues (illness, death and dying, disability, patient-professional relationship) that bridge disciplines and demonstrate how multidisciplinary perspectives must be included in the exploration of such complex issues.

However, this marked expansion has also prompted demands for inclusiveness. As an inter- and multi-disciplinary field, the medical humanities have become increasingly complex with multiple identities and myriad challenges, not the least of which is the demand for measurable outcomes or identifiable competencies. But by its very disciplinary descriptor, *medical*, it retains a narrow frame, largely concerned with the value of history, literature, philosophy, art, and media to medical education and medical practice. Scholars such as Paul Crawford (2010), who has created the International Health Humanities Network, are arguing for a "more inclusive, outward-facing and applied discipline, embracing interdisciplinarity and engaging with the contributions of those marginalized from the medical humanities," such as allied health professionals, patients, and informal caregivers (Crawford et al. 2010, 4). Thus, as we near the half centenary of the discipline, we believe that the original essays and imaginative works in this volume will not only offer readers an engaging and diverse representation of the field but will also persuade them to adopt the more encompassing, contemporary, and accurate label of the current academic enterprise—the *health humanities*.

For some scholars and educators, the terminological shift from *medical humanities* to *health humanities* might feel like just an academic exercise or a mere distraction; while we all know that nomenclature matters, this shift will likely have little effect on our daily work. However, mirroring the dynamic but deliberative process that fostered and shaped the original disciplinary project over forty years ago, timely and robust discussions have emerged about the political, ethical, rhetorical, and cultural implications of such as shift. For example, in a lively and recent conversation on a medical humanities Listserv, reactions to such a suggestion ranged from simple expressions of appreciation for inclusiveness—"This field is important to all professionals including physical therapists, social workers, nurses and not just physicians" (Shirley 2012)—to practical considerations around community engagement and public policy—"The notion encompasses more than the individual's experience of disease, illness and health, but the community perspective of these issues including equity, funding, policy, resources allocation" (Klugman 2012)—to nuanced and informed perspectives addressing a more contemporary focus on global health. For example, one of the contributors to this reader, Daniel Goldberg, shared the following:

> Part of the rationale . . . reflects the critical importance of distinguishing between the delivery of medical care and the pursuit of health. Many sick people are not actively patients, may not engage biomedicine much if ever, and perhaps more importantly, overwhelming evidence suggests that health and its distribution in human populations is mostly not the result of medical care (which is not to deny the myriad ways in which the latter is both meaningful and important). Thus, I would suggest that any definition of the health humanities cannot be limited to the field of medicine, medical care, or medical professionals, and also ought not have as its central goal the advance of the practice and science of medicine. I also believe our primary goal should be directed to health and human flourishing rather than to the delivery of medical care; the two objectives are actually not nearly so tightly interwoven as most tend to think, even if both are independently of great worth. (2012)

The various disciplinary identities and affiliations of all the contributors to this volume meet the objective for inclusiveness and expansiveness; as such, they model the kind of inter- and multi-disciplinary inquiry and innovative collaboration that is the hallmark of health humanities scholarship and education. Represented in this reader are writers from medicine, nursing, pharmacy, and undergraduate education; writers who are clinical practitioners, community health workers, educational filmmakers, and patients; and writers credentialed in history, literature, philosophy, rhetoric, religion, and cultural studies. All are writing across the health professions. Essays such as Felicia Cohn's on religion and end of life, or Rosemarie Tong's on parental responsibility and genetic enhancement, or Allison Kavey's on the history of epidemic diseases would be relevant and meaningful to a physician, physical therapist, social worker, clinical ethicist, or disability studies educator.

With that claim in mind, where is all this diverse content, all this creative activity, located in an already overstuffed health professions curriculum, and how is it taught?

THE HOW

The humanities are found throughout health professions curricula in various forms and with a full range of complexity regarding content and pedagogy. In the most instrumental approaches, humanities content is inserted into lectures for the purpose of illustrating a phenomenon: a film or YouTube clip, an excerpt from a poem or short story, a paragraph lifted from a *New Yorker* article—the genre Charon (2001b) calls the "lay exposition" of narrative writing. The content itself is likely not explored through the methodologies of literary criticism or media studies but more often used to exemplify something, even to liven up a class. Frequently, such an approach finds its way into smaller formats like group discussions, where the aesthetics of a short story or the elements of a film are bypassed for the examination of the clinical or bioethical relevance of its content. There is the tendency here to view the text as an instance of clinical reality—*Away from Her* as a case study of Alzheimer's, for instance—rather than a linguistic or imagistic construct.

Teaching humanities disciplines with increasing complexity involves a fuller engagement with whatever text is under study—a documentary film, an historical essay, a bioethics case, a legal document, or a classic work of fiction, such as *Frankenstein.* This kind of critical practice has the potential to alert students to language in ways they would not have recognized otherwise: the words that caregivers and patients use when attempting to understand each other, the plots of the stories patients tell, the themes and tones of various narratives, the pervasive but unspoken issues surrounding power in healthcare settings, the layers of complexity in seemingly uncomplicated decisions, the unspoken worldviews and values informed by religion and spirituality.

Over the past twenty years, cultural studies and disability studies have influenced many disciplines and pedagogies, including the medical/health humanities. With these orientations, students encounter texts that might be literary, historical, or media produced and that include arts-based and cultural artifacts. These materials raise issues related to power, authority, and justice in health care and challenge the hegemony of a biomedicine that contributes to disparities and the discrimination of persons who don't quite fit the codified and naturalized norms of health. Such approaches offer teachers and students an opportunity to examine critically the origins and nature of their personal beliefs and values, the beliefs and values embedded in the curriculum and the learning environment, as well as institutional policies—all of which intersect and that influence the quality of care they give to patients. Such approaches also require that teachers and students step out of their comfort zone in order to raise difficult and complex issues, scrutinize their own biases and prejudices, and disturb their reliance on a biomedical approach to health care—in other words, a "pedagogy of discomfort" (Boler 1999). The enactment of this kind of fearlessness is dramatically and poignantly represented in the essays of Michael Blackie and Erin Lamb, Sayantani DasGupta, and Rebecca Garden in this reader. Finally, in addition to engaging them in such critical and political inquiry, the materials and methodologies of the medical/health humanities can reinforce students' sense of agency in developing their own professional identities, understanding their own special influence on healthcare practice and delivery, and accepting their own responsibility in how caregiving is both taught and modeled.

The "how" of this section can also refer more specifically and more practically to the design of this particular reader. We recognize that there are multiple organizational strategies for a work of this breadth and depth, and we hope that users will develop their own frameworks and connections within and among the contents. Our own process was simple and straightforward: we first identified a number of common topics in the health humanities and next invited recognized scholar-teachers from a variety of disciplines to address that topic in an original critical essay. Finally, we included an imaginative or reflective piece by an artist, writer, teacher, or scholar that explores the topic. Our goal with each section is to perform a 360-degree examination or expression of a topic and show how different methodologies deployed by scholars and artists compliment and comment on the same theme.

It is our hope that this unique collection of critical essays and creative works by recognized scholars, educators, artists, and clinicians will empower and enlighten students, inspire and support teachers, and advance and focus health humanities study and research.

Part I

DISEASE AND ILLNESS

Chapter 1

BEING A GOOD STORY
The Humanities as Therapeutic Practice
ARTHUR W. FRANK

CERTAIN people remain especially vivid in my memories of the years I spent speaking to illness support groups. One was a man I met at a prostate cancer group. He challenged what I was saying, and I have been trying to respond to him, in different ways, ever since.[1]

I was there to talk about how to make illness something worth living with, which is a notch up from simply living with illness. This fellow was probably the age I am now—mid-sixties—lean and gray, looking like he had lived a physically active life. He spoke without much affect, yet forcefully. His statement was nominally phrased as a question, but it was a form of testimonial. He asked what all this meant when you were in pain all day, scarcely able to move. His life at that point seemed completely rooted in his ill body, and that body offered only pain, little more of capacity or interest.

My response to him tried to tread an ultra-fine line: recognizing the reality of his pain but suggesting that he was well enough to get to this meeting, and so maybe he could find other ways to re-create a life around his pain. One of the most difficult messages to convey without seeming to blame people is that they do have a basic choice: either allow illness to determine their lives, which was the position this man assumed, or seek the energies to sustain a life that is more than illness. That message is all the more difficult to convey because it is much easier to speak from a position of health than to practice while being ill.

Even healthy people who have been ill fairly recently, as I had been when I spoke to that group, risk making it sound too easy to live with illness. We are like skiers standing at the top of an especially steep slope. From the security of that stationary perspective, every turn we plan leads naturally to the next planned turn. It's easy until we're in motion. Then nothing seems as it was when we surveyed the hill as an abstract problem. The man at the meeting who challenged me was actually on the slope; I stood at the top, contemplating it, and there was something pretentious about my shouting down advice to those from whom I stood apart. And yet he needed advice. He was not moving through illness; he was stuck in his pain. A great danger of pain is how it can immobilize a person. Pretentious as advice may be, people sometimes benefit from it. My memory of that man introduces the dilemma of the humanities when they address both those who are ill and those who care for them.

To put the same fable in different terms: perhaps everything I write now, in health, is a message to my future self when he is ill. I hope some of the messages get through when he needs them. I hope they can penetrate the loss and fear, the fatigue and demoralization of illness. I hope they remind me of how I might renew interest in life, find value, even take pleasure in what continues to unfold. That, I believe, is the task of the humanities: to help people find interest, value, and pleasure in words, conceptual schema, images, and imaginations. Illness is one of the ultimate tests of the reach of the humanities to make themselves relevant.

This chapter's title is adapted from one of my favorite lines in any personal illness narrative. Anatole Broyard, writing as he lived with metastasized prostate cancer, describes the relationship he desires with his physician: "I want to be a good story for him" (1992, 45). This chapter asks *how* to do that. The humanities have extraordinary resources that can help ill people first to tell good stories and then in the telling to *become* good stories, not only for their physicians but for themselves, their loved ones, and anybody else they happen to run into. The point, I believe, is not to claim that illness is, in Broyard's title word, *intoxicating*, but to elevate illness above the diminished condition implied by the unfortunate verb *coping*. Stories are good because they are interesting. Illness can be an interesting story.

Or to put the issue differently: "Oh, your poor distracted doctor-ridden carcass," wrote Henry James to his brother William whose health was failing (Richardson 2006, 401). The word that makes this line most memorable for me is *distracted*. Henry James, who spent a great deal of his own life being a doctor-ridden carcass, knew where the true peril of illness lies—in medical distraction from living. This chapter offers ideas about one means of recovery from the distraction that too often attends illness: make the illness a story and rediscover interest in life by making the story a better one.

A few distinctions seem necessary as a preface.

A SPACE FOR HUMANITIES IN ILLNESS

Over two decades ago, when I was struggling to find a voice and a genre to tell stories of several years when I had been critically ill (Frank [1991] 2002), four distinctions emerged as necessary to my clarity about what was happening around me and my capacity to use language truthfully. Even then, none of these distinctions was my original discovery, and today their recognition remains unevenly distributed. I think of these distinctions not as binary polarities but rather as recurring tensions.

The first tension is between *illness* as an experience and *disease* as a condition of the body. Disease can be reduced to biochemistry, while illness involves a biography, a reflective consciousness, multiple relationships, and institutions. By the time disease is imagined, it has already become illness. The humanities become necessary resources as soon as people try to live illness as more than bare disease. At least two qualifications are required. First, imagining disease is a perilous business;

for example, imagination can plunge a sick person into a fearsome future that may never happen or, if it does happen, may not seem as unlivable as imagined. Second, illness and disease are always conjoined: they could be separate only in the impossible condition of the mind locating itself outside the body which is the mind's locus of orientation for imagining, reflecting, and narrating. We tell stories not only with our bodies but equally from our bodies and as bodies. Consciousness of illness is inevitably shaped by being a diseased body, yet consciousness can imagine its body and tell stories about that body.

The second tension is between being a patient and being an ill person. The person who is ill is a patient only some of the time and in certain respects and remains many other things as well. The healthcare professions impose the term *patient* as a total identity; ill people are led to forget that their lives are more than being sick. In Henry James's condolence to William, becoming "doctor ridden" is a condition of thinking of oneself as only a patient, which distracts the ill person from everything else that is going on and its significant value. To risk putting a gloss on what Henry James had the sense to leave open, the patient is distracted from each moment's potential rediscovery of how fascinating life is—a way of living that both James brothers exemplified. Being a patient is a condition of being a character in a story told by an author who has already decided all that any character is capable of being and who requires each to remain strictly within these boundaries.[2] It is a dullness that precipitates fatalism. It is the opposite of health.

The third tension is that the medical history is not the ill person's story. When I was ill and had multiple health professionals taking versions of what they called my *history*, I quickly realized that they suffered from an illusion—that what they were learning about me was equivalent to knowing me as a person. The interviewer who elicits the medical history works within already-set parameters of what counts as relevant, constantly paring down what is told to fit those parameters. The medical patient becomes delimited by his or her history. If the storytelling is truly a relationship, the storyteller is invited to reinvent his or her character.

Broyard exemplifies the distinction between the medical history and the ill person's story by alluding to Marcel Proust's criticism of his doctor failing to "take into account the fact that he read Shakespeare" (1992, 47). I think of *Shakespeare* in this statement as a sort of algebraic x, standing for whatever gives a person his or her unique sense of taste and imaginative possibility. In relations of storytelling, the listener is listening for what counts as that person's Shakespeare—what the storyteller needs the listener to know about him or herself, to appreciate that self.

The fourth tension is between the provision of treatment and the offering of care: treatment is provided as a service; care is offered as a gift. Treatment can be expressed in a monetary value; one can buy more attentive treatment but not true care. The literature on care is overwhelming in its breadth and depth. Let me suggest the care/treatment tension in the following distinctions:

○ Treatment is instrumental; its objective is an end state beyond itself. Care is consummatory; giving and receiving care is an end in itself.

- The provision of treatment requires technical expertise that can be one-dimensional. The giving of care involves the emotions as well as cognition.
- The treatment provider uses his or her body as an instrument. The caregiver's embodiment is compassionate, feeling the suffering of the one who is cared for, while sustaining a boundary that enables the caregiver to act effectively rather than becoming engulfed—another danger of imagination (Frank 2004, 121–122).
- Providing treatment involves a clearly defined boundary between one who provides and one who is treated. The relational nature of care requires a fluid, shifting boundary. Giver and receiver are both subjects, not subject and object.
- Not last but sufficient for this chapter's purposes, treatment is untroubled by its use of power as a resource. Care is endlessly sensitive to asymmetries of power (White 2011).

These four tensions play out on both sides of the street, the side of the ill person who is sometimes a patient and the side of those who treat and sometimes care for this person. People on both sides need the humanities because they are all *disenchanted*, to use a sociological word.[3] Disenchantment, to give it the briefest elucidation, is a condition in which surprise is rarely if ever a good thing and control is always aspired to; mystery represents a failure of rational understanding, adherence to routine trumps any benefit of innovation, and anything worth discussing is measurable, preferably in numeric form. Max Weber (1958) gave disenchantment its classic sociological formulation early in the twentieth century, but his contemporary William James truly evokes the feeling of disenchantment:

The flowers wither at its breath, the stars turn to stone; our own body grows unworthy of our spirit and sinks to a tenement for carnal senses only. The book of nature turns into a volume on mechanics, in which whatever has life is treated as a sort of anomaly; a great chasm of separation yawns between us and all that is higher than ourselves; and God becomes this nest of abstractions. (James 2010, 289)

Disenchanted illness is the body grown unworthy of the spirit, sinking into its own senses, especially the imperialism of pain, and disenchanted treatment reduces life to mechanics.

Disenchantment affects both ill people and healthcare professionals, but on any particular occasion, strategic necessity may require privileging the perspective of one group or the other. In my earlier writing, I addressed ill people's disenchantment by focusing exclusively on their stories when it seemed that ill people's voices were so subordinated to medicine that they needed a venue of their own in order to be heard (Frank 1995). Necessary as it may be to work only one side of the street, this approach risks obscuring the crucial point that storytelling is a relationship. To return to this chapter's title, when Broyard says he wants to be a good story for his doctor, the doctor's participation is crucial. Broyard's particular resource, based on his literary reputation, was that when his physician's participation was not forthcoming, he could publicly imagine that participation before an audience of physicians for whom he could become a very good story.[4]

In health care, this relation of storytelling rests on a fundamental asymmetry. The ill person is the one whose life is being reduced to the bare facts of disease and its progression. Healthcare professionals (a designation that may be the most clunky phrase imaginable, but sorting out any comparable term is beyond this chapter's scope) provide ample testimony how their work often reduces their sense of who they are. But in the relationship at the bedside, the professional has a responsibility to offer care—and then to find other venues for her or his own care. The work of the humanities in illness seems to me to reflect this asymmetry: helping ill people to become good stories and helping professionals to help ill people, which can include telling their own stories but always to the end of participating in their patients' stories.

THE HUMANITIES AS THERAPEUTIC

To open up the crucial issue of how stories help people who are suffering, let me follow William James's argument presented in a lecture given in 1906 in which he described a general human problem in terms that evoke the demoralization of illness: "The human individual lives usually far within his limits; he possesses power of various sorts which he habitually fails to use. He energizes below the maximum, and he behaves below his optimum. In elementary faculty, in coordination, in power of inhibition and control, in every conceivable way, *his life is contracted*" (James 2010, 278; emphasis added). This is illness: the effect of contracting the life of the ill person, narrowing horizons of possibility, filtering and reducing the possibilities for *joy*, to use a word seldom spoken in institutional medicine (Brody 2009, 58–59). It may well be that illness only exacerbates what James maintains is a habitual condition of humans living with their energies "below the maximum," but that further reduction is what is intolerably demoralizing about being sick.

The task, potential, and capacity of the humanities is therapeutic, insofar as the humanities seek to expand what illness has contracted. James called these *dynamogenic effects*, and he located three principal sources: "excitements, ideas, and efforts" (2010, 267–268). *Excitements* include being caught up in events that require extending one's energies to meet the crisis of the moment; James's examples are soldiers' reports of discovering enhanced energies in battle. His examples of *efforts* include ascetic spiritual practices such as self-starvation and sleep deprivation. To illustrate, he quotes a long report by a man who undertook a rigorous program of yoga and reported feeling new and previously unimagined energy within himself. *Ideas* are exemplified by conversions, "whether they be political, scientific, philosophical, or religious," and the energies that attend these (2010, 268).

James is eloquent in his enthusiasm for "dynamogenic" programs, but he is also realistic: "Of course there are limits: the trees don't grow in the sky." Illness is disease, and disease will take its toll; hospitals are institutions, and institutions impose their needs upon individuals, both patients and staff. Yet James refuses to allow these limits to have the last word: "But the plain fact remains that men the world over possess amounts of resource, which only very exceptional individuals push to their extremes" (James 2010, 268). Lest James's historically conventional gender bias of language be distracting, I note that his prime example of such an exceptional individual is a woman whom he leaves anonymous but is likely to be his sister Alice:

The most genuinely saintly person I have ever known is a friend of mine now suffering from cancer of the breast. I do not assume to judge the wisdom or unwisdom of her disobedience to the doctors, and I cite her here solely as an example of what ideas can do. Her ideas have kept her a practically well woman for months after she should have given up and gone to bed. They have annulled all pain and weakness and given her a cheerful active life, unusually beneficent to others to whom she afforded help. (James 2010, 278)

Idealized as that portrait may be, it provides an illustration for what the humanities can offer as a therapeutic in response to the loss of what James calls *energy*, a diffuse term he uses to designate the capacity to live life to the fullest. Contemporary psychological writing seems to use *resilience* in much the same way. Against the contraction brought about by disease and its treatment, the humanities can give many people the often self-reported sense of their lives having become enhanced. James would understand these reports as reflecting the vitality that attends using one's energies at previously unexperienced levels. The ill person comes to realize—if conditions are right and resources are available—how much of his or her life is being lived "with a sort of cloud weighing on us" (2010, 265). One's body may, indeed, be sicker (or disabled or older), but that can make the sense of dispelling the cloud all the more exhilarating.

A note of caution is necessary, however. If the humanities offered only sunlight and flowers, these would be thin offerings. The humanities also offer tragedy and all manner of sufferings made more intense in their aesthetic depiction. They offer the bitter humor of irony and the revenges of satire. They offer *equipment* for surviving illness. The danger of aesthetic depictions of suffering is that the idealized image can displace the reality; the work of art can become a form of denial. That danger seems greatest when those who are not ill or no longer ill wax on about all that illness can offer. Support groups, in particular, suffer from a rhetoric of enforced cheerfulness (Frank 2012). This danger seems minimized when people depict their own suffering while it remains reasonably proximate. The greater benefit of aesthetic depictions of suffering is to make ill people feel less alone. That—*feeling less alone*—requires the increased energy that James wrote about, but once acquired, it enhances people's energy.

STORYTELLING AS EVERYPERSON'S ART OF THE EVERYDAY

I focus on storytelling not because it enjoys any privilege as an art form but because it has a common-denominator status of accessibility. Storytelling certainly can be impaired (Hydén and Brockmeier 2008), but because most people are already equipped to tell stories when they become ill, storytelling may have the most inclusive claim to be every person's art form. Moreover, stories have the capacity to *refocus the everyday*. A great sociologist, who often adopted a cynical stance, once said to me that in order to make grading tolerable, he sent students out to do observations because "even dull students can write interesting ethnography." I suggest that even a dull life can be made interesting when transformed into a good story.

If I wish one thing for myself when I finally do become seriously ill again, it is that I remember, as soon as possible after the initial shock, that my condition has given me access to rich materials for storytelling: people, at moments of crisis, responding to suffering. Awareness of having that material all around me might be what James meant by an idea that can have the "dynamogenic" force of awakening inner energies. The idea can become a practice. For example, do not simply suffer the rudeness of the hospital worker (attending surgeon or admissions clerk); *draw out* that rudeness to its extreme and explore it in order to discover a character about whom a story can be told. Maybe the story will be an Oscar Wilde farce or an Orwellian dystopic fable—or both, at different times, to different listeners with whom the story will be the basis of a relationship that will renew energies.

Lest these projections into the future seem naive, I fully recognize that upon becoming seriously ill again, I will first be submerged in the fear and anxiety of realizing that the nagging symptom is not going to go away; then will come the shock of having some physician confirm (gently, if I'm lucky) that my worst fears are justified; followed by the news of how bad both the symptom progression and the treatment are going to be. This submergence may last a day or a week or a month. But most diseases these days are chronic for some time before they are critical. Sometime, maybe by the second month, the losses will be counted and dealt with (so far as possible), the routine will have become just that, and then I hope to remember that I still can be a storyteller.

If all but the most impaired persons are already equipped to be storytellers of their illness, that does not mean that storytelling to renew energies will occur without specific encouragement. Life-threatening illness—the kind that most needs stories—remains something of a taboo topic, although that has changed enormously in the last two decades. People need models on which to tell their stories, and here we encounter a significant paradox: stories are very much one person's own, but any person's story is also a more or less (often less) creative mixture of previously heard stories. That paradox is crucial: people's claim to the authenticity of their own stories deserves to be honored, but nobody makes up his or her story by him or herself. Birds make their own nests, but neither the materials nor the design are innovations. The stories in which we humans nest our lives are woven in predictable ways from predictable elements. We could not tell our own stories without having others' stories as sources of material and design. The danger of others' stories is that they can colonize the imagination of the person who necessarily borrows from them.

For storytellers of illness today, the good news is that multiple models are available in books, films, newspapers, and perhaps most of all, on the Internet. However, the danger is that those public stories can make too encompassing a claim, imposing themselves as models and crowding out different stories. I see no way to avoid this duality: storytelling needs models, but models risk taking over any person's story. The response, I believe, is not to avoid stories—which would be impossible and utterly self-defeating—but to avoid getting stuck in one niche of stories. The remedy to stories' dangers is more stories (Frank 2010; Lewis 2011).

A principle task of the humanities, then, is to offer ill people the broadest range of stories in as many media and genres as possible. With those models available, the humanities can then work with ill people, supporting the therapeutic potential of stories in three ways: prompting stories, enhancing storytelling, and appreciating stories.

NARRATIVE THERAPEUTICS: PROMPTING, ENHANCING, AND APPRECIATING

Both by training clinical staff—again, either the attending surgeon or the admissions clerk—and working directly with ill people, the humanities can practice a narrative therapeutic. I distinguish this practice from *narrative therapy*, which has a great deal to teach the applied humanities but which has more focused objectives (White 2007, 2011; White and Epston 1990). Applied narrative practice can be segmented into three stages: prompting stories to be told, enhancing how stories are told, and offering appreciations that reinforce aspects of the selves displayed in storytelling. An overarching goal is to connect stories: again, to help people to feel less alone by showing how any person's story, unique as that life is, still has considerable overlap with others' stories.

The idea of *prompting* stories is already familiar from extensive work in teaching physicians reflective writing (Charon 2008). Prompts are general questions—strategically vague—that help a storyteller get a story under way. If the context is a hospital, the prompt gives permission for the ill-person-as-patient to speak in a way with which staff are generally impatient. Permission for storytelling is expected in the context of support groups, but even there, permission may be necessary for topics and emotions that the group more or less avoids (Frank 2012). The crucial point is that the phrasing of prompts be sensitive to local norms of storytelling, recognizing what stories particular people expect to be asked to tell and what stories they expect to be discouraged from telling. As in reflective writing exercises, the prompt can include a suggested time limit. People who are not immediately comfortable with the idea of telling stories can find a boundary reassuring, although, as the story develops, that boundary can be ignored.

Rita Charon (2011a), leading a reflective writing exercise for professionals, uses a prompt that she credits to Kathryn Montgomery: "Tell me about your scars." Part of what makes that such an excellent prompt is that it encourages personal revelation but allows considerable latitude about which scars are told and how they are told. For example, stories can be told in the genre of medical case history, as long-healed personal event, or as unhealed current pain. The story of any particular scar can be shifted and expanded, and one scar story can lead to another. The scar prompt can elicit a more or less medical story; it's the storyteller's choice.

As good as the scar prompt is, the best prompts are those that are most specific to person and occasion. I once interviewed a patient whom the staff experienced as noncompliant with treatment. Receiving in advance a summary of her medical history, I was immediately demoralized, as the description of her was nothing more than a collection of pathologies (with attendant management problems). I then noticed that she was born in 1923, which gave me my prompt. I did not forget the medical history but sent it into deep background, so that I could become happily curious about this woman's life as she lived it.

I began our conversation by noting that when she was six years old, the Great Depression was beginning. Had she been aware of the shifting economy? How did it affect her family? Perhaps she was surprised that I had not asked her anything medical, but with little more participation from me, she told that packed room the rich story of her family, a matriarchy—men did not stay around very long. She talked of her relationships with her grandmother and mother, her work during the war, her various troubles afterward, and the friendships that mattered most. Twenty minutes later, we landed in the present, and her responses to her disease and treatment made a lot more sense as part of this longer story—she was continuing to uphold the person she had always been, including some specific actions that she might not need to continue. Short-term reports were that her behaviors did change, as did those of the staff treating her.

For storytelling at the end of life, an interesting prompt is the invitation for people to think about all the material things they call their own. Everybody has stuff—photographs, letters, things they have made and inherited, pets, tools of their trades, and objects of economic or sentimental value. If scars are on the body, material possessions are projections of the self. Among these possessions, about which is the person most concerned after she or he is gone? What things does he or she want to have dispersed or disposed of in what particular ways? Is she or he worried about where any particular things might end up? Does she or he look forward to other people having particular things, and why (either so the thing will have a good home or so that the recipient will remember the giver)? The prompt opens up questions about what stuff matters, where it came from, and in what circumstances it acquired its value. The question also invites reflection on the person's current network of people who might receive things.

In some storytelling, simply prompting the story can be sufficient; the person's inherent narrative abilities will do very well. However, some storytelling may require further prompting, which I think of as *enhancing*. Follow-up questions can enable the story to develop those elements that narratologists know are essential to good—which in this usage means energizing and relation-building—storytelling. For example, the action in stories always takes place somewhere, but many storytellers omit details of the setting; questions can elicit those details and the memories that go with them. Stories talk about people, but again, descriptions of how people look—their grooming and clothes—are often left out. These narrative enhancement questions lead to more fundamental concerns. The drama of stories depends especially on creating and building suspense (Mattingly 1998), and a narratologist-listener can subtly direct the telling to enhance suspense. The trick is to hear the story that could be told but is not yet being told, suggesting just enough of that potential telling for the storyteller to take it up. A film director might suggest how an actor play the role, but the art of directing is knowing when to step back and allow the actor to create that which has only been suggested. By *directing* storytelling, the listener introduces his or her reactions to encourage ways of telling. For example, a listener who remarks on his or her sense of suspense encourages telling in a way that increases suspense.

Just as James observes that people generally use only part of the energy available to them, so people often tell less of a story than they could about their lives. To enhance the story is to energize the life. I recall meeting with residents of a hospital-based community for the elderly, mostly in their nineties. I encouraged their storytelling, but the occasion bogged down with one resident's long story of some crucial events in her life. After she left, the others complained about how often they had to hear this same story told the same way—they fled from it. I wondered, in a Freudian way, what compelled the woman to keep repeating the story; what might still be lacking that each retelling might replace? If I had had more time, I would have encouraged her to retell the story (a request that undoubtedly would have surprised her, thus opening a potential for change), and I would have asked questions to reanimate it. What was originally a crisis had turned into a chronicle of events; her telling lacked suspense, and her characters were undeveloped. The tragedy of her very old age was that she had now become as bored as her listeners. Remembering her, I have the feeling she was trying, hard but not very effectively, to regain the energy that attended the crisis as it was lived, but the original drama had gradually gotten lost in repeated telling. Her story needed direction in the sense of restaging—her story needed a new production. A great story, but she had forgotten how to tell it, and watching her remember would have been extraordinary.

The contribution of people trained in the humanities is to see that potential for new, restaged productions in what have become tired, dusty stories. Here is a far more vital practice of what is called "active listening," which is unfortunately often reduced to a set of techniques applied with little discrimination. Humanistic active listening requires considerable narrative skill joined to utmost tact and sensitivity. The point is to direct by the selective appreciation of what is not yet there in the story to be appreciated but what the humanistically trained caregiver can sense could be there.

In responding to the ill, the humanistic function academically designated as *criticism* is better reimagined as *appreciation*. Narrative therapists Michael White and David Epston (1990) have developed a specific methodology for writing "therapeutic letters" to clients as a follow-up to sessions. I have suggested the utility of adapting this method as a way of opening up interpretations in narrative analysis (Frank 2010, 109). The essential point is to approach ill people's stories with an emphasis on what is most admirable. In family therapy, that might be how one member of the family is caring for another or how the whole family has organized itself to protect one member. Illness stories often involve acts of caring for others— the story itself is offered as an act of care to those who need its companionship.

My writing about the "generosity of the ill" (2004) could be called narrative analysis, but its objective is to enter into a dialogue with the stories of the ill by articulating what can be appreciated in these stories. Appreciation is due both to the storyteller and, perhaps even more, to the story itself, as it is caring for the person who does not simply tell it but whose life is guided by it (Frank 2010). Appreciations are offered not simply to make people feel good about themselves. The point is to increase people's capacity to tell stories that revitalize their lives. Encouraging such storytelling requires the skills to articulate what *specific* qualities the story displays that the person might want to accentuate in acts that generate future stories. Offering appreciations requires interpretive skill to specify and articulate what is to be appreciated so that the appreciation will be heard as reflecting true recognition, not as a perfunctory gesture. The work—and I emphasize it is skilled work—of articulating appreciations can be therapeutic without becoming formal therapy; that is, there is no contract to work on specific problems and no assessment of progress in that work.

The work of the narrative humanist is midway between the sort of conversation a person might have with an especially caring, insightful friend and therapy with a professional. The singular advantage of this middle position is that the ill person already is, to return to Henry James's phrase, a "distracted, doctor-ridden carcass." There are already multiple professionals defining the ill person in terms of his or her problems. If ill people often do not need a therapist, they do need someone who is more than a friend. The healthcare humanist, which I propose as a professional designation, can play that role in direct engagement with ill people, while the humanist is also training clinicians when and how to relate to their patients on this middle ground between the professional relationship and friendship.[5]

The key humanistic skill, acquired through practicing narratology, literary criticism, folklore, and other interpretive work, is being able to say which parts of a story are doing what. Narrative criticism becomes compelling by how well it demonstrates the method in a creator's art. The objective of appreciative response is to lead people to see the method in their art of living and then to be able to enhance that art, doing more of what they already do best. Against the distractions of illness and treatment, appreciations focus on what people are doing best for themselves and for others.

HOLDING ONE'S OWN

The physician Eric Cassell (2004) is frequently cited for his compelling argument that the suffering of illness is caused by the threat of loss to all or part of what a person most values in her or his existence. Physical pain, especially chronic pain, can certainly cause suffering, but suffering exceeds pain (Frank 2001). The first-person illness narratives that have been my most constant personal and professional companions for many years—especially those of Audre Lorde (1980), Anatole Broyard (1992), and Reynolds Price (2003)—are each written as an act of *holding one's own* in the face of the multiple threats that are the occasion of suffering. Each experiences pain, each finds more degradation than support during medical treatment, and each worries about dying. But more than these, each suffers the threatened loss of who she or he has been, and each writes as a way of sustaining and even enhancing that identity through illness. To hold one's own is to sustain a self that is threatened. Acts of holding one's own attempt to restore the foundation of the dignity that demonstrates the value of the self, at least to itself. Acts of resistance can be ways of holding one's own. In illness, the resistance is against the eroding, demoralizing effects of disease and its treatment. Illness calls upon people to hold their own, demonstrating that they still can be whatever was best about their pre-illness selves.

My appreciation to Audre Lorde is that she finds ways to continue to protest the silences that are invidious assaults on the self. The single line in her writing that I most appreciate is when she tells her readers "your silence will not protect you" (1980, 20). She holds her own by continuing to tell truths, specifically about breast cancer, that others suppress (Frank 2009). Anatole Broyard (1992) seems most threatened not by prostate cancer but by the loss of the personal style through which he defines himself. His writing becomes the means of continuing to display that style—the wit, the properly inserted literary reference, the perfectly phrased observation, the sense of sustaining elegance amid hospital squalor. Broyard fears death less than ceasing to be the persona he has created. He writing is his last, possibly greatest act of self-fashioning.

Reynolds Price (2003) suffers the loss of the body in which he took pride and pleasure, but he holds his own by sustaining two more important identities: one as a person of faith and the other as an artist. His faith is enacted in what may be his memoir's most dramatic scene: the waking vision in which he is transported to the Sea of Galilee and encounters Jesus who tells him he will be healed. Price's paraplegia, an effect of the radiation following the surgery for a malignant tumor in his spinal column, becomes a version of the wound that humans invariably incur when they encounter divine forces. His claim as an artist occurs when he ends his memoir observing that since his illness, his literary productivity has increased. He holds his own on all fronts.

To understand how people hold their own requires asking what is most at stake for them. Ill people's stories are, at first, attempts to sort out what is at stake. Few of us can fully appreciate, while our lives proceed unthreatened, what is most at stake in our sense of self or our dignity—on what do these depend? As illness impairs and threatens, it clarifies what is dispensable and where the stakes truly lie. But that clarification requires saying and being heard; it needs storytelling. And storytelling is progressive because what any story discovers is mobile; in telling the story, the self moves on, assuming an identity more or less continuous with the pervious one, but changed. Price's title, *A Whole New Life*, is surely hyperbolic: his new life after illness depends on his former skills and reputation, but his claim to a new wholeness is well taken.

Humanists in health care have skills and trained sensitivities to support ill people holding their own through storytelling. Their contribution can be extraordinary.

NOTES

1 Although I do not specifically cite "Five Dramas of Illness" (Frank 2007), this chapter is complementary to that article, which also begins with Anatole Broyard.

2 I refer here to Mikhail Bakhtin's distinction between the dialogical and monological novel; see Frank (2004, 2010) for background and discussion.

3 Kleinman (1989) remains the classic statement of how medical care demoralizes both the ill and healthcare workers. In this chapter, my usage of *disenchantment* is effectively synonymous with *demoralization*, although each word reflects a different tradition and emphasis.

4 Portions of what became the text of *Intoxicated by My Illness* (Broyard 1992) were originally presented in grand rounds at the University of Chicago Medical School.

5 On the boundary issues raised here, see Charon (2008).

Chapter 2

ILLUMINATING THE IT, THEE, AND WE OF DISEASE AND ILLNESS

The Metamorphosis and Related Works

DAVID H. FLOOD AND RHONDA L. SORICELLI

D ISEASE is an inevitable part of our human condition. The DNA of our cells may be genetically flawed or mutate spontaneously. Microorganisms invade us; environmental contaminants degrade our systems. Bodies break down from constant use and decay over time; telomeres shorten, impairing the body's ability to repair itself while the quest for the Fountain of Youth remains as elusive as ever. More important than the physiological facts of disease itself, though, is our experience of it—what we call illness.[1] To what extent does disease influence our customary way of living? How does it change the way others respond to us or lead their own lives? How does it alter our perception of ourselves? Our very identities? Do we become "the other," alienated from the world of the healthy and "normal"? Or do we adapt this altered self into a new, positive identity? As John Keats observed, "Until we are sick, we understand not" ([1818] 1958, 279). This revelatory, often transformational aspect of disease on ourselves and those around us will be the focus of our discussion, first of Franz Kafka's *The Metamorphosis* ([1915] 1972) followed by commentary on related works and themes.

THE METAMORPHOSIS

At first glance, the surrealistic story of a man who becomes a giant insect seems to have little to do with medicine. But if we think of the story as a metaphor for the sweeping transformation that disease or accident brings to the patient and patient's family, Kafka's tale provides an insightful exploration of the experience of illness from multiple perspectives. As such, it has become one of the core texts in medical/health humanities education. Uniquely, it provides an opportunity to explore the experience of illness as a generalized concept free from any specific disease. We are not reading a story of cancer or diabetes but a narrative that looks at illness at a meta level, forcing us to confront the existential aspects of this betrayal of the body.

Part I opens with Gregor Samsa waking to discover that he has been transformed into a "monstrous vermin" (3). There is no explanation, no cause given, merely the fact. At least since the book of Job, part of the response to disease has involved the question, Why me? As humans, we need to find meaning in life's experiences and often cope better with even horrendous situations when that meaning is present. But sometimes it is not forthcoming, as in Gregor's case. Like so many other patients, his initial reaction to the inexplicable alteration of self is denial. Surveying his room, he notes that everything is the same as it was; only he has changed, and perhaps that will not matter as this transformation is surely a fantasy. Gregor's initial objective is to cling to the normality he has always known. It is not his affliction—his beetleness—that concerns him but rather its potential impact on his life. Realizing he has missed his train and will be late to the job he detests, he considers using his new infirmity as a reason not to go to work; indeed, for some, disease can provide a useful excuse for avoiding unpleasant responsibilities, and perhaps Gregor's altered state reflects alienation from his core self created by his soul-numbing job.[2] However, his role as financial provider for his family and concern about being perceived as lazy prevail as he decides how he might catch a later train.

As Gregor struggles to leave his room, the office manager arrives. Now Gregor must consider how his boss and family might respond to him. For all patients, the reaction of others can affirm a sense of connectedness with the world of the well or confirm illness as a force of alienation. Believing they are concerned about his well-being, Gregor "felt integrated into human society once again," but when he finally appears at the door, he quickly discovers his mistake: he is greeted by stares and screams of repulsion and is driven back into his room (13). Gregor can no longer deny his estrangement from the healthy, normal world.

Part I began with Gregor waking in the morning; part II begins as he awakens from a "coma-like sleep" at the end of his first day in this altered state (21). Now his focus shifts from maintaining his former existence to adapting to his new life, and he discovers differences and capabilities rather than just losses. He also becomes aware that his condition is gradually transforming his identity, not only externally but also internally. His tastes in food, ideas about comfort, even his vision are changing. He thinks more about the impact of this malady on his family and, as many patients do, experiences guilt about the "inconvenience" he is causing, determining to diminish it as much as possible (23). Gregor's family cannot understand his bug-like noises, though, and assume he cannot understand them, so he is talked about instead of with—the fate of many altered by disease or injury.

While illness is primarily the patient's story, narrative theory and its adaptations in narrative medicine and ethics inform us that we must also consider the multiple points of view from which the story can be constructed by all affected. Hence we turn our attention to Gregor's family.[3] Although concerned about him, they focus mainly on coping with the outcome of the Gregor problem in their own lives. Their maid wants to quit, and they have lost the earnings of the family breadwinner. A caregiver is needed, a role that falls to Grete, Gregor's seventeen-year-old sister. While she genuinely tries to accommodate her brother, her repulsion is evident, albeit less so than that of their parents. But is compassionate duty Grete's guiding force or something else? This question arises as we note the metamorphosis of Gregor's bedroom into sickroom. Grete observes Gregor's preference for crawling

on the walls and ceiling rather than scuttling across the floor and suggests removing the furniture—a practical solution but one that terrifies him. Would this freedom be "at the cost of simultaneously, rapidly, and totally forgetting his human
past" (33)? The presence of familiar furnishings in a sickroom can be a significant
expression of continuity and connection with the world of the well and one's previous identity. And so Gregor resists, battling especially to preserve a picture hanging on the wall—one of little significance in itself but representing the familiar.

The scene is revealing about Grete. We presume she is considering Gregor's best
interest, but the text also suggests that she is attempting to increase his dependence
on her: "to make Gregor's situation even more terrifying in order that she might do
even more for him" and to create a room in which "no human being beside Grete
was ever likely to set foot" (34). Indeed, Grete's motive may be the need for a special identity and a sense of purpose in being Gregor's caregiver, motivation that
quickly becomes detrimental to the welfare of her patient. When Mother intervenes and faints during Gregor's attempt to save his picture, Gregor rushes from the
room with Grete to get help, only to be confronted by Father. This formerly passive,
broken-down man has found a job and now walks with upright posture and determination in his eye: Gregor's illness has wrought a positive change in him. Unfortunately, with his newfound vitality, Father forces Gregor back into his room by
throwing apples at him, one of which sticks in his back, creating a serious wound.
Father exhibits the frustrations of living with a chronically ill patient that can all
too easily lead to abuse in both personal and professional caregiving situations.

By part III of Kafka's novella, Gregor is barely tolerated.[4] In the illness narrative
the family has constructed, although still acknowledged as family, he is "the other"
in their midst who has woefully altered their lives: "They had been struck by a misfortune as none of their relatives and acquaintances had ever been hit" (42). The
effect of their attitude on Gregor is palpable as he becomes "completely filled with
rage at his miserable treatment" and his overall condition deteriorates (43). His
room, now used to store unwanted items (like Gregor himself), becomes a further
symbol of his alienation. Poignantly, although he has lost his appetite and perhaps
the will to live, when he hears Grete play the violin, a hunger of the soul for what
it means to be human overwhelms him. Gregor longs for beauty and compassion,
things absent from the life he now knows.

Life has evolved for Grete just as it has for Father and Mother. She has taken
a job and increasingly shows her displeasure toward her caregiving duties. She
refuses assistance, however, demonstrating how caregivers are often reluctant to
admit that they are not up to the task. No one suggests the obvious—that perhaps
it would be better to relegate Gregor's care to the cleaning woman, who views him
matter-of-factly, with curiosity rather than revulsion. Often the detachment of an
outside professional caregiver is the best solution for families. Although there is no
further overt violence against him, Gregor is nonetheless being abused, this time
through neglect.

To relieve ourselves of moral responsibility to others and to make it easier to act
in certain ways toward them, we sometimes dehumanize them. To insulate ourselves from the unsettling reminder of the relationship of the diseased to us and

to their former selves, we emphasize their difference. Interestingly, caregiver Grete becomes the one most vehemently opposed to Gregor, referring to him as "this monster" and "it" (51). In her need to detach, she sees him as having *been* Gregor but being Gregor no more, mirroring the sentiments of many who are close to late-stage Alzheimer's patients, completing the process of alienation begun at the outset of his disease. His metamorphosis, however, is not yet complete. As Gregor lies dying, his anger fades; his compassion is restored: "He thought back on his family with deep emotion and love," and he accepts his sister's verdict that the only way for him to reclaim his humanity is by exiting their lives—and his (54).

Using *The Metamorphosis* as a metaphor for illness lends itself to seeking meaning in the experiences of Gregor and his family. If we take the existentialist position (with which Kafka is often associated), there is none—life is absurd, and events such as disease are simply random misfortunes to which we respond as best we can. Even so, most people will try to find or at least create some meaning. For Gregor, "illness" forces him to assess his life experience from new perspectives that reveal the fragility of his preconceived notions about both himself and his family. Mr. Samsa's words at Gregor's death summarize the family's position: "Now we can thank God!" (55). While the words may well express relief at being rid of him, they may equally articulate gratefulness that Gregor is spared further suffering—a common response of families of dying patients. As for readers, who co-construct their versions of events, ambiguity prevails. In Kafka's world, the experience of illness by patient and family is at once dehumanizing and life affirming, although little of this is realized by the participants. Disease indeed does have meaning, but in Kafka's world it can be difficult to decipher.

THEMES, TEXTS, AND CONTEXTS

The Metamorphosis works as a teachable text because of its insights into the experience of illness and disease and because of its relatively short length. Beyond convenience, brevity can allow a more extensive sampling than fewer longer readings would allow. With that principle in mind, let us explore some additional works to supplement our discussion of the major illness themes in Kafka's novella: alienation and isolation, the impact of illness on family and friends, and illness as a source of identity and self-awareness.

Alienation and Isolation

John Updike's "From the Journal of a Leper" (1976), a fictionalized autobiographical piece about a man with psoriasis, exemplifies our first theme.[5] While he is not "ill" per se, this condition causes an ugly, red, scaling skin rash over most of the body of our narrator. The opening journal entry of this self-described "leper," tellingly dated October 31, that feast of monsters and of hiding behind masks, sets the tone for a story characterized by intertwined isolation and self-loathing: "The name of the disease, spiritually speaking, is Humiliation" (28). Unlike Gregor Samsa, the leper denigrates self and assumes rejection by others. Even in his environment, he seeks visual connection with his disease so that Boston's Hancock

Building, famous for shedding its windows "as I shed scales" (28), becomes his icon. But, as with the Hancock Building, there is a cure that for him yields a curious transformation. No longer a leper, he becomes self-absorbed with his scale-less appearance: "I am beautiful," he narcissistically declares (32). A potter by trade, he is driven by a fanatical devotion to delicate perfection inspired by his own imperfection. But now his artistic vision changes, and his standards begin to slip: "Notes for a new line of stoneware: bigger, rougher, rude, with granulations and leonine stains" (33). His relationship with his girlfriend loses its passion as he focuses on the flaws of her skin rather than his own. Ironically, while psoriasis had affected his life in negative ways, lack of obvious disease does, too, at a deeper, spiritual level, leaving us to contemplate the ambiguous impact of disease on identity.

Richard Selzer's "Four Appointments with the Discus Thrower" (1987a) likewise vividly portrays isolation and the reactions of others to the diseased, this time in a hospital setting. In the short story's portrait of a blind, legless, dying older man, we are struck by the challenge of empathy that the patient poses: "What is he thinking behind those lids that do not blink?" (94). Observing him through the eyes and ears of the doctor, we search for clues. As with Gregor, his "sickroom" is significant in that its emptiness reveals the depersonalization of its inhabitant. But this patient has been dehumanized even further—nameless, he is referred to only as "Room 542." The head nurse complains about the patient's infuriating habit of hurling his breakfast dish of scrambled eggs against the wall of his room, a ritual that the doctor observes the next morning. To the nurse, this is clearly a "difficult patient" with whom she interacts confrontationally. Rendered helpless by disease, "unheard" by his caregivers, the old man tries to reclaim some sense of control through the only means available to him—throwing the discus of eggs against the wall. Or perhaps the message is even stronger, and he is expressing that this existence is no longer worth living, that he would rather starve to death. What he needs most, his independence, expressed through his request for shoes for his legless body, medicine cannot restore. Compassionate abiding is likewise absent. The nurses avoid his room, and when he dies, the discovery is made "quite by accident" (95). Echoing the final "thank God" of Gregor's father, the head nurse comments that "it's a blessing"—words we suspect are spoken not out of compassion but of relief that he will be a nuisance no more: "Room 542 is deceased" (95).

Alexander Solzhenitsyn's *Cancer Ward* ([1967] 1983), set in a 1950s Soviet Russian hospital, furthers the discussion of alienation and isolation through the experiences of many who, like Gregor, wake up one day to find they have crossed over from health to disease.[6] Excerpts from this long novel provide ready entry into the stories of two patients in particular. Chapters 1 and 2 profile Pavel Nikolayevich Rusanov, a prominent official just entering the hospital, with chapter 1's title, "No Cancer Whatsoever," underscoring Pavel's initial denial of his diagnosis and defensiveness as he gradually acknowledges the full meaning of his illness. For him, the word *cancer* represents a dividing line: "In the space of a few days all . . . had been cut off from him. It was now on the *other* side of his tumor" (16). The idea of a line that has been crossed is a recurring theme in the illness experience with a parallel situation appearing in chapter 32, "The Other Side of the Coin," when Pavel's physician, famed radiation specialist Dontsova, discovers that she herself has cancer. For thirty years, cancer had been the disease of other people, a diagnosis disconnected from any understanding of its individualized human experience. Now she, like Pavel, finds herself cut off from her previous, pre-cancer existence; she will not even look at her own X-rays in her new role as passive patient. Additionally, as she crosses over from being doctor to patient, she finds patienthood incompatible with her role as healer: "She felt as if she had been deprived of her rights as a doctor" (454). Like Edward Rosenbaum, physician author of the memoir of his own cancer diagnosis and treatment (Rosenbaum 1988) made into the film *The Doctor* (Haines 1991), she now agonizes over how she ignored the personal experience of illness in her patients while focusing only on the technological aspects of their care.

Many artworks also illuminate the alienation and isolation caused by disease. Edvard Munch's *The Scream* (1893), an iconic image rich in possible interpretations, portrays a screaming figure caught in a no-man's-land between the stability of the linear boardwalk on which it stands and the swirling chaos beyond. Separated both literally and existentially from the others in the scene, the figure becomes a powerful metaphor for the experience of being swept away from the healthy, normal world into the realm of the sick. Ben Shahn's painting *It's No Use to Do Any More* (1996), portraying a victim of radiation in a hospital room where the major element is the empty distance between patient and caregivers, likewise provides a valuable visualization of the sick person's reality. In contrast, Pieter Bruegel's *Landscape with the Fall of Icarus* (ca. 1558) metaphorically puts the individual sufferer's isolation into a larger context where it sinks into insignificance: Icarus has fallen from the sky into a world where others, unaffected by his plight, ignore it. Like those in the painting, we hardly even notice the drowning Icarus. As W. H. Auden's poem "Musée des Beaux Arts" ([1938] 1991) observes about the scene, "everything turns away / Quite leisurely from the disaster" (170).

The Impact of Illness on Family and Friends

As is typical in our society, Gregor Samsa's care in *The Metamorphosis* falls to a female in his household. Because men now frequently become caregivers, our discussion of the impact of illness turns to portrayals of women being cared for at home by their male partners. In Anne Brashler's compact short story, "He Read to Her" ([1988] 1990), a woman grapples with a recent colostomy, the "brown puckered rose" (68) that has become the focal point of her disease identity. A humiliating indignity, it fills her with self-loathing, especially when the colostomy bag breaks, spewing its contents across the bathroom, and her husband, "gagging from the odor" (68), comes to rescue her. A catastrophic event has led to the colostomy, one that fills her with fear and untold anger that is primarily directed at her husband, one that fills him with guilt and self-loathing as well. Their struggle to negotiate a path through her anger and a new way of relating to each other illustrates the challenges of interacting with a patient whose self-image has been severely undermined by disease. Ignoring her request that he just go away, the man begins to read to her, and we are left to wonder if his choice of *Moby-Dick* indicates his abiding presence at her side or perhaps suggests that they are embarking together on an epic journey into the unknown to confront a new life of moral ambiguity. Jack Coulehan's poem, "Eleven Steps" (1991), also presents an angry, frustrated patient, a stroke victim, and her well-intentioned caregiver. No matter how hard he tries, he cannot grasp the depth of her loneliness and despair. When she attempts the "[t]welve steps from bed to porch" prescribed for her rehabilitation, he instinctively intervenes as she falters at the eleventh step. *"You son-of-a-bitch!* [she] blurt[s]" as he thwarts her feeble effort toward independence (31). For even long-term spouses, the divide between sickness and health often presents a challenge in understanding for both.

"Tube Feeding" (1987b), Richard Selzer's short story about a man caring for a woman with a massive tumor swelling her neck, offers a seemingly different caregiver-patient relationship. This couple has settled into roles with which they both seem comfortable: he interacts with her gallantly, especially during her tube feedings, and she welcomes his devotion as they ignore her disease as much as possible. But these are almost fictional roles that each has accepted as a way of coping with an underlying truth they wish to avoid, "that at the bottom of each of these tube feedings was the sediment of despair" (163). A crisis breaches this facade when, during one of the feedings, the tube dislodges, sending the man into a barely disguised panic: "He senses that a limit has been reached. But he clenches himself" (164). After inserting a new tube with great difficulty, he leaves the room to vomit stealthily in the bathroom, but the woman hears him. When he returns to continue the feeding, she stops him: " 'It is enough,' she says. 'No more' " (165). Both seem to acknowledge that a limit has been reached in the mutual suffering they have been trying to hide. As he puts the feeding utensils "away on the top shelf of the cupboard . . . where he won't be apt to see them again for a long time," we are left to wonder if that limit is temporary or final (166). Even this couple seems ultimately unable to bridge the gap between the healthy and the sick, caregiver and patient.

Susan Sontag has made many significant contributions to the discourse on illness, and here we turn to her short story, "The Way We Live Now" (1986), set during the early days of the AIDS epidemic, for insights on how illness affects relationships with others.[7] In contrast to the patient's perspective in "From the Journal of a Leper," this experimental fiction depicts an AIDS patient exclusively through the eyes of his friends. Unlike the rejection that Gregor receives or Updike's "leper" assumes, this band of comrades shows its concern for and solidarity with the patient, competitively vying for his attention and acceptance into the inner circle of the sickroom. At the same time, they are comforting each other and see themselves in him, the latest symbol of the plague decimating their numbers: "Everybody is worried about everybody now, said Betsy, that seems to be the way we live, the way we live now" (43). He is a member of their besieged community, and the wagons need to be circled. Part of the challenge of illness, as Gregor discovers, is to determine one's new role, and the friends examine closely the patient's behavior as he makes familiar the unfamiliar. But the question of new role equally applies to them. How should these friends act, and why? If they stay away, are they cowards? If they drop by the hospital daily, are they denying their fears of disease and mortality, striving rather "to identify [themselves] more firmly and irrevocably as the well, those who aren't ill, who aren't going to fall ill" (45)? A good companion piece to Sontag's story is Heather McHugh's "What Hell Is" ([1988] 1991), an early AIDS poem that powerfully captures the impact of disease on a family in ways reminiscent of *The Metamorphosis*. The theme of isolation predominates. Hell has become what used to be the family home, that bastion of middle-class safety and security, but now the place where the AIDS-stricken son has come to die. In sharp contrast to "The Way We Live Now," no one comes to visit; the whole family is avoided because of the stigma and fear of this still mysterious disease. Like Gregor Samsa, the patient is increasingly "spoken of / not with" in another room (393). His former self is becoming unrecognizable as is the family's life. Both have been indelibly transformed by the disease and responses to it.

Illness as a Source of Identity and Self-Awareness

Bugness in Kafka, psoriasis in Updike, colostomy in Brashler, tumor and tube in Selzer: for many patients, illness has the potential to shape our sense of self—our very identity—often negatively. For some, however, sickness can be at least partially a positive force for change. We saw an evolution of "self" to some extent in Updike's "From the Journal of a Leper" (1976); we encounter it less ambiguously in Lisel Mueller's poem, "Monet Refuses the Operation" ([1986] 1994). Whereas his doctor assumes that Monet would prefer healthy, "normal" vision to cataracts, Monet vibrantly catalogues his paintings as the rationale for his refusal. Clearly there is a value conflict, as the doctor cannot comprehend the unique artistic vision the cataracts bestow: "Doctor, / if only you could see / how heaven pulls earth into its arms" (122). As we contemplate Monet's incorporation of his impaired vision into his very sense of self, we are powerfully reminded of the body of work of Frida Kahlo whose catastrophic streetcar accident as a teenager and multiple surgeries thereafter provided much of her artistic inspiration.

Oliver Sacks's "Witty Ticcy Ray" (1985), about a man with Tourette's syndrome, furthers our exploration of illness as identity. In this case-based "clinical tale," the interaction between Ray and neurologist Sacks as they work to manage his syndrome is particularly instructive. Sacks, like Monet's doctor, logically assumes that his patient seeks relief from his symptoms and so prescribes Haldol. The drug works—too well. Ray loses the tics and outbursts that were a handicap at work, but he also loses the improvisational quality that made him a superior drummer and ping-pong player as well as the quickness that enabled him to dart in and out of revolving doors. As Ray and Sacks come to understand, Tourette's had become a defining part of Ray's identity: "I consist of tics—there is nothing else" (98). Much like Gregor's adaptation to his beetle existence, Updike's "leper" to his psoriasis, and Monet to his cataracts, Ray has not only accommodated to the limitations imposed by his syndrome but has also incorporated its advantages into his sense of self.

Ethan Frome (1911), Edith Wharton's novel set in late nineteenth-century rural New England, offers an unusual twist on illness identity through the character of Zeena. The central plot involves the sense of entrapment Ethan feels as caregiver first for his parents and then for Zeena, the woman he marries out of gratitude for helping him care for his parents. Throughout the novel, Zeena, whom we might well label a hypochondriac, alternates between the closely intertwined roles of caregiver and chronically ill patient: "[Ethan] soon saw that her skill as a nurse ha[d] been acquired by the absorbed observation of her own symptoms" (72).The opening section of chapter 7 (107–118) is particularly helpful in exploring Zeena's sense of illness. Returning from yet another visit to a doctor, she emphasizes to Ethan the gravity of her "complications" (108). It quickly becomes clear, though, that she relishes the diagnosis as it places her far above her neighbors with their more mundane category of "troubles." In contrast to the stigma some disease labels carry, "complications" confers special status on Zeena, for whom the roles of caregiver and patient mirror each other. Initially, she experienced fulfillment in caring for Ethan's parents and having others depend on her; now she finds similar satisfaction in the sick role that enables her to be the center of attention and control others' lives. By the end of the novel, Zeena miraculously recovers when she is needed as caregiver again, this time for Ethan and the girl with whom he was involved in a serious accident—a role she fulfills for more than twenty years. For Zeena, illness and caregiving are two sides of the same coin, meeting the same basic emotional needs.

No discussion of the experience of illness is complete without reference to Margaret Edson's play *W;t* (1999) and the film of the same name (Nichols 2001). Our protagonist is Professor Vivian Bearing, a woman of giant intellect, impeccable scholarship, and imperious teaching who now has stage 4 ovarian cancer. While the play focuses on the dehumanization of patient as research subject and breakdowns in patient-physician communication, it also powerfully details Vivian's developing self-awareness. As she experiences the alienation imposed by her illness and the hospital environment and the emptiness of her room devoid of visitors, she comes to understand the person she was in the context of who she has become. It is a painful realization—"the senior scholar ruthlessly denied her simpering students the touch of human kindness she now seeks" (59)—and the insight comes too late for her to act on it in any meaningful way, leading us to question its overall value. Does it serve only to augment her physical pain with spiritual suffering or does it add meaningful perspective to her life, a value in itself? In many ways, Vivian's situation parallels that of Leo Tolstoy's dying patient in *The Death of Ivan Ilyich* ([1886] 1981): "The doctor said his physical agony was dreadful . . . but even more dreadful was his moral agony," as he realizes he had lived life falsely (126).[8] In the end, however, Ivan achieves a final peace just as Gregor does in realizing compassion for his family. For Vivian, we are not so sure as there is "not even time for a proper conclusion" to her drama (72).

Disease, as we have seen, frequently brings alienation, often from our former selves. Its impact on relationships is challenging and revealing even if, as in Vivian's case, it simply unveils their absence. But, as our initial quotation from Keats suggests, disease also can bring understanding of what it means to be human. It can throw open a door on our former lives and transform our identities, often in positive ways.

NOTES

1 For a medical discussion of the terms, see Helman (1981, 548–552); for a linguistic discussion and personal account, see Fleischman (1999, 3–32).
2 See Sokel (1988), 105–116.
3 Howard Brody focuses on the family's reaction to Gregor in *Stories of Sickness* (1987, 105–112).
4 Michael Rowe, in "*Metamorphosis*: Defending the Human" (2002, 264–280), discusses the book within the framework of his son's fatal illness to emphasize the challenge of preserving the patient's humanity in the face of alienation all too easily imposed on the sick person, especially by caregivers.
5 For discussions of Updike and the impact of his psoriasis on his life and art, see Tatum (2010), 127–153; and O'Farrell (2001), 133–150.
6 For a discussion of the relation of Solzhenitsyn's own cancer to the novel, see Meyers (1985), 108–119.
7 See, e.g., her books *Illness as Metaphor* (1978) and *AIDS and Its Metaphors* (1989).
8 For other parallels between Edson and Tolstoy, see Jones (2007), 395–409.

Chapter 3

"THIS WEIRD, INCURABLE DISEASE"

Competing Diagnoses in the Rhetoric of Morgellons

LISA KERÄNEN

S UFFERERS' symptoms sound like the stuff of science fiction. As singer-songwriter Joni Mitchell told the *Los Angeles Times* in April 2010: "I have this weird, incurable disease that seems like it's from outer space" (Diehl 2010). Evoking the fantastical plotlines of the hit 1990s television show *The X-Files*, with its creepy alien "black oil" virus, people with self-diagnosed "Morgellons disease" report cutaneous stinging, biting, and crawling sensations; a shedding of black residue and granules; and multicolored, self-fluorescing fibers erupting from lesions on their skin. Patients appear in doctors' offices—especially across Texas, California, and Florida—bearing plastic bags containing fibers, skin debris, and black specks. They often describe "fatigue, mental confusion, short-term memory loss, joint pain, and changes in vision" (Molyneux 2008, 25). For many healthcare practitioners, the condition bears the hallmark signs of delusional parasitosis (DP): "a psychiatric disorder in which patients mistakenly believe that they are infested with a skin parasite" (Savely et al. 2006, 1). Most patients, however, reject the psychiatric diagnosis and insist that their condition is somatic and infectious, making it, as Elizabeth Geddes and Rashid Rashid observe, "one of the more complex management problems encountered in the dermatology clinic" (2008, 16). Facing pressure from members of Congress and the Morgellons Research Foundation (MRF), the Centers for Disease Control and Prevention (CDC) launched an inquiry into the nature and extent of what they term "unexplained dermopathy, aka 'Morgellons,'" and what others call the "Fiber disease."[1] In a move that fueled online conspiracy theories about bioweapons research gone awry, the CDC eventually enlisted the U.S. Army to help with the investigation (Centers for Disease Control 2009b). Thus, at least three groups—citizen advocates, the medical establishment, and the U.S. government—compete for the ability to define what, for some, appears to be a new, unexplained, and poorly understood condition (Savely et al. 2006) and what, for others, constitutes a classic psychiatric condition spreading wildly via the Internet (Vila-Rodriguez and Macewan 2008).

Whatever name it bears—Morgellons, Fiber disease, unexplained dermopathy, or delusional parasitosis—this contested condition provides an opportunity to consider the role of rhetoric in public healthcare exchanges involving emerging illnesses that sit at the intersection of biology and culture (Dumit 2006; Morris 1998). In the absence of mutually acceptable explanations about the nature and cause of this condition, various stakeholders create, deploy, challenge, and extend competing characterizations of the illness that materially affect its meanings, research, and treatment. In this chapter, I use the controversy over Morgellons/delusional parasitosis to explore what a rhetorical perspective offers the medical/health humanities. Morgellons/delusional parasitosis is a particularly instructive case for analysis because it reveals the power of the Internet to shape health consciousness, highlights the significance of patient advocacy in molding medical care, and allows us to examine how patients and practitioners mutually seek to persuade one another about certain aspects of their existential condition. After outlining key features of a rhetorical approach to the study of health medicine and offering a brief history of Morgellons, I track competing characterizations of Morgellons disease, delusional parasitosis, and their sufferers across recently published medical literature produced by dermatologists and Morgellons advocates. I find that, while Morgellons sympathizers appeal largely to visual evidence and adopt a "medical mystery frame," dermatologists and psychiatrists appeal largely to cultural and psychological explanations that identify Morgellons as Internet-fueled hysteria. More significantly, perhaps, the case of Morgellons demonstrates how providers and patients subtly, but mutually, shape the discourse and practices of one another even as they continue to advance radically divergent accounts of the causes and effects of sufferers' complaints.

THE RHETORIC OF MEDICINE AND HEALTH

As a growing interdisciplinary field, the rhetoric of medicine and health shares with the medical/health humanities a concern for the sociocultural, ethical, linguistic, historical, and aesthetic dimensions of clinical medicine (Berkenkotter 2008; Derkatch and Segal 2005; Hyde 1993; Keränen 2007, 2010a, 2010b; Lyne 2001; Scott 2003; Segal 2007, 2009a, 2009b). However, a rhetorical perspective focuses especially on how specific symbolic patterns structure meaning and action in health and medical contexts and practices. Historically, the study and practice of rhetoric flowered in fifth-century Athens when the art of defending oneself in public became a requisite skill for citizens of the budding democracy. Rhetoric, defined narrowly as persuasive speech, became part of the Latin trivium, the core humanities curriculum that required instruction in subjects such as grammar, logic, and dialectic. Contemporary rhetoricians have expanded the focus of rhetoric from oratory to the use of symbols in society more broadly, investigating the role of both verbal and nonverbal symbols in creating social realities, identities, and structures. Judy Segal explains that "the defining feature of rhetorical study is that it isolates the persuasive elements in these [medical and health] texts, genres, and discourses, and seeks to understand something about what they do, how they act in professional and public settings" (2009b, 227). But more than explaining persuasion, research in the rhetoric of medicine and health also involves investigating the role of language in creating biomedical knowledge, structuring health and illness identities, and coordinating patient care (Keränen 2010b).

Many of the earliest studies of medical rhetoric in the late twentieth century come from communication scholars who applied rhetorical theory to medical artifacts (Anderson 1989; Hyde 1993; Solomon 1985). In 1990, Barbara Sharf argued that doctor-patient interaction could be seen as a kind of "interpersonal rhetoric" whereby both parties sought to persuade others using narrative structures (217). Since that time, two developments have expanded the study of the rhetoric of medicine. First, growth in the rhetoric of science, from which rhetoric of medicine emerged in part, became a significant site of scholarly production with studies of medical and health discourse occupying an increasing share of the literature (Segal 2009b). Second, cultural studies configured the human immunodeficiency virus (HIV) as a robust object of study, prompting many rhetorically attuned analyses of HIV/AIDS texts. For instance, Paula Treichler (1999) and J. Blake Scott (2003) examined the cultural and linguistic aspects of HIV/AIDS across a wide swath of texts and practices. Scholarship in the rhetoric of medicine has since blossomed, encompassing analyses of the language of clinical encounters, public discourse about health and medical topics, new media engagement of medical themes, cinematic and popular cultural treatments of medicine, and social movements associated with medicine and health (Leach and Dysart-Gale 2011). A recurrent concern, one that is taken up in this essay, examines how language configures patients, illnesses, and the provider-patient relationship—and with what consequences. The basic premise is that language choices are bound up in knowledge and understanding. Studying differences in framing and characterization can reveal underlying worldviews that shape private life and public thought and action.

In what follows, I apply a rhetorical lens to examine the contest to define Morgellons. In the only published academic, sociological investigation of Morgellons to date, Brian Fair (2010) tracks how the trajectory of Morgellons as an emerging, contested illness became altered as it intersected with the existing trajectory of delusions of parasitosis. I extend this line of thinking by focusing on how the competing rhetorical constructions of Morgellons and delusional parasitosis configure both conditions and how these constructions in turn affect biomedical research and clinical practice. By tracking opposing characterizations of Morgellons, we can begin to grasp the rhetorical obstacles and practical challenges that lie at the heart of this vexing, contemporary phenomenon.

MORGELLONS: A BRIEF HISTORY OF A POSTMODERN CONDITION

The recent rise of what sufferers self-diagnose as Morgellons originates with Mary Leitao, a former laboratory technician whose two-year-old son, Drew, began complaining of "bugs" in 2001 (Atkinson 2006; Fair 2010; Harlan 2006). Leitao became alarmed when she began to pull fibers from lesions on Drew's skin, and she consulted various physicians to no avail; one infectious disease specialist at Johns Hopkins declined to see her, suggesting she had Munchausen's by proxy

(DeVita-Raeburn 2007, 98). Frustrated, she informally founded the Morgellons Research Foundation in 2002, which became a nonprofit in 2004. In the meantime, she established a website about the condition, soon receiving a steady stream of e-mails from those who claimed to be afflicted. According to Fair, "Leitao herself was initially unaware that there were so many Morgellons sufferers nationwide, and she was likewise presumably unaware that her son's Morgellons symptoms were virtually identical to those of DP, as neither she nor her son had elicited that diagnosis" (2010, 602).

Leitao selected the name *Morgellons* from French case history, drawing from descriptions of a condition "that caused considerable interest in the seventeenth and eighteenth centuries" (Kellett 1935). In *A Letter to a Friend*, published posthumously in 1690, Sir Thomas Browne described hairs breaking out in children "called the Morgellons" (Accordino et al. 2008, 9). One 1721 medical treatise notes the presence of "Hairs or Bundles of Hairs" (LeClerc 1715, as cited in Kellett 1935). Yet, between a 1935 medical history written about the oddity of Morgellons (Kellett 1935) and the term's 2002 reappropriation by Leitao, the condition virtually disappeared from medical annals. Moreover, the twenty-first-century version sounds remarkably different from its rhetorical ancestor, and the Morgellons Research Foundation (2011) conceded that there is likely no relation between the two. Instead of the hairs or bundles of hair that marked the French malady, one of the more eerie and credibility-straining facets of present-day Morgellons is the presence of unusual fibers, which are often described as "autoflorescing" (Savely et al. 2006, 1). As Robert Accordino et al. (2008, 8) note: "Descriptions of patients claiming to have the disease are strikingly similar, and their symptoms are consistent with that of those diagnosed with delusions of parasitosis." "Carol A.," spotlighted as a "Morgie of the Month" on the Holman Foundation website (2011), supplies a typical account:

My health had been deteriorating for years, and I was covered on my arms, hands, and legs with horrible lesions which would not heal. Strange fibers emerged from the lesions. . . . My exhaustion was off the charts, my weight soared regardless of diet, my thyroid had been destroyed, depression prevailed, narcolepsy and sleep apnea and night terrors took over my nights and days, my day/night cycle was out of sync, my short term memory and ability to concentrate caused me to doubt my own mind, my mind ruled in a slow-motion fog, and the lesions caused me horror and shame and hopelessness.

Despite the fact that the condition sports few mainstream dermatological supporters, Morgellons gained some traction in the public sphere following several well-publicized analyses of selected patient specimens, which found no match to hundreds of known textile fibers (DeVita-Raeburn 2007, 100; Fair 2010). Moreover, sympathetic practitioners lent their expertise to the case. Oklahoma State University's Chief of Pediatrics Rhonda Casey—whose skepticism turned to support when she realized the patients who self-identified with Morgellons also presented with neurological symptoms—found fibers embedded in unbroken lesions on multiple patients that she believed could not have been self-inflicted (DeVita-Raeburn, 2007, 100). Casey teamed up with colleague Dr. Randy Wymore, who began a series of conferences on Morgellons and who eventually founded the Charles E. Holman Foundation to spread awareness and search for a cause and cure.

Casey and Wymore's involvement catapulted the condition to national media outlets. Fair found that the "vast majority" of television transcripts followed Dr. Wymore's engagement with Morgellons (2010, 604). At the time that CBS aired a news story about Morgellons, Leitao and co-authors published an opinion piece in the *American Journal of Clinical Dermatology* (Savely et al. 2006), and Billy Koch, former pitcher for the Oakland A's, appeared on television claiming to have Morgellons along with his wife and three children (Fowler 2004; *KTVU News* 2006). In the meantime, flooded with constituents' reports, more than forty members of Congress lobbied the CDC for Morgellons research (Molyneux 2008). By July 2011, more than 15,600 people, representing all fifty states and more than fifteen countries, had registered with the MRF; Joni Mitchell and Louise Mandrell had dedicated their time to the cause; and new grassroots organizations—both supportive and debunking—sprouted. Here patient advocacy, the Internet, celebrity culture, and mass media converged to spread awareness and catalyze support for—and castigation of—Morgellons, thus illustrating a typical postmodern configuration: a medical establishment losing control of the discourse and finding itself competing with various lay and professional experts to define and manage contested conditions.

Theories about the cause and origins of Morgellons proliferate on the Internet, ranging from agrobacteria infection resulting from genetically modified organisms to exposure to an infectious element in wastewater or fertilizer, from side effects of airplane chemical trails to artificially intelligent nanotechnology (Smith 2011). While sufferers go to drastic lengths to get providers to take them seriously, conspiracy theories animate websites and lay publications, further diminishing credibility for the already skeptical. Commander X and Tim R. Swartz's publication, *Morgellons: Level 5 Plague of the New World Order* (2007), a collection of verbatim excerpts from websites and news sources, reviews conspiracy theories ranging from Morgellons development in a U.S. biological weapons laboratory to its origin in outer space. The concluding page of the booklet maintains, without evidence, that "CIA informants have revealed that Morgellons could be a manmade disease that is being propagated by the secret elite group that controls the world . . . in order to create panic in the general population" (50). *X-Files* redux! Yet, no matter how vivid the conspiracy theories it has inspired, Morgellons sits at the intersection of a far-reaching contest to define the nature of the condition, its causes, and remedies. Lacking a mutually credible explanation, various stakeholders create narratives about Morgellons that bolster or challenge the biomedical paradigm of delusional parasitosis.

THE POWER OF NAMING: MORGELLONS AS DELUSION, INTERNET HYSTERIA, OR MEDICAL MYSTERY?

Self-identified Morgellons sufferers and their dermatologists often engage in a not-so-delicate dance of persuasion, each trying to convince the other of the legitimacy of their account of the condition. Both groups deploy strategic characterizations in order to maintain their respective views, and the struggle to define the nature of Morgellons pivots on opposing portraits of "dermatopsychiatric disorder" and "medical mystery." In dominant dermatological and psychiatric accounts of delusional parasitosis (DP), the condition manifests as a primary or secondary "persistent delusional disorder" (Bewley et al. 2010, 1), a "monosymptomatic delusional disorder" (Sandoz et al. 2008, 699), a "psychocutaneous disorder" (Dewan et al. 2011, 745), or a "monosymptomatic hypochondrial psychosis" (Accordino et al. 2008, 9). Referred to variously as *delusions of parasitosis*, *Ekbom's syndrome*, and *parasitopobia*, the condition is characterized by "fixed, false beliefs [of infestation by animate or inaminate objects] that patients hold with unshakeable conviction, which are not grounded on a larger cultural, ethnic, or religious set of beliefs" (Sandoz et al. 2008, 699). With its own code in the *Diagnostic and Statistical Manual of Mental Disorders* (*DSM-IV-TR* 2000), DP benefits from institutional legitimacy, an insurance billing code, and privileged status in the published dermatological literature.

Consistent with a psychiatric diagnosis, much of the literature focuses on the mental state of patients, noting a preponderance of females over males. One case history emphasizes "severe anxiety and depression" in a patient who presented as "anxious, tearful, and suffer[ing] from logorrhea" (Sandoz et al. 2008, 699). In another case, "The patient became guarded and hostile when questioned further about the delusional belief and produced a bag containing a small insect that she believed originated from her body" (Sandoz et al. 2008, 698). "The clinical picture is unmistakable," explains Caroline Koblenzer: "The patient is intensely anxious, is obsessively focused on his or her symptoms, brings 'specimens' of the offending agent, or agents, and is unshakable in his or her belief as to the cause" (2006, 920). Obsessive, anxious, and feminized, patients are constructed as suffering first and foremost from a psychiatric condition. One practitioner even opines that his patients with Morgellons disease are "almost uniformly sexually deprived" with "sexual abandonment" serving as the "precipitating factor" (Haines Ely in Fellner and Majeed 2009, 137). In short, the dominant dermatological construction of patients presenting with feelings of formication is that—in stigmatizing lay terms—they are "crazy," despite the fact that a Mayo Clinic study found that half of patients initially diagnosed with DP were later found to have a "very real cause for the itching" (Schulte 2008). In this construction, Morgellons becomes the effect of a psychiatric condition requiring antipsychotics and therapy.

A second major interlocking and more recently emerging characterization of Morgellons/delusional parasitosis by dermatologists and psychiatrists is its repeated dismissal on grounds that it represents Internet-fueled hysteria (see Accordino et al. 2008; Freudenreich et al. 2010; Vila-Rodriguez and Macewan 2008). So prevalent is the role of the Internet in spreading awareness of Morgellons to potential sufferers that some clinicians maintain that self-diagnosis made from the Internet is a diagnostic sign, despite the fact that some Morgellons patients lack computer access (Schulte 2008). Accordino at al. (2008) detail the case of a sixty-year-old patient at the psychodermatology unit at New York Presbyterian

Hospital: "As she continuously excoriated her scalp, arms, and chest while in the clinic," they wrote, "she told us that she was certain of her diagnosis because of reading she had done on the internet describing a disease consistent with her symptoms" (8). "To use the language of infections," explain Oliver Freudenreich et al. in their editorial concerning Morgellons, "the Internet can be regarded as a 'vector' that can spread information—without regard for accuracy or usefulness" (2010, 456). Likewise, two physicians based in British Columbia wrote a letter to the editor of the *American Journal of Psychiatry* outlining an experience with a person who self-diagnosed Morgellons in which they observed the power of the Internet to "spread shared delusional ideation" (Vila-Rodriguez and Macewan 2008, 1612), while Andrew Lustig et al. (2009, 90) opine that the condition is merely "an Internet meme." Similar to the construction of Morgellons as delusional, the prominent dermatological/psychiatric configuration of it as Internet hysteria flattens cause and effect, positioning those seeking solace from unrelenting stinging skin sensations as needing psychiatric treatment.

Although they do not use the term, many dermatologists who discuss delusional parasitosis as an Internet-era effect describe it in terms Elaine Showalter calls *hystories*, "infectious epidemics of hysteria spread by stories circulated through self-help books, articles in newspapers and magazines, TV talk shows and series, films, and the internet, and even literary criticism" (1997, 5). Because she seeks to reclaim the term *hysteria* on feminist grounds, Showalter eschews taking a judgmental stance on stories of hysteria. She instead asks us to analyze the underlying anxieties and fantasies associated with the hysterical epidemics that circulate via new media. In that sense, we can easily read Morgellons as the ultimate dystopian biotechnological fantasy: human immune systems come under attack by an unknown agent that may be the result of post-9/11 laboratory science gone wrong that produces alien, glow-in-the-dark fibers and neurological dysfunction. However, privileging such psychoanalytic readings risks minimizing the suffering faced by the tens of thousands of people looking online for relief of their symptoms, people who often shun the skeptical medical establishment in favor of an active and supportive virtual community.

By contrast to the dominant dermatological framing of delusion, Morgellons advocates frame the condition as a likely infectious but presently unexplainable medical enigma. Spurred in part by a lack of medical interest in exploring the condition, the Morgellons Research Foundation (2011) developed its own case definition, which involves filaments and granules, movement sensations, slow healing and scarring skin lesions, musculoskeletal pain, aerobic limitation, cognitive dysfunction, and emotional effects such as intermittent obsessional states with cause unknown. The "medical mystery" frame, which appears across MRF literature spanning its website through its editorials and scientific papers (Holman Foundation 2011; Morgellons Research Foundation 2011; Savely 2010; Savely et al. 2006), translates well in popular television and magazine coverage garnering popular attention to the condition (DeVita-Raeburn 2007; *KTVU News* 2006). In the standard account of MRF advocates, Morgellons is cast as a "multi-systemic illness that has been presumed as a delusional phenomenon for decades as its obvious and disconcerting manifestations resembled actual (but 'unverified') parasite infection as well as various psychopathologies" (Harvey et al. 2009, 4). The condition is configured as somatic, infectious, and stigmatized (Savely 2010). According to William Harvey et al., "Morgellons manifest[s] as a skin phenomenon, an immune deficiency state, and a chronic inflammatory process" (2009, 4). In this framing, Morgellons requires additional research—something DP advocates generally regard as unnecessary—and antibiotic therapy aimed at staunching the presumed but unknown infectious cause.

Whereas the construction of the DP patient emphasizes psychiatric symptoms, MRF characterizations stress patients' pre-Morgellons normality. In fact, the MRF's Virginia Savely maintains that "its victims have no prior history of psychiatric disorders, the onset often follows an immune suppressing event, it occurs in children and in entire families [and pets], it is more prevalent in certain parts of the country, and its onset is seasonal" (2010, 215). Morgellons Research Foundation publications observe that nurses and teachers constitute two main occupations of those reporting symptoms (Savely et al. 2006, 3). Nonetheless, Harvey et al. concede that "strikingly, most patients in this study (23 out of 25) had prior psychiatric diagnoses" (2009, 3). Although Harvey and colleagues conclude that "Morgellons disease can be characterized as a physical human illness with an often-related delusional component in adults," they also note that "all medical histories support that behavioral aberrancies onset only after physical symptoms" (Harvey et al. 2009, 1). In other words, Morgellons advocates position the symptoms of Morgellons as the effect, not the cause of psychiatric symptoms, thus reversing the accepted dermatological position.

In an largely futile attempt to overcome the credibility gap of symptoms that strain plausibility, Morgellons sufferers frequently enlist visual rhetoric wrapped in a patina of scientific-sounding language—for example, "coenocytic (aseptate), smooth-walled, branching, filamentous objects" (Morgellons Research Foundation 2011)—to make their case. In clinical settings, patients often present fibers and skin debris as evidence of their admittedly bizarre-sounding condition. Many purchase microscopes to study and document the filaments, cataloging them on the web. For instance, the website associated with the Charles E. Holman Foundation, a grassroots advocacy organization dedicated to Morgellons awareness, contains numerous magnified images of Morgellons that constitute a staple component of discourse on the Internet (Holman Foundation 2011; see also Morgellons Research Foundation 2011; Smith 2011). Such fibers attempt to provide solid proof to bridge the credibility gap that lies at the heart of the condition. Yet such efforts to marshal material rhetoric often fail to convince. "You think you are bringing them evidence," explains Leitao, "but you're really just shooting yourself in the foot" (Leitao as cited in DeVita-Raeburn 2007, 99). Here, the "baggy sign" (so named because Morgellons patients often present fibers in plastic bags to healthcare providers as evidence) condemns Morgellons sufferers to the delusional parasitosis paradigm, prompting "doctor shopping," depression, and some reports of suicide (Schulte 2008).

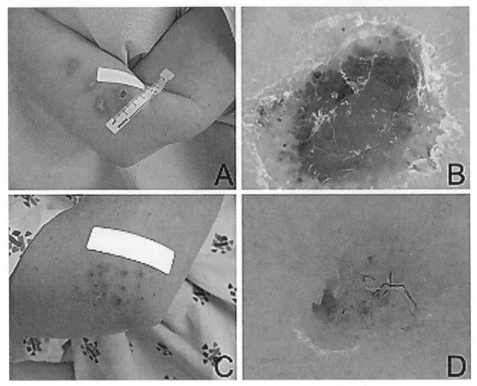

FIGURE 3.1 Morgellons/unexplained dermopathy images, Centers for Disease Control and Prevention, 2012. These images appear in Pearson et al. (2012) and are open access.

DUELING DISCOURSE COMMUNITIES: COMPARING MORGELLONS/DELUSIONAL PARASITOSIS IN MEDICAL PUBLICATIONS

While the contrasting language choices of dermatologists and Morgellons advocates may merely seem to reflect the interested labels of disparate discourse communities, they in fact align with material differences in the approach to studying, treating, and understanding the condition. If we compare the language of two medical journal essays concerning Morgellons/delusional parasitosis, we witness the deep conceptual rift existing between mainstream dermatological community and Morgellons advocates. The first paper comprises a 2009 case report series by members of the MRF in the *Journal of Medical Case Reports*, reviewing physical, medical-historical, and laboratory data for twenty-five consecutive patients with self-defined Morgellons (Harvey et al. 2009; hereafter *CR*).[2] The second paper appeared in the *Archives of Clinical Dermatology* in summer of 2011, authored by clinicians at the Mayo Clinic who sought evidence of infestation in patients diagnosed with delusional parasitosis (Hylwa et al. 2011; hereafter *Archives*). *Archives* received major news coverage in the days following its online release because it found that none of 108 patients with suspected DP had evidence of infestation.

News headlines bearing Morgellons-related articles soon declared that the disease was "An Infestation That Begins in the Mind" (Healy 2011).

Both papers evidence the struggle over naming the condition popularly known as *Morgellons*. "For semantic accuracy," *CR* acknowledges, "there is only one 'proven' MD [Morgellons disease] patient: the child first given that label"; *CR* also acknowledges that Morgellons is a "placeholder" name selected because of the "dermal similarity" to its several-hundred-year-old cousin (Harvey et al. 2009, 8243). Nonetheless, the paper consistently deploys the term *Morgellons disease* in a deliberate effort to reclaim patients' experiences from the psychiatric diagnosis of delusional parasitosis. Harvey et al.'s (2009) use of the term *disease*, as opposed to syndrome or illness, further signifies an attempt to link the condition to an infectious process and to mark it as a legitimate medical problem with biological components.

By stark contrast, *Archives*'s steadfast refusal to use the lay label *Morgellons* in the body of the paper—despite the term's appearance throughout the bibliography and in the study's patient record search criteria—punctuates the preferred interpretation of its authors. Here, not only is delusional parasitosis the favored moniker, but also the entire *Archives* investigation hinges on (not) finding evidence of parasitic infestation, thus betraying a crucial conceptual gap between Morgellons advocates and the dermatological community. Fibers and feelings of formication are not bugs. There is a difference between the sensation that bugs are crawling on your skin and believing that bugs (or, in the case of Morgellons, fibers) are inhabiting your dermis; therefore, the *Archives*'s study design privileges the medical establishment's implicit frame of psychiatric delusion instead of probing for other shared physical explanations for the sensations. Consistent with this frame, *Archives* concludes by advocating antipsychotics and raising the question of whether skin biopsies are necessary for patients suspected of delusional infestation.

Comparing the divergent framings of illness across these two publications helps us to see why Morgellons patients and their providers often find themselves at a rhetorical impasse. On the one hand, Morgellons sufferers are convinced they experience a bizarre and presently unexplained medical mystery, one that is often readily dismissed by the mainstream medical community. On the other, dermatologists portray Morgellons sufferers as difficult "to manage" as "they often take considerable time and other resources to engage in therapeutic management" (Bewley et al. 2010, 1). Beyond the fact that reports of self-fluorescing fibers erupting from unbroken skin strain plausibility, part of the rhetorical burden for sufferers seeking care is that three of the most commonly used persuasive mechanisms available to them are listed as diagnostic signs in the dermatological literature: self-diagnosis from the Internet; presentation of a baggy sign; and refusal to accept a psychiatric diagnosis (Accordino et al. 2008; Robles et al. 2011). Morgellons sufferers face a profound rhetorical quandary in that their appeals index the psychiatric diagnosis they seek to avoid, thus forcing many of them to seek help outside the medical establishment. Providers similarly face a frustrating rhetorical obstacle in that their patients are, by and large, unwilling to accept the terms of a psychiatric diagnosis. And thus we arrive at the crux of the matter: both dermatologists and self-described Morgellons sufferers, in the absence of mutually acceptable proof, engage in ongoing persuasive exchanges in which each attempts to bring the other round to his or her way of seeing the world.

MUTUAL PERSUASION: SHIFTING TERMINOLOGY AND THE THERAPEUTIC ALLIANCE

Despite the shared difficulties of their encounters, the upshot of the interactions between Morgellons patients and their physicians is that—in a world where they are mutually interdependent—each community makes rhetorical accommodations to appeal to the other (Fahnestock 1986). Koblenzer summarizes the clinical challenges:

Clearly, as more and more of our patients discover [the MRF web-]site, there will be an ever greater waste of valuable time and resources on fruitless research into fibers, fluffs, irrelevant bacteria, and innocuous worms and insects. It behooves us, therefore, as dermatologists, not only to be aware of this phenomenon, but also each to develop an effective way to work with these patients, and so enable the patients to be able to accept one of the medications that we know to be effective. This is a challenge indeed—so often the patient, feeling "brushed off" or not understood, simply does not follow through either with medication or with psychiatric referral. (2006, 921)

In light of these challenges, some clinicians are adapting their language to the Morgellons community.[3] To address the lack of trust and the tendency to disavow psychiatric diagnoses, clinicians have maintained that it is important to use the term *Morgellons*, accompanied by a staged approach to therapy, involving more than the traditionally prescribed antipsychotics and psychiatric referrals. For instance, Jenny Murase et al. have advocated using *Morgellons disease* as a "rapport-enhancing term" to overcome the significant obstacles to patient care (2006, 913). Similarly, Accordino et al. advocate a "therapeutic alliance" by "acknowledging that there are skin issues to be treated" and by prescribing a combination of psychiatric, cutaneous, and antibiotic therapy (2008, 11). By "meeting the patient halfway," they hope that patients will comply with medical interventions. Accordino et al. (2008) further detail what amounts to a translation of the physician's desire to prescribe antipsychotics into terms more confirming to Morgellons sufferers:

For the dermatologist treating a patient claiming to have Morgellons disease, there is not only an issue of nomenclature, but also one of action. Regardless of what the disorder is called, dermatologists must acknowledge to their patients that they know that their sensations and suffering are real and that they will do everything they can to help. The physician should then explain that the dysesthesia that the patient is experiencing is mediated, in part, by neuropeptides, and that symptoms are often improved when patients go on certain known medications [antipsychotics] that act on these neuropeptides. (11)

Here, the clinician modifies her appeal from a psychiatric frame into a psychocutaneous frame by appealing to the drugs' effects on skin sensation. As Fair (2010) suggests, such staged efforts at persuasion signify a replacement of the patient compliance model, whereby physicians attempt to gain compliance of patients to biomedical interventions, with a physician compliance model, in which clinicians adapt their treatment and language choices to resonate with the patients. While rhetorically expedient, such accommodations may also raise ethical issues associated with autonomy and truth telling.

Another accommodation occurs at the level of nosology, the classificatory naming of illness conditions. As patients seek out sympathetic practitioners, armed with letters from advocacy groups and the latest research findings, their rising numbers in dermatology offices have prompted proposals for new names in the medical literature. A. P. Bewley et al., for instance, suggest replacing *delusional parasitosis* with *delusional infestation* (DI), which would include "the so-called 'Morgellons syndrome'" (2010, 1). "DI is a more accurate term," maintain P. Dewan et al. (2011, 747), "as it incorporates the spectrum of imaginary pathogens." Moreover, some clinicians have suggested that Morgellons be characterized as subset of delusional parasitosis (Robles et al. 2011, 2). As David Robles and colleagues explain: "In DP the delusional focus is on being infested with parasites, whereas patients with Morgellons disease believe that unusual fibers or other material is in their skin" (2011, 4). Observing that "most patients and family members do not respond well to the implication that they are maniacal, delusional, or psychotic," dermatologists H. W. Walling and B. L. Swick advocate abandoning "outdated, pejorative" terms such as *delusions of parasitosis* and *neurotic excoriation*, the term dermatologists use to index "repetitive, injurious scratching behavior" (2007, 317–318). Instead, these authors advocate terms such as *disorders in cutaneous perception* or *pseudoparasitic dysaesthesis* (318). "These conditions are sufficiently challenging to treat without fabricating a barrier of insensitive language," they explain (319). Such examples illustrate that Morgellons publicity and the rising number of patient complaints about fibers and crawling skin sensations are pushing the medical community to alter its nomenclature.

Morgellons advocates are also being influenced by the DP community. The 251 National Library of Medicine (NLM) references to delusional parasitosis influenced the MRF researchers who noted that their review of these references "leads us to the possibility that Morgellons disease and DP are grossly truncated labels of the same illness but with the reversal of the cause-effect order" (Harvey et al. 2009, 1). Moreover, the MRF casts *delusions*—the key term from the dermatological paradigm—as the *result* of Morgellons, not the cause, and the controversy surrounding Morgellons/DP can be read as pivoting on competing explanations of cause and effect.

The rhetoric reviewed in my analysis thus far confirms that Morgellons patients and dermatologists are in some ways attempting to accommodate each other's discourse and practice. Yet my analysis also reveals the recalcitrance of each discourse community's preferred terms. Morgellons advocates continue to advance labels such as *Morgellons*, *disease*, and *infectious*, even as the dermatology community clings to *delusional* and *psychiatric*. In short, despite modest modifications at the level of clinical interaction, both discourse communities largely retain opposing characterizations and understandings of the illness's nature and causes.

CONCLUSION: COLLECTIVE CONSTITUTION OF AN EMERGING CONDITION

Illness and disease occur in social and historical contexts where prevailing conventions, discourses, and technologies shape the conditions of possibility (Morris 1998). A rhetorical approach to illness and disease calls attention to the role of language in shaping meaning and action. In the case of Morgellons, we witness divergent stakeholder groups competing to define Morgellons as an Internet-era manifestation of delusional parasitosis versus an emerging and likely infectious medical mystery. This debate is unlikely to be resolved in the near future, regardless of the findings of the much-awaited CDC/Kaiser Permanente study (Centers for Disease Control 2009a). Nonetheless, the struggle to define Morgellons affords the opportunity to examine how patient empowerment—in this case, via the Internet and citizen advocacy groups—can shape clinical practice and public biomedical research agendas. Pro-Morgellons websites not only seem to have catalyzed a virtual support community around Morgellons issues but have also helped to force others to take the issue seriously. Segal explains that, "far from being simply an innovation, Internet health is a new iteration of a direct exchange between patients and information, absent the physician" (2009a, 364). In this case, we see that patient advocacy groups move forward with their own case definitions, research projects, and funding streams even as they push for government research, while mainstream medical professionals work to develop responsive modes of persuasion and treatment. But we also see how the Internet allows conspiracy theories and misinformation to flourish in the absence of a patient-accepted clinical paradigm, and we witness how discourse communities make rhetorical accommodations while still retaining their dominant rhetorical characterizations of the condition.

Morgellons advocates pose an interesting challenge to the mainstream medical community: "Does the practice of 'evidence-based modern medicine' come from peer-reviewed literature, or from the actual patient?" (Harvey et al. 2009, 2). This brief examination of the competing rhetorics surrounding Morgellons/DP suggests that peer-reviewed literature, Internet content, and patient testimony interact to modify subtly both lay and clinical pictures of Morgellons/delusional parasitosis—even when the discourse communities otherwise advance radically divergent explanations of the nature and cause of the condition. Whatever "facts" about Morgellons are discernible from published scientific papers and patient narratives, the social reality of Morgellons/DP is continually reshaped in a persuasive dance in which mutually interdependent stakeholders seek recognition and influence. Analyzing the rhetorical interplay between the mainstream dermatological community and Morgellons advocates therefore allows us to begin to understand how stakeholders jostle to co-create evolving characterizations of illness and its effects.

POSTSCRIPT

As this chapter was headed to the editors, the CDC and Kaiser Permanente (Pearson et al. 2012) published their study of unexplained dermopathy/Morgellons.

Their analysis of data from 115 case patients in California found no infectious or environmental explanation for the skin lesions, identified most fibers as compatible with skin fragments or cellulose/cotton fibers, and noted that a substantial number of participants scored highly on measures of co-existing psychiatric conditions. The study concluded that, "in the absence of an established cause or treatment, patients with this unexplained dermopathy may benefit from receipt of standard therapies for co-existing medical conditions and/or those recommended for similar conditions such delusions infestation [*sic*]" (12). Many Morgellons supporters remain unconvinced by the study's conclusions, and the struggle over the characterization and legitimacy of the condition continues. The Morgellons Research Foundation went offline in 2012 and donated their funds to Oklahoma State University, where the Holman Foundation was busy planning "Searching for the Uncommon Thread: The 5th Annual Morgellons Disease Conference" (Holman Foundation 2012). Meanwhile, Morgellons sufferers actively refute the CDC/Kaiser Permanente findings online. In time, we will discover how the clinical and lay pictures of Morgellons/DP will continue to influence one another and whether Morgellons sufferers will someday receive the clinical and public support their advocates so passionately seek.

ACKNOWLEDGMENTS

I thank Yara Youssuf for research assistance during the initial stages of this project and Kirstin Runa for help during its completion. I appreciate conversations about this paper I've had with Tess Jones, Les Friedman, Delese Wear, Sandra Hartnett, Stephen Hartnett, Hamilton Bean, J. Blake Scott, and members of the 2011 Rhetoric Society of America Institute's workshop on "Medicine and Its Publics."

NOTES

1 The MRF became inactive in 2012 after the CDC/Kaiser Permanente study (Centers for Disease Control 2009a) was published and after this essay was written. Some of the MRF's members now serve as advisors or board members of the Charles E. Holman Foundation. A copy of the MRF website as it appeared online in July 2012 is on file with the author. This essay therefore provides a glimpse into the evolving nature of social advocacy surrounding a contested illness.

2 For Harvey et al. (2009) article, I used the page numbers from the online version throughout for convenience. While the authors declare they did not have competing interests, their affiliation with the MRF is muted in the credits except for a note that co-author Mary Leitao created the current Morgellons "label, and concept" (6). Moreover, lead author William Harvey's position as head of research for MRF is conspicuously unstated.

3 As I was completing this essay, I discovered that Fair similarly but independently relied on Koblenzer (2006), Murase et al. (2006), and Accordino et al. (2008) to find that the disease trajectories of Morgellons and DP had an "interactive relationship" (Fair 2010, 598). I maintain, however, that despite these rhetorical accommodations, the broader discourse of each community reveals incompatible underlying beliefs about biomedical knowledge.

Chapter 4

MY QUEST FOR HEALTH

MICHAEL SAPPOL AND SHELLEY WALL

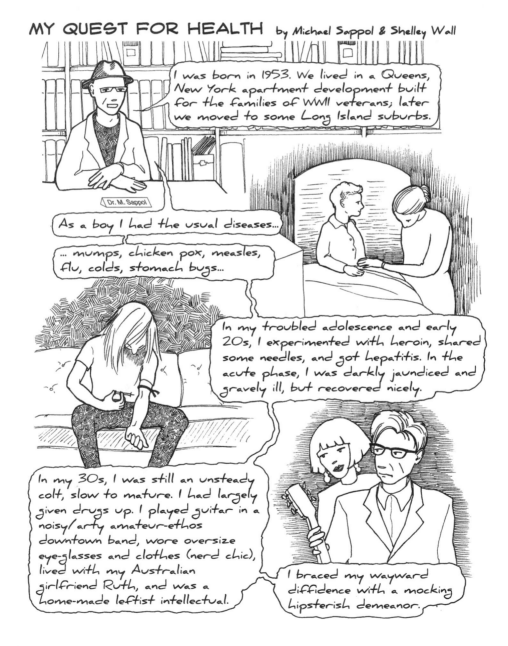

Around 1985, I became ill in a new way.

Even when hospitalized with hepatitis, I had never worried about death—I was too exhausted for that. But this new condition came on me quickly and alarmingly, without the lethargy that makes you feel indifferent to the disease that possesses you. It woke me up (but eventually wore me out).

It began like this:

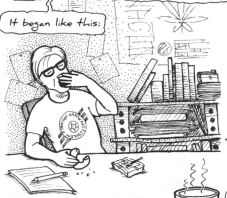

I was in the offices of High Times magazine, where I was a freelance proof reader and copy-editor. It was in the afternoon. I was sitting at my desk, about to doze off.

Suddenly I was caught short, couldn't breathe or swallow, and felt nauseous. Even worse, those operations which had always been automatic now seemed voluntary and hard to coordinate. I was confused about what my windpipe should be doing.

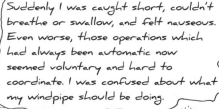

PANIC ATTACK. HAPPENS ALL THE TIME.

My co-workers called for an ambulance.

The paramedics gave me some oxygen, calmed me down. They recommended I see my doctor (I didn't have one), but offered to take me to the hospital. I decided not to go, but was shaken, went home.

The symptoms abated, but quickly recurred.

I was now conscious, in a way I had never been, that my throat had two passage-ways, one for food the other for air, and the two no longer worked together collaboratively. I had trouble breathing, and swallowing food and pills.

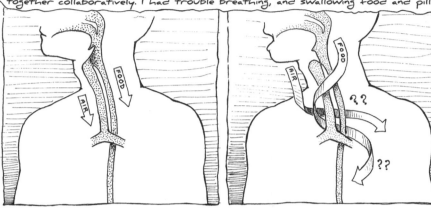

I felt like I had a rock in my throat. After meals, I felt nauseous and my mouth filled up with saliva. It was summertime and Ruth and I started going for evening walks in Tompkins Square Park where I would spit every ten feet or so.

On top of all that, when I was in my greatest distress my chest vibrated: which wasn't an imaginary symptom. Ruth could feel it when she put her hand on my chest, could even see it.

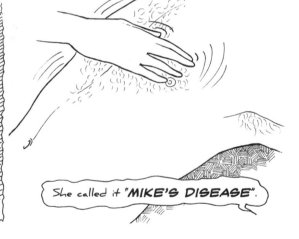

She called it "MIKE'S DISEASE".

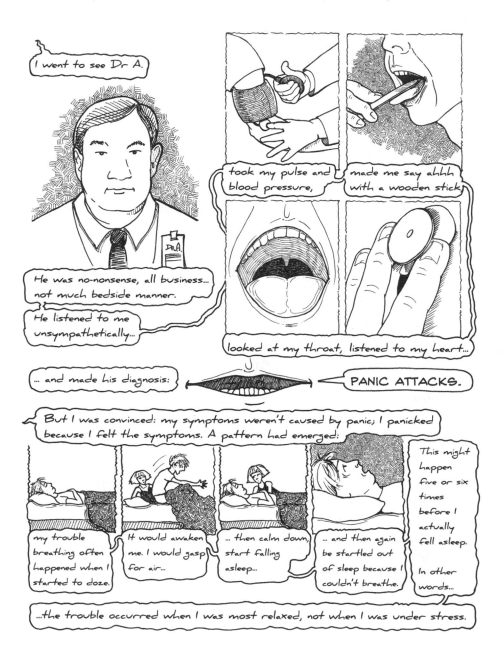

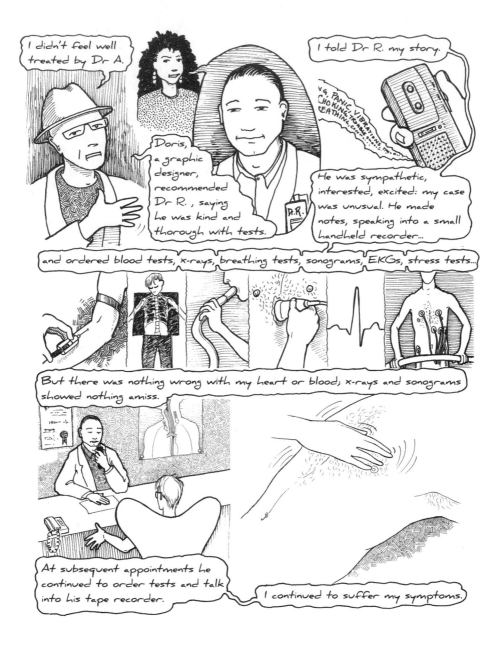

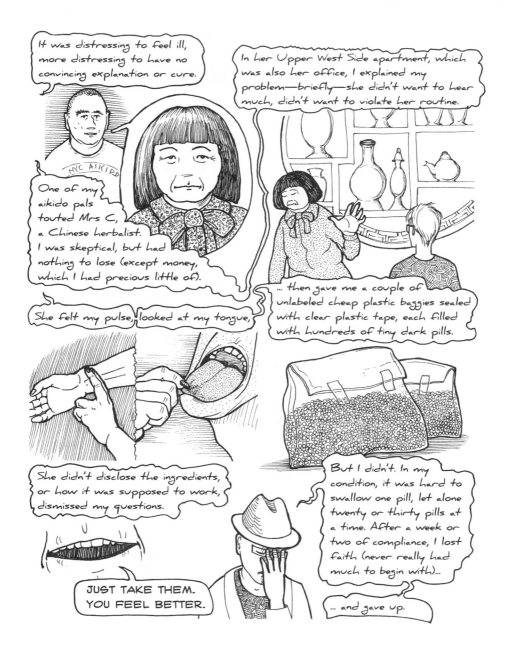

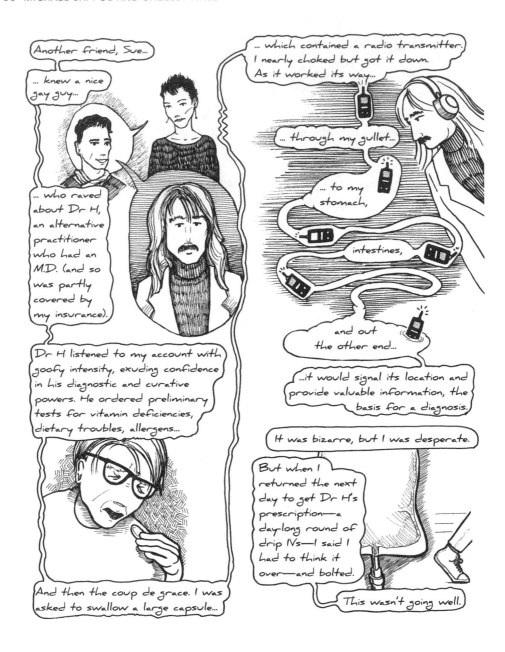

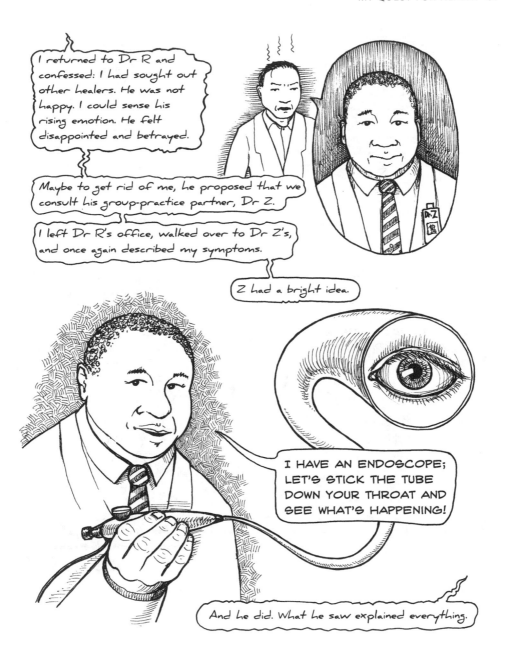

I had a form of esophageal reflux. The stomach acid never went high enough for me to feel heartburn, but contacted my pharynx and made it go into spasms. Which were the vibrations that I felt. And which affected my swallow/gag reflex, caused the rock in my throat, and made me salivate.

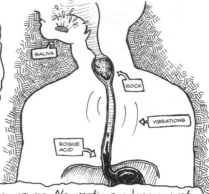

So that was the answer. No exotic syndrome, just something extremely common. Not curable, and undoubtedly made worse by anxiety, but treatable. The explanation was in some ways the main treatment. It reassured me that there was nothing life-threatening.

Dr R was humiliated.
Thereafter, if I tried to make an appointment with him, the receptionist shunted me to Dr Z. If I ran into Dr R at the office, he averted his gaze.

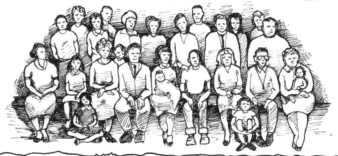

Years later I told the story to my Aunt Raye. She told me that she, my mother, their four sisters, my cousins, and my grandmother—nearly everyone in the family—had all experienced a similar crisis in their 30s.

Mike's Disease was the Family Curse.

I still have it: the Family Curse and I have grown old together. But it has evolved.

The rock in my throat is smaller—or maybe I'm now used to it. I get nauseous after meals, but my mouth no longer fills up with spit. I only occasionally confuse swallowing and breathing, and still sometimes gasp for air as I doze—and also after orgasm—a new symptom! I take medications (which didn't exist in the 1980s) and use two pillows to elevate my head when sleeping. I get periodic checkups for Barrett's Syndrome, which can lead to esophageal cancer. (Last year, my younger brother had cancer and had his esophagus removed. We don't talk much; I didn't know he also had the Family Curse.)

I'm now almost 60 and have to deal with liver disease, cancer, auto-immune problems, fallout from surgeries, and aging—which interact with the Family Curse and confuse me and my doctors.

Gathered together, my health records, scattered among all the doctors over the decades, would run to thousands of pages.

For more than 30 years, Mike's Disease has sickened me, vexed me, medicalized me, re-made me. I've told this story in bits to friends and family. Now, I hope this "quest for health" story will help my daughters if they are someday afflicted by the Family Curse. (Happily, there's no evidence of that yet.)

Part II

DISABILITY

Chapter 5

DISABILITY IN TWO DOCTOR STORIES

MARTHA STODDARD HOLMES

It was already one in the morning; the rain pattered dismally against the panes, and my candle was nearly burnt out, when, by the glimmer of the half-extinguished light, I saw the dull yellow eye of the creature open; it breathed hard, and a convulsive motion agitated its limbs. . . . I had worked hard for nearly two years, for the sole purpose of infusing life into an inanimate body. For this I had deprived myself of rest and health. I had desired it with an ardour that far exceeded moderation; but now that I had finished, the beauty of the dream vanished, and breathless horror and disgust filled my heart.

MARY SHELLEY ([1818] 1994, 39)

THUS unfolds the crisis of creation in a classic "doctor story" involving disability, Mary Shelley's novel *Frankenstein*. The experimental scientist Victor Frankenstein has obsessively focused on his goal of bringing life from death, isolating himself from his family and fiancée to collect and combine raw materials from charnel houses, dissecting rooms, and graves. At the moment of "birth," however, Frankenstein flees his creation, all his anticipation turned to revulsion. When the creature seeks him out, extending its hand and making communicative noises, Frankenstein leaves his own house to escape the "miserable monster" and "demoniacal corpse to which I had so miserably given life" ([1818] 1994, 40).

Shelley's focus on scientists playing god, the "monsters" that can result, and the ethical obligations of creators to their creations make *Frankenstein* a fertile field for meditations on biomedical research ethics, an effective touchstone for ethicists' communication of ideas about science to the public, and a useful text for medical education. This early science fiction narrative seems to be a clear cautionary tale against the dangers of human overreaching through technology. The novel invites reflection and discussion about how hubris combined with a passion for science can lead us astray, because our capacity for medical/technological interventions may exceed our capacity for evaluating their ethical consequences.[1] While he is not any sort of a doctor, Victor Frankenstein is memorialized in popular culture *as* "Dr. Frankenstein" to the extent that he is regarded as a doctor figure, with multiple valences of Ph.D. and M.D.—researcher and physician. In medical education, the instructive value of *Frankenstein* presumes the reader/medical student's imaginative identification with the overzealous researcher seeking to overcome the boundary of death through human knowledge or the physician who pursues futile or otherwise questionable interventions, rather than letting nature take its course.

Despite its sustained focus on the figure of the scientist, however, *Frankenstein* is arguably quite a bit richer as a narrative about the experience of the research subject or perhaps even the patient.[2] Shelley's work devotes substantial narrative energy to rendering the perspective and voice of the creature that is eagerly brought to life and then summarily rejected by his parent, as well as most other humans. In fact, the novel offers a memorable first-person account of the experience of being stigmatized and socially disabled by physical differences considered "deformities." Consider the scene in which the being, at birth, is pronounced hideous by an authority; his repeated exclusion from public spaces because of "ugliness"; Victor's dramatic prevention of the creature's sexual and reproductive agency; and the creature's internalization and ultimate embracing of his "monstrosity" as his only satisfaction. The creature's process of becoming a monster is a harsh but not unimaginable version of what a baby with physical singularities, pronounced "deformed" at birth, might experience growing up in a society that finds him or her monstrous or freakish.[3] While the novel is a provocative "doctor story" with its focus on the researcher and research ethics, I suggest that it may have even greater value for students of the medical humanities as a classic narrative of the social construction of disability—a fiction that might be read in concert with such works as Erving Goffman's *Stigma* (1963) and Lucy Grealy's *Autobiography of a Face* as a classic text on the social body and the individual's assimilation of or resistance to a stigmatized social identity. The scholarly discipline of disability studies offers the tools for such an analysis.

DISABILITY STUDIES VERSUS THE MEDICAL MODEL

Disability studies is a mode of critical thinking about disability beyond the "medical model" that has had significant authority, not simply to diagnose disability, but also to determine its cultural meanings. The medical model usually assumes the perspective of physicians and the able-bodied, seeing disability as a radical and essential human difference and narrating disability as a personal tragedy or (if "overcome") triumph. As Abby Wilkerson notes,

> One of the most important influences of medicine—and the reason it has received so much critical attention in disability studies—is its active shaping of cultural perceptions of disability identity itself, which thereby structures how the nondisabled interact with people with disabilities. . . . It is, of course, medical discourse we usually turn to in order to decide which bodies are sound and even what bodily soundness is, and the reliability of this discourse is seldom questioned. . . . [Disability's] status appears to be incontestable because it is medically certified, with medical evidence regarded as utterly objective, detached from values, emotions, and particular human interests. (2002, 50–51)

Medicine tends to consider disability as a problem that needs repair or cure and locates disability in individual bodies/persons and conditions rather than in a complex of social, cultural, and political relationships.

Disability studies, in contrast, generally draws on some version of a social/cultural constructionist approach: these scholars consider disability as above all, and most powerfully, a set of social and cultural meanings shaped by the popular imagination, by obstructive or welcoming physical and social environments, and by institutions like hospitals and schools as much as—or more than—by the fact of legs that do not walk or ears that do not hear. While individuals have impairments (differences of function), disability is not located *in* those individuals but in the interactions between people and their social and physical environments, which jointly produce ability and disability by degrees.

An impairment only becomes a disability when the environment is one that associates disadvantages with it. Thus, disability can be said to be created by communities that assign impairment disabling and disadvantaging meanings. For example, in a community fluent in sign language, like Martha's Vineyard in the 1800s, as described by medical anthropologist Nora Groce (1985), being deaf or hard of hearing was minimally disabling in comparison to experiencing the same impairment in a non-signing community. Similarly, wheelchair users' degree of disability changes dramatically in a society with—or without—ramps and curb cuts.

As *Frankenstein* illustrates, disability can be constructed even in the absence of physical impairment. The creature is physically able and powerful, "more agile" than the average human, but treated as a monster and denied basic rights because of his perceived hideousness (Shelley [1818] 1994, 96).

The dynamism of the constructionist model directs us to consider disability historically, locally, and specifically rather than as an essential, stable, or generalizable truth. As Lennard Davis argues, "The fact that disability and normality can be looked at as sociohistorical concepts is crucial to disability studies, since the alternative paradigms—the medical and rehabilitation models—presume that disability is a universal constant" (2002, 40). The reality of living disabled, in contrast, involves good days and bad days and accessible and inaccessible environments; disabled people's experiences and situations change through time and across cultures.[4]

Rethinking disability as a construct rather than an essential truth spurs us to think innovatively, overturning as impermanent our assumptions about the meaning of disability. One example of this is the process of thinking *with* disability rather than *about* it. This can mean that disability studies scholarship engages, as central and crucial, the perspectives of disabled people or that it reflects on disability as a generator of insight, aesthetics, innovation, knowledge, pleasure, and desire.[5] While the disabling effects of social and physical environments produce situations of disadvantage and discrimination, from a disability studies perspective, these negatives are not inherent in the experience of impairment—or even in the experience of disability. The realities of impairment and disability can be culturally rich, creative, and communitarian as well as the isolated, sorry states they are in many popular representations.

As an academic field, disability studies originated in the social and behavioral sciences and has in the past quarter century gained recognition in the humanities (including literary and visual studies, critical theory, philosophy, and history) and cultural studies. Increasingly, disability studies scholars have attended to the interactions among disability and other aspects of social identity such as gender, sexuality, race, ethnicity, age, "beauty," class, wealth, and education, since our situations as persons are generally shaped by multiple, mutually inflecting aspects of our perceived or claimed selves.

Disability studies can also be seen as part of a larger field of "body studies," which includes gender studies, queer studies, ethnic studies, age studies, and, arguably, medical humanities. The critical analysis of scientific and medical culture in science studies, as well as the medical humanities more generally, has surely worked in similar terrain to disability studies: after all, the body and its stories are at the heart of all of these disciplines. Conversations between disability studies and medical humanities, however, have been limited and not always satisfactory. One reason for this, as Diane Price Herndl argues, is that "medical humanists (at least those who work in medical schools) . . . find that to be heard at all, their message cannot alienate physicians. Thus, while disability studies takes as its primary goal changing policies, environments, and minds, medical humanities seeks to improve the status quo" (2005, 595).

Disability studies scholars, Price Herndl asserts, have embraced a poststructuralist orientation toward the social construction of the material body, whereas the medical humanities have been much slower to engage postmodern critical theory. Her remarks also remind us that disability studies, like other minority studies movements, has always been linked to social activism, whereas the medical humanities have not. Similarly, Tobin Siebers asserts that a constructionist model "makes it possible to see disability as the effect of an environment hostile to some bodies and not to others, requiring advances in social justice rather than medicine" (2006, 173). The medical model, in contrast, tends to see disability as a problem within individuals requiring medical or psychological adjustment rather than social change.

What both disciplines share, however, is the practice of looking closely at familiar cultural representations, reading them "closely" to unfold how they work to shape the meaning of embodiment. Close reading of representations provides an important way to begin the process of increasing social justice for people of all embodiments by thinking critically about how stories, films, television shows, jokes, comic books, advertisements, and other cultural products shape how we imagine and confer meaning to not only science and technology but also embodiment and disability.

A DISABILITY STUDIES ANALYSIS OF *FRANKENSTEIN*: SEXY MONSTERS OR SEX WITH MONSTERS?

In the case of *Frankenstein*, disability studies extends and refreshes the work done by numerous feminist and postcolonialist scholars who have found that *Frankenstein* is rewarding to reconsider with an emphasis on the creature rather than Victor and to ask what societal or cultural perspectives the creature might represent, such as those of marginalized groups. The creature has been read, for example, as a figure for the women writers who, like Mary Shelley, patched together their narrative voices and selves within a patriarchal society. While such analytical perspectives require a reading of the creature as "like" women or persons of color, the novel's direct plotting as an experience of stigma and rejection on the basis of bodily strangeness and "deformity" doesn't require any metaphorical leaps. The creature's mistreatment by his creator and almost every other human on the basis of extraordinary, visible, physical differences connects quite literally with the varied but universal human experience of disability—no metaphor required.

One of the most complex such conflicts in the plot unfolds from Victor's decisions regarding the creature's desire for a mate. He first accedes to what he considers the creature's reasonable demand for a mate that will allow him to "live in communion with an equal[,] . . . feel the affections of a sensitive being, and become linked to the chain of existence and events, from which I am now excluded" ([1818] 1994, 121). In essence, the creature—having internalized his social treatment as evidence of his own "hideousness"—now desires to live a peaceful (and vegetarian) life with "a creature of another sex, but as hideous as myself" (120–121). Later, however, Victor destroys—in a passion—the half-made female creature, in front of her aggrieved and enraged prospective mate, spurring the murder of Victor's own lifemates (his friend Clerval and his fiancée Elizabeth). Through a judgment that links the creature's deformities to a dangerous or inappropriate sexuality, Victor functions as a paternalistic figure of scientific/medical authority, in effect sterilizing his disabled child. The creature, disempowered of every kind of participation in community for which he is eligible—intellectual conversation, love—is thrown back on the last resort of the massive body, violent power and destruction. There are no other possibilities for the creature either to "escape" the distinctiveness of his appearance and its marking of deviance from normative attractiveness or—even better—to be valued for the beauty and desirability of that atypicality.

Victor's actions are contextualizable within a long history of non-disabled people's reluctance, refusal, or simply inability to imagine disabled people as sexual agents, making the novel an excellent focus for the history of discussions about who should or should not be sexual, what "having sex" is, and who should or should not inhabit the world or reproduce themselves. Such debates are part of a larger cultural picture that interlinks sexuality and personal power. Wilkerson argues that "sexuality . . . is . . . a culturally feared aspect of the body, with especially serious implications for those whose bodies are perceived as falling outside a fairly narrow and rigid norm," and, further, that "erotophobia is a central tool of inequality . . . a very effective means of creating and maintaining social hierarchies, not only those of sexuality, but those of gender, race, class, age, and physical and mental ability" (2002, 33, 41). In short, when the sexuality of disabled people is feared and denied, the effect is tantamount to denying disabled people full personhood and political agency.

A clue to the erotophobia of Frankenstein is in the key passage in which Victor contemplates his creation:

How can I describe my emotions at this catastrophe, or how delineate the wretch whom with such infinite pains and care I had endeavoured to form? His limbs were in proportion, and I had selected his features as beautiful. Beautiful! Great God! His yellow skin scarcely covered the work of muscles and arteries beneath; his hair was of a lustrous black, and flowing; his teeth of a pearly whiteness; but these luxuriances only formed a more horrid contrast with his watery eyes, that seemed almost of the same colour as the dun-white sockets in which they were set, his shrivelled complexion and straight black lips. ([1818] 1994, 39)

The pleasure Victor takes in separating himself from his fiancée and family to secretly piece together an ideal man is thrown back in his eyes as a sense of horror that may not be the horror of the composite (one thinks of Photoshopped fashion shoots) so much as that of the horror of seeing his own desires embodied. The 1994 Kenneth Branagh film, which often gets things right in its very excesses, captures the mixed feelings in this scene by dramatizing the meeting between Victor and the creature as a slippery wrestling match between two men—one a bare-chested, overreaching researcher (Branagh) and the other a naked, full-grown homunculus covered in amniotic fluid (Robert De Niro). The interaction renders a fully embodied, clear view of the homosocial and homoerotic longing that shapes the entire novel *Frankenstein*, in which successive narrative frames feature men longing to find soul mates in other men, as well as dramatizing Victor's disgust regarding so many aspects of the body, from his mother's fatal illness to the creature's imperfections to (perhaps) his own queer sexuality. The resolution to *Frankenstein*, which mirrors the theme of Shelley's father William Godwin's novel *Caleb Williams* (1794), sets Victor to stalk the creature as the creature has earlier stalked him, with no love or happy resolution for either but perhaps with more clarity about the novel's investment in erotic energy between men.[6]

If we consider the creature as a figure of disability and disability's social construction as radical difference; asexuality or deviant sexuality; transparency and concurrency of bodily, mental, and moral deficit; and affective catalyst for pity or fear, new perceptions about disability and social justice emerge from our reading of this canonic novel.

ON DOCTORING, DISABILITY, AND SEXUALITY

Another way to contextualize *Frankenstein* is as part of a long-standing narrative of doctors and patients that necessarily involves illness and disability. Nearly two hundred years after the publication of *Frankenstein*, doctor stories continue to engage disability, increasingly exploring both the erotic energy that circulates between and among doctors and patients and also the interesting (and related) fact of occasional disruptions of the neat equation of doctor = whole, while patient = damaged and disabled.

The television series *House, M.D.* (2004–2012) is an interesting recent example. Consider this scene: the camera fades in on two white-coated doctors tending to two patients on gurneys. As the camera dollies out, we see the bars on the windows and the cuffs on the patients: it's not a clinic but a prison, and these are inmates. A third inmate wheels a cart across the foreground of the frame. A close-up of his face as he listens to the two doctors' shoptalk transforms him into the point-of-view character. "Good catch," one doctor says to the other, who has noticed her patient's high fever. "Thanks," she says, then, "You missed that," to the eavesdropping inmate, a wiry, craggily handsome man with brown-gray hair and large, deepset eyes enhanced by his prison blues. He moves to her station and pauses behind her. "It's not gonorrhea," he says quietly.

Against the doctor's retort that she never said gonorrhea, the worker-inmate clarifies what *she* has missed: the patient has lupus. He also notes the elitism of her surprise on learning that he, too, was once a doctor: "Doctors can be degenerates, too." A bit more cross talk and a shot/reverse shot connecting the eyes of the doctor and this inmate suggest that devoted viewers will get exactly what they are waiting for in this eighth season of the Fox TV series *House, M.D.*: more scenes of disruption, detection, and erotic energy with Gregory House at their center.

By the time the show concluded in 2012, House (Hugh Laurie) was well inscribed in public culture as a beloved reference point for viewers across many demographics—despite or because of being a rude, misanthropic, occasionally lecherous jerk. His acerbic treatment of patients and colleagues, disrespect for protocol and boundaries, and addiction to painkillers seemed to be subsumed or gilded for many viewers by his highly evolved critical thinking ability. House synthesizes left and right hemispheres into the workings of a Sherlock Holmesian "golden brain" that detects the causes of any number of fascinomas, sometimes with minutes to spare before the patient dies. As if modeling the audience's response to House, a series of highly successful and exceptionally beautiful women fall in love with him, and several other highly accomplished but pleasant-tempered physicians of both genders are loyal friends to him despite the cruelty, unreliability, and other classic "addictive personality" traits of this character.

House is an example for students of health and humanities to consider as they explore how a conversation between cultural texts and popular beliefs (neither of which is discretely the origin of the other) generates the cultural meanings of disability. Multiple aspects of the show's production disturb conventional uses of disability in narrative literature or cinema. Some conventions are familiar from *Frankenstein*, such as the supplemental or metaphoric roles disabled characters usually play, the relegation of disabled protagonists to villains, victims, or supercrips, and the portrayal of disabled characters as either asexual or hypersexual and deviant. A visibly disabled protagonist is uncommon in mainstream film and television; disabled characters are usually figures that serve the story in (often limited) emotional and metaphoric ways. As in the history of Western literature, contemporary physically disabled characters may serve to draw out the feelings of characters and audience alike, without being protagonists themselves, just as Tiny Tim in Charles Dickens's *A Christmas Carol* (1843) provokes Ebenezer Scrooge to regain the spirit of charity at Christmas and just as the film *Gattaca*'s bitter, alcoholic, paraplegic Jerome Morrow (played by Jude Law; Niccol 1997) is both physically and thematically instrumental in the success of his genetic inferior, Vincent Freeman. Jerome shares his genetic material (in the form of blood, skin scrapings, and nail clippings) and also imparts and reinforces, for the audience, a new "grand narrative" about the inadequacy of genetics to encompass our full potential for success and misery and a very old one about the inherent misery of paraplegics.

When a story's main character is disabled—such as Shakespeare's Richard III, the intellectually and physically disabled Forrest Gump (Zemeckis 1994), para- plegic Jake Sully in *Avatar* (Cameron 2009), stage 4 ovarian cancer patient Vivian Bearing in *W;t* (1999), or (for part of the movie, anyway) quadriplegic Frankie in *Million Dollar Baby* (Eastwood 2004)—all too often he or she is still created with the interests of others in mind. These protagonists tend to satisfy, emotionally, other characters or the audience by creating a sense of villainy or tragedy and then either being killed off or "triumphing" over disability through death and a range of other plot devices, including cure and species transcendence. These limitations in disabled characterization have a long history; they are partly reflective of centuries of the narrative convention of disability as emotional shorthand or metaphor and well supported by the widespread assumption that some forms of disability consti- tute a state worse than death.

When a character is given little subjectivity, it stands to reason that she or he is rarely developed as a sexual or political agent. Accordingly, while not always the case in the history of stories about disability, sexuality is distinctly missing in nineteenth- and twentieth-century plots for disabled characters (even when they are protagonists) and is only gradually becoming an element of popular narratives in the twenty-first century.[7] When sexuality is part of a disabled person's character- ization, it tends to support either a gothic or a tragic mode for the narrative. While Richard III's sexuality is presented as part of his pervasive deviance, examples of tragic (and unconsummated) disabled sexuality include the ill and intellectually disabled Smike's love for Kate Nickleby in Dickens's 1839 novel *Nicholas Nickleby*, the spinally impaired Philip Wakem's love for Maggie Tulliver in George Eliot's 1860 novel *The Mill on the Floss*, and the disabled servant Rosanna Spearman's love for gentleman Franklin Blake in Wilkie Collins's 1868 novel *The Moonstone*—all situations resolved by a death in the plot. This is not to say that disabled characters' sexuality is always denied or thwarted—resolutions in the nineteenth century, for example, include happy marriages—but the issue of sexuality and particularly reproductive sexuality is handled with great care, possibly because of widespread uncertainty about the nature of heredity and of transmission of disabilities from parents to children.

Narratives about disability and sexuality in the twentieth and twenty-first cen- turies are the focus of several films, many bracketed by fatal illness (*A Walk to Remember*, Shankman 2002), many characterized by bitterness and anger (*Born on the Fourth of July*, Stone 1989), and a noticeable number enmeshed in a theme and plot of deception, suspicion, and crime that supersedes the romance (*Blink*, Apted 1994; *Jennifer 8*, Robinson 1992). Films featuring a voluntary, unvictimized sexual partner who is disabled are rare.[8] As Siebers argues,

the sexual activities of disabled people do not necessarily follow normative assumptions about what a sex life is. [This does not mean] that people with disabilities do not exist as sexual beings. One of the chief stereotypes oppressing disabled people is the myth that they do not experience sexual feelings or that they do not have or want to have sex—in short, that they do not have a sexual culture. (Siebers 2008, 138)

In these contexts, the character House is interesting because he enacts a multi-layered code-scrambling of disabled stereotypes. The medical model often dominates the perspective of "doctor shows" like *House*, even when these shows critique the medical model. In most television shows—dramas and comedies alike—disabled people are generally seen as patients rather than doctors. A disabled doctor upends that premise and is arguably even more disruptive a concept than a disabled king or president.[9] Whereas disabled characters tend to be victims or villains, House is both or neither, depending on the situation. Disabled characters are rarely given a sexual life except in terms of a non-disabled character's willingness to "overlook" disability, and disabled people's sexuality (notably that of people with intellectual disabilities) remains a particularly fraught and disruptive concept for able-bodied people to discuss, in that it forces them to question the very concept of what sexuality is, who can be sexual, and what determines the normativity or queerness of sexual feelings and practices. House is clearly sexual, but his sexuality is made to seem non-normative or queer, almost by definition, through the central focus on disability in the erotics of his relationship with Chief of Staff Cuddy.[10]

In most of the series, House walks with a cane because of an arterial infarction that resulted in the myopathy and excision of his thigh muscle. He is an off-and-on abuser of Vicodin in response to limb pain. In the prison scene that opens season 8, however, thanks to the rolling trash bin he pushes and that also supports him, there are no indications of House's mobility impairment; his visible disability has been "disappeared." As public affection for House grew, the show seemed intermittently to forget his physical disability—and the season 8 preview seems to encourage that forgetting.

Is forgetting House's disability a good thing, a bad thing, or a mix? Again, disability studies offers a tool for critical analysis. The way that House's disability fades in and out of view may be an indicator that this cultural representation of a disabled protagonist has achieved a triumph in terms of social justice and equity, Rather than *seeing* House's disability (but seeing it as an incidental, rather than central, aspect of character), we no longer see House as disabled at all.[11]

From some perspectives, this is the program's greatest failure. Forgetting House's disability is disallowing a significant and valuable aspect of his personhood. House's strategies for claiming or denying a disabled identity are arguably central to his characterization.[12] How do we interpret the dynamic through which the season 8 premiere trailer (if seen by a viewer new to the show) presents a character without a physical impairment? Is it that House is so familiar to so many viewers that it is no longer necessary to reveal his disability because we know it's there anyway (a particularly odd situation of relinquishing "drag" since we also probably know, but choose to forget, that Hugh Laurie is an actor and that he does not have an impaired leg)? Perhaps House's disability—initially the queer element that enhances his facial and intellectual attractiveness—is eventually sidestepped because it can be: Laurie is not physically disabled, and House's psychological disabilities provide rich soil for further character development building on other kinds of "old plots," such as those about attractive, unreliable men who are addicts and the women who are temporarily addicted to them.

Alternately, the increasing development of House as a sexual character is the source of the change, evidence of the show's compliance with resilient cultural scripts that reiterate the message that disabled people are not full protagonists with complex sexual, social, and professional lives. By this logic, characters who develop such lives can no longer be considered disabled.

House, at various stages of the series' development, seemed ready to explore the kinds of transformative questions McRuer and Mollow ask in the introduction to their important coedited collection on sex and disability:

But what if disability were sexy? And what if disabled people were understood to be both subjects and objects of a multiplicity of erotic desires and practices? Moreover, what if examining the ways in which these desires are enabled, articulated, and represented in various contexts—contemporary and historical, local and global, public and private— made possible the reconceptualization of the categories of both "sex" and "disability"? (2012, 1–2)

House (the show and the actor) at times posited—or reiterated—the inherent attraction of a sometimes startling combination of beauty and disability.[13] (By season 8, the show may have abandoned the exploration of these questions and possible answers.)

An even more even more intriguing layer that Altavilla (2010) explores with an historicist approach is the fact that House—sexy, disabled, and untrustworthy—is actually not new but old. He reiterates various Renaissance conventions of disability, including the idea of a corrupt body reflecting a corrupt spirit and the concept of disabled people as hypersexualized. In fact, as Altavilla develops, House is in many ways legible as a descendant of that canonic figure of disability, Shakespeare's Richard III. The fact that his sexual relationship with Cuddy, which verges on the normative, has been derailed indicates not simply good plotting (only conflict is story) but also potentially a nod to older conventions of disability and sexuality, in which House's sexuality *must* remain somehow queer (though heterosexual in practice) as long as he is disabled.

Frankenstein's creature's experience with thwarted sexual agency may actually illuminate *House*. What makes House's sexualization possible is that, in him, the combination of disablement and elements of beauty is effective, possibly because the disability is performative and imagined. Hugh Laurie's attractiveness seems actually to have been increased by the role of House, if we compare his sexualization in this role to his portrayal of silly Bertie Wooster (*Jeeves and Wooster* 1990– 1993) and dour Mr. Palmer in *Sense and Sensibility* (Lee 1995). Is this increase in sexiness predicated on our knowledge that Laurie is only *acting* a physical disability? Alternately, the erotic context of medical practice and medical power is the key to House's sexualization, which combines medical authority with a handsome face, an impaired leg, and the phallic prosthesis of a cane.

Whatever it is, House's sexuality is engaging, while the creature's sexuality seems to be terrifying. Despite the beauty of Boris Karloff's portrayal of Frankenstein's creation in the iconic 1931 movie (directed by James Whale), the reiterated message is that the creature is repellant, and not *jolie laide* but simply ugly. That, in a word, is his disability, whereas House's face is beautiful and his leg impaired. My point is not to argue for any of these as definitive readings of *House* but rather as examples of ways in which this extremely popular doctor story presents an increasingly compelling example of the cultural meanings of disability, one with particular relevance to medical humanities because of the narrative's location in the context of the hospital and its focus on the disabled body of the physician. The scholarship of cultural studies of disability—or simply *disability studies*—can help us to think more critically about House and how he both disrupts and confirms unexamined assumptions about disability, particularly as they function in the key area of sexual agency.[14]

CONCLUSION

As well as yielding theoretical and aesthetic insights unavailable from traditional and stereotypical views of disability, disability studies has much to offer in the realm of ethical and practical considerations that affect or will affect the lives of every human being. Disability is a statistically normal part of every human life and, arguably, the most universal of all human differences. Even if our experiences are only marginally connected to those of Frankenstein's creature or House, we are all likely to experience many forms of disability if we live long enough,

Oddly enough, the public imagination has not generally considered disability in such terms. Most of us encounter physical, cognitive, or affective disabilities in ourselves or in our loved ones throughout our lives, but many of us—especially if we live in environments where we do not encounter disability daily in ourselves and others—enclose disability in a protected compartment of our minds where its assumed strangeness and mystery, hidden away, dig deeper into our imaginations. Stories both popular and classic engrave the idea that disabled people are not only atypical in body or mind, or both, but also radically alien as a result, and in largely negative ways. Yes, there are inspirational "overcoming" narratives of extraordinary disabled individuals like actors Michael J. Fox or Christopher Reeve, athlete and model Aimee Mullins, or scholar Stephen Hawking—who not only surmounted great challenges but also became public figures and activists. The media, however, invites us to share a gaze at these inspirational figures that in its mix of reverence, pity, and relief serves mostly to distance them from us, producing the same effect of narratives of disability as horror.

Further, in focusing on individual stories of tragedy and triumph—the usual model—we may not think about disability as a minority-group, political, or social identity. In fact, we may not think of disabled people as a group that will ever include us. (Thus, the *House* premiere may be argued as a representation of disability that makes disability invisible, thus allowing viewers who identify as nondisabled complete identification with the charismatic House.)[15]

Not surprisingly, given these pervasive cultural narratives of loss and disfigurement, those of us who identify or are identified as disabled often experience disadvantage and discrimination. In fact, many disabled people assert that social and economic discrimination, more than any functional challenges linked to the body or mind itself, is what makes living disabled difficult. Further, since pity and fear are the emotions that most frequently enshrine and enshroud cultural representations, the eventual transformation of all people into disabled people can be unduly traumatic. After all, if we've spent most of our lives learning that becoming disabled means being isolated, neglected, dependent, deficient, asexual, angry, bitter, or dully virtuous, the realization of inhabiting that stigmatized and abject identity is set up to be overloaded with negative affect.[16]

Part of what makes these narratives of the body powerful is their existence as received and unquestioned truths; untroubled, such stories build and bolster the cultural imagination of disability, providing the guideposts for those who have yet to meet a disabled person (or recognize that they have disabled people in their lives already) or become disabled themselves. As central as the medical model has been as a target and focus of activism and theoretical change, other cultural narratives about disability—those we encounter in books, films, television, and advertising—have been at least as powerful as those generated by the medical model. Disability studies can help us ask critical questions about how the meaning of disability is and has been created in specific communities, societies, cultures, time periods, and economic, political, social, and aesthetic climates by looking carefully at pervasive and reiterated messages about disability and the influential cultural artifacts that produce them, asking (for example) how stories of disability in literature, film, television, and other cultural channels pervade our awareness and inform our expectations about the disabled experience. In this context, *House* and *Frankenstein* invite analysis, not because their representations of disability are blatantly reductive and silly, but rather because they are sophisticated, nuanced, and interesting: powerful sites of meaning-making.[17]

One way to think about figures of disability is that they are palimpsests: fabric on which one text is written and erased in order to write a new one that bears the traces of the earlier writing. From Philoctetes and Oedipus through Frankenstein's creature, Tiny Tim, and Quasimodo—from Laura Wingate and Bertha Plummer to X-Men and House—disabled figures bear the traces of earlier cultural representations. *Frankenstein* and *House*, similarly, are two doctor stories in a long history of texts that think through bodily difference in relation to science and medicine: from the deformed body as object/project/patient to disabled body as subject/authority/doctor. It is not, however, a straight trajectory as much as a recursive line that tends to move forward, then loop back to set up parallels and connections between old and new.

Literary and visual cultural narratives of disability are thus more open to dynamism and influence than discourses produced by medicine and other institutions. This may be particularly true of dynamic popular cultural forms such as comic books and fashion, where change not only occurs more quickly but also is even an imperative.[18] If entrenched public narratives of disability are the product of a failure of imagination, thinking critically about these narratives reactivates our imagination. Correspondingly, imaginative visual and textual culture can regenerate our ability to think differently, innovatively, and transformatively about disability—for the benefit of every one of us.

NOTES

1   The Broadview Press Edition of *Frankenstein* (Shelley [1818] 1999), for example, offers as contextual sources both key humanities texts that Victor and the creature read and excerpts from scientific texts by Charles Darwin and Humphry Davy.

2   While it may be more of a stretch to consider the creature in terms of a patient emotionally rejected by the physician whose treatment has been unsuccessful—a "failure" —Kenneth Branagh's (1994) production's use of this word for Victor to express his response to the creature suggests its appropriateness.

3   See Gail Landsman (2005) for a discussion of the impact of medical professionals' pronouncements of disability on mothers' reactions to their infants. For a discussion of the historical use of Ugly Laws to prevent disabled people from appearing in public, see Susan Schweik (2009).

4   In fact, a dynamic model of disability invites consideration of chronic illnesses and thus bridges a conceptual gap sometimes encountered between illness and disability.

5   By "insight" I mean practical, experience-based insight, not the compensatory, magical gifts often featured in recurrent figures in popular narratives such as blind seers/detectives. For a discussion of the centrality of disability to modernism, see Tobin Siebers (2010).

6   For a foundational example of such analyses, see Eve Kosofky Sedgwick (1992).

7   For a historicization of disability and sexuality in the nineteenth century, see Martha Stoddard Holmes (2004). For a recent collection of essays on disability and sexuality, see Robert McRuer and Anna Mollow (2012).

8   Even rarer are narratives in which the sexual partner is intellectually disabled. Wilkerson (2002) notes that "people with developmental disabilities have also been regarded as hypersexual, and in some cases as predators of (nondisabled) children, or as inherently and inevitably victimized—but in any case as possessing a sexuality requiring monitoring and control by others" (43).

9   Consider, e.g., the concealment of Franklin Delano Roosevelt's post-polio disability.

10 In terming House "queer," I reference Gina Altavilla (2010). As Altavilla details, the erotic relationship between House and Cuddy seems to parallel that between Richard III and Lady Anne Neville.

11 For examples of characters whose disabilities are treated as incidental, see, CIA techie Auggie, on *Covert Affairs* (2010–), a blind man (played by sighted actor Christopher Gorham) or hospital chief of staff Dr. Kerry Weaver, on *ER* (1994–2009), who uses a cane for a congenital mobility impairment. Auggie's blindness, like Weaver's disability and queerness, are frequently treated as aspects of identity rather than the only interesting or important things about the characters.

12 See Simi Linton's *Claiming Disability: Knowledge and Identity* (1998) for the foundational discussion of what it means to claim a disabled identity.

13 For an earlier example, see Miserrimus Dexter, Wilkie Collins's double congenital amputee with long, flowing hair and a strong muscular chest in the 1875 novel *The Law and the Lady*.

14 For a provocative and important new discussion of disability and sexuality, see Mollow (2012).

15 A related question, of course, is what happens to the disabled-identified viewer who may already be disrupted in identification because of the knowledge that Hugh Laurie is not disabled in the ways that House is, although he has recently identified himself as experiencing depression. For useful discussions of seeing disability, see Rosemarie Garland-Thomson (2002, 2009).

16 For more on stigma and disability as "rejected" body, see Goffman (1963) and Wendell (1996).

17 Other examples of nuanced and very popular representations that invite critique include the movie *The King's Speech* (Hooper 2010), the animated television shows *Family Guy* (1999–) and *South Park* (1997–), and the television show *Joan of Arcadia* (2003–2005).

18 See, e.g., fashion shoots of Aimee Mullins as analyzed by Garland-Thomson (2001).

Chapter 6

MUSIC AND DISABILITY

JOSEPH N. STRAUS

MUSIC and disability are usually conjoined under three medicalized rubrics: music therapy, abnormal psychology, and medical interventions for music-related injuries. According to the goal statement of the American Music Therapy Association, music therapy "is an established healthcare profession that uses music to address physical, emotional, cognitive, and social needs of children and adults with disabilities or illnesses." Music therapists are medical professionals who seek to cure, remediate, or normalize their patients, and music is their therapeutic tool (Hurt-Thaut 2009; McFerran et al. 2009). In the professional psychological literature, the musical abilities of people with cognitive, intellectual, or sensory impairments are studied in isolation from the normal mainstream, on the assumption that their musicianship is fully circumscribed by their disability and usually defective in some way. Oliver Sacks (2007), in perhaps the best-known and widely circulated current discussion of music and disability from a neurological and psychological point of view, focuses on the musical behavior and abilities of deviant individuals. His case studies of freakish musical talents and activities, although sympathetic, confine people with disabilities to a medicalized intellectual ghetto. In recent years, the medical professions have begun to attend to disabilities and injuries associated with musical performance. Music can be a dangerous business, and musicians frequently have injuries associated with the stress of intensive, repetitive practice, vocal damage, hearing loss from prolonged exposure to loud sounds, and other injuries (Lubet 2011; Stras 2006; Woo 2010).

In contrast to these medicalized approaches, this essay will approach music from the point of view of disability studies, which imagines disability, not as a medical pathology requiring study and cure, but as a social and cultural practice inviting acceptance, accommodation, and appreciation. Within this new social and cultural model, disability is understood as an aspect of the diversity of human morphology, capability, and behavior: *a difference, not a deficit.*

DISABILITY STUDIES AND MUSIC: BEYOND THE MEDICAL MODEL OF DISABILITY

The medical model of disability, prevalent in the West since around 1800 (Davis 2010a; Deutsch 2002), defines disability as a pathology or defect that resides inside an individual body or mind that can be remediated or even cured through medical intervention and personal effort. More broadly, the medical model of disability is an expression of what Rosemarie Garland-Thomson (2004) calls "the cultural logic of euthanasia": disabled bodies should either be rehabilitated (normalized) or eliminated (either by being sequestered from sight in homes or institutions or by being allowed or encouraged to die). While the medical model is itself historically contingent, changing with evolving medical concepts and practices, it is fundamentally characterized by its adherence to what Jackie Scully calls "the deficit/repair paradigm," within which disability is understood as "an abnormality of form or function, the cause of which lies in the biology of the individual" (2008, 3, 23).

Within the past thirty years, a new way of thinking about disability has emerged as an alternative to the medical model. Accompanying the political disability rights movement, the new interdisciplinary field of disability studies understands disability not as a medical pathology but, rather, as a social and cultural construction. A new generation of disability activists has begun to claim disability as a positive political and cultural identity, demanding the right to represent themselves and explicitly rejecting regimes of normalization (Linton 1998; Siebers 2008). In Scully's memorable phrase, disability has "migrated from pathology to ontology" (2008, 4).

In that spirit, this essay will explore three sorts of disability-related ways of making music (including the composition, performance, and comprehension of music): autistic music making (based on local coherence, associative networks, absolute pitch, and prodigious rote memory), deaf music making (based on seeing, feeling, and moving to music), and mobility-inflected music making (in which rolling rather than walking through the world might lead to the perception of music as a continuous flow, rather than as a series of punctuated events). The goal will not be the cure, remediation, or even study of medical pathologies but rather the appreciation of the ways in which disability can shape music. Our interest will be in what sorts of musical activities disability enables.[1]

AUTISTIC MUSIC MAKING

Most discussions of autism take place within a medical model that defines it as a pathology. For example, the description of autism in the *Diagnostic and Statistical Manual of Mental Disorders* (the most current edition is *DSM-5* [2013])—the authoritative manual of psychiatric diagnoses—describes autism as involving impairments in social interaction and communication together with abnormally restricted or repetitive behaviors.[2] Recently, a nonmedical counternarrative has arisen that describes autism as a cognitive and behavioral difference, not an illness. This counternarrative has its roots in the disability rights movement and, specifically, in the movement toward "neurodiversity." People writing from this point of view, including many individuals who are themselves on the autism spectrum, have identified a number of components to what they think of as an autistic "cognitive style." I will review three salient features of that style, which I will refer to as "local coherence," "private association," and "imitation." For each of these attributes of autistic cognitive style, I will discuss how it might shape the creation, performance, and comprehension of music (Headlam 2006).

One prevalent theory of autism considers it a disorder characterized by "weak central coherence"—an abnormally weak tendency to bind local details into global percepts (Frith 2003; Frith and Happé 1999). In this view, the deficits in social relatedness, considered one of the three defining characteristics of autism in the *DSM*, as well as other intellectual deficits associated with autism, are manifestations of an underlying inability to create larger meanings or patterns from discrete elements. To recast the same notion as a cognitive difference rather than a deficit, we might say that people with autism are often richly attentive to minute details with an unusual and distinctive ability to attend to details that are not subsumed into a larger totality. Autistic cognition is thus based on *local coherence* (Belmonte 2008; Mills 2008).

How might an autistic cognitive style based on local coherence play out in music? In the domain of pitch perception, absolute pitch (AP)—the ability to name a pitch or produce a pitch identified by name without using an external source—is significantly more prevalent among people with autism than in the general population.[3] As a nonrelational strategy of pitch perception, one based on the internal qualities of a tone without respect to other tones, AP would seem to epitomize an autistic cognition of music, based on local rather than central coherence. More generally, we might speculate that autistic musicianship emphasizes the integrity of the discrete event, an orientation toward the part rather then the whole.

A second prevalent theory of autism contends that the central deficit is a lack of a "theory of mind," that is, a deficiency in the ability to attribute intentions, knowledge, and feelings to other people (Baron-Cohen 1993, 1997, 2001, 2004; Frith 2003). As a result, people with autism have difficulties both with social relatedness and with communication (two of the three principal markers of autism, according to the *DSM*).

We can recast these apparent deficits as differences characteristic of a distinctively autistic cognitive style, one based on locally coherent networks of private associations. Like poetry, especially modernist poetry, autistic language often involves unusual, idiosyncratic combinations of elements and images, with as much pleasure associated with the sounds of the words as with their meaning (Chew 2008; Grandin 1995).

In relation to music, we should thus imagine an autistic musician as someone more attuned to private, idiosyncratic associations than larger shared meanings. Individual musical events are not so much clumped together to create larger patterns as they are appreciated both for their own sake and for the associations they may evoke in relation to other individual events, in rich networks of private associations and meanings.

A third prevalent theory of autism relates autistic behavior to deficiencies in the brain's "executive function." People with autism often manifest "restricted, repetitive, and stereotyped patterns of behavior, interests, and activities" (*DSM*), which, according to this theory, result from difficulties in modulating mental focus or in shifting attention easily from task to task.

Autistic fixity of focus is a quality that enables another characteristic of autistic cognition, what Sacks refers to as a "gift for mimesis" (1995, 241). People with autism, especially those with so-called savant skills, often have prodigious rote memories.[4] We might thus imagine an autistic musician as someone with a preference for repetition and with the cognitive capacity for recalling extended musical passages in full detail. Prodigious rote memory, absolute pitch, focus on discrete musical events in all of their concrete detail (i.e., local coherence), preference for the part rather than the whole, and rich networks of association (often involving private or idiosyncratic meanings) thus epitomize autistic musicianship.

All of these aspects of autistic musicianship are evident in the music making of Glenn Gould (1932–1982), widely acknowledged as one of the greatest pianists of the twentieth century (Bazzana 1997, 2004). Gould performed and recorded widely, both as a soloist and with major orchestras, and left a legacy of audio and video recordings that are still very much in demand. As a pianist, he is best known for the astonishing clarity of his playing—each line and each note sharply etched —and for the shocking originality of his musical interpretations. As a performer, he is at least equally well known for his many eccentricities: he sat very low at the piano and accompanied his playing with constant singing and humming, as well as unusual hand gestures; he was a germ-phobic hypochondriac who always wore an overcoat, even in the summer; his personal grooming was below normal standards. He disliked the give and take, the socially interactive nature of live performance and, at a relatively early stage in his career, he permanently left the concert hall for the privacy and seclusion of the recording studio. For many critics, their annoyance at Gould's unusual behaviors engulfed their response to his music: they found it impossible to talk about the music without reference to the behavior. Even among Gould's supporters—and he has by now achieved something like cult status among classical music lovers—a big part of the allure was his obvious deviance from normal standards of behavior for pianists.

It has recently been argued, convincingly in my view, that Gould belongs on the autism spectrum and that his autism provides a common source both for his personal eccentricities and his distinctive musical interpretations (Maloney 2006). His profound social disengagement—the central hallmark of autism—isolated him not only from the live concert audience but also from the community of past and present pianists. This may thus have contributed to the astonishing originality of his musical interpretations.

Specific aspects of Gould's playing may also be related to his autism, including his preference for extreme isolation of individual tones through persistent staccato articulation. One of the distinctive features of Gould's playing is separation and detachment: he separates the lines within a polyphonic texture and within each line, he separates the notes from each other. The detachment of lines from other lines and notes from other notes is a striking musical affirmation of an autistic preference for "local coherence." In this sense, Gould's autism provides a way of understanding his life and his art in an integrated way. Instead of seeing his famous "eccentricities" as distracting, inessential personal mannerisms, we can see them as part of an autistic worldview.

The most common narrative frame for disability involves *overcoming*. Through heroic personal effort, often depicted as the triumph of the human spirit over adversity, the disability is transcended. Such a response seems inappropriate for Gould and other autistic music makers. Instead of focusing on what they do in spite of their disability, we should shift our attention to what they do through, with, and because of their disability. Similarly, it is important to resist the therapeutic impulse. Instead of fantasizing about normalization or cure, let us accept that autism and the sorts of music making it enables are desirable and enriching aspects of naturally occurring human diversity.

DEAF MUSIC MAKING

At first blush, deaf people might be thought to have no music at all—the prevalent view of deafness is that it involves an absolute inability to hear, a life of total silence. But this is mostly false. The large majority of people classified as deaf, and most people who identify themselves as Deaf, have some degree of hearing (Padden and Humphries 1988).[5] What is most distinctive about Deaf musicianship, however, is the extent to which Deaf people use senses other than the auditory to make sense of what they hear: they see and feel music.

The visual plays a central role in Deaf culture (Baumann 2008). As George Veditz, a president of the National Association of the Deaf, famously observed in 1910, Deaf people are "first and foremost and for all time, people of the eye" (quoted in Bauman 2008, 12). Although the common understanding of music is that it is something taken in exclusively through the ear, in fact music can also be seen. When sighted people go to a concert or play music themselves, they see music being made or see themselves making music. They see the choreography of musical performance, the bodily gestures involved, and can thus see musical relationships. A visual listener will be attuned to musical features that might otherwise be ignored by nonvisual listeners: a seeing listener—and Deaf people are primarily seeing listeners—will hear and make sense of music differently.

Deaf hearing involves the tactile as well as the visual. H-Dirksen Bauman describes the Deaf as "visual-tactile minority living in a phonocentric world" (Bauman 2008, 4). As Carol Padden and Tom Humphries observe, "For many deaf people, the lower frequencies are the most easily detectable, creating not only loud sounds they can hear but vibrations on the floor and furniture" (1988, 94). Within the Deaf cultural world, music is often performed so as to maximize its felt vibrations (audio speakers placed face down on the ground, so that vibrations can be felt by dancing feet, or balloons held in hands to enhance sonic vibration).

Hearing music by feeling it may extend beyond the tactile to the kinesthetic. One can hear music and make sense of it by moving or dancing to it. A listener who is also a dancer is likely to be more attuned to musical rhythm than the normal listener. The Deaf relationship to music thus involves sensory input from a variety of sources—it is not confined to the ears.

Deaf music making may also be silent and inward. Inner hearing—the ability to conceptualize music in its full particularity in the absence of audible sound—is a distinguishing ability of trained musicians and a central focus of musical education. It is obviously a crucial ability for performers (who need to know, silently and in advance, what sound they are to produce) and composers. It is also characteristic of a certain mode of contemplative hearing in which music, in either the presence or absence of musical notation, is appreciated silently in the musical mind.

All of these aspects of Deaf music making—visual, tactile, kinesthetic, inward, and silent—are apparent in the artistry of the widely acclaimed Scottish percussionist Evelyn Glennie. Glennie's deafness has shaped the way she makes sense of music and produces music, causing her to attend to the tactile and visual aspects of sound: she feels and sees the music:[6]

Deafness is poorly understood in general. For instance, there is a common misconception that deaf people live in a world of silence. To understand the nature of deafness, first one has to understand the nature of hearing. Hearing is basically a specialized form of touch. Sound is simply vibrating air, which the ear picks up and converts to electrical signals, which are then interpreted by the brain. The sense of hearing is not the only sense that can do this, touch can do this too. If you are standing by the road and a large truck goes by, do you hear or feel the vibration? The answer is both. With very low frequency vibration the ear starts becoming inefficient and the rest of the body's sense of touch starts to take over. For some reason we tend to make a distinction between hearing a sound and feeling a vibration, in reality they are the same thing. . . . There is one other element to the equation, sight. We can also see items move and vibrate. If I see a drum head or cymbal vibrate or even see the leaves of a tree moving in the wind then subconsciously my brain creates a corresponding sound. (Glennie 1993)

Glennie's deafness is integral to the way she understands and makes music; it is not a barrier or deficiency to be overcome, but an enabling difference:

I never hoped that they would discover some miraculous cure for my hearing. . . . It didn't disappoint me to learn that no surgery or hearing aid currently available was going to restore me to good hearing. I had learnt to cope with my silent world, and felt that my own ways of listening to music gave me a sensitivity that I far preferred to the "normal" way of hearing that I had experienced as a tiny child. Because I had to concentrate with every fiber of my body and brain, I experienced music with a profundity that I felt was God-given and precious. I didn't want to lose that special gift. (Glennie 1990, 125–126)

A similar sense of deafness as a valuable musical gift has long played a role in discussions of the music of Beethoven, especially the music he composed late in his life, when his hearing loss was increasingly profound. Critics commonly divide Beethoven's music into three periods and have often observed how closely these are correlated with his experience of deafness: an early, exuberant period before he became aware of his incipient deafness; a "heroic" middle period replete with narratives of overcoming during a time of deepening hearing loss; and a late period of remarkable innovation coincident with increasingly complete deafness (Kinderman 2009). During Beethoven's lifetime, his late works were seen as artistically inferior and defective, the direct result of his inability to hear (Wallace 1986). In the generation immediately after Beethoven's death, critics tried to distinguish the apparently defective final works from the healthy ones that came before. They tamed the problematic late music by finding its origins in physical pathology and segregating it from the rest (Knittel 1995).

However, beginning with Richard Wagner in the later part of the nineteenth century, critics again sought to distinguish the late period music on the basis of Beethoven's deafness, but now in order to valorize rather than pathologize it. Wagner "glorified Beethoven's deafness as a trait of enhanced interiority—the deaf composer forced to listen inwardly" (Burnham 2001, 111). Rather than a personal affliction, Beethoven's deafness seemed a mark of divine inspiration—by cutting him off from the conventional and the quotidian, deafness enabled him to ascend the spiritual heights. Whether or not one accepts the Romantic myth of the tortured creative genius, the inwardness of his late music has been universally acknowledged, as has its frequent dance-like qualities. In this sense, Beethoven's late music can be understood as emblematic of Deaf music making. In contemplating Beethoven, Glennie, or Deaf music making generally, both the usual medicalized language of normalization and remediation and the familiar trope of disability as an obstacle to be overcome seem out of place. Instead, deafness is better understood as an enabling difference.

MOBILITY-IMPAIRED MUSIC MAKING

How might a non-normative way of moving through the world, either with a halting gait or with a wheelchair, affect the way people compose, perform, or listen to music? If people understand the world, including the musical world, through their prior, intimate, concrete experience of their own bodies (Johnson 1987; Lakoff 1987; Lakoff and Johnson 1980), then it stands to reason that different experiences of moving through the world—the jerky motion through a series of near falls (i.e., walking) versus a smooth glide—may lead to subtle shifts in perception.

The brilliant young pianist Stefan Honisch suggests a number of ways in which his wheelchair use, coming after years of increasing difficulty walking, has shaped his musical perceptions and his musical performance. His remarks, offered before a concert, are evocative and worth quoting at some length:

Each of the works which I will perform for you tonight has been part of two very different time-periods in my life, past and present: the period, long past, in which, as a high school student, and then an undergraduate, I was still walking, albeit with a noticeable lack of fluency, and the present, in which as a doctoral student, I use only a wheelchair to move through the world. My interpretive view of these works has changed considerably, not only as a result of further study, but also, it seems to me, as a result of my changed perspective of the world as seen from a wheelchair. I now experience musical time in these works as much smoother, much less laborious, characterized by a hitherto unfamiliar kind of momentum. I find that the sensation of "rolling" along the ground on wheels shapes the circular motions which my hands describe at the keyboard in the search for a legato sound. . . . When I was still walking, my perception of motion as goal-directed was almost constantly undermined by the sheer effort of moving. In order simply to remain upright, I had to focus awareness on what I was doing, with a consequent ignorance of where I was starting and where I was going. . . . Knowing that physical movement is not necessarily painfully laborious, I can draw on my embodied experience of flexible pacing in a wheelchair, to inform the ways in which I rhythmically inflect the music I perform. I have recently begun to question whether my experience of moving through the world in a wheelchair might somehow be at the core of my preference for matters of detail in musical interpretation. Does viewing the world from the ground up, or more accurately, near the ground and looking up translate, musically, into an embodied inclination toward viewing works of music from a near-the-ground perspective, as opposed to a "bird's eye view" to invoke another common metaphorical formulation? This question remains unanswered for the present. (Honisch 2010)

For Honisch, then, the experience of moving through the world in a wheelchair shapes his music making in a variety of ways, creating a sense of smooth motion through time—a continuous flow, rather than a series of punctuated events—with more focus on long-range goals, and possibly greater attention to detail from a "near-the-ground perspective."

Bass-baritone Thomas Quasthoff was born in 1959 as, in his words, "one of twelve thousand thalidomide children" (2008, 35). In a cultural environment hostile to people with visible physical disabilities (Poore 2009), Quasthoff's short stature, mobility impairment, and vestigial arms limited his early musical opportunities and have continued to shape his career even after he achieved international renown. In discussing Quasthoff, music critics have often invoked the familiar trope of disability heroically overcome as a "triumph of the spirit" (see, e.g., Gleick 1997). Some critics further imagine that Quasthoff's disability somehow elevates and ennobles him—they see him as one whose obvious bodily differences and presumed suffering have conferred upon him a superior, visionary knowledge and a deeper wisdom (see, e.g., Gereben 2002). Quasthoff himself has resisted having his artistry and his disability endlessly juxtaposed (2008). Like many artists with disabilities (and like artists belonging to any oppressed minority group), he has frequently expressed the desire to have his art appreciated on its own terms: he wants to be known as a singer, not as a disabled singer.

At the same time, Quasthoff has openly acknowledged the ways in which his disability has shaped his career and quality and nature of his music making. The most obvious effect has been on his choice of operatic roles. Because of his unusual appearance, short stature, and mobility impairment, opera houses were extremely slow to offer him any roles at all. That has changed a bit in recent years, but the roles offered most often have been those of disabled operatic characters, like Verdi's Rigoletto. In a world of operatic casting that is willing to suspend disbelief when it comes to race, age, and various other physical characteristics, one would like to see Quasthoff offered the full range of operatic roles to which his voice is suited.

In the absence of suitable operatic roles, Quasthoff has built his reputation largely as a singer of art songs. In this domain, where mobility is not required, he has suggested that his disability may actually confer interpretive advantages: "I am in the good position of not being able to make gestures with my hands so my voice is the only form of expression that I have. This forces a huge concentration on the part of the audience. If you remain still and have only the face and the voice, the audience has to concentrate, much more so than for those who use gestures. So maybe it is also an opportunity" (Quoted in Moss 2000).

Itzhak Perlman occupies an almost unique position in our culture, a classical musician (acknowledged as one of the greatest violinists of our time) and a popular celebrity. He also has a visible disability, namely a mobility impairment resulting from polio, which he contracted at the age of four. Since then, Perlman has worn leg braces and has generally gotten around using crutches (he plays the violin in a seated position). In more recent years (Perlman is now in his sixties), his mobility has become further impaired by post-polio syndrome and he has come to rely more on a scooter or wheelchair, although usually not in a public performance.

As with Quasthoff, early critical responses to Perlman placed his music in relation to his disability and traced a familiar narrative of overcoming, with the brilliance of his playing understood as a triumph over disability. Perlman has reacted strongly against critical reception in this vein. For a long time, he considered it demeaning to be identified in terms of his disability and resented any inference that his successes came either in spite of or, even worse, because of his disability. He did not welcome discussions of his disability, which he considered peripheral to his core concerns as a musician.

More recently, as he has become increasingly active as an advocate for the disabled and especially for architectural accessibility, Perlman has changed his attitude. Now, instead of attempting to distance himself from his disability, he actively claims it as a core part of his identity: "At the beginning of my career, the critics always mentioned my disability—the headlines would say something like, "Crippled Violinist Plays Concerto"—and that made me mad. Now they never mention it and I *want* them to. I think it is important to identify myself not only as a violinist but as one who has a disability" (Quoted in McLellan 1981, D1). For Honisch, Quasthoff, Perlman, and other mobility-impaired musicians, medicalized language of deficit and repair or pathology and cure seems utterly inappropriate. They are not sick and they are not suffering. Their bodies are not deficient or defective, just different from the norm. But, as with all bodily differences, these mobility impairments may shape the way music is performed and heard. Rather than concerning ourselves with normalization and cure, we will find it more productive to attend to the distinctive artistic vantage point conferred by disability.

CONCLUSION

Rosemarie Garland-Thomson offers a relevant typology of disability reception, which she calls "a taxonomy of four primary visual rhetorics of disability: the wondrous, the sentimental, the exotic, and the realistic" (2001, 339). Each of these rhetorics suggest a way in which we might respond to a visibly impaired musician: "The wondrous mode directs the viewer to look up in awe of difference; the sentimental mode instructs the spectator to look down with benevolence; the exotic mode coaches the observer to look across a wide expanse toward an alien object; and the realistic mode suggests that the onlooker align with the object of scrutiny" (2001, 346).

Response to musicians with disabilities has often fallen into the first three of Garland-Thomson's categories. In the wondrous mode, we imagine the musician on a remote pedestal, and cut off from us by disability. In the sentimental mode, we pity the poor sufferer. In the exotic mode, we treat the disabled musician as a case study, a medical specimen. These three modes all create insuperable barriers between a presumably able-bodied "us" and a visibly disabled "them."

In Garland-Thomson's realistic mode, however, the barrier between us and them dissolves, and we recognize that all music making is shaped by bodily experience, with disability understood not as a medical pathology or defect, but as a naturally occurring and enabling difference.

NOTES

1 A note about essentialism: I am not suggesting that all people who are autistic, deaf, or mobility impaired make music in the ways I describe or that to make music in these ways one needs to be autistic, deaf, or mobility impaired. Disability and music are both, in a sense, performed, and individuals, both disabled and nondisabled, have a range of choices in their performance. The disability-inflected music making I describe here is a matter of elective affinity, not essential identity.

2 The history of rapidly expanding autism diagnoses is traced in Gil Eyal et al. (2010) and Roy Grinker (2007). For a vigorous critique of the *DSM* as more a pragmatic, social document than a scientific one, see Herb Kutchins and Stuart Kirk (1997) and Bradley Lewis (2006). On autism as a cultural practice rather than a medical diagnosis, see Joseph Straus (2010). See also Stuart Murray (2008); and Majia Holmer Nadesan (2005).

3 For a survey of work on absolute pitch, including the autism connection, see W. Dixon Ward (1999). Laurent Mottron et al. (1999, 486) suggests "a causal relationship between AP and autism," which they relate to an "atypical tendency to focus on the stimulus rather than its context."

4 The literature on musical memory in people with autism, often referred to in the past with the offensive label *idiot savant*, includes Beate Hermelin et al. (1987), Leon Miller (1989), Adam Ockelford (2007), Geza Révész (1925), John Sloboda (2005), and Darold Treffert (1988).

5 Following increasingly standard usage, I use lower-case *d* (deaf) to refer to a condition of sensory impairment and upper case *D* (Deaf) to refer to a linguistic and cultural minority group.

6 A tactile way of hearing is reflected in the titles of a documentary film about Glennie, *Touch the Sound* (Riedelsheimer 2004) and her autobiography, *Good Vibrations* (Glennie 1990).

Chapter 7

AMERICAN NARRATIVE FILMS AND DISABILITY

An Uneasy History

MARTIN F. NORDEN

How and from where do members of mainstream society get their ideas about disability and people with disabilities (PWDs)? What sources do they turn to, consciously or not, for information about them? How are their resulting impressions and opinions reinforced or contradicted?

These are questions of central concern to scholars and activists engaged in a relatively new field of inquiry—disability studies (DS)—and the answers are complex and not easily teased out. For starters, it is reasonably clear that majority members get precious little of that information directly from PWDs themselves; social psychologists and communication scholars have observed for decades that able-bodied people often do not know what to say or do in the presence of PWDs and tend to avoid interacting with them as a result (Braithwaite 1994; Thompson 1982a, 1982b; Yamamoto 1971). Bluntly put, majority members would rather not encounter living, breathing reminders of their own fragility as human beings. There is more than a little truth to disability author Nancy Mairs's trenchant observation, born from firsthand experience, that "most nondisabled people I know are so driven by their own fears of damage and death that they dread contact, let alone interaction, with anyone touched by affliction of any kind" (Mairs 1996, 100).

If able-bodied people seldom derive their opinions about PWDs through direct interaction with them, from where do their opinions arise? Schools, multiple levels of government, religious and charitable organizations, and other social institutions provide various frameworks for understanding disability, but there is little question that popular culture, which envelopes us, plays a critical role in shaping the ways that people think about disability and other aspects of the world around them. As postmodern theorist Jean Baudrillard suggested, "We forget a little too easily that the whole of our reality is filtered through the media" (1993, 90)—an overstatement, surely, but one with enough weightiness to give us pause.

Practitioners in the DS field investigate and deconstruct media representations of disability precisely because the images, which have often gone unquestioned, are so widespread and presumed to be influential (e.g., Snyder and Mitchell 2010). In pursuit of this research, DS scholars have repudiated the two paradigms that have long contextualized the thinking about disability: the moral and medical models. The former paradigm, which has existed for centuries, if not millennia, treats disability as a moral shortcoming of the person bearing it, typically framing it as a sin, a manifestation of evil, or punishment from a divine source. The latter, which began displacing the moral model in the wake of medical and surgical advances during the nineteenth and early twentieth centuries, privileges medical and rehabilitative authorities over their disabled clients and regards disability as an individual's pathological problem to be overcome mainly through sheer strength of character. Disability studies scholars have instead promoted a third paradigm—the social model—which contextualizes a person's disabled status not as something inherent in that person but as a social and cultural construction. Instead of regarding PWDs as reflectors of sinfulness or divine retribution, or as hard-luck individuals bitter about their misfortune and woefully in need of guidance from well-meaning physicians, advocates of the social model argue instead that PWDs are a significant minority group that, like other minorities and women, has been subjected to abuse, prejudice, and gross misrepresentation.

Disability studies authors have been particularly keen to deconstruct images from the seemingly all-pervasive medium of film; indeed, with the social model guiding their approach, they have been investigating film representations of PWDs at least since the early 1980s, and have uncovered a glaring paradox: though people with disabilities are among society's most marginalized and invisible constituents, filmmakers have populated their productions with hundreds, perhaps even thousands, of disabled characters since films first flickered across music hall screens in the late 1890s. Their fascination with disability, however, has hardly been problem-free. The film industry has relied heavily on, and perpetuated, long-standing stereotypes to inform its characterizations, mainly to generate feelings of pity, awe, humor, or fear among able-bodied audiences. There is little question that the industry has played a central role in "Otherizing" PWDs—keeping them in their place, in a sense, while pandering to the presumed tastes of mainstream audiences.

In the belief that many majority members have drawn on the "reality" of the movies for their ideas about disability and PWDs, I propose in this chapter to sketch the historical representational trends and highlight one or two films that reflect each tendency. The trends may offer some insight into a number of areas: namely, the nature of the film industry's long-term interest in disabled figures, and the ways that able-bodied persons have historically thought about disability.

As I have suggested elsewhere (Norden 1994), the history of disability film depictions can be readily divided into three reasonably distinct periods of approximately equal lengths: the late 1890s to the late 1930s, the World War II years into the 1970s, and the 1970s through today. Though it would be a mistake to assume that these periods are rigidly discrete, the following discussions should make clear that certain disability types have dominated each division.

Films that marked the first period tended to feature highly exploitative portrayals, with a major strand centering on the representation of children and young women. In almost all such cases, filmmakers inscribed these PWDs—whom I have labeled "Sweet Innocents"—as good and worthy characters. Anchoring one end of the disability stereotype spectrum, the Sweet Innocent typically exhibits such traits as purity, wholesomeness, asexuality, godliness, and meekness. In a belief, perhaps guided by the moral model, that "good" and "disabled" are contradictory values, filmmakers almost always rewarded such characters with a miracle cure by the films' conclusions. Films that featured the Sweet Innocent include the many movie adaptations of Adolphe d'Ennery and Eugène Cormon's nineteenth-century stage play *Les Deux Orphelines* [*The Two Orphans*]—most notably, D. W. Griffith's *Orphans of the Storm* (1921)—and numerous adaptations of Charles Dickens's 1843 novel *A Christmas Carol*.

The most famous Sweet Innocent film of the lot is undoubtedly *City Lights* (1931), a film produced, directed, co-written, and co-edited by Charles Chaplin, who also starred in it and composed much of its musical score. An early synchronous-sound era film that presented a disabled character in a prominent role, *City Lights* features a young impoverished blind woman (played by Virginia Cherrill) who sells flowers for a living on a congested street corner. One of the people she encounters is Chaplin's iconic "Little Tramp," a down-on-his-luck fellow whom she erroneously assumes is well to do. Smitten by the nameless young woman and not wishing to spoil her image of him, the Tramp secretly sets off on a series of ill-considered ventures, including stints as a street sweeper and a prizefighter, in order to raise funds for an operation that would restore her sight.

City Lights follows in the tradition of the many disability-themed films of the 1910s and 1920s in that its flower seller is sweet, pure, docile, and spiritual. In addition, Chaplin insisted that the performer who played her had to be pleasant to look at. One of his greatest difficulties as the film's producer was, in his words, "to find a girl who could look blind without detracting from her beauty. So many applicants looked upward, showing the whites of their eyes, which was too distressing" (Chaplin 1964, 326).

In addition, *City Lights* was hardly unique in its view that a "good" PWD should be rewarded with a miracle cure. In fact, the Tramp's quest to raise money for a corrective operation is the main force that propels the movie's narrative. And, after the young woman has undergone a successful surgical procedure, the film implies that something else has been restored along with her eyesight: her sexual drive. Reinforcing the widespread belief that PWDs are sexless, the film portrays the flower seller pre-operation as a demure and child-like ingénue and post-operation as a spirited soubrette.

Filmmakers represented disabled men in notably different ways during this time. Adult males were constructed in the earliest silent films as "Comic Misadventurers," fellows who cause supposedly humorous problems for themselves or others because of their impaired status. Given to pursuing others or, more likely, being pursued themselves, the disabled men appearing in films with such titles as *The Legless Runner* (1907), *The Invalid's Adventure* (1907), and *Don't Pull My Leg* (1908) were designed as comic Others, their physical differences serving as the differentiating markers to audiences.

As questionable and insulting as these figures were, filmmakers supplanted them with an even more repugnant character type as the medium matured during the 1910s and 1920s: the "Obsessive Avenger," a wronged Ahab-like figure who doggedly seeks revenge on those he holds responsible for his disabled status or some other moral-code violation. (Indeed, two movie versions of *Moby Dick*—both starring John Barrymore as the obsessed, one-legged Captain Ahab—appeared in 1926 as *The Sea Beast* [Webb] and 1930 as *Moby Dick* [Bacon].) Two men in particular shared the responsibility for developing this character type: director Tod Browning and actor Lon Chaney. Separately and in several notable collaborations, Browning and Chaney breathed life into the Obsessive Avenger in such films as *The Penalty* (Worsley 1920), *The Hunchback of Notre Dame* (Worsley 1923), *The Unknown* (Browning 1927), *West of Zanzibar* (Browning 1928), and *The Devil-Doll* (Browning 1936). Cut off from society and consumed by a pathological desire for retribution, the monstrous Obsessive Avenger simultaneously borrows from and supports two of mainstream society's most deeply held beliefs about PWDs: "deformity of the body is a sure sign of deformity of the soul" and "disabled people resent the nondisabled and would, if they could, destroy them," in the words, respectively, of Joanmarie Kalter and Paul Longmore (Kalter 1986, 42; Longmore 1985, 32). Not all films of the time represented disabled males in this way, of course. *The Big Parade* (Vidor 1925), for instance, was a box-office hit about a severely injured but non-vengeful World War I serviceman and was written by Laurence Stallings, himself a disabled World War I veteran. Such productions, however, were overshadowed by the work of Browning, Chaney, and their like-minded peers.

Browning's notorious film *Freaks* (1932), which depicts an entire colony of Obsessive Avengers, remains one of the most disturbing disability-themed movies ever made. Loosely based on the 1923 Tod Robbins short story "Spurs," this rather crudely made film presents a troublesome mixture of mawkishness, low-grade humor, and sideshow-like exploitation in its representation of disabled carnival performers who transform themselves from benign to homicidal with relative ease.

Featuring a traveling circus as its context, *Freaks* unfolds the story of Hans (Harry Earles), a short-stature sideshow performer mesmerized by Cleopatra (Olga Baclanova), an able-bodied trapeze artist. Cleo finds the little man laughable until she discovers that he is about to inherit a fortune. She talks the all-too-willing Hans into marrying her, and after the ceremony she and her lover, the circus strongman Hercules (Henry Victor), act on their plan to dispatch Hans by poisoning him. Hans learns the truth in time, however, and his fellow carnival "freaks," galvanized by Hercules and Cleo's attempt to swindle and murder one of their own, wreak unspeakable revenge on their two able-bodied colleagues.

Unlike other early-1930s horror films with which *Freaks* was intended to compete, Browning's untidy little film did not use any trick-effect cinematography, atmospheric settings, or creepy prosthetic makeup. Instead, it relied mainly on the unadorned imagery of actors with highly visible bodily differences for its chilling effects. The disabled sideshow performers recruited by Browning included John Eckhardt (a.k.a. "Johnny Eck"), whose body ended slightly below his ribcage; Frances O'Connor, an armless woman; conjoined twins Violet and Daisy Hilton; Prince Randian, a limbless man variously billed as the "Human Caterpillar" and the "Living Torso"; and Simon Metz (a.k.a. "Schlitze"), a cross-dressing performer with microcephaly. Audiences could not reassure themselves so easily that "it's only a movie" while watching *Freaks* as they could with *Frankenstein* (Whale 1931), *Dracula* (Browning 1931), *Mystery of the Wax Museum* (Curtiz 1933), and other Hollywood horror movies of the period.

Seldom rising above a comic-book level of complexity, the disabled characters in *Freaks, City Lights,* and other such films defined the Hollywood perspective on disability during this time. After about four decades' worth of such problematic imagery, however, a change was under way. Influenced no doubt by the legions of disabled veterans returning to the United States during and after World War II, and perhaps inspired by *The Big Parade* and other poignant disabled-veteran films of a previous generation, Hollywood began offering more sensitive and enlightened portrayals. Movies took on more of an exploratory quality during this time, as images of heroic people "struck down" by disabling circumstances only to make awe-inspiring comebacks began displacing, but not entirely replacing, the older stereotypes. Disability, which filmmakers had used during the first period mainly to symbolize some aspect of a person's character or simply trigger a primitive plot, was now treated as a major issue to explore and overcome. Such an approach was not without its problems; most notably, the resulting movies often placed the burden of "overcoming" squarely on the shoulders of the PWDs while refusing to address or even acknowledge problems of social prejudice and access. Nevertheless, they represented a major step forward.

The first wave of the exploratory films focused, appropriately, on a group we might call "Noble Warriors": severely wounded veterans either on their way back to the United States or already home. These figures appeared in a long line of films, including *Thirty Seconds over Tokyo* (LeRoy 1944), *Since You Went Away* (Cromwell 1944), *The Enchanted Cottage* (Cromwell 1945), *Pride of the Marines* (Daves 1945), *The Best Years of Our Lives* (Wyler 1946), *Till the End of Time* (Dmytryk 1946), *Bright Victory* (Robson 1951), and *The Men* (Zinnemann 1950). There was little mistaking the message borne in these and other Noble Warrior movies: these newly disabled ex-servicemen, each cloaked in the mantle of heroism, deserve support as they ultimately overcome physical and psychological readjustment problems.

These films, in turn, began giving way to biographical accounts—*biopix*, in Hollywood parlance—of famous artists, politicians, and athletes who "triumphed" over disabling circumstances. These larger-than-life figures—"Civilian Superstars"—included professional baseball player Monty Stratton (James Stewart) in *The Stratton Story* (Wood 1949), songwriter Cole Porter (Cary Grant) in *Night and Day* (Curtiz 1946), singer Jane Froman (Susan Hayward) in *With a Song in My Heart* (Lang 1952), a pre-presidential Franklin D. Roosevelt (Ralph Bellamy) in *Sunrise at Campobello* (Donehue 1960), and world-renowned author Helen Keller (Patty Duke) in *The Miracle Worker* (Penn 1962). Late films in this cycle include *The Other Side of the Mountain* (Peerce 1975) and *The Other Side of the Mountain, Part 2* (Peerce 1978), both of which follow the story of Olympic skiing hopeful Jill Kinmont (Marilyn Hassett) and the changes in her life after a disabling accident.

Often heavily fictionalized, these biographical films suggested that the same spirit and tenacity that drove these Civilian Superstars to the top of their professions also led to their ultimate "conquest" of their disablements. Designed to be inspirational, the movies promoted several unfortunate perspectives: (1) that disabilities are personal problems, not socially constructed ones; (2) that, to succeed, PWDs need only absorb the wise words of sympathetic family, friends, and physicians and develop the right attitude; and (3) that PWDs must "pass" as able-bodied before their reintegration into society is considered complete. Their implied message is clear: the burden is on PWDs to make that lonely and heroic effort to "overcome." If they do not succeed, they have only themselves to blame.

An exemplary film from the period is *Interrupted Melody* (Bernhardt 1955), which tells the story of Marjorie Lawrence (Eleanor Parker, in an Oscar-nominated performance) and her rise from Australian farm girl to world-class operatic singer. The film manifests a conspicuous disability theme: Marjorie's "melody" is "interrupted" when she collapses during a rehearsal and later learns that she has contracted a case of poliomyelitis. She becomes extremely depressed and rebuffs the attempts of her physician husband Thomas (Glenn Ford) to have her begin physical therapy. When he tells her he only wants to help, she exclaims, "You're a doctor. Help me to die." Her explanation reeks of an all-too-common Hollywood perspective on disability: that recently disabled people are filled with self-loathing and believe that their lives are now worthless. As she later says to her husband, "I can't go on anymore. Not like this. It's no marriage, no life, nothing! I can't give you anything: home, children, family."

Thomas eventually convinces her that life is indeed worth living, but there is yet another adjustment problem; Marjorie believes her professional singing career is over. An army doctor asks her to sing at a nearby veterans' hospital, but she tells him she does not perform in public anymore. He asks, "But if your voice is OK, why not?" She replies, "Well, you see, I—I'm in this thing all the time," in reference to her wheelchair. After reflecting on the physician's response—"So are a lot of the boys"—she decides to go through with it. She warbles the Judy Garland signature tune "Over the Rainbow" while wheeling through a hospital ward full of severely wounded veterans, and she finds the experience so gratifying that she decides to return to the professional stage. When she does, however, the filmmakers added one final twist very much in line with many other Civilian Superstar films: she props herself up against the stage scenery in order to pass as able-bodied before she sings. Perhaps believing that audiences were no longer accepting the miracle cure, so common in pre–World War II movies, as a viable outcome, the filmmakers turned to the obligatory "passing" scene as the next best thing.

The third general period of disability depictions, which began around the start of the 1970s and overlapped for a few years with the previous period, began featuring movies that treated disability in more of an incidental fashion. Rehabilitative struggles, which were the main focus during the second period, began giving way to other concerns: pursuing a career, fighting for social justice, sexually expressing oneself, simply living everyday life. In other words, filmmakers were now contextualizing the characters as people who happened to be disabled and have a wide range of concerns like anyone else.

One of the first films in this tradition was *Tell Me That You Love Me, Junie*

Moon (1970). Directed by Otto Preminger, *Junie Moon* is highly unusual among disability-themed films in that it not only presents a community of PWDs living on their own—the title character (Liza Minnelli), who bears prominent facial scarring; Arthur (Ken Howard), prone to epileptic-like seizures; and Warren (Robert Moore), a wheelchair-using man—but does so without any pity. The film examines a number of important disability-related subjects that were emerging during the 1960s, including deinstitutionalization, the independent living movement, and strategies for coping with ableist prejudice.

Tell Me That You Love Me, Junie Moon is admirable for its willingness to address issues that have been almost completely invisible in popular culture. It presents the positive image of three profoundly ordinary PWDs leading independent lives yet does not ignore the difficulties that many disabled people face daily: discrimination and bigotry, lack of access, the elusiveness of good jobs, poverty. These subjects are of vital importance to the PWD community but had been virtually unexplored in American mainstream cinema up to that point.

Junie Moon differs sharply from the Civilian Superstar movies and others governed by the medical model of disability in another respect. Unlike films such as *Interrupted Melody*, in which paternalistic physicians set all the agendas and provide all the answers, *Junie Moon* rather subversively presents doctors as unfeeling and ignorant. A scene early in the film in which a physician discusses the situations of Junie, Warren, and Arthur with a group of interns is a case in point. The scene's primary purpose is to provide background information about the trio to the audience, but it does something else; it reveals the physician as exceptionally impersonal and condescending. He even refers to the threesome in the third person, even though they are immediately present in the scene. In addition, the *Junie Moon* physicians, in contrast to their counterparts in the second-period films, seldom have the answers. As Arthur notes to Junie and Warren, his doctors are completely bewildered by his neurological disorder, and he therefore has to advocate for himself.

Though disparaged by critics at the time for, among other things, relying too heavily on Broadway and off-Broadway actors for its cast, *Junie Moon* ushered in a most welcome trend: films that began treating its disabled characters as complex and well fleshed out. Movies that represented disabled war veterans were on the leading edge of this movement, just as they were during the second period of disability depictions. Films such as *Coming Home* (Ashby 1978), *Cutter's Way* (Passer 1981), *The Big Chill* (Kasdan 1983), and *Born on the Fourth of July* (Stone 1989) dealt with disability, masculinity, notions of heroism, and the legacy of the Vietnam War in varying and highly compelling ways. They were quickly matched by such resonant disabled-civilian films as *Inside Moves* (Donner 1980), *Children of a Lesser God* (Haines 1986), and *The Waterdance* (Jimenez and Steinberg 1992), all of which feature communities of PWDs in support of their disabled lead characters.

Since those early years of the third period, a number of movies have dealt with disabling circumstances in ways that are both incidental and quite welcome. In the American-British co-production *Notting Hill* (Michell 1999), for instance, the relationship of wheelchair-using Bella (Gina McKee) and her husband Max (Tim

McInnerny) provides a refreshingly down-to-earth counterpoint to the fairy-tale romantic entanglement of the film's lead characters. In *Runaway Jury* (Fleder 2003), a blind man named Herman Grimes (Gerry Bamman) is elected foreman of the film's eponymous group. The 2004 romantic comedy *Garden State* (Braff) features Sam (Natalie Portman), a young woman who happens to be epileptic, while Todd Solondz's 2004 film *Palindromes* includes a fundamentalist Christian family made up of two able-bodied parents and about a dozen adopted disabled children. In the religious satire *Saved!* (Dannelly 2004), Macauley Culkin played the wheelchair-using brother of one of the film's lead characters. In all of these examples, the films do not handle the disabling circumstances in a syrupy way and do not dwell on them as problems to be overcome. Instead, each film simply acknowledges disability as a typical part of the human condition and then moves on.

Though the general movement from exploitative to exploratory to incidental treatment might suggest a slowly developing enlightenment on disability issues, it is important to note that this period has been marked by a frequent return to the older stereotypes. Such movies as *Hook* (Spielberg 1991), *The Fugitive* (Davis 1993), *Speed* (De Bont 1994), *Forrest Gump* (Zemeckis 1994), Disney's *The Hunchback of Notre Dame* (Trousdale and Wise 1996), *Wild Wild West* (Sonnenfeld 1999), *Unbreakable* (Shyamalan 2000), and *Hannibal* (Scott 2001) have all fallen back on the age-old practice of linking disability with evil or innocence. In addition, *Million Dollar Baby* (Eastwood 2004), a high-profile film about an up-and-coming boxer (Hilary Swank) who suffers a traumatic injury during a title match and is left a quadriplegic, presented a highly problematic and contentious message: that the lives of severely disabled people are not worth living. Sadly, the screen continues to be haunted by negative and regressive imagery of PWDs.

Despite these setbacks, the movie image of PWDs has generally exhibited a sense of progress. I would argue that this progressiveness is due at least in part to the more direct role that PWDs themselves have taken in the creation of popular culture since the latter decades of the twentieth century. For example, Ron Kovic, a disabled Vietnam veteran, co-wrote the screenplay for the autobiographical *Born on the Fourth of July*, a film starring Tom Cruise and directed by fellow Vietnam vet Oliver Stone in 1989. Three years later, Neal Jimenez wrote and co-directed *The Waterdance*, a film modeled partially on his own experiences as a newly disabled person. Christopher Reeve, who became the world's most famous PWD in 1995 after an equestrian accident left him paralyzed from the neck down, served as an executive producer for *Rear Window* (Bleckner 1998), a TV-movie remake of the Alfred Hitchcock classic, and also played the leading role of a wheelchair-using man who believes he has witnessed a murder across the courtyard of his apartment building.

The gradual rise of disabled writers, directors, and producers in the entertainment business is an important factor in the growth of positive representations, but it is not the only one; the movie industry's increased use of actors with disabilities has had an impact as well. Though most disabled characters have historically been played by able-bodied actors—a practice that many disability activists have likened to the long-disparaged and disreputable practice of having white actors perform in blackface—the situation is changing for the better.

Peter Dinklage, an actor with achondroplasia, has been at the forefront of disabled movie actors in the United States. Dinklage has appeared in numerous movies and television programs beginning with *Living in Oblivion* (DiCillo 1995), a film about low-budget filmmaking in which he fittingly played an actor who objects to being exploited because of his size. In perhaps his most famous film, *The Station Agent* (McCarthy 2003), Dinklage played Finbar McBride, a train buff who inherits a dilapidated train depot in rural New Jersey. The film does not shy away from the various kinds of prejudice directed toward Fin and other short-stature people (people often gawk at him; a cashier literally overlooks him; a youth taunts him with "Hey, buddy—where's Snow White?"), but it does not place them at center stage. Instead, the film is primarily about the bonds of friendship that develop among initially mismatched people who find themselves coming together in the most unlikely of circumstances.

The mid-1990s emergence of Bobby and Peter Farrelly as major filmmakers in the United States has had an effect on the movie representation of disability through their employment of disabled actors. Though their over-the-top humor in such films as *Dumb and Dumber* (1994), *There's Something about Mary* (1998), and *Me, Myself, and Irene* (2000) is decidedly not for all tastes, the Farrelly brothers have committed themselves to hiring disabled performers. Danny Murphy, an actor who has used a wheelchair since a 1974 diving accident, has been a Farrelly favorite, having appeared in at least eight of their films. In *Shallow Hal* (2001) and *Stuck on You* (2003), the Farrellys also gave hefty secondary roles to Rene Kirby, an actor with spina bifida, and gave him a number of choice lines of dialogue. In *Shallow Hal*, for example, his character, named Walt, happily tells a friend that he has just sold his company to Microsoft and then says, "Let's just say if I had an ass, I'd wipe it with twenties."

The employability of actors with disabilities received a significant boost in 2008, when the Screen Actors Guild, the American Federation of Television & Radio Artists, and Actors' Equity Association—the three unions that represent most professional actors in the United States—launched a civil rights campaign designed to draw attention to issues of media access, inclusion, and accuracy as they relate to disability. Dubbed "Inclusion in the Arts & Media of People with Disabilities," or I AM PWD for short, it was conceived specifically to improve the employment opportunities for performers with disabilities. As Robert David Hall, national chairman of the tri-union I AM PWD committee, put it, the typical career struggles encountered by any performer

are complicated ten-fold by our industry's reluctance to include people with disabilities in the full landscape of entertainment. In the twenty-first century, media is the world's common cultural environment. Society's values and priorities are expressed and reflected in film, television, theatre, news and music. If you aren't seen and heard, you are invisible. People with disabilities are largely invisible within the arts and media landscape. I AM PWD will awaken the general public to the lack of inclusion and universal access for people with disabilities by uniting with a network of industry, labor, community and government allies. (Cited in "SAG, AFTRA" 2008, 1)

Hall's views were echoed by Screen Actors Guild national president Alan Rosenberg, who said that SAG "is committed to inclusion of all actors, and will work tirelessly to advocate and seek visibility and equal employment opportunities for performers with disabilities as they are an integral part of the diverse landscape of the Guild membership and the American Scene" (cited in "SAG, AFTRA" 2008, 1). It is reasonable to expect that actors with disabilities will continue to appear before the camera lens in ever-expanding numbers and that their presence will have an increasingly positive influence on the movies to come.

The films noted in this chapter make up only a small fraction of the disability-themed movies produced in the United States, but I believe they are representative of their times. I also think it is fair to say that, despite such retrograde Hollywood fare as *Forrest Gump, The Hunchback of Notre Dame,* and *Million Dollar Baby,* the movie depiction of people with disabilities has moved forward overall and has gravitated toward the incidental and the unsentimental. "It's clear that familiar stereotypes continue to endure," wrote disability commentator Jeff Shannon in a 2003 issue of *New Mobility* magazine. "It's equally evident, however, that Hollywood's acceptance of disability is running parallel to society in general; as the mass public grows more familiar and comfortable with disabilities of all kinds, that gradual integration is reflected in mainstream entertainment" (Shannon 2003, n.p.). As American filmmakers continue to explore the richly varied experiences of PWDs, there is every reason to have cause for hope.

Chapter 8

STANDOUT

LISA I. IEZZONI

A FEW years ago, an intern sent me an indignant e-mail recounting her conversation with a senior physician at her academic medical center. When my name
came up, the physician succinctly summarized his opinion: "Lisa would have been
a standout if only she hadn't been disabled." The intern was outraged, but my first
response was to laugh. Having used a wheelchair for more than two decades, I rel-
ished the artful metaphor—"standout"—with its unintentional irony.

My second reaction was to worry for the intern. She'd had a spinal cord injury
shortly after becoming an intern and now uses a wheelchair. What message was the
senior physician sending to her?

But my third reaction was to recognize that I am finally safe from the hurt of
those words. They just rolled off my back. How had I come to this point?

Before considering this question, I must note the critical backdrop for my comments: the reassuring presence of the Americans with Disabilities Act (ADA),
which celebrated its twentieth birthday on July 26, 2010. If the ADA had existed
when my career began, I (ironically) might not have achieved the success that I
did. Nonetheless, today I am constantly, albeit generally subliminally, aware of and
bolstered by the ADA's existence. It is my touchstone, my backstop.

When I was diagnosed with multiple sclerosis (MS) at the end of my first semester at Harvard Medical School, in December 1980, I felt like a deer caught in the
headlights. I knew nothing about MS except the prevailing fundraising slogan—
"MS, crippler of young adults"—intended to evoke pity and make donors open
their wallets. I rapidly learned one tough lesson. The medical profession I had
wanted so badly to join, yes, "to help people," vigorously enforced an unspoken
rule: "able-bodied only admitted here." Three examples from dozens of my medical
school experiences exemplify this view.

First, during my third year medicine clerkship, I'd look up from writing notes on
patients to find the chief resident peering around the corner at me. I found out later
that my supervisor, the fearsome attending physician, had accused me of being
lazy although I'd worked up my full quota of patients. The clerkship director had
deployed the chief resident to spy on me, to assess the attending's claim. Second,
during my surgery clerkship in the operating room, an attending surgeon told me
that I had no right to become a doctor. I lacked the primary quality required in a
physician: complete 24/7 availability. Finally, at a dinner for medical students with
senior Harvard faculty, I asked the CEO of a major academic medical center advice

about an internship. Maybe I could share a position or do it half time. "There are too many doctors in the country right now for us to worry about training a handicapped physician," he said. "If that means someone gets left by the wayside, that's too bad."

It didn't come as a surprise when during my fourth and final year, my internship advisor told me that the deans had discussed my case. They had decided to pass the hat to department of medicine chairs at the Harvard teaching hospitals to get donations for a salary. They thought they could offer me a position, but it would not be board eligible (i.e., I could never get that essential credential of board certification). Furthermore, they'd only pay me $3,000, although starting salary at that time was $26,000. That was an offer I could only refuse, so I had to look for a job.

One man who interviewed me paused, steepled his fingers, and said. "I have three choices. Hire you because I feel sorry for you, or not hire you because I don't want to deal with your MS, or look at your CV and see if you're qualified." Another said he'd offer me a job but only at half pay, because he was sure I would only work forty hours per week and full-time with his group was eighty hours. I finally got a job, as a research assistant, because a local physician leader who knew me telephoned a friend.

Once I got that job, I worked with a frenzy to ensure that I would keep it. Fortunately, though, I loved most of what I did. The mid- and late-1980s were a fertile time for the type of work I do (evaluating health policies), and much of my success came from riding that lucky wave. But my early academic recognition also likely resulted from my response to profound fear: fear of being fired, dismissed because of my disability. I worked incessantly, classic overcompensation. My behaviors certainly burdened my tolerant colleagues, who simply shook their heads at the list of "manuscripts in progress" I kept on my whiteboard.

I also followed other rules. Medical school had taught me another big lesson—never, ever talk about my MS. It can't be cured, so don't mention it. And for a dozen years, I virtually never, ever talked about it. Six years after graduating, I was welcomed warmly back to Harvard as a faculty member by some of the very people who had quasi-offered me jobs only those half dozen years previously, although it was clear they didn't remember a word of those conversations. In my new incarnation as a successful academic, I found a supportive environment and wonderful colleagues.

Nonetheless, I learned that disability stigma remained, post-ADA, more subtle and hard to combat. In the late 1990s I traveled to a large university to be interviewed for an endowed professorship. A few days before the trip, I telephoned the administrative assistant who had arranged the meeting logistics just to make sure the locations were wheelchair accessible. The assistant paused, a lengthy silence, before responding, "We didn't know you use a wheelchair." I made the two-day visit, and the physician who led the recruitment rarely looked me in the eye and did not say goodbye at the visit's end. I never heard another word from them. But how could I complain that Dr. So-and-so never made eye contact and didn't say goodbye? I'd sound like a fool saying that.

I only started talking about my wheelchair because other people talked to me about it. The day of Oprah had dawned, and people had intimate conversations with strangers. In airports, shops, and other places, people came up and asked me how to get a scooter wheelchair for themselves, their parents, other relatives, or friends. They told me details about their lives and difficulties walking. With recognition of the irony, I felt I could do good for other persons with disabilities precisely because I had authority from that medical degree. So I shifted my research focus to disability, trying to inform the physician community through my work.

Things are still complicated—even success can come with its little zap, maybe not outright discrimination but something that makes me nervous, vigilant, slightly on edge. I was promoted to full professor at Harvard Medical School in 1998, when it was relatively rare for women to obtain that rank. The man who promoted me, my imposing department chair, patted me on the head when he saw me at the annual departmental dinner shortly afterward. I continue to encounter difficulties getting my disability-related work published in some medical journals. Editors have sent rejection letters openly saying, "Our readership is not interested in this population."

Circling back to the story from the start—the physician leader's comments that I would have been a standout if only I hadn't been disabled—let me acknowledge that the ADA can't mandate attitudes. Perhaps the next generation will see things differently. I am hopeful it will. But as we enter the third decade of the ADA's protections, it is helpful to remember a major reason that it passed: that over their lives, everyone is touched at some point in some way by disability—in ourselves, a parent, another family member, or dear friend. Disability rights thus aren't something we seek only for others. We must also seek them for the ones we love and for ourselves.

Part III
DEATH AND DYING

Chapter 9

WHEN THE DOCTOR IS NOT GOD

The Impact of Religion on Medical Decision Making at the End of Life

FELICIA COHN

RELIGIOUS and spiritual beliefs are well recognized and important influences in an individual's life. As an individual approaches death, these beliefs may affect not only how he or she lives, but also how he or she dies. In this context, religious values may become especially important to the patient and family but also may complicate medical decisions. Such complications may be ignored, addressed based on stereotypes, or relegated to the purview of the hospital chaplain, rather than included among the factors pertinent to medical decisions.

Physicians offer treatment choices and make recommendations based on standards of care, the evidence base, prognostic statistics, and their experience. They are concerned with the potential for a treatment to work, the likely benefits and harms associated with a treatment, the effect of a treatment on a patient's illness and life expectancy, and the patient's ability to endure a treatment. Medical decisions require informed consent from patients or, when patients are unable to make decisions, from loved ones patients have trusted to make decisions on their behalf. For physicians, the primary question is, "Do you accept the treatment plan I am offering?" The physicians' goal is to treat their patients to the best of their abilities and to avoid treatment that will be more harmful than helpful.

For the patient and the patient's family, other factors may be as important as the medical considerations. Although most people value health, for many other values take priority in decision making. For patients, the primary question is, "How do my illness and the proposed treatment fit into my life?" Their goal is to live and die in a manner consistent with their values. Families, in the role of making decisions for patients, will similarly seek to determine how best to care for their ill loved ones.

This divergence of priorities may result in conflict about treatment decisions among healthcare professionals and patients and their families. It is not that physicians believe that individual values are irrelevant to decision making; rather, they may not be aware of or understand these values and are unprepared to account for them in proposing care plans. Family members may also not know a patient's values, or they may not understand the importance of those values to a patient, or they may hold contrary beliefs.

Three patient narratives demonstrate the impact of religious beliefs on medical treatment with implications for life and death.[1] While religious beliefs are just one category of values that may affect medical decisions, they often emerge powerfully in the end-of-life context. These cases provide insights into addressing conflicts that involve deeply held values and perceptions about the role of religion in medical decision making. In the first, a Jewish woman's treatment decisions are confounded by the beliefs of her Orthodox son. In the second, a patient's written preferences conflict with his wife's interpretation of his Catholic beliefs. In the third, an elderly patient's daughter accuses the physician of religious bias in his treatment recommendations. Each story addresses the religious beliefs involved, the effect of those beliefs on medical treatment, and the conflicts those beliefs produced. The stories describe patient/family conflicts with the treatment proposed by the involved physicians, conflicts among family members with different belief systems, and conflicts resulting from conjecture about religious beliefs. The narratives reveal the importance of addressing religious beliefs in the clinical setting, the dramatic influence of religious beliefs on medical care, and the need for compassionate and tolerant communication.

"ACCORDING TO JEWISH LAW, WE CAN'T WITHDRAW TREATMENT"

Janey Steinberg was a sixty-five-year-old woman who was brought unconscious to the emergency room of the local Jewish hospital by her son Joshua after collapsing at home. The emergency physicians determined that she was bleeding in her abdomen and immediately sent her to surgery. The surgeons diagnosed a blood clot in her mesenteric artery, which caused ischemia in the ascending colon. As they worked to remove necrotic colon, the surgeons observed that the remainder of her colon and her stomach had turned gray. The perplexed surgeons then determined that surgical intervention was no longer beneficial and sent Janey to the intensive care unit. After several days of observation, tests, and supportive treatment, her physicians believed her prognosis to be poor. She remained on a ventilator to support breathing, was unable to be nourished effectively, had unstable blood pressure, and her kidneys were starting to fail. Her physicians were pessimistic about recovery and noted that, if she survived, she would require lengthy hospitalization, extensive rehabilitation, and permanent colostomy. The physicians asked what Janey would want.

Janey intermittently regained consciousness but appeared confused when awake. When asked by physicians and family members, she sent mixed messages about her treatment preferences. The physicians determined that Janey lacked capacity for decision making and turned to the advance directive she had written following her mother's death from Alzheimer's disease. She and her brother Aaron had fought for weeks over whether to continue their mother's artificial nutrition and hydration. Though Aaron ultimately left the decision to Janey, the conflict haunted her. Janey had prepared a very specific advance directive with the hope of sparing her four children the turmoil she and Aaron had experienced.

Utilizing common language found in advance directives, Janey stated her desire not to have her life prolonged artificially if she were suffering from an incurable condition, if her death were imminent, or if she were unable to interact with others meaningfully. She named her oldest child, Joshua, as her primary decision maker but wrote into the document a preference that "all of my children be informed and in agreement about my medical treatments."

Janey had been a vibrant woman, active in her community and with her family. She remained involved with the Orthodox synagogue where she had been a member since getting married after high school and chaired the sisterhood organization. Janey kept a kosher home and attended services weekly. She spent much of her time visiting her children, caring for her grandchildren, and traveling with friends.

Joshua reflected on his mother's experience with his grandmother, their discussions about the death of his grandmother and father, and the treatment preferences expressed in her advance directive. He believed his mother had selected him to serve as her decision maker because of their close relationship and shared values. He painfully came to the conclusion that his mother would not wish to continue to receive the medical interventions that were sustaining her life and was prepared to stop treatment as the physicians had recommended. Yet, also based on her advance directive and his knowledge of the importance of family to her, Joshua refused to make any decisions without agreement from his siblings.

Despite her goal to ease the decision-making process for her family, Janey had inadvertently created conflict. She trusted Joshua to make the decisions she would have made but did not want Joshua to bear the burden alone. Yet the involvement of his siblings ended up increasing his burden. The four children did not agree, each convinced they understood Janey's values and unable to get beyond his or her own needs. The second child, Bea, was convinced her mother would be angry that her wishes were not being respected and demanded that all treatment be stopped. The younger daughter, Katy, was distraught and insisted her mother would not want to leave them. The youngest, Noah, a physician and the most religious of the family members, stated: "According to Jewish law, we can't withdraw any treatments." He claimed that Judaism was a central part of their mother's identity, and had she understood the Jewish views on end-of-life care, she would have acted accordingly.

Interpretations of Jewish beliefs and law (*halacha*) vary widely among and within the different Jewish traditions. The Torah and the Talmud provide the principles and laws that guide Jewish people, but Rabbinic interpretation allows for adaptation to the changing situations of Jewish people. Generally, ancient sources and modern interpretation suggest that Judaism views every moment of life as sacred. The Talmud emphasizes the concept of *pikuach nefesh* ("saving a life") and instructs that only the prohibitions against murder, idolatry, incest, and adultery cannot be violated to save a life. Preserving life, even for another hour is considered a *mitzvah* (good deed). A physician has the responsibility to treat a patient even when death is anticipated soon and may not withhold food, fluids, or oxygen, even if these need to be delivered by artificial means (Abraham 2000, chap. 30). Acts or interventions intended to hasten death are considered murder.

Yet Judaism also recognizes death as a part of life, as the Torah says, "For everything there is a season. . . . A time to be born and a time to die" (Eccles. 3:1–2; *Holy Scriptures* 1955). *Halacha* recognizes and addresses the terminally ill (*trefa*) and the imminently and inevitably dying (*goses*). Within the Talmud are stories of the dying that have been interpreted to suggest that medical treatment cannot be stopped if doing so will hasten death but also that it should not be initiated if it will result in suffering.

Joshua believed Janey was more socially than theologically committed to Judaism and was concerned that Noah favored treatment that was contrary to their mother's stated preferences. Yet he recognized that his mother presented herself differently to each of her children and that their expectations of her varied with their own beliefs. He respected Noah's commitment to Judaism and his mother's devotion to each of her children and their family.

With the family unable to make a decision, the hospital's ethics committee got involved. The physicians were frustrated with what they perceived to be the family's confusion and internal battling. The religious issues seemed irrelevant to them in the face of the patient's clear decline and suffering. The hospital had a policy that allowed physicians to act on a patient's advance directive to forgo life-sustaining treatment over a family's objections if two physicians had determined a patient was terminal. The physicians were ready to withdraw what they considered to be unbeneficial treatment. The family requested more time to do as their mother had asked—to reach an agreement. The ethics committee had correctly identified the conflict over the decision to forgo life-sustaining treatment, but it failed to address the sources of that conflict. Until the religious issues were addressed and the siblings could come together, there could be no decision. The default was to continue treatment, despite hospital policy.

The ethics committee recognized the need for a different approach to address the conflict rooted in varying degrees of religiosity. They called Janey's rabbi to help. The rabbi declared it wrong to withdraw the ventilator, even for a *goses*, as doing so would hasten death. He turned attention to the dialysis offered as Janey's kidneys failed. Though the treatment had been initiated, it was not continuous and need not be started again if the likely result would be an increase in suffering. The family agreed to no more dialysis. Their final decision turned on a technical religious distinction that offered a compromise between Janey's stated values and presumptive religious values and that was acceptable to all four siblings.

"SHE IS USING CATHOLIC BELIEFS AS AN EXCUSE"

Alberto Montez was an eighty-year-old male who had been happily married to his second wife, Rose, for twenty-nine years. They had no children together, but Alberto had two sons and Rose had three daughters from their first marriages. By all accounts the blended family got along well. Alberto had been receiving treatment for a metastatic brain tumor during the last year, but the disease was progressing. His oncologists described his prognosis as poor and had recommended only supportive care. Alberto was able to remain at home and engage in most of his activities of daily living.

One evening, Alberto fell while in the shower. In the emergency room, physicians diagnosed a left-sided subdural hematoma and admitted him for surgery. Neurosurgery performed an emergency craniotomy that went well. Postoperatively, he was treated for seizures and persistent hypertension. Over the next two days, his mental status improved slightly, and Alberto was able to breathe on his own, open his eyes, and respond to simple questions with intelligible words. However, his physicians believed further progress was unlikely and determined him incapable of making complex medical decisions. The family believed Alberto would not want aggressive medical interventions and agreed to hospice care.

When awake, Alberto would point at his mouth, and Rose believed that Alberto was asking for food. Because he was unable to swallow, Rose requested a feeding tube. She believed Alberto wanted to eat and was concerned about "starving him to death." A nasogastric tube (NG tube) was inserted through his nose down his esophagus to his stomach to provide feeding. The next day, Alberto pulled the NG tube out. The tube was reinserted, and Alberto's hands were put into mittens to decrease the risk of another self-extubation. Alberto managed to pull the tube out again. Rose insisted that it be reinserted, but multiple efforts to do so failed. At this point, Rose requested a gastric tube (G-tube) to be inserted directly into his stomach, which she believed would be a more comfortable means of nourishing Alberto.

The physicians resisted this request, believing it would be harmful, of limited benefit, and contrary to the comfort care plan. Alberto had significant ascites, or accumulation of fluid in the peritoneal cavity, which would require treatment before the surgical procedure and would increase the risks. Diuretics to decrease this fluid had not been effective. The gastroenterologist was concerned about doing a paracentesis to remove the fluid by needle, given the patient's overall tenuous state.

Recognizing a conflict over the treatment plan, the physicians called for an ethics consultation. On review of the chart, the bioethicist discovered that the patient had an advance directive (AD). The AD, which was prepared as part of an estate-planning process ten years prior, stated a preference to forgo life-sustaining treatment, including artificial nutrition and hydration, in the event that two physicians agree that Alberto had an irreversible and incurable condition that would be likely to result in his death in a short time. The physicians believed this statement applied to the current circumstances. The hospital policy on advance directives required that the patient's expressed preferences guide treatment for patients without decision-making capacity unless the patient's surrogate decision maker could produce either a more recent document or evidence that the patient's current preferences would be contrary to the written statements.

At that point, Rose stressed that the patient had designated her as the decision maker because he trusted her to make decisions for him and that based on their Catholic beliefs, it would be morally wrong to "starve Alberto to death." Rose insisted on feeding by whatever means possible. Her grandson, Robert, noted that the AD was dated 2001, three years prior to Pope John Paul II's 2004 statements that continuing artificial feeding and hydration are morally obligatory. The pope had declared feeding to be "basic care . . . not a medical act" and called withholding a feeding tube "euthanasia by omission" (John Paul II 2004). Robert used the word "murder." Though the pope's statements referred to feeding patients in persistent vegetative state, a condition his grandfather was not suffering, Robert convinced Rose it applied.

Alberto's son, Eduardo, objected to this treatment. He believed that his father would consider artificial nutrition and hydration under the current circumstances to be extraordinary treatment. He argued that his father, in keeping with the way he had lived, had been very purposeful in documenting his specific wishes to preclude tube feeding. He was distressed that his father's wishes were not being respected and believed his father would be angry if he understood the treatment being imposed on him. He further expressed concern that Rose was exploiting his father's religious beliefs to justify her own discomfort about forgoing feeding.

The ethicist requested that the family contact Alberto's priest, consult with the hospital chaplain, and review Catholic moral teachings. A fundamental precept of Catholic beliefs is that direct and voluntary killing of an innocent human person is always wrong (John Paul II 1995). Robert understood these teachings to mean that withdrawing or withholding life-sustaining medical treatment with the intention of allowing death, therefore, is unethical, regardless of motive, and is considered the moral equivalent of euthanasia or suicide. He acknowledged that the Church recognizes the human condition and advises that there is no obligation to accept treatments that are futile or overly burdensome. The principle of proportionality, used to weigh treatment benefits and burdens, includes assessment of the patient's condition and potential for improvement, pain and suffering, physical and psychological effects, the impact on liberty, the patient's beliefs, and resources. Treatments of great benefit and limited risk are considered ordinary and are therefore obligatory, while those of limited benefit and great risk are extraordinary or heroic and optional (U.S. Conference of Catholic Bishops 2005).

Rose concluded that continued feeding was ordinary treatment that would have been acceptable to Alberto and demanded that the physicians find a way to feed him. Rose asserted that the benefits of addressing her perceptions of hunger and maintaining life outweighed the possible harms and restrictions on liberty. The physicians presented various options for feeding, describing the risks and benefits of each. The NG tube remained a possibility but moved beyond ordinary treatment as insertion would require interventional radiology and would likely necessitate burdensome restraints. A G-tube was also possible, but given the risks due to the patient's ascites could be viewed as extraordinary treatment. Ultimately, Rose elected to attempt to treat the ascites to determine if a G-tube could be provided. When that did not work, an NG tube was reinserted at her direction, and the patient's wrists were placed in soft restraints to prevent self-extubation.

Eduardo remained concerned that his father's wishes were not being respected and accused Rose of "using her Catholic beliefs as an excuse" to impose treatment on Alberto that he would not have wanted. However, as his father declined, he reconciled himself to his father's selection of surrogate decision maker and decided not to contest her authority. He also admitted that Rose may have understood his father's religious beliefs better than he. While he remained convinced his father would be angry and that the feeding tube was of no benefit to a dying man and that Robert was imposing Catholic beliefs his father had rejected, he did believe the treatment would benefit Rose and respected the trust his father placed in her.

"THE DOCTOR IS PERSECUTING US"

Ali Asadi was a ninety-two-year-old male with an extensive medical history that included heart disease and chronic obstructive pulmonary disease. He and his family had immigrated from Iran decades before, but Ali spoke little English. He was hospitalized with pneumonia, and his family hoped he would return home quickly, but his difficulty breathing increased. He agreed to intubation, believing his need for the ventilator would be temporary. When his kidney function declined, his mental status was affected. A nephrologist, Dr. Mahdavi, an Iranian who spoke fluent Persian, included a mental status assessment in his examination to confirm Ali's decision-making capacity. In addition to the usual questions about location, date, and current events, the physician also asked, "Who is the president of Iran?" and "Who is the spiritual leader in Iran?" To that last question, the patient responded, "He is not worth mentioning." Dr. Mahdavi concluded that the patient was able to understand and make complex decisions. He also determined that Ali was a poor candidate for dialysis and then explained Ali's condition and his treatment recommendation to Ali and his family. Dr. Mahdavi told them that he believed Ali was dying. He also stated that he believed that dialysis could result in a life-threatening drop in blood pressure and otherwise would only prolong dying. The family declined aggressive treatment and agreed to comfort care, and Ali was discharged to a skilled nursing facility on a hospice program.

After Ali's death, his daughter Maryam contacted the hospital to express concerns about Dr. Mahdavi's professionalism. She was dismayed that Dr. Mahdavi did not offer any hope of recovery and that he spoke to Ali directly about his prognosis. She and her family believed that Ali's negative comment about the Islamic spiritual leader during the capacity evaluation had turned the doctor against the patient. They assumed that the physician was a Muslim, had recognized that they were not, and refused to provide dialysis on that basis. Maryam threatened to sue for unprofessional behavior and religious persecution.

After much discussion with the involved parties, it appeared that the family's concerns resulted from their expectations and perceptions. The family described their view of how a physician should address an elderly patient. Though they were not Muslims, they drew on the Islamic beliefs they assumed the physician held. In Islam, caring for one's elderly parents is considered an honor and opportunity for spiritual growth. Maryam believed that Dr. Mahdavi's behavior was disrespectful and lacked the compassion and selflessness that is owed to the elderly (based on Quran 17:23–24; see Ali 2001). She speculated that either the physician was punishing them for not being Muslims or that he did not believe her grandfather deserved the same kind of respect that would be accorded to an elderly Muslim man. She further suggested that her grandfather might have received more aggressive treatment if he and the physician shared religious beliefs. The physician had sensed the family's change in demeanor during his visits but attributed this to distress that Ali was dying. Dr. Mahdavi believed he was acting in a culturally appropriate manner in respecting an autonomous patient who he identified as the family patriarch. Reliance on stereotypes and assumptions about religious and cultural belief systems created problems that might have been avoided with more direct discussion about beliefs and values.

CONCLUSIONS

Each of these narratives demonstrates how religious beliefs and values influence medical decisions. In the context of death and dying, these beliefs may be a critical factor in decision making, a significant influence on perceptions about the quality of care, or a determinant of patient or family satisfaction. In each case, the treatment plan was better understood in terms of religious values.

For Janey's and Alberto's families, discussion involved reconciling the documented treatment preferences with religious beliefs. Despite seemingly clear advance directives, treatment decisions were ultimately guided by religious values that had not been explicitly addressed. It seemed in each case that the treatment decisions were complicated by the existence of the advance directive, and it would be easy to fault the document for not specifically including attention to religious beliefs. However, the more significant problem was the inadequate understanding of those written preferences in the context of the patient's larger worldview and belief system.

Varying interpretations of religious principles may be at the root of conflict about end-of-life treatment. In Alberto's situation, the patient's blended family all professed to be practicing Catholics, yet the children from his first marriage perceived him to understand religious principles differently from his second wife and her family. Though they shared beliefs, they differed on the application of those beliefs to the situation. Robert prioritized the physical effects of the treatment and hoped the treatment might extend the patient's life. Eduardo prioritized the psychological effects of treatment and the impact on the patient's autonomy, and did not believe that his father accepted the pope's comments as authoritative. It was not clear whether Rose's religious beliefs dictated her treatment preferences or were merely used as a basis for asserting her position. Either way, introducing the patient's religious beliefs changed the focus of the discussion from the meaning of the statements in the advance directive to varied understandings of what was most important to the patient. The different interpretations of the importance and practical applications of the patient's religious beliefs created conflict.

Even within families in which religious beliefs are shared, treatment decisions may be complicated by varying degrees of religiosity, which will again alter interpretations. The extent to which Janey embraced Orthodox Jewish beliefs, her expectations that her religious beliefs would guide treatment decisions, and her understanding of Jewish views on end-of-life care were unknown. For Noah, religious beliefs functioned as action guides and were prioritized above most other values. He believed his mother shared that construct. While Janey's other children shared the belief system, they did not prioritize religious values in the same way. They were not as religious and did not believe their mother to be, either. However, it was not the religious beliefs themselves that were the problem but the degree to which each family member believed them to be normative.

In Ali's story, the family did not disagree with the treatment recommendations but with their presentation. The family expected different behavior, based on their assumptions about how an Islamic physician should behave toward an elderly patient. The physician's and family's understanding of respect differed and appeared predicated on unarticulated perceptions and assumptions. While the physician may not have recognized religion as a relevant factor, he introduced its consideration when he asked about Iran's spiritual leader. For the physician, this was merely a question to which he thought the patient could relate, part of a culturally sensitive exam. Yet the family interpreted this question differently, found it offensive, and assumed that the patient's religious orientation was affecting treatment recommendations. As in the other two cases, it is not the religious beliefs that were the problem but the perceptions about beliefs and their role in medical decisions.

In each case, discussion of patient and family values might have improved the decision-making process. Patients may draw on religion specifically and explain their decisions based on religious laws or specific guidance from spiritual leaders regarding issues such as the afterlife, the sacred nature of existence, or human relationships. Religion may also shape worldviews and conceptions of right and wrong and subconsciously or subtly influence treatment decisions. Surveys have consistently found over time that most Americans believe in God and identify with a particular religious denomination. A majority report that religion is among the most important influences in their daily lives (*Gallup Daily News* 2011). It should not be surprising that this influence extends to medical decisions and may emerge as a dominant influence in the end-of-life context.

Discussion about religious beliefs can serve to open dialogue about the factors relevant to making these decisions. The families in each of these cases raised religious issues explicitly, but often the influence is more subtle. Dialogue between healthcare professionals and patients and families is needed to elicit important values, religious and otherwise, that will affect medical decisions. Religious beliefs represent what is important to individuals and families and provide well-recognized points of diversity and therefore potential conflict. Underlying the diversity of views, however, are the values embedded in religious beliefs that may provide commonalities or at least starting points for discussion. Though overly simplified, Janey's story involves the family as a decision-making unit; Alberto's, a conflict between respect for patient autonomy and nonmaleficence; and Ali's, stereotyping, professionalism, and tolerance. Religious beliefs added specific substance and meaning to those values. Respect for the values expressed is essential for addressing conflicts and considering treatment decisions. Communication, using the patient's or family's reference terms, can help address or even avoid conflicts.

NOTES

1 Each narrative is based on a real situation. The names and details have been changed to protect privacy.

Chapter 10

POSTMODERN DEATH AND DYING
A Literary Analysis

MARTHA MONTELLO AND JOHN LANTOS

IT is impossible to think seriously about the ethical issues surrounding death and dying without looking to the reflections of great poets, novelists, and playwrights. From ancient times until the present, writers ranging from Aeschylus, Seneca, Confucius, and Solomon, to Shakespeare and Montaigne, to Philip Roth and David Foster Wallace have meditated on the meaning of mortality. Doctors and bioethicists who want to deepen their own thinking about human finitude might start with such masterpieces of European fiction as Thomas Mann's (1912) *Death in Venice* or Leo Tolstoy's *The Death of Ivan Illych*. They might consider an absurdist satire like Evelyn Waugh's (1948) *The Loved One*, or philosophical inquiries such as Philippe Ariès's ([1981] 2008) *The Hour of Our Death* or Ernest Becker's (1973) *The Denial of Death*.

While these books and stories are essential reading, we suggest that they all work from what might be called a premodern notion of death and dying. Becker's 1973 work might be considered the last great work of that premodern era. The defining features of the premodern era were the lack of life-sustaining technologies such as mechanical ventilation and renal dialysis. Before such technologies became a fixed feature of the end-of-life experience, death was an involuntary event. It was something that happened to people. After the introduction of these technologies, death became voluntary in a new and important way. It became something that had to chosen, then planned and implemented. Only now are we beginning to appreciate the implications of the change.

This new era has begun to produce literature that reflects and considers this changed experience. One of the first books of the new era was Elizabeth Kübler-Ross's unlikely best-seller, *On Death and Dying* ([1969] 1997). Though it was actually written before Becker's *The Denial of Death*, Kübler-Ross's book was the first to appreciate the profound implications of our new ways of death and dying. Interestingly, it did so almost accidently. Kübler-Ross is famous not just for her insights about the dying process but also for an astounding lack of analytic rigor, methodological sophistication, or historical awareness. In the early pages of her classic book, she recalls how, in the fall of 1965, she began to work with four theology students at the Chicago Theological Seminary who wanted to write about dying as "a crisis in human life." She and the theology students decided that "We would observe critically ill patients, study their responses and needs, evaluate the reactions of the people around them, and get as close to the dying as they would allow us. . . . The whole project seemed rather simple and uncomplicated" ([1969] 1997, 35).

One must take Kübler-Ross at her word. At first glance, there is something mind-bogglingly naïve about a trained psychiatrist, working with theologians, who might imagine that talking to dying patients about their thoughts and feelings would be simple and uncomplicated. But was she truly that naïve? Or was she striking a deliberate authorial pose? Or was she, as she suggested, trying to find a way to clear her mind of preconceptions so that she could focus on what people were actually saying and feeling? She believed that the latter explanation grounded her methodology, noting they wanted to conduct this experiment without any "preconceived ideas." Thus, she claims, she and her graduate students steadfastly did not read any papers and publications on the topic of death and dying before they began their work. They claim that they did not even review the medical records of the patients whom they interviewed.

They then made a curious decision that would be far more controversial today than it seems to have been in their day. They decided that the interviews with dying patients should be semi-public. They conducted them in a room with a one-way mirror, so that others could observe the interviews without being seen by the patients. The patients, of course, knew that they were being observed but couldn't see their observers. It was an oddly theatrical contrivance, raising questions about whether the patients' self-reports would have been different if they had been elicited in a different context. We will never know. Of course, this was before the days of either institutional review boards (IRBs) or the Health Insurance Portability and Accountability Act (HIPAA), so the issues of research ethics, privacy, and confidentiality were not explicitly addressed.

After recording, transcribing, and analyzing the interviews, Kübler-Ross developed her now famous five-stage framework for describing how dying patients understand and process the realization that they are dying. The methodology and the conclusions raise so many more questions than they answer that it is not surprising that the book went on to become an international best seller. It is also, perhaps, unsurprising that Kübler-Ross's research has never been replicated or validated. Perhaps this is because her interviews were so quirky, so personal, that the five stages do not reflect the raw experiences of dying patients so much as they reflect the results one might obtain through a very structured approach to interviewing and counseling dying patients. Kübler-Ross was, after all, an old-school psychiatrist, trained both to elicit people's emotional responses to psychologically difficult events and to interpret those events.

The interactions with patients were dramas of conversation and compassion, of shared insights and overlapping interpretations. Most important, they reflect the relationship between the dying person and a health professional, a researcher, a member of the healthcare team, a part of the healthcare system. This feature of the experience of dying patients—the idea that a person's understanding of death and dying can best be achieved in the context of a formal therapeutic relationship with a health professional—is what makes *On Death and Dying* the first truly modern book on death and dying. It posits a process by which patients are offered a kind of control over their own deaths.

The fact that the five-stage schema has never been empirically validated doesn't matter. This is, after all, not a scientific book. It is a literary one. This is illustrated by the fact that the schema has become a shorthand way of describing human responses not only to dying but to a wide range of psychologically traumatic events, including grief, divorce, and drug addiction. In a brilliant parody that highlights both the intuitive appeal of the five-stage schema and its inherent absurdity, the comic Larry David uses it to describe his approach to golf, "Finally, after years of pain and struggle, I had accepted the fact that I would *never* be a good golfer. Acceptance is the final stage of grief. I was in the final stage, not as a terminal patient but . . . as a golfer" (2011).

Kübler-Ross was writing her path-breaking book at the time when the experience of death and dying was changing dramatically. Intensive care units were becoming common, treatments for cancer were just beginning to show some efficacy, and life-sustaining technologies like mechanical ventilation and renal dialysis were becoming widely available. Such developments made it essential for people to approach their own deaths with deliberation.

Susan Block, director of Harvard's Center for Palliative Care, says, "No one wants to think about the stuff I do—death, suffering, pain, heartache, grief, sorrow" (Block 2011). In fact, the opposite seems to be the case. In recent years, it seems everyone wants to think about these things. Bookstore shelves are full of memoirs by people who are dying and by their friends, spouses, parents, or children. Plays about people dying of cancer or degenerative neurologic disease have been hits on Broadway. Books of poetry by and about a woman caring for her dying father or another struggling with breast cancer have wide following. Myriad memoirs and novels about critically ill babies, critically ill spouses, and critically ill parents sit beside legal, sociological, theological, and philosophical treatises about death and dying and have a wide following.

But do we need a new understanding of dying? How different, really, is the experience of dying today from that of the past? Do these contemporary books actually help doctors or patients to understand what they are facing? Or are we still where Tolstoy was when, as he lay dying, he reportedly said, "I don't understand what I'm supposed to do."[1] Or where Walt Whitman (1855) was when he noted, more whimsically, that, "to die is different from what any one supposed."

Entwined with these inquiries is a central mystery: accounts of dying itself are all written from the perspective of those who are observing the process of dying. The person who dies can report on the process only up to the moments before death, at which point the testimony necessarily ends. We can only imagine what the moments of dying are like. If we experience them, we cannot report on them.

Many works are then inevitably about death and dying as experienced by the observers, the people who are not dying. The survivors need to imagine the subjective world of the dying person, piecing it together from a word or phrase, a facial expression, an empathetic response. As with fantasy or science fiction, the writers have never been to the worlds they describe. But, like the best science fiction, they require both imagination and a sense of where we are heading.

It is not easy to figure out where we are heading. We have so many more ways to go toward death today than ever before. One can choose hospice and palliative care. Or one can choose mechanical ventilation and dialysis in the intensive care unit. One can travel to Oregon for assisted suicide or to Switzerland for euthanasia. One can go to free-standing, for-profit chemotherapy centers in Houston or Phoenix for an unapproved cocktail of cancer chemotherapy or have one's heart augmented by a shiny Berlin heart or the tiny Impella LVAD (left ventricular assist device) from the Boston-based Abiomed Corporation. More and more often, death seems almost optional, more of a creative act than an inevitability.

Given all these developments, we believe that the necessity for advance planning and the possibility of making choices have changed the experience of people who are dying and of the doctors and family members who care for dying people. We all must make choices that we never before had to make in more circumstances than ever before. Often the choices must be made in circumstances of extensive prognostic uncertainty. People must decide whether to continue or forgo potentially life-prolonging interventions without knowing precisely how imminent death might be or even whether death is inevitable. They often don't know whether or not interventions will be beneficial, harmful, or simply ineffective.

One of the consequences of such choices is that people—that is, patients, family members, and healthcare professionals—must live for extended periods of time in what Barbara Sourkes has called "the living-dying interval." She notes,

In the past, the illness trajectory moved directly from diagnosis to death, with little intervening time or space. This "new" middle phase can unfold in many guises: a cycle of remissions and relapses, a gradual downhill course, or prolonged remission implying a cure. . . . The challenge which faces the patient and family is to maintain a semblance of normal life in the "abnormal" presence of life-threatening illness. (1982, 55)

The patients whom Dr. Kübler-Ross interviewed were living in that interval. She notes that, among her interviewees, "survival ranged from twelve hours to several months. Many of our more recent patients are still alive and many of the very critically ill patients have had a remission and have gone home once more. Several of them have had no relapse and are doing well. I emphasize this," she writes, "since we are talking about dying with patients who are not actually dying in the classical sense of the word" (39).

That period of time—between diagnosis and death—has always existed, of course. In the past, though, it was not often the occasion for explicit discussion or deep reflection of options and decisions. Now those discussions and reflections can be of central importance to those going through the interval. Although we have more choices than ever, more freedom, we most often lack a philosophy or a theory to guide our decisions as we confront the end of our lives or that of someone to whom we are deeply connected. Bioethics has largely failed to provide a coherent theory. Instead, it offers primarily a neutral and nonjudgmental stance about the value of alternative theories. Any choice can have value, as long as the

decision maker can be deemed autonomous and competent by whatever definitions are in play for the theorist. What we need, though, is a guide to our thinking
about death and dying in this changed world.

LITERATURE'S CONTRIBUTION

Literature fills the void with memoirs, fiction, drama, and poetry about different
ways of dying, various ways of seeing what matters at life's end, and of understanding what it means to witness and survive the death of someone deeply loved. Those
who write about their experiences with death sometimes do so from a "desire to
face illness and death and bring them into the fabric of life," as Anatole Broyard
did in *Intoxicated by My Illness* (1992, xvii). They respond by writing about their
predicament, to give their experience a specifically narrative shape. Making narratives, Broyard insisted, rescues the ill person from the unknown, demystifies it by
describing it. "It may not be dying we fear so much," he avers, "but the diminished
self." As illness threatens "to diminish or disfigure you," Broyard says, shaping a
narrative of the experience brings the ill person to the center of his own life, finding
a way to be alive until he dies (25).

READING A LIFE

Each individual who faces her own death or the death of a loved one lives it as if
for the first time. Each family's encounter with the process of end-of-life decision
making seems to be about that particular family, that disease, that certain set of circumstances. Literature enables us to become familiar with events, emotions, and
moral questions they have arisen for others but that we have not yet experienced.
Thus, for a physician or bioethicist who helps care for dying people and their families, reading a story can, in literary critic Roger Shattuck's words, "acquaint us with
specific and intensified repertories of emotions, experiences, and possibilities such
that later, coming upon an event, we have a counterpart at hand . . . available. And
the movement of our minds is to say, 'This is it.' For we have lived it once already"
(1963, 134).

By reading about the experience of another person, fictive or real, we integrate
his or her moral questions, values, and responses with our own experience and discover a sense of "having been here before." This way, Shattuck tells us, we "achieve
personal experience sooner, more directly, and with less groping" (1963, 134).

TWO LITERARY EXAMPLES

To read Raymond Carver's "A Small Good Thing" (Carver 1989) for instance, is to
gain a privileged glimpse of a young mother's thoughts and emotions as she loses
her only child. The short story is about the tragic death of eight-year-old child,
Scotty, who is hit by a car on his birthday as he is walking to school. For the next
twenty-four hours, Scotty is in the "living-dying interval," but, as is so often the
case, nobody is quite sure whether he will recover or die. His parents try to get

answers from the doctors, try to understand what is happening, and, through the author's description of them, begin to reflect on their own lives. Describing the father, Howard, Carver writes: "Until now, his life had gone smoothly. So far, he had kept away from any real harm, from those forces he knew existed and that could cripple or bring down a man if the luck went bad, if things suddenly turned. He pulled into the driveway and parked. His left leg began to tremble" (1989, 379). The mother, Ann, starts to pray for the first time in many years: "I almost thought I'd forgotten how, but it came back to me. All I had to do was close my eyes and say, 'Please God, help us—help Scotty,' and then the rest was easy. The words were right there" (384). Later, as Scotty seems to be getting worse, Carver writes, "She knew in her heart that they were into something now, something hard. She was afraid, and her teeth began to chatter until she tightened her jaws" (387). The story twists and turns after that but what sticks with the reader is Carver's evocation of the first vague and desperate recognitions by both Howard and Ann of the possibility—and then, ultimately, the reality—of losing their son. In both cases, the recognition is visceral before it is cognitive. Howard's leg begins to shake. Ann's teeth begin to chatter. Their bodies understand the fear, even before their minds accept it.

To read Katherine Anne Porter's "The Jilting of Granny Weatherall" is to imagine what the moments right before death might be like for an old woman with strong grievances, regrets, and longings. As Granny lies dying in her bed, her family around her, she gives orders to her children and to the doctor attending her. The mastery of the story lies in the way Porter has conveyed the way the demarcation of Granny's inner and outer life dissolves as she moves closer to death. The reader becomes as unsure as Granny herself of the point at which she can no longer communicate with the others and her words only turn inward. At the end, she speaks only to herself. Fusing memory with fantasy, she comes to realize that she is dying, leaving them all. With the same resolve and sense of control she drew on to live her life, "She stretched herself with a deep breath and blew out the light" ([1930] 1958, 136).

Certainly, each story told or each vignette rendered is unique to its particular characters. No singular experience described is generalizable in its specifics to all people going through a similar event. Part of what literature offers is the uniqueness of each person's story as a valuable insight in itself.

By entering the life of a protagonist in reading a narrative, we increase our competence in shifting our perspective from our own way of seeing to that of another person. Reading someone else's story requires that we adopt the singular frame of reference from which the narrator perceives his or her world. In doing so, we hone a narrative skill that can be of central importance when we are confronted in our lived lives with the kind of experience rendered in the poem, play, short story, or novel.

With each narrative we read, we alter our view of the world, our perceptual stance, at least for the period of time we are drawn into the text. Each story we encounter demands that we relinquish our hold on our usual view of reality. At least for the moments of reading, we adopt the unique frame of reference from which another person perceives and interprets the world. By shifting our perceptual stance, we gain access to unfamiliar reality. Old boundaries can give way to new understandings, so that when we later face a similar experience for the first time, we have that sense of having "been here before." We're on familiar ground, somehow. A moral path has already been broken, and we may find our way more easily and, as Shattuck concludes, with less groping.

READING THROUGH GRIEF

In the same way, reading literature can yield a sense of familiarity when life confronts us with the imminence of death. It offers a guide. In her critical book on grieving and loss, Sandra Gilbert (2006) reveals what literature gave her as she groped for a way to survive the death of her husband. In *Death's Door*, she describes how returning to certain stories and poems guided her through an entirely new and disorienting experience. Looking back on the moments just after her husband died, she says, "I now realize that what I experienced, gripping the iron hospital bedrail and gazing in shock at my husband's body, was a sensation Lawrence had often explored in the wake of his mother's death" (6). Providing markers along the way as she came upon the unfamiliar ground of profound sorrow, familiar works of literature helped her interpret what was happening to her.

More than anything, Gilbert tells us, returning to certain works of literature helped to give shape to her grief, to "formulate the loss . . . to name its particulars" (xx). She read the words of others who had struggled to describe the experience of confronting the reality of death. In *A Grief Observed*, C. S. Lewis's description of his feeling of separation from the world when he was grieving the death of his wife gave Gilbert a way to make sense of her own inability to connect with others after her husband's death. For her, the sense of isolation she felt had been exacerbated by her inability to name this disorienting experience. Reading poetry and fiction provided a guide through this new territory. Shelley, Milton, and William Carlos Williams give voice to her silent feeling that she must protest against death, even as her certainty of its injustice is "impossible to tell" (98). Sylvia Plath and Reynolds Price give shape to her inchoate sense of the way the technologies of modern death in a hospital transform our much-needed belief in the soul's journey to a welcoming heaven.

WHAT SHOULD WE READ?

If reading can help in this way, if poets and storytellers can be our Dante, our guide through terrible ordeal, what should we read? Though each reader might respond with a different list of works of literature, some are becoming touchstones along the way. The play *W;t* (1999) by Margaret Edson has garnered not only critical acclaim but passionate, widespread gratitude from those who see or read the play. Its enactment of a middle-aged professor's illness and death from ovarian cancer captures many people's yearning for human connection at life's end, especially as dying takes place so often in institutions where technology and research seem to take center stage.

In *Intoxicated by My Illness* (1992), Anatole Broyard chronicles the final months of his life with prostate cancer. With wit and intensity applied to a remarkably sharp self-examination, he creates a "narrative" of his journey from the moment of diagnosis up to two weeks before his death. He faces illness and the prospect of dying by drawing them right to the center of his life.

Readers who are connected to the world of health care, especially the realm of serious chronic illness, often find a gem in Franz Kafka's *Metamorphosis* (1915). One of the most famous works in Western literature and subject to endless interpretation since it was written, the story has been read as everything from a religious allegory to psychoanalytic case history. Notable for its clarity of description and attention to detail, the story nevertheless begins with a fantastic premise—a man awakes one morning to find himself transformed into a giant insect—and describes the events that lead to his death. Many readers discover profoundly moving parallels to the experience of dying patients and their families. In particular, the story somehow conveys the confluent senses of disorientation, anguish, and loss that both family and patient might feel when the patient can no longer communicate and seems less and less like the person they knew.

Many valuable works of literature portray the experience of being with a loved one who is dying. Each in a unique way gives the reader a view of what the narrator endures when of losing someone central to his or her life. But these works also open a window into the narrator's sense of what dying is like for the one he or she is losing. In *Patrimony* (1991), Philip Roth describes his father's struggle with the brain cancer that will kill him. With unrelenting tenacity, the son accompanies his father through the emotions and memories—and medical choices—along the way of his ordeal. Throughout, many readers recognize the particular kind of ordeal that dying has become now that technology is a fixed feature in medical care at the end of life.

In the same way, Donald Hall describes his wife's illness and dying and his grief during the following year. In the series of poems that comprise *Without* (1998), the technology of her medical care appears as a given: "The ship's massive engines kept its propellers turning" (15). At each step on her daily ordeal of dying, the choices that needed to be made by the poet, by his wife, and by her doctors were most often woven through their attempts to fight, then accept her dying. The beauty of the collection, however, rests on the poignancy of the individual poems, for their celebration of love and their rendering of the ravages of loss.

CONCLUSION: THE STORY ENDS

Although each reader resonates with individual works in his or her own way, there are commonalities in our human responses to the moral questions and suffering that surround the experience of death. In poems, novels, stories, memoirs, and plays, writers have rendered both the uniqueness of each experience of death and the common sense of bafflement, disorientation, and grief we share at life's end. Whitman (1855) wrote, "The smallest sprout shows there is really no death." Edna St. Vincent Millay (1921) echoed these feelings: "It is apparent that there is no death." Both were talking about life in the abstract, life in the world, rather than about the certainty that every individual and particular life will certainly come to an end.

Broyard wrote eloquently about making choices about how he wanted to spend his last days. "The space between life and death is the parade ground of romanticism. A critical illness is like a great permission, an authorization or absolving. It's all right for a threatened man to be romantic, even crazy, if he feels like it. As a first step toward evolving a strategy toward my illness, I've taken up tap dancing" (1992, 23–24). Those who have the privilege of caring for and accompanying the dying as they leave this world should recognize that they are confronting something that is, at one and the same time, the greatest mystery and the only certainty of life. Reading what others have written about death and dying cannot demystify the experience. In a certain way, the experience is like love, Gilbert tells us, a private madness that no one else can hope to penetrate. Every death is also intensely private. But privacy need not be isolation or loneliness. The privacy of death allows caregiving and comfort. Literature can help equip us to travel with those who are dying, right up to the last moments, and to live beyond the loss.

NOTES

1   This quote is cited by Anatole Broyard in a review essay on books about illness and dying (Broyard 1990). Other sources disagree. The "Last Words of Real People" website has a listing of famous last words by famous people. They claim that Tolstoy's were, "But the peasants, how do they die?" (Tolstoy n.d.) And Dr. Wayne Dyer (2006) claims that Tolstoy's last words were, "What if my whole life was wrong?" However, this reported rhetorical question is nearly identical to that by Ivan Ilych, one of Tolstoy's most famous literary characters ("What if my whole life has been wrong?" [Tolstoy 2001, chap. 11]).

Chapter 11

SECOND DEGREE BLOCK
Poem and Commentary

AMY HADDAD

SECOND DEGREE BLOCK

For more than three decades, I have saved
the fine etching of your dying
in a recipe box where I kept 3 × 5 cards
on which I painstakingly printed
words like *antiarrythmic* and *cardiotonic*.
I used the cards to tell my instructor
about the drugs I would give
and why even though
I didn't really know.

The EKG strips are pale green graph ribbons
clipped to the drug card for digoxin
to "slow and strengthen the heart."
I have underlined these words.
The problem was with conduction
not the muscle, I see now.
The electrical circuits of your heart were faulty,
like old, stripped wires
the message haphazardly getting through to the ventricles
as the spaces between the spidery spikes grew wider.

As we stared at the bank of monitors in the nurses' station,
I only had eyes for the one labeled "Room 4."
When your heart misfired, I would freeze the screen
and hit the print button.
I learned to measure the length of your failure
with a ruler to place tiny precise marks
between the QRS peaks and valleys
and the roll of the t wave.
Dutifully, I counted the miniscule squares,
noted the times on the back of the strips,
each hour the rhythm a little worse.
I took them home to practice measuring,
never tracing them back to you.

The recipe box is a tin one that I painted cobalt blue when I was in high school. The blue is luminous, and on the lid I painted a tiny house on a green hill with an even tinier clothesline with sheets blowing in the wind. It was one of many things I painted during this time of my life when I thought I might be an artist.

Later, when I was in college and nursing school, I used the box to store my "drug cards." In the days before computers and handheld devices that provide instant information, we had to write up basic actions and side effects on all of the drugs we gave to our patients. When we moved to a new house a few years ago, I found the long-forgotten recipe box of cards and was flooded with memories of the time when I first learned about drugs, what it meant to take care of patients, and basically how to be a health professional. As I flipped through the index cards, I found the slightly dog-eared one for digoxin. Paper-clipped to the back were EKG strips that belonged to one of my long-ago patients. Gently unfolding the strips, I found myself back in the cardiac care unit standing with my instructor and other students in a circle around the monitors with our backs to the patient rooms that lined the hall.

The inspiration for the poem arose from these recollections of my novice self, what the language of the EKG was telling me then and what it says to me now. Even as I write this, I am struck by the difficulty in finding the right words to talk about what these artifacts of healthcare technology mean. For example, do the EKG strips belong to the patient or to me? It is the rhythm of her dying heart that is inked onto the green graph paper. It is my handwriting, in pencil, that added tiny marks and numbers including the date and time that situated her dying and tried to discern the cause. As I looked at the strips, I was struck most of all by the literal and figurative distances or spaces between us.

There is the distance between dying on graph paper and actually dying. I think the patient was a woman, but I am not sure anymore. I certainly don't remember her name or age. I do remember that this patient died. Maybe that is why I saved the strips. I know I spent most of my time hypnotized by the EKG monitor rather than at the bedside. I watched her dying on the monitor. Unfortunately, I suspect that health professionals today are even more under the spell of monitors to tell them how their patients are doing. I know patients, too, will often look at the monitors in their rooms to gauge how they feel rather than trust what their bodies tell them.

There is the distance between my young, healthy self and the patient who I recall as being "elderly." I don't know how old she really was, but when you are twenty, anyone over fifty looks elderly. Was it because of my age and inexperience that death seemed so unreal and, yes, distant? I don't recall being scared, but maybe that was part of it. The nurses' station was safer and more predictable than a dying patient's room.

There is also the distance between my young, healthy self and the woman I am now, not so young and healthy but hopefully wiser. I can look at the EKG strips now and understand the story they tell regarding the patient's cardiac condition. But does knowing the diagnosis help me understand what was most needed by the patient? Clearly, my priority then was to learn how to translate what the EKG said so that we could treat the problem before an irregular rhythm became life threatening. I was not only seeking answers in the EKG but also trying to find my place in the grand scheme of the life and death dramas that were playing out daily at the hospital. I am impatient with my younger self, wasting time on technology when something so much more important was literally happening in the next room. I believed then that my place was in the nurses' station interpreting EKGs. Perhaps that was the only way I could see my role at that time in my life when there was so much to learn.

Hindsight and experience now offer me some clarity about place that is drastically different from my early days as a nurse. There is nothing more important than being present to a person who is dying. There is nothing more important than holding a patient's hand and reassuring her that she is not alone. Someone else can take care of the technical details and, rest assured, there is always someone who is more than willing to do this. There aren't as many people who are willing to walk into a dying patient's room and stay there.

Finally, I generally resist this kind of analysis of my own poetry. There is a lot of intuition and instinct in my writing, and I always feel that tinkering with it too much in this analytical way will eventually break it. My reading is only that, *my* reading. I encourage other readers to find meaning in the distances that are embedded in the poem.

Part IV

PATIENT-PROFESSIONAL RELATIONSHIPS

Chapter 12

SOCIAL STUDIES

The Humanities, Narrative, and the Social Context of the Patient-Professional Relationship

REBECCA GARDEN

> Poetry is produced for purposes of comfort. . . . It is undertaken as *equipment for living*, as a ritualistic way of arming us to confront perplexities and risks. It would protect us. . . . Poetry is "medicine," therapeutic or prophylactic.
>
> KENNETH BURKE, *The Philosophy of Literary Form* (1973, 61)[1]

L ITERARY theorists like Kenneth Burke have long recognized that literature (not simply poetry) and other artifacts of creative cultural production can protect and restore our well-being. Burke says that literature can "immunize us by stylistically infecting us with the disease" and nurse us with an "'allopathic' strategy of cure" (1973, 65). Health humanities scholars bring this recognition of literature's curative and immunizing power to bear on health care itself. They see literature as a necessary counterpart to a scientific and evidence-based medicine. Literature and the arts do more than protect and mend the soul; they generate the insights that are a necessary social supplement to medicine, a means of moving beyond treatment to healing. The health humanities draw on creative fiction, nonfiction, poetry, and other "texts"[2] as well as theories of language, ethics, embodiment, and power that have developed through an engagement with literature and representation. One critical function of these texts in health professions education and practice is to represent patients' perspectives of illness, disability, and health care. These texts can also describe patients in broader and more complex contexts than the healthcare setting, contexts often artificially and troublingly obscured in the clinical encounter.

In this chapter, I argue for the health humanities as a critical means of developing a fuller understanding of patients in social context, particularly the power relations and social norms in the clinic that contribute to disparities and discrimination, as well as the social factors that contribute to disease and disability.[3] Focusing on autobiographical narratives, I discuss a range of texts that illuminate the social factors and relations often obscured by a biomedical approach to health care. These texts confront the complex sociocultural forces that undermine the power of people who do not fit social norms, and they educate us about perceptions and assumptions that can further diminish patients' power in the healthcare setting.

By recognizing difference and the social forces that marginalize those viewed as different, by tolerating the discomfort that difference may cause, and by acting to recalibrate the power imbalance by making patients' stories, experiences, and insights central to the healthcare encounter, clinicians can provide better care to *all* patients.

SOCIAL CONTEXT AND SOCIAL RELATIONS

Influenced by natural science paradigms, contemporary medicine has focused primarily on disease and deviations from average ranges of function that have been, over time, codified and naturalized as the norms of health. Following this model, clinicians identify and treat disease agents, narrowing attention to the scope of pathophysiology and thus essentially fragmenting people—who exist within a web of complex sociocultural interconnections—into biological systems and functions. The biomedical model excludes social issues, social relations, and social factors in illness and disability, narrowing the focus to the individual patient's biological and/or personality issues (Engel et al. 2008, 25–35; Lorber 2000, 1–2). This overly narrow focus has overlooked social factors—such as class, age, gender, and ethnicity—that contribute to disease and differences in function, thus neglecting potential causes of illness and disability. It also fails to recognize the impact of socially constructed barriers to functionality and well-being, whether they are physical, attitudinal, or institutional obstacles. Increasingly, health care has recognized the importance of sociocultural factors in disease and disability and has developed new standards for knowledge and approaches to care that draw on the work of social scientists and researchers in the humanities.[4] Clinicians are learning how not only to look at the physiological causes of illness but also to work with patients in a "participatory" way, beginning with listening to patients' accounts, their stories of what brought them to health care (Lorber 2000, 99–100). This attempt to address the power imbalance in the clinical encounter and to develop the skills for understanding the patient's sociocultural context can lead not only to more ethical and interpersonally rich interactions but also to better medical outcomes—particularly in cases of chronic illness where habits, traditions, and sociocultural practices are involved.

NARRATIVE AND HEALTH

The health humanities build on the argument that Arthur Kleinman and many other humanities scholars, social scientists, and clinicians have made, that "it is necessary to make the patient's and the family's narrative of the illness experience more central" to clinical practice and education (1989, 255). Physician-ethicist Howard Brody (1994) argues that the physician's role in healing involves participating in a "joint construction of narrative," that is, listening to the patient's story of illness and developing it through the interview to build a more full account, rich in data that are both medical and sociocultural. Nursing scholar Bernie Carter (2004) proposes that nurses who care for children with chronic pain draw on children's narratives to better understand their experiences of pain and to more fully recognize children's agency. Physician-educator Arno Kumagai (2008) educates students in empathy and perspective taking by having people tell their stories of illness to students and also by assigning published narratives. These individual instances are part of an ever-growing study and pedagogy of a health humanities approach that focuses on narrative, sometimes called "narrative medicine." This approach to research, education, and practice makes the patient's narrative central but involves narrative in a number of ways, including qualitative analyses of patients' stories, the study of published narratives of illness and disability, and clinicians' narratives.[5] The focus on narrative complements a broader humanities approach to health and the health professions.[6]

REPRESENTATION AND SOCIAL CONTEXT

Literature and other creative texts represent the "psychosocial" in a biopsychosocial approach to health care, the "whole" person in holistic approaches, and the "social" in concerns about the social factors that determine health and illness. Literary approaches address *illness* as opposed to the biomedical focus on *disease*, following Kleinman's distinction between *disease*, an "alteration in the biological structure or functioning," and *illness*, "how the sick person and the members of the family or wider social network perceive, live with, and respond to symptoms and disability" (1989, 3, 5–6). Because sociocultural forces shape the development and experience of illness and disability—as well as medical research, education, and practice— healthcare professionals need to analyze and comprehend the patient-provider relationship through training in social and cultural issues. Literary and cultural studies approaches to literary and other cultural texts can provide this training.[7]

Disability rights advocates and their colleagues in the academy, disability studies scholars, have developed a body of theory that analyzes the social factors that contribute to illness and disability and often intensify suffering (or, in the case of those who are disabled and completely healthy, create suffering where it does not otherwise exist). This "social model of disability" describes disability as the interrelationship of physiological and/or mental impairment and social factors, ranging from biases that influence the built environment (stairs instead of ramps and elevators in public buildings; the lack of medical equipment that accommodates different bodies, such as those using wheelchairs) to biases that play out socially, such as discrimination against disabled people in education and the workplace (Iezzoni and Freedman 2008; Shakespeare 2010).[8] This model applies to those who are ill as well as disabled people (and in fact, chronic illness and disability are overlapping categories). Literature and other cultural productions can illuminate the sociocultural context that is often artificially absent from the patient-provider encounter.

NARRATIVE AND AUTOBIOGRAPHY

First-person narratives have the potential to inform the patient-provider relationship by representing the subjective experience as an overtly political act of looking back at and speaking to a diagnostic gaze, whether that is leveled by a clinician or by those who think of themselves uncritically as "normal." Whether short—even one-page—accounts, essays, blogs or vlogs, video, graphic (comic-book-style) memoirs, or book-length accounts, the first-person narrative of the experience of illness, disability, and other sorts of difference often explicitly conveys a challenge to a normative observation.[9]

The title of Kenny Fries's collection, *Staring Back: The Disability Experience from the Inside Out* (1997), confronts the encounter in which the ostensibly "normal" person's objectifying observation of the other, the one who is somehow different, becomes in itself a kind of marking, a stigmatization. "Staring back" is a reversal of the power dynamic that is at once claiming the power to define and even stigmatize while also assuming the role of observer and author, of subject rather than object—a kind of social relation that often typifies the clinical encounter. In Joan Tollifson's essay in that collection, the narrator, who was born without an arm, explains her realization, in a support group for disabled women, that "my supposedly private hell was a social phenomenon. . . . We discovered, for example, that we had all had the experience of being patronized and treated like children even though we were adults. . . . This was part of a collective pattern that was much larger than any one of us. . . . Suddenly disability became not just my personal problem, but a social and political issue, as well" (1997, 107).

In her memoir *Sweet, Invisible Body*, Lisa Roney describes how she felt that she was accepted only when she concealed her diabetes:

When you have a disease that no one can see, you are alone with it in a peculiar way: the more obviously ill and handicapped may be rejected out of hand, but with diabetes you are accepted, to the extent that you can "pass." And, I might emphasize, *only* so far as you seem "normal." What this creates is a division of self, the "abnormal" hidden within the "normal," the body primed to betray its secrets, the rejections delayed but looming. . . . I am always a guest in the good graces of others, and, directly or indirectly, it is my body that will turn them away from me. (1999, 32–33)

Through narratives like Roney's, clinicians can learn about the suffering that disabled and ill people experience, not only because of the biological effects of their impairments or illnesses but also because of the pressure they feel to pass for normal or, failing that, to "cope" and "overcome" and even "triumph" over difficulties—as individuals pitted in isolation against the odds, rather than as members of a society that recognizes difference and accommodates it.

Narratives can redefine a world peopled with a range of abilities, bodies, and experiences, rather than one that is destructively divided into the overly simplistic categories of healthy/unhealthy, able-bodied/disabled. Nancy Mairs's *Waist-High in the World* (1996) and Stephen Kuusisto's *Planet of the Blind* (1998) represent ontologies shaped by using a wheelchair and being blind. Simi Linton's *My Body Politic* (2005) makes explicit the interconnectedness of the personal and the political, the individual and the historical, in her account of the development of her disability cultural awareness in the context of the emerging disability rights movement. Narratives of illness and disability can stare back at assumptions of what constitutes normalcy until those assumptions become obvious, which may lead to defensiveness and a standoff or may open up a space for redefining and growing comfortable with difference.

Narratives can reorient the reader to new subject positions, whether waist-high or seeing through the "frosted windows of my cataracts" on a *Planet of the Blind* (Kuusisto 1998,186). And what these non-normative subject positions help us to see is less the experience of paralysis or blindness or cancer or diabetes than a dismantled illusion of normalcy. Meri Nan-Ama Danquah's memoir, *Willow, Weep for Me* (1999), describes her experience of depression as a middle-class, well-educated, African American, urban woman. Lucy Grealy's *Autobiography of a Face* (2003) is not only an account of a child's experience of cancer and an adult's experience of facial difference perceived by our culture as deformity. It also situates those experiences within community (white, suburban, middle-class, U.S. American) and family (Irish immigrants, well-educated but struggling financially).

Dagoberto Gilb's short story, "please, thank you," represents the recovery of a Mexican American man who is hospitalized following a stroke. His somewhat paranoid confusion about the bigotry of the health professionals who care for him is difficult to disentangle from their actual assumptions and attitudes. His gradual return to his previous cognitive status, represented as his painstakingly typed reorganization of consciousness, reveals not only a point of view that readers can come to recognize and accept but also his own developing empathy for nurses and therapists who care for him, even the detached nurse who responds "thank you" at inappropriate moments: "he is strange, my daughter says quietly as he leaves. very odd character. but you know, i say, i think hes harmless. hes here. doing this" (2010, 69).[10]

Terry Tempest Williams's *Refuge: An Unnatural History of Family and Place* (2001) represents not only her own experience of breast cancer and treatment but also that of nine other women in her family. Moreover, it explores the environmental and social context of breast cancer in its engagement with "place," her family's home on the plains of Utah, exposed to radiation during atomic bomb testing in the early in 1960s. The book focuses not only on an individual "patient" but also on the impact of illness on family and community more broadly: Illness is represented as a communal rather than individual experience. Narratives that contextualize disability and illness in terms of family, community, culture, place, and in terms of health care—and critical frameworks that emphasize this contextualization—help clinicians to recognize the social determinants of their patients' suffering, including the patient-professional relationship.

STARING BACK: FAT, DISABILITY, AND BEAUTY

Literature can allow clinicians to look with fresh eyes at the habit of profiling and stereotyping, which can function as a necessary means of managing complex data but can also lead to misperceptions and clinical as well as social forms of medical error. The broader social stigmatization of what is described in medical terms as *obesity* and in activist terms as *fat* (and I use *fat* in the spirit of this activist reclaiming) likely contributes to the high rates of negative perceptions of fat people among healthcare providers.[11] Fat is often treated as if it were a disease in itself, rather than correlated with disease under certain circumstances, and healthcare providers often communicate their disapproval and even disgust of fat people, viewing them as weak willed and self-indulgent, attitudes that drive people away from the medical care they need. Narrative accounts like Judy Freespirit's short story, "On Ward G" (2003), represent a fat person's experience of health care, looking back from the inside out. The narrator must negotiate staff who are "fat phobic" and engage in intensive "emotional labor" in order to get good clinical care: "It's as important for the patient to have the right bedside manner as it is for the staff. Even more important since we're talking about survival here. . . . So I straighten my own sheets, push the red button on the IV machine when it starts beeping, get myself water, things like that. The other thing is that you have to be polite, but not too polite, or they'll ignore you" (156–157). The narrator is hungry, especially when the staff are microwaving fried chicken and the smells torment her, but she refuses to ask for food: "I didn't want to provide them with a funny story about the fat lady who wanted their food" (155). Texts like Freespirit's hold up a mirror to the stigmatization and stereotyping that contribute to disparities in care and discourage many people from seeking health care, particularly when their experiences of stigmatization are more disabling than their illness, physiological or mental difference, or impairment.

Narratives supplemented with critical discussions of social factors that construct disability can begin to address the disparities that many disabled people experience in the clinic.[12] In his narrative *The History of My Shoes and the Evolution of Darwin's Theory*, Kenny Fries describes an encounter with a physician in which the physician's reaction to his differently formed limbs is more disabling than Fries's impairment: "In this situation I must act as if my disability is the worst thing that ever happened, when the truth is, this examination, Dr. Mendotti's stare, are much more difficult to endure" (2007, 1). Because most clinicians see disabled people when they are sick and need medical care, health professionals often perceive life lived with a disability more negatively than disabled people do. In U.S. culture, there are very few representations and reflections of disabled people who live, create, interact, and express fully and richly, as opposed to narratives that construct disability as a tragedy (Couser 1997; Garden 2010). Given that clinicians may have little firsthand experience with disabled people, popular cultural representations tend to reinforce rather than correct the assumption that life with disability is not worth living. The health humanities offer critical analyses of stigmatizing representations of illness and disability that train clinicians to recognize and resist these stereotypes (Gilman 1988; Price Herndl 1993; Lupton 2003). Counternarratives like Fries's educate readers and viewers about assumptions and the nature of representation itself.

Dance, video, and other forms of performance arts also offer compelling counternarratives that resist reductive stereotypes and illuminate the possibilities and limits of representation. A short video excerpt of a dance called "The beauty that was mine, through the middle, without stopping," produced by the AXIS Dance Company (AXIS 2009), a mixed-ability group, represents dance as performed by dancers who use wheelchairs as well as those whose bodies conform to traditional expectations of dancers. Nondisabled dancers pair off with two dancers in wheelchairs, one manual and one motorized. One dancer uses his upper body to roll his wheelchair and the other, nondisabled dancer over onto the floor, and he dances with her, supporting her and following her movements on her legs with movements of his arms. They move in tandem, echoing and playing off of each other while expressing the forms of the movements through different parts of their bodies. The nondisabled dancer lies and spins herself on the wheel of the sideways-tipped chair while the disabled dancer rotates himself in the opposite direction beneath her. They move in synchronicity through their duet, mirroring each other's directions and forms through the different modes of different bodies, one of which extends itself into space through an assistive device, the wheelchair.

A text like a dance performance (or a video clip of one) can thus represent information that may be critical to a clinical assessment and to clinical care: the broader context of life with illness or disability, or, more specifically, as in this case, the potential for a rather extraordinary quality of life lived through what Rosemarie Garland-Thomson (1997) calls "extraordinary bodies." Clinicians may see people who use wheelchairs primarily or exclusively in the clinic when they are sick or need some sort of care or treatment. This compounds the lack of exposure that nondisabled people have to disabled people in general and to the goodness of life that disabled people experience. Nondisabled and disabled people have markedly different perceptions of the quality of a life lived with a disability, a fact that has a significant impact on medical decision making (Gill 2000). The AXIS dance is a powerful representation of quality of life: movement with paralysis, beauty, creativity, complex social relations—between the dancers and between dancers and audience—work and productivity, and so on. It is also a representation of functionality across difference, disabled and nondisabled dancers achieving a shared goal through interdependence.

Later in the clip, a nondisabled dancer holds a large picture frame in front of a dancer with prosthetic legs. The dancer in the frame says, "This is me. This is me walking. This is me stopping. Walking . . . walking . . . stopping. This is me. Nothing much to look at." She reaches up and touches the frame and continues: "A picture of me, but not *really* me—in the end." With this verbal recitation, the piece thus explicitly addresses the issue of representation itself. Dance, like language, is a representation of "me" or some other subject, but, in the end, representations are mediations of selves and experiences, "not really me." If language and other sorts of self-presentation are not "really me" or "really you," is "real" communication possible? The AXIS performance raises important questions that are integral to patients and clinicians' relationship: What is "really me"? How well can I really know the other? What is really happening to this patient? What do her or his words mean? What does this clinician understand about my experience of illness? What is he or she thinking? What do her or his words really mean? And how can we find a shared and even healing mode of communication and understanding? Engaging critically with literature and the arts through the health humanities does not necessarily engender empathy for patients' perspectives (Garden 2007); however, it establishes the foundations for that empathic understanding, as well as a respect for patients' authority, by raising questions about assumptions, stereotypes, language, and the nature of representation itself.

NARRATIVE, INTERSECTIONAL IDENTITY, AND DIFFERENCE IN THE CLINIC

In another counternarrative that invites reassessment of categories of health and of gender and sexuality, Eli Clare grounds his autobiographical writing, *Exile and Pride*, in a merging of body and place: "Home starts here in my body, in all that lies imbedded beneath my skin. My disabled body: born prematurely in the backwoods of Oregon, I was first diagnosed as 'mentally retarded,' and then later as having CP [cerebral palsy]" (2009, 10). Clare's narrative weaves together his intersectional (that is, mutually constructing) social identities with a complex sociocultural context: "Rural, white, working-class culture that values neighbors rather than anonymity, that is both tremendously bigoted—particularly racist—and accepting of local eccentricity, that believes in self-sufficiency and depends on family—big extended families not necessarily created in the mold of the Christian right" (2009, 38).

Clare is "queer"—a transgender and former lesbian. He is "crip"—disabled. The degree to which he embraces aspects of the rural, white, working-class community where he grew up correlates with the ways in which that community "accepted eccentricity," that is, difference. While Clare rejects that community's bigotry and, elsewhere, their unwillingness to take responsibility for the integrity of their fragile environment, he is equally critical of many environmental activists for *their* bigotry: when stereotyping those who live in rural areas or when making assumptions of able-bodiedness in regard to other activists. Clare's intersectional identities reveal the range and diversity of ways of being that are excluded from social norms. His sexuality, queer and transgender, and disability are forms of difference that medicine has and continues to constitute as either disease or abnormality. (Homosexuality, for example, was, in the nineteenth century, increasingly viewed as deviant behavior, and medicine began to classify it as a psychological disorder; until 1973, it was included in the American Psychiatric Association's *Diagnostic and Statistical Manual of Mental Disorders* [Terry 1999].)

Clare's terms (*queer* and *crip* as opposed to *homosexual* and *handicapped*) represent a rejection of dominant culture's designation of LGBT (lesbian, gay, bisexual, transgender) sexuality and disability as abnormal or aberrant. He expands on his critique of the medicalization of disability:

For me having CP is rather like having blue eyes, red hair, and two arms. . . . The biggest difference is no one gives me grief, denies me employment, treats me as if I were ten years old, because of my blue eyes. My CP is not simply a *medical* condition. I need no specific medical care, medication, or treatment for my CP. . . . Some disabled people, depending on their disabilities, may indeed have pressing medical needs for a specific period of time or on an ongoing basis. But having particular medical needs differs from labeling a person with multiple sclerosis as sick, or thinking of quadriplegia as a disease. (2009, 122)

Clare's narrative reveals disabling social problems experienced by those who are different: because of his CP, he is "given grief" and infantilized and discriminated against in employment, conditions that may prove as much or more of a barrier to realizing his potential than the impairment of CP itself. His narrative also describes discrimination and infantilization due not only to his disability but also to his sexual identity and, in some cases, his working-class and rural background. *Exile and Pride* defamiliarizes what has been naturalized by privilege and sensitizes readers to the ableist and classist assumptions of, for example, the predominantly white, urban, middle-class LBGT community and the predominantly white, middle-class environmental activist community.

By reading narratives like Clare's, clinicians can learn to deconstruct and denaturalize norms. Critical theory further develops the awareness that bodies and identities are not predetermined, universal, and able to be objectively classified by science as normal or abnormal, healthy or diseased—or definitively classified in terms of gender, ethnicity, or race. Feminist, queer, and critical race theories have challenged categories that are taken for granted in science as biologically marked and static. For example, by questioning the medicalization of stages of female life— menstruation, childbirth, and menopause—feminist and queer theorists have illustrated the degree to which all aspects of biologized identity are constructed by culture and shaped by power and authority through knowledge and the regimented management of bodies and behaviors (Butler 1993; Fausto-Sterling 1992; Lorber 2000; Price and Shildrick 1999). Disability and Deaf studies scholars and activists like Clare have deconstructed the medicalization of disability and deafness, for example, arguing for a reconsideration of prenatal testing to eliminate the births of children with impairments (Parens and Asch 2000) and for the designation of Deaf people as not impaired but rather a linguistic minority (Ladd 2003).[13]

Clinicians can improve their care of patients by studying theoretical arguments that challenge the authority of medical science and its control and management of patients' bodies and minds, particularly those patients already disenfranchised by minority group status. Reading analytical accounts such as Clare's (a sort of merging of first-person narrative and sociocultural criticism that can be understood as a kind of autoethnography) can help healthcare providers recognize the potential to deconstruct or subtly to construct and reinforce norms. Clare's representation of his intersectional identity—queer, lesbian, working-class, white, rural, environmentalist, and crip—challenges appeals to empathy as a means of fostering greater justice in health care. If empathy involves being able to imagine the perspective of the other, Clare's complex subjectivity may elude the clinician's experience and thus ability to imagine. The narrative thus educates clinicians in both the importance of learning about the point of view of others and also a kind of humility that recognizes the difficulty of assuming complete knowledge of that point of view (Garden 2008, 124). Narratives invite understanding through rich representations of experiences and perspectives. However, clinicians must respect the alterity—or inability to be fully known—of the other. Respect for alterity reiterates the centrality of the person who seeks clinical care as a critical if not the primary source of information about the medical issue and its sociocultural dimensions.

CONCLUSION

Analyzing, discussing, and writing about narratives and other arts and humanities texts (including theoretical texts) develops essential critical thinking skills involving imagination, reflection, and emotional reasoning. These skills are essential to the best clinical care and yet are often neglected in traditional medical and nursing training and practices. The compelling need to focus on the mastery of pathophysiology—that is, the biomedical model—all too often eclipses an engagement with texts and issues that develop critical thinking about the sociocultural, ethical, and representational dimensions of the patient-professional encounter.

Clinicians have the power to construct or reinforce norms to the detriment of the patient: a smile or chuckle when describing a case involving two mothers; obvious discomfort when discussing a transgender patient considering sex reassignment therapy; reluctance to provide a sign language interpreter for a Deaf person; or impatience with a person considered obese whose body does not conform to standard medical equipment. Through training in the health humanities, clinicians can deconstruct norms. Clinicians may or may not be able to address the biological factors involved in patients' illness, injury, or impairment, but they can help patients and even heal them by recognizing and reassuring them as individuals with complex identities embedded in networks of friends and family, community, culture, and society. Clinicians can tolerate their own discomfort and develop a respectful curiosity about patients, recognizing them as authorities on their own experiences of illness or disability and on their unique identities. They can also recognize that their training and the biomedical model are only one source of knowledge about illness and disability and only one source of authority—even while it remains the dominant source of power in the clinic. Bodies are not only biological; they are also sociocultural. Healing people (rather than just bodies) involves "social studies": sociocultural and narrative knowledge and skills, as well as skill in medicine.

NOTES

1 Diane Price Herndl discusses this passage in *Invalid Women* (1993, 4).
2 The expansive term *texts* refers to not only published narratives, poetry, stories, and novels but also film and video, blogs and vlogs, visual art, television, and other creative modes of cultural production.
3 The term *health humanities* reflects a critical focus on physicians' power that was often absent from the first wave of the *medical humanities* and marks the second wave's commitment to expanding patients' power and also to a leveling of interdisciplinary relations.
4 See Arno Kumagai and Monica Lypson (2009); Stephen Murphy-Shigematsu (2009); Conny Seeleman et al. (2009); Cayla Teal and Richard Street (2009); Delese Wear (2003); and David Williams (1999).
5 For examples, see Einat Avrahami (2007); Alan Bleakly (2005); Howard Brody (1987, 1994); Rita Charon (2006); Jack Coulehan (2003); Thomas Couser (1997); Sayantani DasGupta and Rita Charon (2004); John Engel et al. (2008); Frank (1997); Rebecca Garden (2010); Trisha Greenhalgh and Brian Hurwitz (1998); Anne Hunsaker Hawkins

(1999); Seth Collings Hawkins (2004); Arthur Kleinman (1989); Arno Kumagai (2008); Arno Kumagai et al. (2009); Bradley Lewis (2011); Hilde Lindemann Nelson (2001); Cheryl Mattingly (1998); Cheryl Mattingly and Linda Garro (2000); Femi Oyebode (2003); Hedy Wald and Shmuel Reis (2010); Delese Wear (2002); and Delese Wear and Julie Aultman (2005).

6 See Catherine Belling (2006a, 2006b, 2010); Jeffrey Bishop (2008); Marcelline Block and Angela Laflen (2010); Rafael Campo (2005); Cheryl Dellasega et al. (2007); Martyn Evans (2002); Kleinman et al. (2006); Allan Peterkin (2008); Suzanne Poirier and Daniel Brauner (1990); Susan Squier (2007); and Delese Wear (1992, 2009).

7 "Literary and cultural studies approaches" is shorthand here for a broad range of theoretical approaches that includes literary studies, ranging from literary criticism to language and social theory or philosophy; feminist and gender studies; disability and Deaf studies; critical race theory and ethnic studies; medical sociology and anthropology; and queer theory, among others.

8 I use the term *disabled people*, rather than a term like "people with disabilities," as a way of reiterating the social relations that construct disability; disability is thus the discrimination that results in segregation and diminished rights, rather than a quality or defect inherent in an individual.

9 For short accounts, see Tony Gramaglia (1996); for essays, see Fitzhugh Mullan et al. (2006). Blog and vlog examples include *Bad Cripple* (Peace, n.d.); *First, Do No Harm: Real Stories of Fat Prejudice in Health Care* (Barbara Benesch-Granberg, n.d.); *Being Mentally Interesting* (Molloy, n.d.); *Inflamed: Living with Rheumatoid Arthritis* (Angela, n.d.); and *Lenois* (Savage, n.d.). Video examples include Amanda Baggs (2007); and Tricia Pil (2011). For graphic (comic-book-style) memoir examples, see David B. (2005); and Harvey Pekar et al. (1994).

10 The absence of capital letters and punctuation in the story function as a "reality effect": the narrator is typing the story as an exercise for occupational therapy.

11 See Mary Margaret Huizinga et al. (2009); Josephine Kaminsky and Dominick Gadaleta (2002); Rebecca Puhl and Kelly Brownell (1991); Rebecca Puhl et al. (2009); Marlene Schwartz et al. (2003).

12 For examples, see Gary Albrecht et al. (2001); Jean-Dominique Bauby (1998); Lennard Davis (2010b); Anne Finger (1990); Terry Galloway (2010); Temple Grandin (1996); Leah Hager Cohen (1995); Susanna Kaysen (1994); Harlan Lane (1999); Simi Linton (1998, 2005); Carol Padden and Tom Humphries (2006); Ralph James Savarese (2007); Marsha Saxton (1997a, 1997b); and Mark Vonnegut (2010).

13 See also Bauman (2004); Lane (1999); and Linton (1998).

Chapter 13

HUMANITIES AND THE MEDICAL HOME

MARK CLARK, HOWARD BRODY, AND REBECCA HESTER

Patient-professional relationships have always been a principal focus of consideration for the medical/health humanities. Indeed, a major impetus for the emergence of humanities' engagement with health professions education in the 1960s and 1970s was a concern that, in an age enamored with and devoted to technological advance, the central significance of inter*personal* engagement— relationship—in health care was becoming dangerously overlooked (Fox 1985): such relationship was, humanists recognized, at the heart of the healthcare endeavor. One group of experts in medical and nursing education has argued that *relationship* is so basic to health care that it ought to be the very organizing principle of all health professions education (Tresolini and the Pew-Fetzer Task Force 1994). The prospect of regarding relationship as such an organizing principle, furthermore, points to the value of the humanities' interdisciplinary perspective and methodology as a means of understanding the dynamic nature of the relationship in the contexts of cultural change. As an illustration of the ways that an interdisciplinary humanities approach can be both theoretically rich and practically useful, we consider here a health policy proposal that has recently attracted great interest among policy makers, large employers, patient groups, and organized medicine: the patient-centered primary care medical home.

The medical home has been proposed as a viable option to reorganize the primary care office in order to improve access to quality health care for more Americans at a lower cost (Backer 2007; Grumbach et al. 2009; Martin et al. 2004; Rosenthal 2008; Sia et al. 2004). The *medical home* suggests a convenient, friendly point of entry into the healthcare system, where the vast majority of medical problems can be handled directly and services that must be referred elsewhere can be coordinated. *Primary care* physicians are trained to care for most common conditions; a higher percentage of primary physicians serving a population has been correlated with both lower costs and improved quality of care (Fisher et al. 2003a, 2003b; Starfield 1992; Welch et al. 1993). Primary care physicians are also commonly trained to work comfortably in multidisciplinary teams that include nurses, nutritionists, mental health counselors, and so forth: the ideal way to staff a medical home. A *patient-centered* practice implies policies that directly address patient concerns, such as ease of access, same-day appointments, and waiting areas well-stocked with patient education materials. More than just a comfortable setting, however, the success of the medical home hinges on the patient-professional relationship.

The popularity of this model sparks numerous questions that the humanities can help to address. What sorts of relationships should patients have with health professionals in such a home, and what are some challenges to developing these relationships? What skills and attributes ought to be taught to professionals to best prepare them to work in such a setting? What areas of knowledge, especially within the humanities, might expand our understanding of these relationships? How can we strike the right balance between building useful competencies in our students, instilling in them the humility necessary to remain open to unpredictable developments in dynamic relationships within ever-changing environments?

An interdisciplinary humanities approach facilitates a comprehensive view of the patient as a person, foregrounds the importance of care, and considers the contextual and cultural factors that shape the healthcare relationship. All of these concepts are important if the medical home model is to live up to its potential.

DISCIPLINARY AND INTERDISCIPLINARY APPROACHES

If the development of the medical home ultimately requires an interdisciplinary humanities approach, one might begin by asking what the various individual disciplines within the humanities—ethics, religious studies, literature, history, and the social sciences—have to offer as raw material for the inquiry.

A good deal of ethics literature addresses aspects of professional-patient relationships and offers broad ethical categories to better understand them (Emanuel and Emanuel 1992). Yet many ethical models neglect important aspects of the patient's experience by focusing solely on the patient as a decision maker. The centrality of the primary bioethical principle of respect for patient autonomy reinforces this view, although patient-provider relationships find useful analogies within the world of religious thought (Barnard 1985; Beauchamp and Childress 2008). Authors coming from a religious ethics perspective, such as Paul Ramsey and William F. May, stress a better-rounded view of the person (May 1991; Ramsey 1970). Similarly, many literary works often focus on patients' perspectives (Edson 1999; Quindlen 1994; Solzhenitsyn 1974; Tolstoy 1960), and historical studies disclose how these relationships have changed over time (Shorter 1985). The social sciences study how public status and culture affect these relationships, often revealing how idealized models proposed by ethics and humanities are incomplete or flawed (DeVries and Subedi 1998).

Given the breadth of perspectives on the healthcare relationship, where should we focus our energies, particularly with respect to exerting positive influence over the emergence of the medical home and other practice modalities? A humanities approach emphasizes care—over cure or cost—as the principal value in the patient-professional relationship. But humanities must also grapple with the complexities of the different meanings of apparently simple concepts like "care" and "hope" in different social and cultural contexts.

CURE AND CARE

In a typical primary care medical home, the health team will *cure* very few patients. Many patients will come with self-limited problems that would cure themselves with or without help. Many more patients will be dealing with chronic illnesses that can be managed but seldom completely cured. Yet all these patients will require *care.* How can professionals best understand the difference between curing and caring and apply that understanding to their patients' needs?

In 1927, Francis W. Peabody spoke with a voice quite prescient from the standpoint of today's medical/health humanities. This highly regarded Harvard physician, who knew that he was terminally ill, addressed his students on "The Care of the Patient" (Peabody 1927; see also Tishler 1992). This article is known best today for its culminating aphorism "The secret of the care of the patient is in caring for the patient" (Peabody 1927, 882). The entire article, however, offers a complex argument that deserves careful reading. Peabody employs a perspective that informed much later work in psychosomatic medicine: "Disease at once affects and is affected by what we call the emotional life" (1927, 882; see also Harrington 2008). Peabody argues, "The physician who attempts to take care of a patient while he neglects [the emotional and personal] factor is as *unscientific* as the investigator who neglects to control all the conditions that may affect his experiment" (1927, 882; emphasis added). "The good physician," Peabody adds, "knows his patients through and through, and his knowledge is bought dearly. Time, sympathy, and understanding must be lavishly dispensed, but the reward is to be found in that personal bond which forms the greatest satisfaction of the practice of medicine" (1927, 882). By claiming that medical *science,* and not merely the vague "art of medicine," requires addressing the whole person in this manner, Peabody anticipates influential later work such as George Engel's biopsychosocial model (1977).

In more recent times, physician-philosopher Edmund Pellegrino (2001) has addressed the evolution of the patient-professional caregiver relationship. He argues that biomedicine has come to envision "cure" as the principal aim of the therapeutic encounter. Pursuit of cure has led to undeniable benefit, but the biomedical model conceptualizes medical treatment "simply as applied biology," where caregivers are required to function primarily as scientists who focus "on *things* to do for a particular disease that are measurably effective" (2001, 167; emphasis in original). In the history of medicine, "cure" was an elusive ideal. If it occurred, notes Pellegrino, cure "resulted largely from the body's self-healing powers and the physician's compassion, caring engagement, and emotional support" (2001, 167). The "ancient grounding of medicine" lay in "care and compassion," and biomedicine has, with its concentration on the goal of cure, displaced the ancient conception of the caregiver's role in the therapeutic process. Pellegrino argues for a reaffirmation of the ancient grounding. Without rejecting biomedical advances, he proposes that we seriously consider the ways in which care affects the quest for health, well-being, and the alleviation of suffering, even as we reaffirm care as the foundational interpersonal dynamic defining the patient-professional relationship.

"Care," Pellegrino argues, "is the moral base upon which our professional obligations, our ethics, are to be re-formed" (2001, 178).

THE COMPLEXITY OF CARE

But what does care in the ideal medical home involve, and how does one go about exercising it? If Peabody and Pellegrino are right, the exercise of care begins with the conviction that the therapeutic or clinical encounter is an interaction of persons, not merely a scientist making observations about a biological phenomenon. But once one accepts the notion, with Peabody, that competent care involves "insight into the patient's character and personal life" (1927, 882), one begins to comprehend the complexity of care and the challenge it presents to the conscientious caregiver.

Physician and humanities scholar Eric Cassell addresses this complexity (1982, 1991) via the concept of suffering, contending that this emotion "is experienced by persons, not merely bodies, and [it] has its source in challenges that threaten the interactions of the person as a complex social and psychological entity" (1982, 639). Cassell illustrates this point by describing a "35-year-old sculptor with metastatic disease of the breast" (1982, 639). Adverse reactions to her disease and its treatment included hirsutism, obesity, loss of libido, and worst of all, loss of strength in the hand she used to create her artwork. Because her physicians failed to apprize her of what was and would be happening to her, "she became profoundly depressed. . . . . She feared the future. Each tomorrow was seen as heralding increased sickness, pain, or disability, never as the beginning of better times. She felt isolated because she was no longer like other people and could not do what other people did. She feared that her friends would stop visiting her. She was sure that she would die" (1982, 639).

Cassell argues that physicians can comprehend neither the nature of this woman's suffering, nor what it might take to relieve it, unless they understand the many dimensions of her personhood. To begin this task, Cassell offers "a simple topology" of personhood (1982, 641), including the dimensions of

- personality and character (potentially altered by an illness, for example, or found to be inadequate in confronting the illness)
- a past (including previous experiences with illness and physicians)
- life experiences and meanings attached to them
- family ties
- cultural background
- familial and social roles
- relationships with others
- connectedness on the basis of political beliefs
- proficiencies
- customary ways of doing things—familiar ways of living in the world
- corporeal uniqueness and equilibria of bodily comfort
- a "secret life" of aspiration and dreams

- a "perceived future"
- a "transcendent dimension" or "a life of the spirit." (1982, 642–643)

Within any one of these various dimensions of personhood, one may feel relatively whole or relatively fragmented. The degree of fragmentation that would cause suffering in one individual might be the normal, everyday experience of another. The sculptor with breast cancer appears to be suffering because many dimensions of her personhood no longer cohere. Instead of being a part of her personhood, they have become threats to her very survival. Even if her cancer is beyond cure, caring professionals can do something to ameliorate these threats to various dimensions of her personhood. They can restore effective communication, address her fears, assist in finding support among her friends and family, and focus on treatments that might restore for a time some of her ability to be creative as an artist.

Cassell's "topology" should not be viewed simply as a checklist or as an excuse to ascribe pathology to others without listening to their understanding of their own experiences. Moreover, even though health professionals may occasionally be able to relieve suffering, some distress cannot be relieved by any handy interventions. In these latter cases, the professional still contributes to the patient's well-being by witnessing and acknowledging the suffering without attempting to make it go away (Frank 1995).

NARRATIVE, CARE, AND HOPE

Cassell believes that "asking the sufferer" is the best way to recognize what dimensions of personhood have been injured and to respond with effective care and compassion (1982, 643). In asking the patient for an account of his or her personhood and its injuries, the caregiver in the medical home setting invites the patient's self-interpretation and the construction of a life story. By means of this story, the patient may attempt to find meaning in the present experience of illness and suffering—to interpret the bewildering event so that it makes sense in the plot of the patient's life and may serve as a sufficiently stable platform from which to launch a future.

As medical/health humanities scholars have observed, the caregiver and the patient can do narrative work, and this process forms a central method to understand the patient-professional relationship (Brody 2003; Charon 2006; Hunter 1991b; Kleinman 1988). Narrative blends insights from many disciplines—including literature, philosophy, religious studies, and the social sciences—into its essential nature and function. Arthur Frank, a sociologist, contends that "the voices of the ill are often faltering in tone and mixed in message" (1995, 25), for "seriously ill people are wounded not just in body but in voice. They need to become storytellers in order to recover the voices that illness and its treatment often take away" (1995, xii). The caregiver occupies a unique position that can enable patients to become these storytellers—to construct the story needed to restore hope and light the path to what well-being is possible. Professional knowledge can and must contribute to the story's construction, drawing on and integrating the dimensions of personhood that Cassell's topology spells out while also reflecting on the cultural and social differences between physician and patient. Consequently, one of the most important roles that a caregiver plays is as an active listener. Because the stories of the ill emerge, at first, from a state of bewilderment, chaos, and pain, they are often fragmentary and broken, so that, as Frank recognizes, "one of the most difficult duties as human beings is to listen to the voices of those who suffer" (1995, 25). As a result of their brokenness, despair, hesitation, and faltering, "the voices of the ill are easy to ignore" (1995, 25), in part because those voices speak of a mutual vulnerability to illness and suffering that most would rather not acknowledge. Difficult as listening may be, however, "it is also a fundamental moral act" (1995, 25) that is at the heart of quality care.

The construction of the life story is intimately connected with hope. Even where hope of a cure and of prolonged survival is no longer realistic, one's ability to tell a meaningful story about one's present and immediate future remains critical to finding meaning in the life that remains (Brody 1981). As Václav Havel, Czech politician and playwright, puts it, "Hope . . . is not the conviction that something will turn out well, but the certainty that something makes sense, regardless of how it turns out. It is . . . this hope, above all, which gives us the strength to live" (1990, 181–182).

Physician Jerome Groopman has concluded after many years of practice that hope "is as important as any medication I might prescribe or any procedure I might perform" (2004, xiv). "Hope," he has come to believe, "is as vital to our lives as the very oxygen that we breathe" (2004, 208). Research indicates that

a change in mind-set has the power to alter neurochemistry. Belief and expectation—key elements of hope—can block pain by releasing the brain's endorphins and enkephalins, mimicking the effects of morphine. In some cases, hope can also have important effects on fundamental physiological processes like respiration, circulation, and motor function. During the course of an illness, then, hope can be imagined as a domino effect, a chain reaction in which each link makes improvement more likely. It changes us profoundly in spirit and in body. (2004, xvi–xvii)

The physiologic changes Groopman alludes to have been studied under the rubric of the *placebo effect*. A useful metaphor for this effect is the *inner pharmacy*— the idea that the human body is preprogrammed to secrete healing substances when affected by the right sorts of stimuli (Brody and Brody 2000). Stimuli that appear to activate this inner pharmacy include several dimensions of an optimal patient-professional relationship. The professional who listens to the patient and who demonstrates caring, who offers meaningful explanations, and who helps the patient feel more in control of the illness or its symptoms seems more likely to turn on the inner pharmacy (Brody 2000). Recent research has identified the neural mechanisms that allow our beliefs and emotions to trigger the release of chemicals that can promote healing, placing our understanding of the placebo effect on a stronger scientific footing (Benedetti 2009). These data reinforce the insight Peabody had back in 1927—that the caring professional who uses narrative approaches to better understand the patient's emotional and social life is simultaneously the *more scientific* practitioner (Peabody 1927).

Yet our scientific lens can be clouded by our own visions and understandings of hope. Insights from social scientists (Good et al. 1990) demonstrate that cultural meanings associated with hope vary as much for patients as for practitioners. Good and her colleagues state

The American discourse on hope incorporates popular and professional dimensions of our culture of biomedicine. Its emphasis on "will"—if one has enough hope, one may *will* a change in the course of the disease in the *body*—articulates fundamental American notions about personhood, individual autonomy, and the power of thought (good and bad) to shape life course and bodily functioning. (1990, 61)

These insights demonstrate that discourses of hope are not universal. The challenge for the health professional, therefore, is to listen for the ways that the patient understands and operationalizes hope to deal with suffering and illness. Physician and literary scholar Rita Charon stresses the importance of professionals' exercise of "narrative competence," which she defines as "the set of skills required to recognize, absorb, interpret, and be moved by the stories one hears or reads. This competence requires a combination of textual skills . . . creative skills . . . and affective skills" that "together . . . endow a reader or listener with the wherewithal to get the news from stories and to begin to understand their meanings" (2004, 862). The skills used by literary scholars to understand the intricacies of stories—including the ironies, the indirection, the evasion, the silences, the ambiguities, the figurative language that, in part, comprise them—can assist the caregiver to listen well and to help patients construct their stories.

Charon's insights also expose a tension that arises when a caregiver listens well. "When a doctor practices medicine with narrative competence," says Charon, "he or she can quickly and accurately hear and interpret what a patient tries to say." Busy, harried professionals are prone to fall into the trap of seeking greater efficiency, reducing the patient's narrative to a tool or protocol to facilitate medical decision making—threatening to undermine the spirit of listening. "The doctor who has narrative competence," writes Charon, "uses the time of a clinical interaction effectively, wringing all possible medical knowledge from what a patient conveys about the experience of illness and how he or she conveys it" (2004, 862).

The need to address patients' narratives of illness, suffering, and hope highlights both the opportunities and challenges faced by the team in a medical home. What happens when the cultural and linguistic divides between patient and practitioner remain so great that the intricacies of stories are lost in translation? How does a desire for efficient use of clinical time square with the faltering, confused attempt of patients to construct a story? Will patients encountering a physician devoted to such efficiency feel listened to carefully enough? Can the physician's and patient's understanding of the perplexing experience of an illness merge and result in a helpful course of action if efficiency is the higher goal?

CULTURE AND NARRATIVE

In the context of globalization and population mobility—where diversities of culture become increasingly apparent across any geographic region—the challenge of listening and exercising narrative competence increases. Merely renaming the primary care office a "medical home" does nothing to assure that these challenges will be adequately addressed.

The metaphors by which a person from one culture attempts to understand an illness may be quite different from those from a different culture. Notions of plot, the meaning of illness emergence within a life plot, and the meaning of silences will vary. Cassell's topology of personhood remains germane, but identifying each dimension of the person and its relation to suffering becomes more complex as each party brings different expectations and knowledges to the medical encounter.

As with narrative skills, busy professionals are tempted to reduce optimal cross-cultural understanding to a simple cookbook formulation, often advertised as "cultural competence." Bullet lists of supposed cultural characteristics attributed to various ethnic groups more often reinforce false stereotypes than engender real understandings of patients' experiences and beliefs (Kumagai and Lypson 2009; Wear 2003). Several studies have pointed to the communicative disconnects between African American and Native American patients in encounters with white physicians (Cooper and Powe 2004; Cooper et al. 2003; Cooper-Patrick et al. 1999; Johnson, Roter, et al. 2004; Johnson, Saha, et al. 2004). These studies advocate increases in minority student enrollment in medical schools in order to offset these racial and ethnic disconnects. Yet insights from critical race and ethnic studies have stressed that racial and ethnic concordance alone does not guarantee mutual understanding and agreement between individuals.

To complicate further the cultural complexity, H. Jack Geiger (2001) suggests that physicians themselves are members of two cultures: that of the mainstream society, in which some degree of bias is always a component, and the culture of medicine itself, which has its own values, assumptions, and understandings. As Renée Fox points out, "There is . . . a detectable 'Americanness' in the optimistic belief in medical science and technology, in their limitless progress and promise, their vigorous application, and their power to 'overcome' disease, that pervades our society and is pronounced in medical training" (2005, 1316). Every encounter between professional and patient can, therefore, usefully be viewed as a cross-cultural exchange, and lessons from ethnographic and cultural research can be applied to all such encounters (Kleinman et al. 1978). These ethnographic tools require listening to patients' narratives and asking questions without entrapment in cultural stereotypes. Tervalon and Murray-García's concept of cultural humility is useful: "Cultural humility incorporates a lifelong commitment to self-evaluation and self-critique, to redressing the power imbalances in the patient-physician dynamic, and to developing mutually beneficial and nonpaternalistic clinical and advocacy partnerships with communities on behalf of individuals and defined populations" (1998, 117).

Clearly, however, many challenges remain in achieving this goal. A literature review on culture, language, and the doctor-patient relationship in the United States has found that minority patients, especially those not proficient in English, are less likely to engender empathic responses from physicians, less likely to establish rapport with physicians, less likely to receive sufficient information, and less likely to be encouraged to participate in medical decision making (Ferguson and Candib 2002). Another review notes that blacks and Hispanics are more likely to be undertreated for pain than whites (Bonham 2001). Stereotypes, prejudices, and language barriers inhibit good physician-patient relationships (Smedley et al. 2003; Woloshin et al. 1995). Limited time and other institutional barriers also prevent physicians from meaningful engagements with their patients (Dugdale et al. 1999). Cultural and institutional barriers to care must be addressed from within the cultures of biomedicine in order to achieve the goal of patient-centered communication. There have been many attempts at teaching cultural competency but with little demonstrated impact on patient adherence to treatment, health outcomes, and equity of service across racial and ethnic groups (Beach et al. 2005; Beagan 2003; Flores et al. 2000). Medical-cultural issues represent one of the most long-standing challenges in medical education—how medical schools can augment their efforts to teach what they have variously called the "social," "psychological," "humanistic," "behavioral," "nonbiomedical," and "ethical" components of health and illness (Fox 2005).

THE MEDICAL HOME FROM A HUMANITIES PERSPECTIVE

Listening carefully to various people's life stories illustrates that "home" means many different things. For some, such as victims of domestic violence, its connotations are terribly negative; for others, it may sound oversentimentalized. Let us accept that the "medical home" is intended to convey a place devoted to the care and well-being of patients who are to be respected as individual persons while also acknowledging that care is complex and personal and that institutional and cultural barriers may prevent us from caring in meaningful ways. What does the interdisciplinary humanities vantage point suggest about the medical home?

The Swedish philosopher Fredrik Svenaeus offers a promising point of departure. Drawing on the phenomenology of Martin Heidegger and the hermeneutics of Hans-Georg Gadamer, Svenaeus suggests that we conceive of "the phenomena of health and illness as, respectively, homelike and unhomelike ways of being-in-the-world" (1999, 178). Similar to Cassell, Svenaeus views health or homelikeness as a state of equilibrium among all the various dimensions of personhood and illness as a state of disruption or disequilibrium. The goal of professional health care is, therefore, the restoration of homelikeness. Frank would ask further that health professionals aspire to include in the "home" a true sense of welcome, generosity, and even joy (2004).

The idea of the "home" that reflects the ideas of Cassell, Svenaeus, and Frank contrasts with a solely technological and efficiency approach. Some physicians and policy makers view the medical home in ways that stress its technical features— electronic medical records, quality audits, and efficient scheduling systems. As important as these features are, exclusive attention to them threatens our appreciation of the basic idea of "home"—a place where patients should feel welcomed simply for who they are and where they should be taken in even when the rest of the world seems against them (Brody 2009, 53–59). As two of Robert Frost's characters struggle, through conversation, to discover, "Home is the place where, when you have to go there, / They have to take you in"—or home is "Something you somehow haven't to deserve" (Frost 1915).

If busy professionals constantly recall the *patient-centered* aspects of the medical home, instead of focusing too much on its technical bells and whistles, what sort of education must they receive? A couple of humanities electives in medical school or a couple of seminars on cultural diversity are insufficient (Fox 2005). This education must be intellectually sophisticated and integrated substantially throughout healthcare education, as well as carried over into the medical home through ongoing training and dialogue with community members and families (Palfrey et al. 2004). Ideally, foundations in narrative and cultural understanding would begin with an undergraduate liberal arts experience and then be suitably reinforced and expanded in medical school (Doukas et al. 2010). Besides improving the practice of medicine, this extended development will open students' eyes to new paths of research and inquiry. In what way, for example, do elements of narrative, culturally inflected, engender hope that has real physiological and neurological effect?

One worry regarding the medical home is that groups now underserved by the present American health system will be excluded from its potential advantages (Beal et al. 2009). A related concern is that a medical home designed for the middle-class majority will poorly meet the needs of minority and other vulnerable populations. Some developments provide at least limited reassurance. Existing practices modeled on the medical-home concept have been shown to be effective in reducing racial and ethnic health disparities where most other interventions aimed at reducing these disparities have been disappointing (Beal et al. 2007). Pediatric care and family satisfaction were improved in one medical home demonstration (Palfrey et al. 2004). A type of practice specifically designed and successfully implemented to meet the needs of low-income communities, the federally qualified community health center, already contains many of the important elements of the medical home model (Rieselbach et al. 2010), a fact that speaks to its viability and reach.

The communicative skills necessary for an unbiased patient-centered practice must be taught on an ongoing basis in the medical home and must reflect the local social and cultural context. Given that the current healthcare system makes efforts to be culturally competent, while evidence of racial and ethnic disparities in health abounds, there is no reason to assume that a medical home will be more sensitive to the causes of these disparities unless addressing disparities directly is an explicit and well-conceptualized part of the model. The medical home must incorporate meaningful patient-provider exchanges, extended time periods for such exchanges to occur, and the use of interpreters when necessary. Family and community members must be meaningfully and consistently incorporated in the design and development of local medical homes, for, as Palfrey and his co-authors (2004, 1515) found, "a critical element in ensuring the successful operation of the medical home is family buy-in." These reforms would represent a countercultural move from current biomedical practice, which de-emphasizes care and focuses instead on the dual imperatives of cost and cure (often in that order). In addition, some form of reimbursement system that "makes care pay" through a cost-sharing scheme between the primary care physician and specialists would make the medical home concept more viable.

It is not enough to teach that "care" should take priority over technology. Professionals must be sufficiently self-reflective to acknowledge the cultural beliefs that they bring to their relationship with patients, even as they maintain an awareness of and respect for the patients' contributions to the relationship. Instead of relying on a model based solely on a competency that suggests that "caring" will be achieved so long as the professional brings the right skills to bear on the interaction with patients, professionals must possess the humility to allow open-ended and dynamic relationships to evolve, even if the direction those relationships take go beyond the professionals' existing skill set. Professionals need also to monitor the environment within which the dyadic relationship is evolving, to identify factors that either nurture or impede the development of the relationship.

CONCLUSION

The medical home model is a potential mechanism for a more humanistic and scientific way of practicing medicine. While the medical home model is promising as a matter of health policy, our main concern is using it to illustrate in a *practical* way in which the healthcare humanities might approach the development of the patient-professional relationship in a particular cultural and institutional context. If insights from the humanities are used to develop further the medical home concept and to educate its participants, then we can have increased confidence that the model will realize its promise. Since the model will not achieve what we hope from it if we ignore its complexities and ambiguities, humanists must continue to urge a deep exploration of the model along with the larger social, cultural, and economic environments within which it functions.

Chapter 14

OCCUPATIONAL MEDICINE

JACK COULEHAN

As a student in college, I never once shadowed a physician or volunteered in a hospital. There were no doctors in my family. Our general practitioner, who looked like Ernie Kovacs, was intimidating and thoroughly uninspiring. In fact, my only medical role model was Albert Schweitzer, whose memoir, *Out of My Life and Thought* (1933), had given me a serious case of hero worship but no practical information about the medical life. Despite all this, I did have one point in my favor when applying to medical school. I was convinced that I knew what it *felt* to be a doctor because of two summers I spent as "Doc," an informal medical advisor to my co-workers in the general labor pool at the Wheeling Steel plant in Steubenville, Ohio.

In the early 1960s, if you were a college student in Steubenville, summer employment at Wheeling Steel was a real plum. Wages were much higher than you could expect elsewhere. The mill's coveted summer positions were normally reserved for steelworkers' sons. Since my father was in the retail business, I could never have gotten a job there, if Hook, my best friend's dad, hadn't been a big shot in the steelworkers' union. After our sophomore year, my friend decided to stay in Detroit for the summer, so Hook sponsored my application.

College students were sent to the general labor pool where men who had no regular position in the mill were assigned jobs on a day-to-day basis. These were the employees most recently hired, as well as those who for some reason, often alcohol or disorderly conduct, had been demoted from a better position elsewhere. In the locker room at the beginning of each shift, we gathered around a raised platform where the foreman stood, cigar in mouth, clipboard in hand, and called out the name of each job available that shift, starting with the most desirable, and men bid on it. The bidder with the most seniority won the job, gathered his lunch pail, and took off. When all the good jobs had been assigned, the low-paying scut work was divvied out among new hires and college students. Scut work included jobs like sweeping the warehouse, cleaning the johns, and picking up trash in the railroad yards. A few higher-paying jobs were sometimes available because regular steelworkers found them too loathsome to bid on. Among these were emptying grease pits under the rolling machines in the cold rolling mill and shoveling cinders onto conveyor belts at the coke plant where the air looked and tasted like ashes.

On my first day at the mill, my job was to sweep the floor in a section of warehouse where they stored steel coils awaiting shipment. The foreman carefully defined my territory: from the central corridor to the east end of the building. "Okay, kid, no slacking," he said. Then he punched my shoulder and took off. The warehouse was relatively quiet, with only a smattering of forklifts and guys carrying this and that and the distant rumbling and snapping of machines. Dutiful as always, I pushed the broom briskly up and down between stacks of coils. Up one row and down another. Up and down. I finished in about an hour, shoveled the piles of debris into a bin, and set off to find out what I was supposed to do next. There was a guy sitting on some bags of concrete.

"Where's the foreman?" I asked. He looked at me with a peculiar expression.

"Why, kid?"

"I'm finished sweeping. I need another job."

The guy mumbled something unpleasant and turned away. Next I went to a forklift operator and asked the same thing. He spit tobacco juice.

"Kid," he said. "You sweep. You do it slowly. You do it over again. You take breaks. You get lost. Anything. But what you *don't* do: you don't look for the foreman, and you don't ask for more work."

My day's assignment had been to sweep a specific area. The only other requirement was not to be caught napping if and when a superintendent—easily identified by his yellow hardhat—happened to walk by. Many labor pool jobs were like that. An hour or two's work in an eight-hour shift. You could pass the time playing cards, reading the newspaper, or listening to a transistor radio—as long as you were skillful enough to look busy at a moment's notice.

In the caste system of the mill, college students were Untouchables. Nobody wanted to have anything to do with us. First of all, because our positions were temporary, we weren't required to join the union. In our co-workers' eyes, this made us scabs. Second, there was a widespread belief that we were shirkers, since we had chosen to sit on our asses in college, rather than making an honest living. Finally, some college kids had proven to be wiseasses who looked down their noses at regular employees. Thus, the steelworkers shunned us.

However, sometimes we had to eat lunch in close proximity. Perhaps an overheard conversation caused the word to get out that I was studying to become a doctor. Everything changed almost immediately. I told the guys I had two more years of college to complete and then four years of medical school, which meant I knew literally nothing about medicine, but this seemed to make no difference. I turned into "Doc," while my peers rarely made it beyond "Hey, you" or "Kid." An older fellow named Riel, who had been sent back to the labor pool because of unfortunate incidents involving his foreman, explained the situation. While college was generally considered a waste of time, and college students were pampered brats, everyone understood the value of doctors. Thus, though my medical background consisted of a course in invertebrate zoology and another in comparative anatomy, the men soon were soliciting my advice: "Hey, Doc, my wife's gall bladder is acting up." "Hey, Doc, my youngest boy, he's been coughing all night." "Listen, Doc, Brick's got the clap again. He says penicillin doesn't work. What do you think he should do?"

I was conscientious about this new role, mostly because I desperately wanted to fit in. Thus, I'd go home and try to learn something about gallbladder disease, gonorrhea, or whatever the topic might be. There was no Internet in those days, but Steubenville did have its own college, and I heavily relied on its library. I'd find out what I could, then go back to the questioner with some bits of information, like the foods you were supposed to avoid if you had gallbladder disease. Diet was a big topic because half the steelworkers suffered from ulcers and wanted to know whether it was true that alcohol makes an ulcer worse.

The highest-paying job I worked at Wheeling Steel was on a team that knocked down the brick lining in open hearth furnaces. After a certain number of charges, each furnace had to be shut down, allowed to cool, and the refractory bricks that lined the interior replaced. In the first stage, several men climbed inside the chamber, wearing helmets and space suits lined with asbestos. They knocked down the bricks with wooden mallets and shoveled out the debris, after which a team of bricklayers relined the flues. The job paid over three times our base wage. The schedule, too, seemed fairly attractive, alternating twenty minutes inside with a forty-minute break. However, since downtime was lost money, they sent workers into the furnace as soon as the temperature came down to 130 degrees. The light was poor. Ventilation, nonexistent. The air, reddish dust. It was almost literally hell.

I first heard about Dwayne, who was one of Wheeling Steel's "ghost" employees, during a break from the furnace. Dwayne was a tough little man who drank. Since he rarely came to work sober, he usually slept through his shift in one of the locker rooms, while others covered his job. This practice had gone on for years. Everyone knew about Dwayne and a number of other "ghosts" that haunted the mill, but the guys protected them. Dwayne had recently been transferred from his old job in the foundry to the open hearth. This change seemed to have upset his ecology and, according to my co-workers, was responsible for a recent decline in health.

"Doc, he's got yellowing of the liver," they told me. "They say he's not right. Do you think you could take a look?"

We were on the midnight to 8:00 A.M. shift, and it turned out that Dwayne was resting in a corner behind some barrels. He had a sad, sallow face, massive ascites, and was well on the road to hepatic coma, although I had no idea what that was at the time. I sat down on the bench beside him. "How're you doing, Dwayne? Some of the guys are worried about you." He muttered something I had to strain to hear. He didn't seem opposed to my staying around for a while, so I asked what he thought about the Pirates. At the time the Pittsburgh Pirates were sitting in the cellar, which wasn't unusual. "Damn the bastards," he whispered. We went back and forth like this about baseball a couple of times before Dwayne nodded off.

After that, I stopped to see Dwayne every night but didn't learn much, except that he lived with his sister on Railroad Street, and she kept badgering him to get himself admitted to the V.A. hospital. When he got fed up with her yakking, he'd spend his off hours in a booth at Mazzini's Bar. I'd tell him he needed to get his strength up, and the hospital might not be such a bad idea. He said he had tried a bottle of Geritol to build up his blood, but it hadn't worked. He was thinking of trying vitamins. I encouraged him and said maybe he ought to lay off the booze until the vitamins had a chance to work. Then he'd clam up, and I'd go back to the furnace. The guys would ask me how Dwayne was doing. "What do you think, Doc?" Most of them were reluctant to go anywhere near Dwayne, even though they apparently cared about him.

"I just wouldn't know what to say," Riel said.

It wasn't long—maybe two weeks—until Dwayne stopped coming to work, and before the summer was out we heard that he had vomited blood one day at Mazzini's and was rushed to the hospital, where he died.

After that, the guys were solicitous to me. A few of us got assigned to the grease pits for several days. It was my first time. Naturally, as the one with least seniority, I had the dirtiest job, climbing into the pit under the rolling machine in hip-length waders and scooping the grease into a large bucket attached to a rope and pulley system. A co-worker would raise the full bucket, empty the grease into a wheeled vat, and feed the bucket back down. The sweet, piercing odor of grease, a smell thicker than cheesecake, was overpowering. For the first few minutes in the pit, its odor was treacherously pleasant. Scoop, signal, wait. No one was in a hurry, I could set a slow pace, not bad at all. Scoop, signal, wait. Scoop, signal, wait. Then suddenly, my stomach turned.

It turned violently. I crashed on a tide of nausea, vomiting once in the pit and again at the top of the ladder. How feeble! Just what you'd expect from a college kid. I was so embarrassed. But surprisingly, the guys didn't make jokes at my expense. In fact, Brick insisted that I stay on the bench with my head down and worked the pit himself for the rest of the shift. After a while, Art, who always brought a thermos of hot soup in his bag, came over and offered a cupful, assuring me the soup would help settle my stomach. As I sat there for the next few hours, gradually feeling more like a human being, three or four guys stopped by offer encouragement.

"Take it easy, Doc."

"Thumbs up."

"You want an aspirin?"

I hadn't exactly become one of the gang. It never reached that point, but at least I had earned—well, not earned, but rather stumbled into—a place in the labor pool. Riel once explained what the men felt about my therapeutic role with Dwayne: "You did good, Doc, you treated him real good."

Part V
THE BODY

Chapter 15

THE VIRTUES OF THE IMPERFECT BODY

ROSEMARIE TONG

THERE are many ways to approach the topic of the body, but after considerable reflection, I have decided to focus almost exclusively on one question about it: Do parents have either a right or a duty to use the new genomics to procreate babies with perfect minds and bodies? This question is not entirely speculative. Our knowledge about genes linked to human disease and to physical, intellectual, and even moral characteristics is exponentially increasing. Currently, it is possible to test prenatally embryos and fetuses for serious genetic diseases such as cystic fibrosis, Duchenne muscular dystrophy, Tay-Sachs disease, hemophilia A and B, beta-thalassemia, sickle-cell disease, alpha-antitrypis deficiency, and Lesch-Nyhan syndrome (Handyside 1995, 985). In the near future, it will also be possible to test for minor genetic defects such as myopia, for propensities for conditions such as autism, and even for non-disease traits such as longevity and height (Gray 1994, 38). In fact, there are predictions that within a decade, primary care physicians will be able to do a whole genome screen of patients in their office for around $499 (Pollack 2010). Scientific developments such as these transform science fiction into science fact. For example, the society described in the film *Gattaca*, which I first viewed in 1997, no longer seems like a futuristic society to me (Niccol 1997). Rather, much of it seems like a commentary on our present society.

Gattaca presents a society in which the genetic engineering of human beings is routinized and people's genetic heritage determines their social class. In this society, a child named Vincent is conceived the old-fashioned way (in the heat of sexual passion, no doubt) and is born without genetic enhancements. Suffering from myopia, a congenital heart defect, and an accompanying 30.2-year life expectancy, Vincent faces genetic discrimination and prejudice as a result of his parents' impulsive action. The only way for Vincent to achieve his dream of orbiting the Earth is for him to purchase a new DNA profile and identity from someone with better genes.

Vincent buys blood, tissue, and urine samples from Jerome, a silver-medal athlete paralyzed from the waist down as the result of a car accident (actually, a botched suicide attempt). Importantly, Vincent buys *more* than genetically superior bodily materials from Jerome: he buys Jerome's identity. Vincent undergoes painful orthopedic surgery in order to add several inches to his body height. In addition, he gets contact lenses to correct his myopia and audio tapes of a strong-beating heart to mask his heart condition during mandatory exercise sessions. Finally, Vincent has to practice hard to overcome his left-handedness, which is also considered a flaw in Gattaca.

The inspirational message of the film is that the "imperfect" underdog Vincent can overcome his genetic deficiencies through willpower and spirit even as the "perfect" Jerome fails to succeed—that is, get a gold medal—despite his excellent genetic endowment. Although the film's moral is clear, what is unclear is why Vincent's parents set him up in the first place for a life of struggle. Is it really better to be "imperfect," as the film suggests? If so, why did Vincent's parents make sure their second son, Anton Jr., was genetically engineered? In short, didn't Vincent's parents fail him by having him with his genetic "imperfections" instead of having a different—that is, a genetically designed "better"—first son? Is Vincent's life a wrongful life? That is, is Vincent's life worse than no life at all?

PARENTAL RIGHT TO PROCREATE A "PERFECT" BABY?

In trying to answer these questions, it helps to turn to the work of John A. Robertson, a lawyer who believes that parents have a right to select their offspring's characteristics (1994, 149–172). As he sees it, parents' specific right to select their children's characteristics is linked to two general rights: (1) parents' general right *not to procreate* children because of the burdensome aspects (physical, psychological, and social) of parenting, and (2) parents' general right *to procreate* a child with characteristics they value because of their "natural" desire to have a biological legacy, a chip-off-the-old-block, to live on after them. Because carrier screening, pre-implantation genetic diagnosis, prenatal screening, gene therapy, sex selection, and selective reduction enable parents to procreate children with traits they value, Robertson concludes that these activities are usually protected by people's procreative rights (1994, 151–159; see also Tong 2007, 204).

People's procreative rights are not absolute, however. According to Robertson, they probably "protect only actions designed to enable a couple to have normal, healthy offspring whom they intend to rear" (1994, 167). He speculates that genetic interventions that aim to produce subnormal children or clones may "deviate too far from the experiences that make reproduction a valued experience" (1994, 169) to be protected by constitutionally protected liberty rights. However, Robertson also opines that some genetic interventions—those aimed at enhancement, for example—might be viewed as part of "parental discretion in rearing offspring" (1994, 167).

To defend his view that genetic enhancement may be viewed in favorable ways, Robertson points out that parents presently seek to improve their children in a variety of ways. For example, some parents send their children to elite schools; hire specialized tutors for them; give them music, art, and drama lessons; enroll them in debating teams and sports programs; take them to dermatologists to rid them of acne; and so on (1994, 169–171). Other parents go even further than this. In the quest to make their children better, they submit them to cosmetic surgeries, non-therapeutic injections of human growth hormone, non-therapeutic doses of Ritalin (a medication for attention deficit hyperactivity disorder), and non-therapeutic doses of Prozac (a medication for clinical depression). So long as parents are able to show that such interventions are safe, effective, and likely to benefit rather than harm their children, the state will permit parents to shape their children as they please. Therefore, says Robertson, there is no good reason for the state to interfere with safe, effective, and beneficial *genetic* interventions either.

Implicit in Robertson's view is the commonsense idea that trying to make a fetus or a child "better" is good and beneficial but that trying to make a fetus or child "worse" is bad and harmful. Enhancements are permitted; diminishments are not. Lawyer Dena Davis agrees with Robertson that parents should not be permitted to diminish their children because what parents think is in the "best" interests of their child may, in fact, make their children's lives very bad or difficult. For example, Davis says she is a vehement opponent of the U. S. Supreme Court ruling in *Yoder v. Wisconsin* (1972). This ruling permitted the Dutch Amish religious community to limit their children's education to elementary school only. The court determined that

the State's claim that it is empowered, as parens patriae, to extend the benefit of secondary education to children regardless of the wishes of their parents cannot be sustained against a free exercise claim of the nature revealed by this record, for the Amish have introduced convincing evidence that accommodating their religious objections by forgoing one or two additional years of compulsory education will not impair the physical or mental health of the child, or result in an inability to be self-supporting or to discharge the duties and responsibilities of citizenship, or in any other way materially detract from the welfare of society. (*Yoder v. Wisconsin* 1972, 229–234)

Not one to be intimidated by the U.S. Supreme Court just because it is "supreme," Davis claims that it is very harmful for Amish parents in essence to confine their children to two jobs: farmer for men and housewife or domestic worker for women. She predicts that Amish children who get the inner strength to move beyond the Amish way of life will find themselves without the tools they need to pursue careers in one of the major professions, athletics, or music, for that matter. In other words, Davis claims that Amish parents, however well intentioned, nonetheless *harm* their children by substantially limiting their right to control the course of their own destinies. Davis then reasons that if Amish parents harm their children by denying them high school educational opportunities (a lack that Amish children can later repair), parents would more egregiously harm their children by using genetic therapies to deprive them permanently of some basic function such as hearing, for example. She writes:

Deliberately creating a child who will be forced irreversibly into the parents' notion of "the good life" violates the Kantian principle of treating each person as an end in herself and never as a means only. All parenthood exists as a balance between fulfillment of parental hopes and values and the individual flowering of the actual child in his or her own direction. . . . Parental practices which close exits virtually forever are insufficiently attentive to the child as an end in herself. By closing off the child's right to an open future, they make the child an entity who exists to fulfill parental hopes and dreams, not his own. (Davis 1997, 551)

Although Davis's arguments are directed against the practice of genetic diminishment (making a normal child less than normal), we may nonetheless ask whether her arguments would also apply to making a normal or less than normal child more than normal. For example, parents might want their child to be a musical genius like Mozart, or a basketball player like Michael Jordan, or a Nobel Prize–winner like Albert Einstein. Intuitively, it seems that an extraordinarily enhanced child would have a very open future. Normal children cannot write operas so beautiful that people shed tears, nor can they jump high enough and quickly enough to win one basketball competition after another, nor can they solve physics problems that literally change the way we think. In other words, highly talented children seem to have more opportunities and richer experiences than less talented children have.

Still, there are ways in which more than normal children may have fewer doors open to them than normal children have. People like Mozart, driven to write one opera after another, do not get to have a full family life; they are under enormous pressure to perform excellently all of the time and cannot contemplate alternative lives for themselves, such as being a medical researcher, a farmer, or a dancer. Moreover, as children and adolescents, they do not get the opportunity to try several paths in life before deciding which one may lead them to human happiness.

Building on Davis's argument, philosopher Margaret Little fears that parents might use genetic therapy to fit their children to societal standards of perfection. She believes these reigning norms are a largely media-driven set of criteria for human value that generally reflect some of the worst features of an unjust society that remains racist, sexist, homophobic, ableist, ageist, and so on. For example, consider African American parents who might request geneticists to give their children light skin or Caucasian parents who might request thin bodies, blue eyes, and blond hair for their daughters. Little regards such requests as morally suspect because "the norms of appearance at issue are grounded in or get life from a broader system of attitudes and actions that are in fact unjust" (1999, 161). In other words, for African Americans to want their children to be white skinned rather than black skinned is probably not "some aesthetic whimsical preference" (1999, 161) but instead a reflection of a racist history in which being black is devalued and being white is valorized. Similarly, for parents who want their daughters to look like fashion models or movie stars, this is probably not some idiosyncratic choice, either. More likely, the request is a reflection of a sexist history in which obese women or otherwise physically unattractive women are penalized economically and emotionally and thin and physically attractive women are rewarded with good jobs and good mates (Tong 2007, 206).

Rather than welcoming and encouraging diversity and change, many enhancement choices would, in Little's estimation, aim instead for homogeneity and the further ossification of an unjust status quo. The line of reasoning behind Little's thinking has come under fire, however. Her critics claim that many people are more likely to disobey societal norms than to obey them. For example, white parents might want a child who looks multiracial, or a quirky couple may want a gray-haired daughter who is chubby. Or, as Davis points out above, they may want a child just like them with the same flaws and narrow range of talents they have. In other words, Americans' obsession with individuality and, to some extent, idiosyncrasy may shape their efforts to create what they think is basically a "perfect," absolutely unique baby. Although it is hard to prove whether Little or her critics are right, chances are that Little has the advantage in the debate since most people try to conform to social norms overall. Rebellious phases in life are generally short-lived.

PARENTAL DUTY TO PROCREATE A "PERFECT" BABY

Perhaps the greatest concern some people have about genetic testing and screening is that it may lead to a program of eugenics aimed to eliminate so-called unfit people by permitting only "fit" people to be produced. Many healthcare ethicists and practitioners fear that the new *genomics* will make the same mistakes that the old *eugenics* made during the first half of the twentieth century. The eugenics programs that thrived in the United States from about 1890 to 1940, for example, grew in response to several misguided assumptions, including the assumption that the population of "unfit" people was growing at far faster rates than the population of fit people and the assumption that social woes and economic woes such as poverty, criminality, alcoholism, and prostitution were inheritable genetic traits (Kevles 1995, 766).

In *The Black Stork: Eugenics and the Death of "Defective" Babies in American Medicine and Motion Pictures since 1915*, Martin S. Pernick tells the tale of Dr. Harry J. Haiselden, who in late 1915 examined a baby boy born with multiple "deformities" in a Chicago hospital. Even though life-saving surgery was available, Haiselden withheld it, publicly admitting that he routinely withheld treatment from infants he and other "progressive" minds regarded as "defective" (1995, 12–13). Although other physicians practiced infant euthanasia behind closed doors, Haiselden was the first physician to expose his "letting die" policy openly to the general public. He displayed dying infants with defects to reporters, wrote articles on eugenics for a leading Chicago newspaper, gave talks on "eugenic euthanasia," and wrote, produced, and performed in a feature-length motion picture, *The Black Stork* (Wharton and Wharton 1917). The film was screened in American theaters under a variety of titles from 1916 through the early 1940s. Thousands of people attended it and agreed with its message, namely, that infants with severe disabilities should be left to die (Pernick 1995, 150–158).

Advertised as a "eugenic love story" (Pernick 1995, 10), *The Black Stork*, summarized by Pernick, stars Dr. Haiselden as Dr. Dickey and contrasts the lives of two couples: Claude and Anne and Miriam and Tom. Claude has a mysterious genetic disease, the result of his grandfather's affair with an African American slave. Despite a "stern warning" (Pernick 1995, 144) from Dr. Dickey, Claude marries

Anne, the love of his life, with the intention of having children. In contrast, Miriam, who thinks her mother suffered from hereditary epilepsy, refuses to marry her boyfriend, Tom. She fears having a baby with epilepsy. The product of Claude and Anne's marriage is a baby with serious defects who will die without an operation. Dr. Dickey refuses to operate on the baby, stating that "there are times when saving a life is a greater crime than taking one" (Pernick 1995, 144). His decision not to treat the baby aggressively results in a sharp argument with two representatives of the local medical society who think he should operate. They wear "old-fashioned frock morning coats" (Pernick 1995, 144), whereas Dr. Dickey wears a stylish suit to symbolize his progressive, forward-looking thinking, according to Pernick.

Unlike Dr. Dickey, Anne is conflicted about letting her baby die and wonders whether she should get another physician to save her baby. Her question is answered in a premonition from God, says Pernick. If her baby survives, he will experience a childhood filled with "misery and rejection" and an adult life of "poverty and crime" (Pernick 1995, 144). Anne also envisions her defective son transmitting his bad genes to several defective offspring, contributing little if anything to the commonweal. Finally, Anne sees her defective son snapping and killing the physician, who had, by operating on him, "condemned [him] to life" (Pernick 1995, 144). Scared by this awful premonition, Anne obediently follows Dr. Dickey's recommendation. Her baby dies, and his soul ascends to heaven where Jesus awaits him. Even better, says Pernick, the U.S. Congress passes "a national premarital inspection law" (Pernick 1995, 144). Meanwhile, Miriam is rewarded for her noble decision not to marry her true love, Tom, on the basis of her supposed bad genes. She discovers, however, that the woman whom she thought was her biological mother was really her genetically unrelated stepmother. Realizing her genes are "good" after all, Miriam marries Tom. In no matter of time, they have a very healthy baby, every bit as cute as the smiling Gerber baby.

The twofold moral of *The Black Stork* is obvious, according to Pernick: do not reproduce if you know you have bad genes, for you will produce a defective child, and if you do reproduce and have a defective child, let that child die. It is the most compassionate thing to do. Interestingly, mainstream Americans were not upset by *The Black Stork*. On the contrary, they affirmed its message, espousing many of the doctrines of eugenics according to which it was "good" to produce healthy babies with superior genes—that is, the kind of genes that came on ships such as the *Mayflower*—and "bad" to produce defective babies with inferior genes—that is, the kind of genes that came to America on slave ships from Africa or steamers from Central, Eastern, and Mediterranean Europe.

Toward the beginning of the eugenics movement in the United States, Supreme Court Justice Oliver Wendell Holmes ruled in *Buck v. Bell* (1927) that "three generations of imbeciles is enough." Holmes believed that Carrie Buck was a feebleminded white woman who was the daughter of a feebleminded mother and herself the mother of an illegitimate feebleminded daughter. The grandmother and mother lived in the State Colony for Epileptics and Feeble Minded in Virginia, and the daughter was adopted by her foster parents. In the 1920s, *feeblemindedness* was a catchall label that included not only people with low IQs but also poor people, illiterate people, people who depended on state support, prostitutes, promiscuous women, and so forth. In other words, *feeblemindedness* was often synonymous with being a member of a marginalized or stigmatized minority. Between 1924 and 1979, the state felt free to sterilize thousands of "feebleminded" American men and women for the good of society. In this respect, Holmes's words about the justifiability of involuntary sterilization merit a lengthy citation:

We have seen more than once that the public welfare may call upon the best citizens for their lives. It would be strange if it could not call upon those who already sap the strength of the State for these lesser sacrifices, often not felt to be such by those concerned, in order to prevent our being swamped with incompetence. It is better for all the world if, instead of waiting to execute degenerate offspring for crime or to let them starve for their imbecility, society can prevent those who are manifestly unfit from continuing their kind. The principle that sustains compulsory vaccination is broad enough to cover cutting the Fallopian tubes. (*Buck v. Bell* 1927)

Sadly, Holmes's words were not really applicable to the Buck women. As it turns out, they were not "feebleminded." Evidence shows that the two women and little girl were at least of average intelligence. According to Andrea Pitzer, "Carrie Buck had been passed each year with 'very good' marks in deportment and lessons. Vivian had made the honor roll. There was nothing to suggest any mental deficiency in either of them" (2009).

Significantly, the popularity of the U.S. eugenics movement began to decrease in the early 1940s, as the horrors of Germany under Hitler were revealed. Under the Nazis, Germany used the ideas of eugenics, some of which it had borrowed from America, to justify its atrocities against humanity and particularly the Jews. By 1945, very few Americans wanted to be linked to the likes of "fit" Aryans who pushed Jewish people into gas chambers, lethally injected "useless eaters," and involuntarily sterilized countless men and women for reasons even more dubious than the reason of "feeblemindedness" (Tong 2007, 193).

Because of the ways in which people misunderstood and misapplied genetic information in the past, we should have worries about the new genomics. Is the new genomics really less problematic than the old eugenics was? We seek to reassure ourselves that our worries are probably unnecessary, and we reason that, compared to the kind of pseudoscience that produced eugenics, the kind of science that guides the new genomics in general is bona fide science (Juengst 1991, 71). Today's geneticists seem intent on improving humankind's health status, irrespective of individuals' race, gender, ethnicity, or wealth. They do not seem driven by the desire to eliminate certain groups of people. In fact, geneticists would be horrified if their work were used by governments intent on genocide, the expungement of certain people from humankind. The old eugenics was about eliminating "unfit" people and reproducing "fit" people. It was a mean-spirited, arrogant, and wrongheaded movement. Social prejudices fueled the fires of the old eugenics. In contrast, the new genomics seems to be about voluntarily procreating healthy and happy offspring (Tong 2007, 193).

In the ideal, the new genomics is the implementation of views expressed by Marge Piercy in her 1976 science fiction novel, *Woman on the Edge of Time*. Piercy sketches the outlines of a futuristic, genetically savvy society that has opted to breed for diversity instead of uniformity. One of the main characters in the novel explains that the Grand Council had decided

to breed a high proportion of darker-skinned people and to mix the genes well through the population. At the same time, we decided to hold on to separate cultural identities. But we broke the bond between genes and culture, broke it forever. We want there to be no chance of racism again. But we don't want the melting pot where everybody ends up with thin gruel. We want diversity, for strangeness breeds richness. (103–104)

Thus, in Piercy's futuristic society, there are "black Irishmen and black Jews and black Italians and black Chinese" (104). There is even a tribe call "Harlem-Black" (103). Everyone is permitted to change cultures or racial and other identities whenever they feel a switch is in order. Moreover, people do not overly value their genetic links to their families; rather, they treasure their emotional connections to those people dearest to them. In addition, men as well as women are mothers. Comments one character in the novel:

It was part of women's long revolution. When we were breaking all the old hierarchies. Finally there was that one thing we had to give up too, the only power we ever had, in return for no more power for anyone. The original production: the power to give birth. Cause as long as we were biologically enchained, we'd never be equal. And males never would be humanized to be loving and tender. So we all became mothers. Every child has three. To break the nuclear bonding. (105)

As appealing as the ideal of the new genomics is, when it falls short of that ideal, it reveals some ugly spots. For example, consider the large number of men in China where there is an extraordinary preference for sons. In 2009, there were thirty-two million more Chinese men under twenty than Chinese women (LaFraniere 2009). This situation leaves many Chinese men single. Involuntary bachelors often turn to prostitutes or even steal young girls to be their brides (Bureau of Democracy, Human Rights, and Labor 2008). There is also concern that a society with a dramatic sex ratio favoring men is more likely to be aggressive and bellicose. At present, the Chinese government is recruiting men for public work projects, the military, or the police in order to structure single men's lives so that they do not turn their unharnessed energies to destructive activities (Tanner 2005).

Supporters of sex selection claim that, although the practice may be harmful in countries like China where almost everyone wants boys, it should not be considered harmful in countries like the United States where blatant gender discrimination against women is not a major issue. Specifically, the majority of Americans want both girls and boys so as to constitute a family in which parents and children can enjoy the traits and behaviors associated with both sexes. Still, a minority of Americans want an all-girl family or an all-boy family. An all-girl family may be preferred by a single mother who thinks that girls are easier to raise than boys. Similarly, an all-boy family may be preferred by a gay couple who think it would be easier for them to raise boys instead of girls.

Genomics enthusiasts often claim that the aim of reproductive genetic testing and screening is simply to inform prospective parents about the genetic health status of their future child, not to prompt prospective parents to eliminate so-called defective fetuses. In point of fact, however, a high percentage of parents do choose to abort their fetuses if they test positive for a serious genetic disease like Tay-Sachs disease (Mahowald 1997, 144). They certainly do not request that the embryo be inserted into the woman's uterus subsequent to pre-implantation genetic diagnosis. Moreover, a high percentage of couples abort fetuses with Down's syndrome, despite the fact that people with Down syndrome generally lead meaningful and happy lives (McGuire 2005). Adding to the ambiguity of the situation are studies such as one reported by lawyer Lori B. Andrews that asked young American adults about their interest in prenatal genetic diagnosis for a number of behavioral attributes and psychiatric conditions. Under the assumption that curative gene therapies were not available, almost 80 percent thought prenatal testing acceptable for alcoholism, 65 percent for obesity, 70 percent for attention deficit and hyperactivity disorder, 27 percent for homosexuality, 25 percent for short stature, and 18 percent for the absence of perfect musical pitch (Andrews 1999, 154). In a similar vein, a very recent British study found that even higher percentages of couples would abort their fetus if it has club feet, an extra digit, or cleft palate, yet all of these conditions are very treatable ("Babies Aborted for Not Being Perfect," 2006).

Given the outcomes of studies like these we can expect to find ourselves increasingly torn between two lines of diametrically opposed reasoning with respect to procreating children with genetic diseases and disorders. Proponents of not procreating defective children will insist that it is emotionally draining and economically costly to bring such children into the world, especially if they have a serious genetic disease or disorder; furthermore, they will argue that it is not in the best interests of a child to bring it into the world for a life full of pain and suffering. Comments philosopher Laura Purdy:

When I look into my heart to see what it says about this matter I see, I admit, emotions I would rather not feel—reluctance to face the burdens society must bear, unease in the presence of some disabled persons. But most of all, what I see there are the demands of love: to love someone is to care desperately about their welfare and to want for them only *good* things. The thought that I might bring to life a child with serious mental problems when I could, by doing something different, bring forth one without them, is utterly incomprehensible to me. (1996, 58)

In contrast to Purdy, those who oppose her line of reasoning stress that the concept of "normality" is a moving target. For example, Andrews claims that, as genetic testing "becomes routinized for minor as well as major disorders" (1999, 162), our understanding of what is normal will become exceedingly high. As I stated above, in the film *Gattaca*, people who are not healthy, beautiful, and smart are confined to lowly occupations and a generally unfulfilling lifestyle. Vincent's relationship with his parents is ruptured because he has dreams of becoming someone better than they think he is. Vincent may think his parents failed him by giving into passion and not genetically engineering him as they did in the case of his younger brother. However, if his parents had used genetic technology to have their first child, Vincent would not have been born; instead, another, "better" child would have been born. The question then becomes whether Vincent would prefer nonexistence to the life he has.

Like others who wish to slow the march toward what they view as genetic perfectionism, Andrews is particularly concerned that, increasingly, pregnant women may feel they have not simply a right to test their fetus for genetic disorders and diseases, mild as well as serious, but also a *duty* to do so and to consider seriously aborting their fetuses, should they prove to be less than completely normal. Many people claim that it is not fair to a child to bring it into the world if it is defective. Moreover, some people claim that it is simply "irresponsible and immoral" (Andrews 1999, 134) to knowingly give birth to a defective child, especially if one does not have the time and funds to pay for the child's care. They say it is not fair for these parents to ask the state to pick up the bills for a child society thinks they should not have had.

In view of these last considerations, disability rights advocate and bioethicist Adrienne Asch advises pregnant women to withstand perfectionists' pressure tactics and decide for themselves whether they want to abort a fetus that *perfectionists* find lacking. Asch claims that if it is wrong to abort a fetus solely because it is a female, then it is also wrong to abort a fetus solely because it has the gene for Down's syndrome, spina bifida, cystic fibrosis, or muscular dystrophy (four genetic diseases that do not usually prevent those who have them from leading meaningful lives). Ableism is no less wrong than sexism in Asch's opinion (1995, 386–387; Tong 2007, 195).

Considerations about the right to have the best possible baby as well as the duty to terminate a pregnancy that will result in less than a normal baby play a great role in so-called wrongful-birth and wrongful-life civil suits. In a wrongful-life suit, the child claims that it would have been better not to be born than to live with his affliction. In a wrongful-birth suit, parents claim they were wronged when health-care practitioners failed to provide enough accurate and timely information to empower them to avoid the conception or birth of a defective child. On the whole, courts are more receptive to wrongful-birth cases because it is easier to assess damages, especially economic damages. For example, Weil recalls a case where geneticists' failure to tell a pregnant woman that her age (over thirty-five) put her unborn child at risk for Down syndrome. When she gave birth to a child with Down syndrome, the court could calculate in monetary terms the medical costs of rearing and maintaining a child with Down syndrome, but the court could not calculate in dollar terms the emotional costs of parenting a child with Down syndrome. Perhaps the joys of parenting the child far outweigh the sorrows and hardships of doing so. This last consideration helps explain courts' near rejection of wrongful life suits where it is nearly "impossible to weigh suffering versus nonexistence" (Weil 2006b).

REFLECTIONS ON MEDICINE

Aware of court cases like the ones above, practitioners of in vitro fertilization, especially those who work in tandem with geneticists, try to give couples as much information as they need to proceed confidently and knowledgably with a pregnancy.

Many geneticists and genetic counselors emphasize that couples' views about the seriousness of genetic diseases vary in many ways. They also point out that if a woman wants to exercise her right to have an abortion in the first trimester of her pregnancy, it matters not to the law whether she does so because her healthy fetus is female, or because she and her husband do not have the means to rear a child, or because her fetus has tested positive for Tay-Sachs disease. Finally, they reason that if one group of healthcare practitioners prevents prospective parents from learning everything they want to know about the genetic status of their child, the prospective parents will simply turn to another group of healthcare practitioners or even the Internet for more information. Better, they say, for prospective parents to be counseled properly and advised by conscientious geneticists and genetic counselors than to leave them to the vagaries of individuals eager to simply make money off of them.

Because many healthcare practitioners are increasingly inclined to give as much genetic information about a fetus to its procreators as possible, critics fear that healthcare practitioners will soon become employees of the "designer child" industry. Critics also fear that medicine will no longer be a practice with ends or aims of its own. Instead, it will be little more than a set of instrumental means that physicians can use to attain whatever ends their patients may want. Thus, physicians and other healthcare practitioners may simply become technicians who exist to please their customers or clients, taking from them whatever amount of money they are willing to pay.

We see evidence of this instrumental view of medicine in some infertility practices and, to a great extent, in cosmetic surgery practices. Who has not heard of Octomom or the sixty-six-year-old Romanian woman who had a child? Nadya Suleman, Octomom, had used in vitro fertilization (IVF) to conceive some of her six children. She then requested that all six of her remaining frozen embryos be inserted into her uterus. Her physician, Dr. Kamrava, obliged despite the prevailing assisted-reproduction norm about implanting only two or at most three embryos in a woman of Suleman's age. After the six embryos were implanted, two of them split into twins, making for a total of eight embryos. In June 2011, a California Medical Board investigation found that Dr. Kamrava had been practicing IVF in an irresponsible manner. He had gone so far as to once implant twelve embryos in a woman. Because of his worrisome track record, the board voted to revoke Dr. Kamrava's medical license in 2011; his manner of doing IVF was viewed as an "extreme" departure from the standard of care (see "Nadya Suleman" 2011).

There has been much controversy about Suleman's decision to have octuplets. Many expressed concern that her decision for more children would burden taxpayers with huge medical bills (most of the octuplets were born very low weight or with some medical problem or another). Raising a total of fourteen children is very expensive, and Suleman had already been on disability for a back injury ("Nadya Suleman" 2011). Others supported Suleman, arguing that if a woman had eight embryos naturally, no one would force her to undergo selective reduction for the common good. They claimed that Suleman had a right to bear as many children as she wanted so long as she was willing to rear them in a caring fashion.

Although most of her children do have medical problems, none of them is devastatingly diseased or defective ("Nadya Suleman" 2011).

No less controversial than willfully having a multi-fetal pregnancy is postmenopausal women using IVF to get pregnant. Adriana Iliescu, a Romanian professor, was sixty-six years old when she used IVF with donor egg and donor sperm. Iliescu had spent her younger years focused on her career, so much so that she had no time for a baby. When she received her doctorate, IVF was still not available for women like her, but as soon as it became available in Romania for older women, she entered an IVF program. Doctors used medications to get her womb properly functioning, and in 2005 Iliescu gave birth to a 3.9-pound daughter, the sole survivor of a triplet pregnancy. She named the baby Eliza and is caring for her alone. Iliescu is not bothered by people who think she is Eliza's grandmother, and she has told her daughter that although she has no rearing father, people love her very much. Interestingly, Iliescu's infertility specialist, Dr. Marinescu, will serve as Eliza's guardian if Iliescu dies before Eliza reaches adulthood (Weathers 2010).

As might be predicted in the United States, a culturally and politically diverse society, the public is divided about postmenopausal pregnancies. There are those who insist that if a postmenopausal woman wants to get pregnant and physicians have the means to help her, they should help her, even if the health risks of extending such help are high. She, not they, should decide whether the health risks of IVF treatment do or do not outweigh the overall benefits to her. In contrast, others do not support IVF for postmenopausal women, arguing that it is irresponsible for a woman in her fifties or sixties to undertake a high-risk pregnancy that may result in serious harm to her. If she does give birth a child, she will be in her late seventies or early eighties when her child graduates from high school. Should that child, they ask, be expected to care for her elderly parent if she gets Alzheimer's disease, for example? As compelling as this last point may be to some, proponents of postmenopausal IVF respond that nowadays many people live not only longer but also healthier lives and that many grandparents rear their young grandchildren successfully (Department for Children and Families, Region IV 2009). They also stress that, if it is socially permissible for men to "father" children in their sixties, seventies, and even eighties, then it should be socially permissible for women of the same age to "mother" a child. Comments Robert Edwards, one of the founders of in vitro fertilization: "If a man of 60 fathers a baby, then we buy him a drink and toast his health at a pub. But it is totally different with a woman of the same age" (Hewitt 1994). To refuse to help infertile older women get pregnant simply because they are older may be a sexist response to a group of women's legitimate treatment needs (Appel 2009).

The notion that medicine is simply an instrumental means to serve people's desires is also present in cultural phenomena such as the human Barbie doll, and Orlan, a French artist, who engages in carnal art. Some women are so taken with Barbie that they employ cosmetic surgeons to give them a Barbie-like face and body for as much as $800,000 (Arthurs 2011). This is no easy or painless task, for Barbie's proportional measurements have been estimated at thirty-six inches (chest), eighteen inches (waist) and thirty-three inches (hips). Moreover, scaled from doll to human size, Barbie would be five feet nine inches and would weigh an anorexic 110 pounds. Yet some young girls and even older women would do anything to resemble Barbie, even though her figure is an unrealistic, even harmful ideal. Interestingly, Sarah Burge, the "Human Barbie," thanks to numerous cosmetic surgeries, recently gave her seven-year-old daughter a £6,000 voucher for "boob implants." The daughter, who was celebrating her birthday, said: "I wanted a new computer, a holiday and a voucher for surgery. When I got it all, it was a dream come true. I can't wait to be like Mummy with big boobs. They're pretty" (Arthurs 2011).

Even more controversial than the Human Barbie is Orlan, the French artist, who uses her body as a "painting" canvas. One of her most famous projects is a series of cosmetic surgeries called *The Reincarnation of Saint-Orlan*. In this series, Orlan uses her body to become the ideal of female beauty as constructed by the male gaze and aesthetics. Among the new features on her face, Orlan has the chin of Botticelli's Venus, the nose of Gérôme's Psyche, the lips of Boucher's Europa, the eyes of the goddess Diana, and the forehead of Da Vinci's Mona Lisa (Pescarmon 2003). Most recently, Orlan has had cosmetic surgeons put two bumps on her temples that look like small horns or "nascent antlers" (Jeffries 2009). Using the operating room as a stage, Orlan wears sexually provocative clothes, while her surgeons are dressed in designer gowns. She is conscious throughout the surgeries but not in pain. Most controversially, the surgeries are videotaped and sometimes broadcast live to audiences around the world. Orlan then sells the bodily materials extracted from her surgeries as relics of her flesh. She views her work not as body art—which can be quite violent and masochistic, as when Chris Burden "had himself nailed through the hands to a VW Beetle" (Jeffries 2009)—but as *carnal art*. Carnal art is about "pleasure and sensuality," according to Orlan, who also views it as "feminist." She uses her body not to conform to traditional Western views of the female body or the pornographic gaze of men but to comment on male constructions of female beauty and to create the kind of idiosyncratic face she wants (Jeffries 2009). She has plans to get a bioreactor "to culture her cells among those of other humans and animals" (Jeffries 2009) and says she is against God, religion, and nature but absolutely in favor of women.

Is Orlan where American medicine is headed? Should American medicine simply meet the American mind and do its bidding in the cause of life, liberty, and pursuit of happiness? Is it hopelessly old school to think that medicine is more than a set of skills that can be taught, bought, and sold any which way for the right price? Is it totally unfair to think that, to the degree that medicine has helped create the enhancement-obsessed American mind, it is guilty of betraying its Hippocratic oath?

The point of grouping together Octomom, Adriana Iliescu, the Human Barbie, and Orlan is that each woman is using her body to serve her own interests, however idiosyncratic and potentially harmful they may be to self or others. The Octomom case is worrisome because multi-fetal births often threaten the woman's health and the medical condition of her newborns. For example, the strain on the woman's heart can be considerable, and bed rest may need to be prescribed (American College of Obstetricians and Gynecologists 2004). In addition, it is hard to care for multiples who are at increased risk for low birth weight, premature delivery, and disability (Roberts 2006, 776–792). Many couples' marriages dissolve because of the wear and tear caused by continuously having to do diaper or feeding duty, to say nothing of paying all the child care and physician bills.

The Adriana Iliescu case is problematic for all the reasons given above and for the additional reason that now at age seventy-two, she is courting the idea of having another child (Weathers 2010). Should her desire trump the psychological well-being of a young child who knows her mother may die before she goes to high school? Although some single mothers die when they are still young, they do not deliberately have a child who will almost surely be an orphan. In contrast, Iliescu realized that she might be dead before her child graduated high school or reached maturity, and she arranged for her physician to rear her daughter if necessary. However, the physician would have to legally adopt the daughter.

The Human Barbie and Orlan cases are particularly worrisome because each time these women submit to elective cosmetic surgery, they compromise their bodies not for health purposes but for very idiosyncratic purposes. Very problematic are the healthcare practitioners who enable these women to achieve their goals. Although the physician who helped Octomom ultimately lost his medical license, other physicians like him continue to practice reproductive medicine irresponsibly. Some of these physicians try to justify their actions on the grounds of patient autonomy, that if a woman knows the health risks of repeated elective cosmetic surgeries and she is competent, then physicians should do her bidding. Others merely excuse their work on the grounds that, if they do not do as patients request, the patients will simply take their wallets to another group of cosmetic surgeons willing to give them the bodies they want. Think here of the patients who go to Mexico or other countries for inexpensive cosmetic surgery, many of whom come home displeased or damaged by the physicians who worked on them. Comments Steven Victor, a cosmetic dermatologist in New York: "We need to regulate this kind of activity better and educate the public. We've been seeing this for years. We've seen faces, lips, breasts, and buttocks injected with unknown substances. In one case, a woman came into my office after she had her lips injected with an unknown substance, which turned out to be a peanut oil mixture. We had to surgically remove it" (Yancey 2011).

RETURN TO *GATTACA*

With respect to bodywork, especially bodywork on potential or actual children, several issues need to be examined closely. The first issue is maintaining "open future(s)" for one's progeny. Davis's arguments about letting children decide who they want to be is hammered home in *Gattaca*. By failing to give Vincent the best of their genes, his parents seem to close doors for him. He is myopic, so jobs that require 20/20 vision are out of the question for him; he has a weak heart, so heavy-duty exercise and athletics are not an option for him. The only work he qualifies for is light cleaning of facilities, ironically including the building where present and future astronauts live. Vincent's brother is a different case, however. Apparently disappointed with their first son, Vincent's parents use their best genes to produce their second child, Anton Jr. He has many more doors open for him, but despite the fact that he has been genetically engineered, Anton is not among the very best and brightest characters in the film. After all, his *parents'* egg and sperm were used and, therefore, Anton Jr. is limited by the limitations of his parents' gametes. If his parents had wanted an even better child, they would have had to use donor egg and donor sperm from the genetic material of two of the best and brightest people available. And although Anton Jr. becomes a professional police investigator—a respectable job, but nothing extraordinary—it is Vincent, despite all of his genetic imperfections, who achieves his dream of becoming someone extraordinary, an astronaut.

The second issue to examine is the motivation behind wanting a "perfect" child. Clearly by the time they wanted a second child, Vincent's parents were motivated to make a "better baby." No mention is made of how much they needed to pay to have Anton Jr. genetically engineered, but as they are depicted as people of modest means, Vincent and Anton's parents likely spent their life savings to make sure their second child would not suffer the fate of their first child. Similarly, people of modest means are spending their limited funds on expensive cosmetic surgeries or on high-priced infertility treatments like IVF. Neither money nor their own well-being seem to be a matter of concern in pursuit of a perfect body or a perfect baby.

No wonder, then, that concerns about justice occupy Maxwell Mehlman and Jeffrey Botkin in their analysis of both somatic cell and germ-line gene therapy, an analysis that could be easily applied to elective cosmetic surgery and assisted-reproduction services. As Mehlman and Botkin argue, gene therapy would be accessible only to those individuals who have adequate insurance coverage or who can raise the money to pay for it out of pocket. They speculate that, as a result of this state of affairs, society would gradually separate into two classes, a "genetic aristocracy" and a "genetic underclass," and comment that the former group

> would be virtually free of inherited disorders, would receive powerful genetic therapies for acquired diseases, and would be engineered with superior physical and mental abilities; [and that the latter group] would continue to suffer from genetic illnesses and would have to content itself with less effective, conventional medical treatments. Its members would be able to improve the mental and physical traits only through comparatively laborious traditional methods of self-improvement. (Mehlman and Botkin 1998, 99)

As bad as the consequences of this divide would be for the individuals in the genetic underclass, Mehlman and Botkin think its worse consequence would be the disintegration of democratic society as a whole. As they see it, a genetically stratified society would undermine the American concept of social equality in a threefold way. First, it would increase actual inequality by enabling genetically privileged people to secure greater genetic health and talent than genetically unprivileged people. Second, a genetically stratified society would erode the belief in equality of opportunity by enabling genetically privileged people to pass on their best and brightest genes to succeeding generations. Finally, it would destroy the hope for social mobility in the genetic underclass by making it increasingly difficult for them to improve their lot in life (Mehlman and Botkin 1998).

The third issue to examine is the role of physicians and other healthcare practitioners in the construction of perfect babies and perfect bodies. In *Gattaca*, parents use physicians to get perfect babies, and, increasingly, in the real world, at least some infertile people in IVF programs are doing the same. It seems like only a matter of time before people—fertile or infertile—will have the option (costly though it may be) of designing their own children. Similarly, in the real world, all sorts of people are using physicians to get the body of their socially determined or idiosyncratic dreams. But why use physicians for this task? Presumably, concepts like "healing" and the physician-patient relationship are becoming obsolete. All we postmodern folks seem to need are technicians willing to do our bidding for the right price, of course. No matter where we look, we see people using clothes, tattoos, hair extensions, cosmetic surgery, and gene selection either to conform to social standards or rebel against them as much as they can. Our bodies have indeed become ourselves. But one wonders whether bodywork is really making people, especially women, happy. Bodywork is good as far as it goes, but if we want to be more perfect people, mind work is also essential. Rather than only focus on how we look to ourselves and others, we also need to focus on who we are for ourselves and others. Whether we use the mind or the body in our quest to be perfect, we cannot really escape the limits that make us human. In the end, we must all still must die. Nature—whatever the word may signify—still sets limits on us, reminding us that our autonomy is not absolute.

ACKNOWLEDGMENTS

Some sections of this chapter are excerpted, revised, or reorganized versions of pages 193–194 and 204–207 in Rosemarie Tong, *New Perspectives in Healthcare Ethics: An Interdisciplinary and Crosscultural Approach*, 1st edition, © 2007 (Upper Saddle River, NJ: Prentice-Hall, 2007). Reprinted by permission of Pearson Education, Inc.

Chapter 16

SEEING BODIES IN PAIN

SANDER L. GILMAN

WHY DO WE CARE ABOUT MEDICAL IMAGES?

Why is it important for students of the medical/health humanities to learn about how we imagine bodies? Isn't medicine about real bodies, not merely about pictures of bodies? Of course medical practice engages with real bodies, yet the pictures or representations of bodies that we conjure up in our minds influences our experience of the real bodies (including our own) that we come upon in life. One of the cornerstones of the humanities is that the study of the body, its processes and illnesses, is pervasively affected by our own cultural presuppositions about bodies. The study of representations of the body, therefore, is linked to ideas of health and illness in direct and unmistakable ways, up to and including diagnosis and treatment.

Many studies within the field of the medical/health humanities focus on the ill body and its representation through actual images (visual or verbal, real or imagined), as well as the ways that such images are given meaning. For example, W.J.T. Mitchell observed in the 1990s that "representation (in memory, in verbal descriptions, in images) not only 'mediates' our knowledge (of slavery and of many other things), but obstructs, fragments, and negates that knowledge" (1994, 188). For him representations are *not* merely "objects representing" but an index (in the sense of C. S. Peirce) of the means by which representations are produced and received. Thus they may reflect the reality of an audience's expectation; may be shaped by the ideological context in which they are generated or received; may reflect individual, cultural, or disciplinary idiosyncratic understanding; and/or may be an artifact of the technology that generates the image of the body. In other words, they are never simply unmediated.

Such a broad and subjective conception of representation comes into direct conflict with the medical sciences that claim to represent the body objectively through brain imaging and the neurosciences or evolutionary biology or psychology, approaches that offer a single, unambiguous pathway without much attention to who sees and what is claimed to be seen. Medical science presupposes that representations within the practice of health care have to be mimetic. Representing the world, therefore, is a function of training to see accurately rather than an artifact of perception. When you look at an X-ray, the image represents a real body, and its meaning is fixed no matter who looks at the X-ray, although the actual practice in medicine seems to undermine such one-to-one interpretive claims: there is a constant, ongoing correction of the reading attached to such images both in the moment and over time.

SEEING IMAGES CAN ALSO MEAN SEEING PAIN

A critical space, a fundamental conflict, exists between representational theories in the humanities and those in the medical sciences. Today's new functionalism in science stresses the "real" aspects of representing the body in ways questioned by the very premises of theories about representation in the humanities. Medical images claim to mirror aspects of the body, whether imaged externally by photographs or internally by X-rays or fMRIs, and thus they claim to represent bodies as they actually are. How the study of the body is represented remains an essential part of this debate about the claims of "seeing the body" in medicine and in the humanities. This dichotomy has existed, at least in Western thought, from the ancient world. Michel Foucault, in *The Order of Things* ([1966] 1994), argued that the classical world saw representation as tied to experience and that only in modernity (which for him begins in the seventeenth century) was there the growing assumption that representations follow, in complex ways, their own rules and may or may not have any relationship to the experienced world. In other words, these rules that define the episteme change over time and from system to system of representation. "Pain" is a litmus test for such claims about how we imagine what we are seeing when we see the body. David Morris argues, following Foucault, that medicine by the eighteenth century stressed the interiority of pain in a "new way of seeing and of speaking" about pain (1993, 226). Yet the claim was one that was understood as coming from an empirical point of view. There was a way of understanding the interior process of the body in an objective manner, though the clinical gaze.

Certainly the problem of "seeing the body" is one that haunts medicine beginning with the Greeks. Greek medicine looks at the body, correlates the signs and symptoms found there and their expression, with pathologies within the body. The physician Hippocrates (or at least the Hippocratic corpus) states that one must both ask the patient about his or her status as well as observe the patient's body. What is learned is the basis for all diagnosis:

> When you examine the patient, inquire into all particulars; first how the head is . . . then examine if the hypochondrium and sides be free of pain, for . . . if there be pain in the side, and along with the pain either cough, tormina or bellyache, the bowels should be opened with clysters. . . . The physician should ascertain whether the patient be apt to faint when he is raised up, and whether his breathing is free; and examine the discharges from the bowels. . . . Attention should also be paid to the hands . . . and observe the nostrils . . . if the tongue be rough, and if there be swoonings, it is likely to be a remission of fever. (Porter 1997, 61)

There is no question that observing, including observing the fleeting physiognomy of illness, is the core of differential diagnosis in Greek and then Roman medicine. And so it should be, says modern medicine. We know intuitively what a healthy expression is and thus are attuned to the face of illness. Such awareness captures a wide range of expressions of illness and their manifestations. I wish to focus in this chapter on that human experience of illness evoked by Hippocrates, pain, and its most recent function in the debates about the representation of the body.

A SUBJECTIVE WAY OF SEEING PAIN

One of the most remarkable factors in any medical discussion of pain, at least from the Enlightenment to the present, is the contradictory assumption of its immeasurability coupled with the claim of its innate visibility (Mann 1988; Pernick 1985; Rey 1993; Thernstrom 2010; van Dijkhuizen and Enenkel 2009). Some scholars view scales of pain, by definition, as subjective, especially the self-reporting scales that are now used to measure pain (the Numerical Rating Scale [NRS-11, NRS-101]; the Visual Analog Scale; the Brief Pain Inventory; among others). Pain is inherently subjective, as doctors have stated over the past half century, as evidenced in this editorial from the *Lancet* in 1940:

When the little girl said tearfully to her sister, "My toothache is worse than your toothache" she put her finger on the crux of the matter; for who shall say her nay? Pain is one of the phenomena that defy measurement, so many are the variables. Some will maintain that there is a wealth of diagnostic information contained in terms commonly applied to pain: gnawing, aching, pricking, stabbing, boring, tingling, cutting, shooting, starting, cramping, agonising, oppressive, bearing down, and many others; and the practitioner may never get the help from his scientific colleagues which will enable him to be more precise. ("The Measurement of Pain" 1940, 167)

But the subjectivity of pain is even more recently described as an artifact not only of the patient's comprehension of it but equally of a reflex of those attempting to measure pain through whatever scale applied: "How a physician thinks about pain affects the way in which he or she assesses a patient who presents with pain" (Turk and Okifuji 1999, 1784). Not only is the patient's account of his or her pain subjective but so also is the reception of such an account by the physician. It is evident that character plays a major role in reporting pain. People are, following Richard Riding and Indra Cheema's dichotomy of "cognitive styles," either "levelers" or "sharpeners." Some understate the intensity of their pain for personal, cultural, or perhaps even physiological reasons; others exaggerate it ("This is the WORST pain I've ever had!"). In addition, the context of the questioner/examiner always plays a major role in self-reporting of cognitive style (Riding and Cheema 1991, 202). But few self-reporting scales build this complexity into its evaluation.

Such descriptive representation of pain is not truly measurable even as medical science begins to attempt to measure pain because "progress in measurement has been slow because pain is a complex perceptual experience that can be quantified only indirectly. Since pain has been operationalized in different ways in animal, human laboratory and clinical arenas of investigation the integration of knowledge across studies has been limited. The last decade has witnessed considerable innovation in pain measurement" (Chapman et al. 1985, 2).

David Morton's notion that pain has objective, visual clues in other higher mammals has been dismissed by researchers who find the human/animal analogy of visibility faulty:

[Yet] many of the reflexes measured in animals are not found in man and this makes it difficult to draw strong, clinically relevant conclusions from experimental observations. The jaw opening reflex observed when dogs or cats are subjected to dental stimulation is not seen in the human although an inhibition of jaw closing muscles occurs. No human analogy to the tail flick response can be found, and human withdrawal latency when a hand is placed on a heated plate is vastly different from that of animals. Few investigators would agree with [L.] Vyklicky that the rodent writhing response captures the essence of the human experience of visceral pain. (Chapman et al. 1985, 2)

Animal models are different from human experiences, it is argued, but as is often the case, humans project their own subjective experiences of pain into specific animal responses and see analogies between them and their own expression of pain. One can add here that, given our understanding of "pain, " human beings can experience pain in ways that other mammals cannot in that not all physical pain may have a physical cause—but more about that later.

AN OBJECTIVE WAY OF SEEING PAIN

There are those, however, who claim quite the opposite: that there is a scientific, universal objective expression of pain that can provide access to its quantification in all human beings but even more so in new claims about judging children's pain (observer-rated pain scales such as the FACES Pain Scale—Revised; CRIES Pain Scale for neonatal health care; Coloured Analogue Scale, FLACC Scale). These scientists agree with those who see any sort of self-measurement as difficult, flawed or impossible, as those in pain cannot adequately describe their own experiences:

People in pain convey their distress to others through a remarkably rich variety of expressive actions. These may include verbal report, paralinguistic vocalizations, withdrawal reflexes, palliative behavior, and changes in facial expression. Most systematic descriptions of pain, whether observed in the clinic or in the natural environment, have been devoted to verbal report. Self-report has numerous advantages for pain assessment, including methodological simplicity, apparent direct access to qualities of subjective experience, and evidence of empirical validity, because self-report commonly varies with tissue pathology and is responsive to healing. On the other hand, self-report indexes of pain may often be inadequate. The impact of situational and contextual variables raises doubts concerning the validity of self-report as a direct index of experience. Self-report is subject to voluntary control and hence to faking. In addition, children and many adults do not have the verbal skills needed to convey their distress effectively. Nonverbal expression provides an alternative source of pain information that would be expected to supplement and complement self-report measures for a variety of reasons. There is evidence that the impact of pain displays on others may be mediated by qualities of nonverbal expression. (Craig and Patrick 1985, 1080)

Only the scientist can claim any type of objective assessment of the patient's pain, and that assessment may be used to correct or negate any subjective statements about pain coming from a patient. Patients misconstrue; observers never do.

At the same time, psychologist Paul Ekman and his collaborators in the 1970s (and their FACES [facial expression; awareness; compassion; emotions] project) presented the idea, now a commonplace, that the emotions can be seen and cat-alogued by trained observers through visual expressions. Ekman's core emotions were anger, disgust, fear, happiness, sadness, and surprise; this list was substantially augmented later (Ekman and Friesen 1969, 1971). Pain, too, is to be seen and there-fore measured, even though pain is not one of Ekman's primary states of emotion:

Is there a consistent set of changes that occur in facial expression when pain occurs, regard-less of the nature of the pain involved? . . . [Is it] possible to discriminate spontaneous from deliberate pain expressions on the basis of facial action? . . . Whether the topography of facial behavior changes when people try to suppress or exaggerate the expression of pain. . . . When pain is expressed some four facial actions are likely to occur. The various analyses reported in the study support the assertion that the actions are cohesive, related to pain experience, and may properly be described as a "pain expression." . . . There maybe a universal expression of pain. (Prkachin 2005, 202)

The "face of pain" seems to be an objective reality whatever the motivation of the sufferer and, perhaps, whatever his or her cultural location. Specific actions of the muscles of the face occur with pain, and these are observable, recordable, analyz-able, and irrefutable.

Underlying such claims are the findings of linguistics that other semantic fields in addition to articulated speech are part of the totality of communication. Gesture and expression (facial as well as bodily) are an intrinsic part of communication. This is seen as hardwired in the development of the brain as part of a physiology of expression. In the case of pain, the body speaks more honestly that does the patient, as its communication is understood as unmediated and unmistakable (at least to the trained observer):

The facial expression of pain has recently attracted considerable interest in experimental and clinical research based on an increasing awareness that it supports the communication of pain as a second signal system besides the verbal one. In line with this, facial activity provides the possibility to develop pain assessment tools in individuals with limited abili-ties to communicate pain verbally (e.g. newborns, individuals with pronounced cognitive impairments and dementia). An early and very important observation as regards facial responses associated with pain was that there is a subset of key facial muscle movements that are displayed consistently across different pain modalities. This subset of pain-relevant facial responses includes brow lowering, orbit tightening, levator contraction and eye clo-sure. Although there is convergent evidence that these facial responses constitute the core of the "pain face," there are also other facial muscle movements that have frequently been observed in the context of pain. (Kunz et al. 2009, 273)

The "pain face" can be read, can be the basis for evaluation, and can provide the sort of instrument for representing the body that self-reporting can never be. Indeed, the lines between self-assessment and seeing are often blurred, as in the Wong Baker Faces Pain Scale developed by the pediatric nurses Donna Wong and Connie M. Baker in 1981. Using the Ekman FACES scale for self-assessment, we can assume that patients are not staring at a mirror but rather reporting the way they imagine their pain to look.

EMPATHY AND SEEING PAIN

Yet the dichotomy between immeasurability and perception is not only a feature of the medical literature. The question of immediate response to pain as a philosophical problem of empathy (what Ekman and the Dalai Lama call "compassion") demands the unmediated "seeing" of a subjective category (Dalai Lama and Ekman 2008). Even Elaine Scarry, whose seminal book, *The Body in Pain*, first raised the question of pain as a social phenomenon for the humanist, seems to see pain's perception as unmediated:

If one imagines one human being seeing another human being in pain, one human being perceiving in another discomfort and in the same moment wishing the other to be relieved of the discomfort, something in that fraction of a second is occurring inside the first person's brain involving the complex action of many neurons that is, importantly, not just a perception of actuality (the second person's pain) but an alteration of actuality (for embedded in the perception is the sorrow that it is so, the wish that it were otherwise). (1985, 289)

Pain can—indeed, must—be seen for us to be empathic to those who are in "discomfort."

Those who argue against such reductionism of the act of seeing (even with its concomitant empathy) call for our awareness that seeing is always a form of cultural mediation with so-called display rules developed within any given culture. Psychologists such as Alan J. Fridlund (1994) and James A. Russell (1994) see an absolute link between pure experience of emotions and its physiological expression as unsupportable. They argue, against the theories put forth by Ekman et al., that cultural rules govern how emotions are expressed, but there is no question that they are expressed and that they are always expressed. Thus Russell notes in 1994 that pain is *not* one of the "basic" emotions to which the observers of emotion, such as Ekman, have reduced facial expression:

Facial movements include not just the 7 ± 2 "facial expressions of emotion," but laughs, pouts, yawns, winces, grimaces, and all manner of actions difficult to describe. In our culture, people use facial cues to infer sleepiness, relaxation, puzzlement, confusion, pain, boredom, interest, attention, and other states besides seven "basic" emotions. An understanding of facial expressions would be helped by integrating studies over the full range of facial movements and inferences from them. . . . Rather than ask whether a given culture agrees with one preformulated hypothesis, we might more usefully ask how members of that culture conceptualize emotions and facial behavior. There may be no short cut to obtaining the needed information. Although the task is great, what we know about the peoples of different cultures suggests that carrying it out will be fascinating. (Russell 1994, 141)

But seen pain must be, even if only within the norms of the culture in which it is experienced, since the "black box" of the expression of emotions is hardwired even if their specific expressions may not be.

The nuances of representing the body are determined in this view by the culture, but the body will express a range of emotions even if the expression differs from culture to culture and from time to time. This is an evolutionary fact; only the expression and perception of states such as pain (and its construction from other forms of emotional expression) are culturally determined. This is the view of the work first undertaken by the Dutch phenomenological psychiatrist Henricus Cornelius Rümke in the 1940s on the so-called praecox feeling ([1941] 1990). Experienced mental health professionals who work with the mentally ill are able to see "intuitively" those who suffer from schizophrenia, or so it has been claimed. In doing so, they lose any sense of "empathy" with the patient. What is actually "seen" are the subtle shifts in non-verbal communication in certain manifestations of the schizophrenias. What is learned is that empathic identification with such patients does not elicit any appropriate affective response. After having seen enough patients, one becomes subconsciously attuned to this expression. Neither the expression of the illness nor its perception is in any way "hardwired." It is a purely learned awareness, and it may even be a learned awareness not of a specific pathological presentation of schizophrenia but of the cultural patterns by which those suffering from mental illness can express their symptoms (Gilman 1983).

Both the schools of Ekman and Russell are biologically grounded. Pain and its expression are reflections of the workings of a black box of emotions. The former assumes that the categories of expression are fixed and are mimetic of an underlying scale of emotions; the latter sees these fixed forms as culturally selected. The scale of the expression of pain in the former are fixed because of the relationship between emotion and expression; in the latter, they are fixed because a given culture has selected from among the widest potential means of expression and underlying emotions those that articulate pain best. The true alternative to both would be that we are born with facial muscles and that these muscles develop over time as we learn the scale of emotions in our world. A radical cultural theory of pain would see our adult projection of pain into the actions of the infant as a loop by which we train infants to express pain.

THE NEWEST TECHNOLOGY OF SEEING PAIN

We might imagine that the most recent advances in medical imaging would resolve this conundrum, but an fMRI today is no more a simple reflection of underlying realities than were X-rays a century ago. While there has been a great deal of work done on pain and its representation in images of the living brain, most of it has been aimed as researching the nature of brain responses to painful stimuli, rather than developing a diagnostic tool for representing pain (Schweinhardt and Bushnell 2010). Recent studies have attempted to distinguish the psychological impact of expectation of pain on its mental representation, and studies of brain scans now evoke the "biopsychosocial" nature of pain (Kong et al. 2009). The problem even with such sophisticated studies that take the totality of experience under consideration is that they assume the more or less uniform representation of complex mental states in fMRIs. Thus, in one recent study, there is an attempt to tease out the difference in pain sensitivity based on the model of self-reporting. The researchers sought objective criteria (as does the Wong Baker test) to measure the accuracy of such self-reporting. They claim that there are objective correlates between the image of complex brain activation and the self-reporting of levels of pain and that this correlation could be used to determine levels of medical intervention. They register differences in individual response to identical stimuli but postulate that these differences may well lie in earlier experience of pain, the emotional state of the subject as well as the expectations of pain (Starr et al. 2010). Yet the idea that one can "see" the totality of such experiences relative one to the other seems illogical. If individuals have a wide range of experiences that shape their own sense of what is painful, and if these experiences are diverse and are located in complex ways in the brain, each scan must be unique and thus would tell us even less than asking "how much does it hurt?"

Even the question of empathy to pain has been explored using brain scans. One recent study claims that when children see an image of a person in pain, the portions of their brain that would have registered that pain on an fMRI scan respond. While the children see a person intentionally hurt, portions of the brain associated with "moral reasoning" are also activated (Decety et al. 2008). The idea that empathy means an affective identification with the experience of the pain of another based on one's own prior experience of pain demands some qualification. Do all individuals respond to all manifestations of pain in the same way? Certainly a "biopsychosocial" approach would argue that they do not. At least one study thinks that one needs to have already had some type of empathic relationship with the person in pain. "Our ability to have an experience of another's pain is characteristic of empathy. Using functional imaging, we assessed brain activity while volunteers experienced a painful stimulus and compared it to that elicited when they observed a signal indicating that their loved one—present in the same room—was receiving a similar pain stimulus" (Singer et al. 2004, 1157). This claim evokes echoes of the infamous (and now oft-rebutted) Stanley Milgram (1963) experiment in which pain was inflicted on a third person while the "scientist" observed and ordered increasingly painful shocks. Here anonymity is replaced by emotional connection. Do we always respond as the researchers here indicated? And what is the nature of the brain coordinates for "moral reasoning"? Indeed, can we even through brain scans distinguish empathic pain from the pain of a "broken heart"? At least one brain neuroimaging study claims to show that that the brain areas that are activated during the distress caused by social exclusion are also those activated during physical pain (Eisenberger et al. 2003).

All of these studies and a much wider range of brains scans representing "pain" in all of its multitudinous forms fall into the pattern of errors of their predecessors. They elide our Western, popular understanding of "pain" and "empathy." They do not attempt to ask how much of the very experience of "seeing" pain is formed by the cultures of pain in which each of us as individuals mature and that seem to each of us "natural." That such patterns would be found in pain is obvious, as it is the brain that catalogues and records, for better or ill, such experiences. But as Eric Racine, Ofek Bar-Ilan, and Judy Illes noted in a major study of the popular reception of such studies, brain imaging experiments "can make a phenomenon uncritically real, objective or effective in the eyes of the public." They described this phenomenon as *neuro-realism:*

Many occurrences of neuro-realism deal with the effectiveness of health-related procedures such as acupuncture. For example, "Patients have long reported that acupuncture helps relieve their pain, but scientists don't know why. Could it be an illusion? Now brain imaging technology has indicated that the perception of pain relief is accurate." Another headline: "A relatively new form of brain imaging provides visual proof that acupuncture alleviates pain.'" The underlying claim is that "the brain can't lie: brain scans reveal how you think and feel and even how you might behave." (2005, 160)

Often such neuro-realism haunts the very science that is received by the public. It is the basis for many of the biological approaches to seeing pain. While it may be believed that brain imaging provides visual proof that certain interventions ameliorate pain, the simple reality is that only the subject can state whether pain has been relieved or not. And self-reporting is a slave to the context in all of its complexity in which the report is made and in which the individual experiences pain. All of the images of relief are useless unless the individual feels relief. And relief may have more to do with the experience of pain and its relief (as in a placebo) than with any mimetic representation of pain in the brain.

Thus we are struck by a conundrum: the more subjective pain is from the standpoint of the sufferer, the more objective it is from the standpoint of the observer unless, of course, the observer too is subjective. "Seeing is believing" unless we don't believe in seeing. Or at least believe that seeing is unmediated.

A SHORT, MODERN HISTORY OF SEEING PAIN

This problem is, not surprisingly, not a new one. Scientists in the Enlightenment came to doubt the efficacy of unmediated seeing in diagnosis. How much of what we see is an artifact of who were are? asks the American physician Benjamin Rush (1746–1813) in the eighteenth century:

Physicians by reviewing the history of complaints from their patients will often have them exaggerated but by frequent visits you cannot be deceived. . . . Endeavor to get the history of the disease from the patient himself and do not interrupt him till he has finished as he will always give the best symptoms tho' he may give the worst causes. Begin to interrogate your patient. By how long he has been sick? When attacked and in what manner? What are the probable causes, former habits and dress; likewise the diet, etc., for a week before especially in acute diseases. . . . In chronic diseases enquire their complaints far back and the habits of life. . . . Pay attention to the phraseology of your patients, for the same ideas are frequently conveyed in different words. A pain in the precordia is called by an Englishman a pain in his stomach, by a Scotchman in his breasts, an Irishman in his heart and by a Southern man mighty poorly. Enquire of your patients the diseases of their ancestors, the age to which they lived and the remedies which relieved them. It is of consequence because there is a hereditary idiosyncrasies [sic] in some families. Patients often conceal the cause of their disease—therefore interrogate them particularly when you suspect intemperance as the cause of disease. (Porter 1997, 257)

Pain is for Rush the exemplary case of patient misunderstanding; only the physician trained in taking a history can comprehend it. The patient's language is insufficient or perhaps too local to communicate his or her experience. Culture articulates pain; one trained in observing the variations in its expression can interpret it.

It was the Scottish physician/anatomist Charles Bell (1774–1842) who put forth perhaps the clearest claim to representing bodily pain in his 1806 *Essays on the Anatomy of Expression in Painting*, later republished as *Essays on the Anatomy and Philosophy of Expression* in 1824. Bell claimed that the very structure of the musculature of the face was solely present in order for man to expression emotions. Aimed at art students, the task of his study was to provide them with the visual vocabulary of human expression generated by those muscles, including that of pain:

In bodily pain the jaws are fixed and the teeth grind; the lips are drawn laterally, so as to expose the teeth and gums; the nostrils are distended to the utmost, and at the same time drawn up; the eyes are largely uncovered, and the eyebrows elevated; the face is turgid with blood, and the veins of the forehead and temples distended, the breath being suspended, and the descent of the blood from the head impeded. Much of the expression results from the strong action of the muscles closing the jaws, and the strong action and consequent stringiness of the cutaneous muscles of the neck R, plate II, which at the same time draws down the corner of the mouth. (1824, 96)

Bell's claim is that such expression is both universal and mechanical. But Bell, prefiguring Scarry's understanding of empathy, also speaks of the internal state of the psyche that is readable through the transparency of the "face of pain." It is a readability that cannot be obfuscated or denied:

In pain, the body is exerted to violent tension, and all the emotions and passions which are allied to pain, or have their origin and foundation in painful sensations, have distinctly this character in common, that there is tension, or a start into exertion, or tremor, the effect of universal and great excitement. It must at the same time be recollected, that all the passions of this class, some more immediately, others more indirectly, produce in the second stage a loss of tone, exhaustion, and debility, from over exertion. . . . Pain first rouses the faculties both of the body and of the mind, and from a dormant state gives us consciousness and real existence. It is bestowed upon us as a perpetual guard, forcing us to watch continually for the safety of the body and the preservation of life. From the expression of pain as a centre we may trace the indications of many of the mixed passions. (1824, 96)

Pain is a safety mechanism to protect our bodies from damage, and its expression allows others to see it.

Bell's work is evoked by the most important scientist to deal with the visibility of pain. Charles Darwin (1809–1882), whose *Expression of the Emotions in Man and Animals*, published in 1872, saw expression and its recognition as a means of the survival of the fittest. Many contemporary scholars of emotions, including Ekman (1973), consider Darwin their major precursor. For Darwin the evidence for universals of expression is to be found in the continuity between human expressions of emotion and that of other mammals. Thus the snarl and aggressive posture of the suspicious dog is a prototype of the same types of posture and expression in a suspicious human being. Darwin observes emotions in the physiological response of all animals, higher and lower. Such claims, as we have seen, are rejected by those who see pain as subjective and advocated by those who claim that they can see and catalogue pain and thus claim Darwin's work as their primary scientific source. Darwin, too, has his models for seeing emotions. Thus he looks to Bell for his argument about seeing pain and continues Bell's argument half a century later:

The long-continued habit of attempting by struggling to escape from the cause of suffering—and the consciousness that voluntary muscular exertion relieves pain, have all probably concurred in giving a tendency to the most violent, almost convulsive, movements under extreme suffering; and such movements, including those of the vocal organs, are universally recognised as highly expressive of this condition. (Darwin 1872, 73)

But like our contemporary "seers of pain," Darwin, too, relies on the response of the observer to document Bell's accuracy rather than simply relying on the scientist's observation:

Sir C. Bell remarks that "horror is full of energy"; the body is in the utmost tension, not unnerved by "fear." It is, therefore, probable that horror would generally be accompanied by the strong contraction of the brows; but as fear is one of the elements, the eyes and mouth would be opened, and the eyebrows would be raised, as far as the antagonistic action of the corrugators permitted this movement. Duchenne has given a photograph of the same old man as before, with his eyes somewhat staring, the eyebrows partially raised, and at the same time strongly contracted, the mouth opened, and the platysma in action, all effected by the means of galvanism. He considers that the expression thus produced shows extreme terror with horrible pain or torture. A tortured man, as long as his sufferings allowed him to feel any dread for the future, would probably exhibit horror in an extreme degree. I have shown the original of this photograph to twenty-three persons of both sexes and various ages; and thirteen immediately answered horror, great pain, torture, or agony; three answered extreme fright; so that sixteen answered nearly in accordance with Duchenne's belief. (Darwin 1872, 305)

Darwin draws not just on Bell's theory but also on the photographs of Guillaume-Benjamin-Amand Duchenne de Boulogne (1806–1875) as Bell's romantic engravings were clearly "art" while Duchenne's photographs gave Darwin (he believed) an unmediated representation of pain (Duchenne de Boulogne 1990, 60). As is clear today, Duchenne's photographs, posed by well-known actors of the day, reflected less a true expression of pain than rather the musculature needed to create the impression of pain for the theatrical audience (Gilman 1982, 164). Darwin's idea of pain as readable in the human physiognomy depends on the consensus of observer and patient as to how pain is to be legibly expressed. But Darwin draws what is expressed into question. Bell believes you have to experience "real" (i.e., physical) pain to have the face of pain; for Darwin it is the expression of the musculature in pain that mirrors that in other animals that shows the continuity of pain expression across species. Yet Darwin understands, following Duchenne, that one does not have to experience pain to express it.

Darwin acknowledges that the *belief* that one is in physical pain is equivalent to being in pain. He approached James Crichton Browne, director of the West Riding Asylum and a passionate photographer, for images of the mentally ill (Gilman 1982, 179). In turn, Darwin sent him a copy of Duchenne's studies of the electrical stimulation of the facial nerves in 1869. Darwin then incorporated Crichton Browne's photographs of the mentally ill into his study:

I begged for information from Dr. Crichton Browne with respect to the insane. He states in answer that he has repeatedly seen their hair erected under the influence of sudden and extreme terror. For instance, it is occasionally necessary to inject morphia under the skin of an insane woman, who dreads the operation extremely, though it causes very little pain;

for she believes that poison is being introduced into her system, and that her bones will be softened, and her flesh turned into dust. She becomes deadly pale; her limbs are stiffened by a sort of tetanic spasm, and her hair is partially erected on the front of the head. (Darwin 1872, 295)

Unlike Bell's study, the very connection between the observable external state of the body and the internal source of that state is drawn into question. Pain may be imagined and be expressed as accurately as if it were "actually" experienced.

A HISTORICAL MEDIATOR: FREUD

It would seem that the question of an unmediated representation of pain, if one reads Paul Ekman, is uncontested after Darwin, yet it is in the work of Sigmund Freud (1856–1939) that Darwin's idea of pain as physical and psychic was confronted in the early 1890s. His teacher, Theodor Meynert, had made reference in his 1884 textbook to Darwin's theory of expression as "through such movements as are involved in expression we obtain a clue to the inner life of others" (Ritvo 1990, 172). Freud, who remained a classic Darwinian his entire creative life, was thus early trained to "see" those afflicted with pain. When he went to Paris in 1885 to study with the neurologist Jean-Martin Charcot, he was confronted with a scientist who relied on the photograph to document states of psychic (rather than physical) pain and had his view that "seeing is believing" reified (Hodgkiss 2000, 64). In an essay in 1890 entitled "Psychical (or Mental) Treatment," he wrote in a pure Darwinian way that

the commonest, everyday example of the mind's action on the body, and one that is to be observed in everyone, is offered by what is known as the "expression of the emotions." A man's states of mind are manifested, almost without exception, in the tensions and relaxations of his facial muscles, in the adaptations of his eyes, in the amount of blood in the vessels of his skin, in the modifications in his vocal apparatus and in the movements of his limbs and in particular of his hands. These concomitant physical changes are for the most part of no advantage to the person concerned; on the contrary, they often stand in his way if he wishes to conceal his mental processes from other people. But they serve these other people as trustworthy indications from which his mental processes can be inferred and in which more confidence can be placed than in any simultaneous verbal expressions that may be made deliberately. (Freud 1955–1974, 7:285)

At the same time, Freud had been obsessed with the phenomenon of physical pain and its amelioration, experimenting with cocaine as a local anesthetic in the early 1880s.

But it is only after he returned to Vienna from Paris in the mid-1880s that he began to become fascinated by Darwin's claim that one can have physical pain caused by a psychological cause as there may be "a 'symbolic' relation between the precipitating cause and the pathological phenomenon—a relation such as healthy people form in dreams. For instance, a neuralgia may follow upon mental pain or vomiting upon a feeling of moral disgust" (Freud 1955–1974, 2:1). Not just a lesion in the nervous system, which could not be seen by contemporary means of visualization, as Charcot claimed, but underlying psychic causes could also cause physical pain. Here we can return to the question asked earlier: what happens when not all physical pain has a physical cause? Conversion disorders translate psychic symptoms into physical ones, including pain. But, as Freud came to understand, such physical pain that is caused by psychic mechanisms such as repression is rarely linked to a specific form of remembering as representation. It is not simply the direct translation of one (the cause) into the other (the symptom), and thus such pain is quite different from the idea of the symptom as developed in *Studies on Hysteria* (1895), in which, for example, the anxiety surrounding seeing a dog drinking from a glass becomes expressed by a patient as the inability to swallow (Freud 1955–1974, 2:1–305). Physical pain becomes for Freud a clinical "compass" to understand more complex psychic mechanisms.

Freud was anxious at the time that focusing on the psychological function of pain may have caused him to overlook some physical cause, as he recounts in his "Dream of Irma's Injection" in *The Interpretation of Dreams* (1955–1974, 4:106). Yet he applies Darwin to his cases of hysteria as in the case of "Emmy von N":

Some of the striking motor phenomena exhibited by Frau von N. were simply an expression of the emotions and could easily be recognized in that light. Thus, the way in which she stretched her hands in front of her with her fingers spread out and crooked expressed horror, and similarly her facial play. This, of course, was a more lively and uninhibited way of expressing her emotions than was usual with women of her education and race. Indeed, she herself was restrained, almost stiff in her expressive movements when she was not in a hysterical state. Others of her motor symptoms were, according to herself, directly related to her pains. She played restlessly with her fingers (1888) or rubbed her hands against one another (1889) so as to prevent herself from screaming. This reason reminds one forcibly of one of the principles laid down by Darwin to explain the expression of the emotions—the principle of the overflow of excitation, which accounts, for instance, for dogs wagging their tails. (Freud 1955–1974, 2:90)

By this point, Freud had broken with Charcot's understanding of representation, dismissing him in 1893 as "not unduly reflective, not a thinker: he had the nature of an artist—he was, as he himself said, a *'visuel,'* a man who sees. Here is what he himself told us about his method of working. He used to look again and again at the things he did not understand, to deepen his impression of them day by day, till suddenly an understanding of them dawned on him" (Freud 1955–1974, 3:10). But, of course, this was a false "seeing," and Freud replaces seeing in his mode of representation (and therapy) with listening. Yet it is also the case that his idea of representing psychic pain is one still very much in the Darwinian mode with an added understanding of the deformation of symptoms in their very expression:

What could be more probable than that the figure of speech "swallowing something," which we use in talking of an insult to which no rejoinder has been made, did in fact originate from the innervatory sensations which arise in the pharynx when we refrain from speaking and prevent ourselves from reacting to the insult? All these sensations and innervations belong to the field of "The Expression of the Emotions," which, as Darwin has taught us, consists of actions which originally had a meaning and served a purpose. These may now for the most part have become so much weakened that the expression of them in words seems to us only to be a figurative picture of them, whereas in all probability the description was once meant literally; and hysteria is right in restoring the original meaning of the words in depicting its unusually strong innervations." (Freud 1955–1974, 2:180)

Freud is able to depart from a strict reading of Darwin's model to understand that the representation of pain may well be tangential to a "real experience," which is, of course, Darwin's own view on his analysis of mental illness and pain.

While Freud initially believes that listening is a means of representation that is objective, he eventually becomes aware of countertransference, that the therapist too is subjective in listening in the analytic situation. As he writes in 1928 to Sándor Ferenczi concerning the question of countertransference:

All those who have no tact will see in this a justification of arbitrariness, i.e., of the subjective factor, i.e., of the influence of one's own unrestrained complexes. What we undertake in reality is a weighing out, which remains mostly preconscious, of the various reactions that we expect from our interventions, in the process of which it is first and foremost a matter of the quantitative assessment of the dynamic factors in the situation. Rules for these measurements can naturally not be made; the analyst's experience and normality will have to be the decisive factors. But one should thus divest "tact" of its mystical character for beginners." (Freud and Ferenczi 2000, 333)

To this, we should certainly add the need to divest representations and their observation of all sort of their "mystical character." But also, following Freud, we should be very careful of "empathy" on the part of the observer, for empathy (that force that thinkers from Bell to Scarry associate with seeing pain) may well be a reflection, not of our comprehension of the Other, but of our own projection onto the Other. Seeing may be the creation of a false empathy of the Other's pain.

PAIN AS A MEANS OF LEARNING ABOUT HOW WE LEARN ABOUT THE WORLD

Seeing pain has a history. It also has a practice in the science of medicine, both ancient and modern. Medicine "sees" pain or at least its representations. But how this act of seeing is understood is part of any epistemology of medicine. Pain becomes a vital site for the meanings attached to conflicting systems of representation. Karen Barad in her *Meeting the Universe Halfway* dismisses the "Cartesian distinction between objects and agencies of observation" to suggest that "measurement practices are an ineliminable part of the results obtained" (2007, 120–121). Pain measurement of both types demand an act (self-reporting or observation or both) that is part of the boundaries drawn, so that "method, measurement, description, interpretation, epistemology, and ontology are not separable considerations" (121). If measurement cannot be separated from what is being measured, Barad concludes, "measured properties refer to phenomena" (197):

I argue that phenomena are not the mere result of laboratory exercises engineered by human subjects; rather, *phenomena are differential patterns of mattering* ("diffraction patterns") produced through complex agential intra-actions of multiple material discursive practice or apparatuses of bodily production, where *apparatuses are not mere observing instruments but boundary drawing practices—specific material (re)configurings of the world—which come to matter.* (Barad 2007, 140; emphasis in original)

Pain is such a "diffraction pattern," which is bounded as a representation by its very examination.

The debates about pain and its expression are ongoing. In the end, however, these debates are about the most efficient manner of representing the body. How one sees and understands the body is an artifact of the theories one has about the very nature of seeing. Dealing with categories such as pain illustrates that even what may seem obvious in representing the body demands complicated means of understanding the very nature of representation and its claims.

Chapter 17

PUBLIC FETUSES

BERNICE L. HAUSMAN

HUMANISTS studying medicine have focused, in part, on how advancing medical technologies profoundly affect experiences of embodiment, health, and illness. Once reliant on the phenomenological expression of the patient and direct physical examination, contemporary healthcare workers now routinely utilize a wide range of technologies to identify problems, screen patients for disease, and pinpoint appropriate diagnoses. In particular, the pervasive use of modern visualization technologies, ultrasound especially, has dramatically transformed customary care in obstetrics and generated far-reaching implications for a wide spectrum of healthcare workers who also rely on a variety of technologies in patient diagnosis and care. Responding to this technological evolution, feminist scholarship has often focused on obstetrical technologies, for example, looking at how the introduction of forceps allowed male obstetricians to squeeze out midwives as trusted overseers of the birthing process. This chapter introduces feminist debates about the impact of visualization technologies in obstetrical care as one way of understanding how medical technologies and their meanings—for both healthcare workers and patients—remain inextricably linked to social conditions and political controversies, underscoring how such technologies crucially affect and significantly alter the phenomenological experiences they are meant to manage.

Over the past two and a half decades, a number of feminist scholars have investigated pregnancy and the evolving imagery around the fetus in an effort to track an increasingly regulatory climate concerning the unborn. The highly politicized abortion debate in the United States has motivated a complex and wide-ranging feminist discussion about the meanings of fetuses and the relation of the political debates and fetal images to the routine, medicalized experiences of pregnancy. As Rosalind Petchesky wrote in the article that has become the touchstone for all subsequent feminist treatments of fetal images, "the 'public' presentation of the fetus has become ubiquitous; its disembodied form, now propped up by medical authority and technological rationality, permeates mass culture. We are all, on some level, susceptible to its coded meanings" (1987, 281).

In focusing on how fetuses have become public through now-routine technological practices in prenatal care, feminist scholars reveal how women become invested in material practices that limit their freedoms. The modern medical regulation of pregnancy is enacted, in part, through the commonplace use of visualization technologies and other technical assessments that mark the fetus as a separate entity. Women develop diverse responses to obstetric technologies, depending on their own personal histories, political beliefs, and sociocultural circumstances, but obstetrics as a whole has come to depend on patients' investment in these technologies as a way to ensure successful pregnancies and healthy babies. In this way, obstetrical technologies operate as ideological practices suturing mothers to hegemonic perspectives on their fitness, capabilities, and embodied risks.

This chapter provides a very selective overview of feminist approaches to the visualization technologies that accompany gestation in modern society. Rather than surveying the whole field of feminist scholarship on reproductive technologies, I characterize predominant positions within the field in relation to the impact of visualization technologies on women's experiences of pregnancy, focusing on a limited number of texts in order to draw out significant contrasts. The title, "Public Fetuses," brings attention to the way in which these technologies publicize the contents of women's wombs and alter their gestational embodiment as well as their authoritative relationship to their own experience. The chapter as a whole provides significant insight into how technological advancements within medicine meant to enhance health and well-being *also* serve to transform human experience, change power relations, and privilege forms of relationship (e.g., visual over embodied) that produce knowledge about the bodies of patients.

FEMINIST THEMES: SEEING AND SPACE

Of the various themes that emerge in feminist discussions of the fetus, I focus on (1) the relation of maternal bodies to technologies that measure, assess, and "see" the fetus, and (2) the womb as a public space. The second theme is made possible, in part, by the visualization technologies suggested in the first theme. Both lead to the purposeful absence of the mother as the site for gestation and fetal development, the larger body within which the fetus not only finds a home but in relation to whom the fetus cannot be separated. But Petchesky argues that the second theme, or at least the way in which pregnant women experience their subordination to the public fetus as the womb becomes a public space, is not the inevitable result of particular visualization technologies: "Technologies take on the meanings and uses they do because of the cultural climate of fetal images and the politics of hostility toward pregnant women and abortion" (1987, 271). Carol Stabile continues this approach by arguing that to investigate "visual representations of fetal autonomy in the service of New Right politics" is to "analyze the conditions that have made possible the ideological transformation of the female body from a benevolent, maternal environment into an inhospitable waste land, at war with the 'innocent person' within" (1992, 179).

In this analysis, visualization technologies do not produce determinate meanings about the pregnant female body and its cargo. Instead, the technologies and their representational products garner meaning through the ideological contexts within which they operate. According to this view, the technologies are ciphers of the larger political world, only technical passive reporting machines. For those who believe the technologies to be formative of the ideological context, that illusion is part of their cultural power. Feminist scholarship thus exhibits a consistent tension concerning obstetrical technologies—either these technologies enforce ideologies that already exist and operate to displace women's central role in pregnancy and childbirth, or they create the very ideologies that they seem to emerge from and reflect. This second position can be perceived to be technological determinism, and many authors are reluctant to give credence to such a view. Nevertheless, the power of obstetrical technologies in and of themselves, and especially visualization technologies, is a constant theme in this literature.

Feminist scholars generally agree that the field of obstetrical medicine tends to imagine (and portray) the womb as a risky environment. Yet the maternal body has not moved, historically, from being perceived as an idealized, safe space to one of unalterable danger; rather, it oscillates between these two views because pregnant bodies are regulated by pollution taboos that demarcate social boundaries and distinguish the proper from the improper (Douglas 1966). As indeterminate bodies in touch with marginal, not-yet-humans, pregnant women negotiate identities in the context of an explicit cultural ambivalence about whether they are to be despised and kept apart or embraced through idealization. To a certain extent, the technologies that regulate pregnancy are engaged as a hedge against this very ambivalence, charting the physiology of pregnancy as an assurance of normalcy (see Hausman 2011, 98–113, for an extended discussion).

By and large, feminist approaches to these issues demonstrate skepticism at the medical control of women's bodies and a desire to return to an alternative norm of pregnancy and maternity that acknowledges women's greater contribution to the forms of knowledge produced from their experience. For many feminist scholars, visualization technologies represent all obstetrical technologies that alienate women from their own pregnancies and produce the fetus as the subject of gestation. Yet even in 1987, Petchesky was careful to observe that many women themselves welcome the use of obstetrical visualization technologies because they seem to offer some control in the context of multiple pregnancy losses or histories of difficult fertility experiences.

Nevertheless, an underlying assumption of many feminist critiques of obstetrical visualization technologies is that they inculcate in women a relationship to the fetus that is like the doctor's and thus like men's in general—not embodied but mediated externally by technologies. In this view, the mediation by technology represents a disruption of women's autonomous experience of pregnancy and their right to a unique existential experience as mothers. This perspective is forcefully articulated by German historian Barbara Duden and, while challenged by scholars like Meredith Michaels, represents a significant trend in feminist scholarship on the fetus.

What feminist scholars like Duden focus on is the transformation of the existential experience of gestation and childbirth due to the introduction of technologies that define pregnancy and motherhood through scientific categories, measurements, and practices. In addition to addressing what it means to be a pregnant woman in the industrialized global north today, this perspective gestures toward a premodern past in which women retained some sort of autonomy and power concerning the social and medical meanings of their embodiment. While such a perspective can be criticized as nostalgic, it nevertheless contributes important insights to debates about the meaning of fetuses in public culture today. Even if there is no "going back," there can be significant lessons to be learned about what "going forward" has meant for women and their babies.

BARBARA DUDEN AND THE PRODUCTION OF "LIFE ITSELF"

Duden's short monograph, *Disembodying Women: Perspectives on Pregnancy and the Unborn*, addresses how the fetus displaces women as the source of aliveness and the unborn. "Life," Duden argues, is the concretization of the concept of the fetus, which is itself an abstracted understanding of the unborn in women's wombs made possible through the visualization technologies that provide access to it. "Life," in this sense, displaces aliveness, which is one way to interpret quickening, the process through which women historically announced their state of being with child. Duden believes that women should resist this displacement: "One can speak an unconditional NO to life, recovering one's own autonomous aliveness" (1993, 110). A defining aspect of this recovered aliveness is a repudiation of scientific perspectives on women's bodies as the truth of their embodied experience.

The public fetus, she argues, is partly an effect of nineteenth-century changes in women's status and public identity and emerges historically when quickening declines in significance:

I understand the demise in the social status of quickening as an event that brings an important paradox to the surface: in the course of the nineteenth century, female innards and interiority become medically, administratively, and judicially public while, at the same time, the female exterior is privatized ideologically and culturally. These opposed but linked tendencies are both characteristic moments in the social construction of "woman" as a scientific fact, as well as in the creation of the citizen in industrial society. . . . Her flesh becomes the forum whose proceedings are of immediate interest to the state and society, to public health and the church, and also to her husband. (Duden 1993, 95)

For Duden, the technologies that visualize the fetus and thus bring us the unborn *as a fetus* end up deadening the experience of pregnancy. The technologies take this experience out of women's hands to define and put women in the service of "life." This historical shift subordinates women to the technologies that define what is in them. And each woman "must decide whether to be the guardian of a public image, whether to share responsibility for its protection and development with representatives of the law" (1993, 54).

Yet Duden acknowledges that women today cannot "put [themselves] outside the framework" of modern medicine, a framework that demands their participation in the "series of unavoidable 'decisions' that lead from amniocentesis to the interiorization of eugenics to the scientifically guided care of a modern infant." Such a refusal of contemporary practices puts women at risk for being bad mothers, either "primitive," "romantic," or "utopian." In any case, Duden suggests, modern women "live in the age of the public fetus. . . . There is no way back to the unborn below the horizon" (1993, 54–55). The place we are now is the result of a momentous change in the way that women experience pregnancy; contemporary experience stands opposed to a longer history of women's greater autonomy: "I want to examine the conditions under which, *in the course of one generation*, technology along with a new discourse has transformed pregnancy into a process to be managed, the expected child into a fetus, the mother into an ecosystem, the unborn into a life, and life into a supreme value" (1993, 2; emphasis added).

Elsewhere, Duden writes, "Motherhood, pregnancy, and birth are no longer somatic experiences of women expecting a child that will come, but the result of acceptance and interiorization of biomedical measurements" (1999, 24). This is a common argument in feminist scholarship on the fetus: that technological approaches that visualize, assess, identify, operate on, or otherwise address the fetus independent of the mother actually produce a historically new subject (or object) of analysis and render it identifiable as a singular being, a person-like being. In part, this new scientific object, the fetus, is an effect of the introjection of scientific measurement into the womb that grounds the modern demand for purity in pregnancy.[1]

Meredith Michaels argues that Barbara Duden "charges the phantom-producing machine with appearance-mongering. I charge her with reality-mongering" (1999, 124). Expanding on this claim, she writes: "Duden asks us precisely to reject the 'medical definitions of the developing young,' to revert to a conception of pregnancy centered on the epistemic privilege of women. I am arguing that we *cannot* reject such definitions, that they indeed define the terms of our culture's procreative economy. Our inability to reject them, however, does not entail that we must accept the position of 'life's passive instrument'" (1999, 131; emphasis in original). This argument with Duden demonstrates a central tension in feminist approaches to the fetus, which can be captured in the question: "To what extent do visualization technologies concretize the fetus and make it real?" Duden consistently refers to another reality that she argues is historically available. Michaels suggests that we live in a transformed reality constituted, at least in part, through the images that Duden rejects.

Feminist philosopher Rebecca Kukla, author of *Mass Hysteria: Medicine, Culture, and Mothers' Bodies* (2005), would not agree with Duden's claims of historical uniqueness. Kukla points to late eighteenth-century France and demonstrates continuities with the Enlightenment concerning the role of women's bodies in shoring up the body politic with their purity and social function as mothers. There seems to be little question of whether significant historical shifts have occurred in the experience of pregnancy; the issue is whether there are continuities of meaning attached to gestation and the unborn that persist through these changes and with the advent of new technologies of visualization and fetal assessment. Duden seems convinced that it may be possible to resist the implications of the new technologies; Kukla believes that they create a new moral reality demanding our attention.

Kukla and Michaels agree that visualization technologies constitute the new normal of fetal existence. Valerie Hartouni suggests that acknowledging the new normal of public fetuses does not suggest an acceptance of the meanings seemingly attached to technological advancement—fetal personhood, or at least viability beyond the maternal body: "The fetus-as-social-subject does not retire the controversies in which it appeared to play to pivotal a part. It leaves unanswered the many obvious moral questions commentators seemed to assume its status as subject would swiftly settle and forcefully reiterates a central problem of determining what significance to attach to it as a social subject, indeed, of determining what exactly its status as subject 'means'" (1999, 302). In this analysis, the technological enters the public domain like any other discursive practice, without predetermined meaning or consequences. Because "no image simply speaks for itself in a clear, unmediated fashion," visualization technologies that make the fetus public only do so in the context of other practices, beliefs, and circumstances (1999, 300). Like many feminists, Hartouni consistently points toward the "messy set of problems" posed by "fetuses in the flesh, embedded in social life and relations, and embodied through both as well" (1999, 302–303). Duden might argue back that "fetuses in the flesh" are the result of historical developments that have transformed both the "unborn" and women's wombs; to highlight their discursivity and contingency is not to challenge the way they have transformed pregnancy to women's detriment.

What most warms me to Duden's argument is her insistence that "NO" is an option. It is, perhaps, too late for many women in industrialized countries to fashion for themselves a maternal subjectivity completely outside the contours of technically mediated experiences. Given the global unevenness of modernity, however, there are many women whose relationship to the interventionist and regulatory apparatus of obstetrical medicine is tenuous, contested, or challenged. Cultural differences also mean that there are many women in the world for whom the fetus does not exist or exists differently than it does in wealthy countries (see Morgan 1997). Duden recalls that period in Euro-American history when the unborn literally took on a different conceptual shape, reminding us that the embodiment of gestation is not static and that changes that seem to offer greater control (through knowledge) may lead to increased subordination. Her work also reminds us that prenatal care does not have to be synonymous with women's subjugation to medical authority.

REBECCA KUKLA AND THE MORAL EFFECT OF OBSTETRICAL TECHNOLOGIES

While Rebecca Kukla finds that women today experience an intensification of expectations in pregnancy and new motherhood, she argues for deep historical continuities in beliefs about mothers-to-be in the Western world since the late eighteenth century. In *Mass Hysteria*, she analyzes the pregnant body as it is figured as permeable and thus liable to imperfection through its corruptibility: "Concerns with the permeability of the maternal body and with its appetites and cravings have . . . been partnered with concerns about the potential for corruption of the pure space of the womb through ingestion and permeation across the boundaries of this body" (2005, 6; see also Keane 1996). Attending to discourses concerning pregnant women and breast-feeding mothers in the late eighteenth and late twentieth centuries, Kukla argues that maternity in Europe and North America has been perceived through the iconic figures of the "unruly mother" and the "fetish mother," the first a "capricious, improperly and porously bounded body, easily corrupted and driven by cravings and passions," and the second a "well-ordered 'natural' body enjoying perfect unity and reciprocity with its child" (2005, 67). Through the course of the twentieth century, the introduction of technologies to manage pregnancy and motherhood has exploited this dichotomization of maternity. As an example, Kukla writes: "Infant formula manufacturers sought to broaden their market, *not* through the rhetoric of replacing nature with superior science, but rather through working to effect a proliferation of ways in which maternal bodies could be special 'problem cases' for which their product was suitable" (2005, 96; emphasis in original). Within the context of this binary opposition between the bad mother and the good one, the uterus becomes "a public theater": "the womb has become a public, rigorously regulated space" in the context of which "pregnant women use a set of public rituals and images to forge and personalize a mediated, third-person relationship with the contents of their own displaced, shared insides" (2005, 109).

Identifying a "mass hysteria" about what pregnant women ingest, Kukla argues that the "logic of the maternal imagination, which turns pregnant women's skins into fully permeable media, ready to transmit directly to the fetus the substances that the pregnant woman ingests, still governs our cultural imagination. We take the womb as a space that must be kept pure in order to perform its task of producing well-ordered nature, and we also take this space as easily corrupted from without, and thereby transformed into a dangerous laboratory of monstrosity," adding, "as in premodern and modern eras, it is still women's cravings and passions, as well as the transparent openness of her womb to disordering influences, that are feared as the sources of deformed human nature" (2005, 106). Later in the text, she notes that medicalized perspectives on pregnancy, accepted in the general populace, try to "control for what we have perceived as the ever-present potential for the mother's body to *turn against* its child—to provide a 'poison environment' during pregnancy and to separate and abandon the child after birth" (2005, 221; emphasis in original). In her view, breast-feeding advocacy materials that invoke the necessity of mother-infant proximity fetishize nearness as a hedge against mothers' impulses to leave, which are figured as similar to mothers' improper cravings— they are actions that endanger babies through the desire of the mother for something other than her child.

For Kukla, the contemporary "ideological practices that constitute and manage the pregnant body" offer women mixed blessings. On the one hand, "our surveillance and discipline of pregnant bodies has upheld an ethos of these bodies as the privileged, even exclusive sites of civic responsibility, often at the direct and tragic cost of sufficient attention to the many other crucial determinants of maternal and child health that lie outside of the boundaries of the pregnant body, such as domestic violence, environmental damage, and the ravages of poverty." On the other hand, "they are not the kind of practices we can simply or morally think our way out of. . . . The transformation of the uterus into a public theater and of the fetus into its canonical lead actor has come along with the availability of a wealth of information that can help us to improve the capacities and chances for [the] flourishing of our future children" (Kukla 2005, 136). At this point, Kukla challenges Duden's repudiation of interventionist obstetrical technology with a strong argument for the alterity of fetuses themselves: "Our fetuses are not independent agents, but they are not simply more of us either" (2005, 137). For Kukla, this means a more measured assessment of what women might do in the current climate of disciplinary fetishization of purity and the proper womb, arguing that the new regulatory environment of pregnancy makes specific moral demands on mothers, who are particularly vulnerable given the "unavoidable volatility and uncanniness of the pregnant body and self" (2005, 139).

Kukla is, of course, echoing Duden's own understanding that women today cannot simply refuse participation in the technic of modern medicalized pregnancy, even as she offers a lengthier, philosophical justification concerning the existential specificity of new motherhood and its ambivalent moral imperatives. Kukla's argument about the ideological work of visualization and other technologies of modern maternity care suggests that women must be careful to understand their effects at a time when they are themselves in the process of monumental changes in embodiment and subjective experience. Overall, she is less sure than Duden of the detriment of the technologies themselves.

Kukla's attention to the continuities in historical views of gestating and breast-feeding women, rather than to the changes that Duden emphasizes, reveals an abiding cultural skepticism about women's capacities as mothers. To a certain extent, for Kukla, the problem of the fetus is not dependent on specific technologies through which the fetus emerges as an entity with particular force. Instead, the problem of the fetus is the result of a long-standing wariness about mothers' bodies imagined as easily corruptible. In this view, technological advances only change the nature of the media that regulate women into particular, socially prescribed behaviors as mothers. Because of this, the technology itself is not Kukla's target. The perception of women as unruly or ideal and the consequences of such a bifurcated view on women's concrete experiences of mothering constitute the focus of her critique.

PROMISCUOUS PLACENTAS AND THE ABSENT FEMALE BODY

The visualization technologies that isolate and create "the fetus" and distort women's moral priorities also operate to absent the pregnant woman from the scene of her own activity. In an essay called "The Promiscuous Placenta," Jane-Maree Maher (2001) suggests that one function of the now-ubiquitous pregnancy ultrasound is to "refigure the work and meaning of pregnancy for the pregnant embodied subject and the others" away from the nonintentional activities that the pregnant body engages in and toward the purposeful management of both the pregnant woman and the medical institution that supervises her. In part, this is accomplished through the foregrounding of the fetal body and the backgrounding of the mother's body and the placenta. Maher writes:

The placental body, with its uncertain edges, its fluidity of constitution and its complex mixture of subjective intent and bodily activity, cannot fit comfortably within these frames where subjective intention and the instrumentality of the body are central. In an "ideal" pregnancy, the potential contaminants of alcohol, coffee and other substances are not allowed to cross into the placenta for fear that they will affect the foetus. In the ideal image of pregnancy, the placenta is not allowed to cross into images of pregnancy for fear that its unsecured edges could destabilize the important boundaries secured in the visual field. (Maher 2001, 212)

In other words, through visualization practices that identify the fetus, the active processes of medical regulation and the technological framing of intentional activity as the important work of the pregnant woman obscure the non-intentional activity of the mother's body in pregnancy. Advice discourses concerning diet that stress control and rational decision making function similarly. For Duden, the non-intentionality of pregnancy is recognized by the woman's statement at quickening that she is with child, that the operation of her body, heretofore unknown to her, is that of pregnancy. This action of the maternal body moving forward with gestation without the intentional participation of the mother is circumscribed or repudiated in the regime of medical management.

For Maher, the placenta itself represents contagion between the maternal body and the fetus, demonstrating the alterity of pregnancy in a kind of necessary, unaccounted-for porousness and mutual contamination. Medical oversight and technological interventions like ultrasonography operate to "still" the "actual and potential seepage, across the pregnant body and the foetal entity, across all bounded bodies produced in this process. . . . The productive communication of fluid, matter and subjectivity is erased—the contagion implicit in the construction of the embodied self is displaced through the visual disciplining of the pregnant body" (2001, 213). While the "contagious nature of the 'placental body' is recognized already in medical and cultural discourse," such recognition generally occurs through "identification of the placenta as the site for the transmission of alcohol and drugs" as well as caffeine, folic acid, and other substances either desired or decried. Maher notes, citing Cynthia Daniels, that "this recognition of the complexity of the pregnant body has always been used to confine and constrain the pregnant woman," not to enable "new definitions of subjectivity to become possible" (2001, 214; see also Daniels 1997).

CONCLUSION

Feminist perspectives on fetal subjects illuminate the complex, cultural ambivalence felt about women's seeming control over gestation as a unique facet of female embodiment (see also Daniels 1999). This ambivalence plays itself out as a desire to regulate women through advice and technological practices during pregnancy. With Kukla, I understand this ambivalence to be one facet of persistent perceptions of mothers as "unruly" and thus not susceptible to commonsense self-regulation of their practices. The other facet is the idealization of mothers, which Kukla identifies as fetishization. This idealization underscores a deeply troubling view of maternal fitness that relies on a belief that mothers must be pure in order to be good. In the context of an impure and dirty world, this means that mothers must display enormous self-discipline—and act in culturally anomalous ways— to be worthy of the fetuses within them and the babies that emerge from their all-too-public wombs.

Obstetric technologies do not operate in a vacuum; they are utilized within an ideological context that confers meaning upon them and is influenced by their use. In the United States, feminist debates about ultrasound use in prenatal care have been influenced heavily by public and politically divisive abortion controversies, in part because the technologies themselves have been utilized in the campaign against legal abortion. Ultrasound renderings of fetuses appear in the consultation room as well as the picket line; in some states, ultrasounds are required prior to legal abortion by state mandate rather than medical protocol.

Visualization technologies that have brought us the "public fetus" have also transformed women's experiences of pregnancy and motherhood, changing expectations of "good mothers" as the fetus has become more and more separate from the gestational maternal body and subjectivity. Women themselves have varied responses to the technological aspects of obstetrical practice. Healthcare practitioners should understand the cultural context influencing their own expectations of medical regulation and routine care, attending especially to the ways in which their patients might resist or be ambivalent about the meanings ascribed to them through the practices they engage. Feminist approaches to the "public fetus" highlight its ambivalent cultural effects, as well as its reflection of cultural ambivalence about mothers and babies, demonstrating how technological advances are never politically neutral.

NOTES

1 Demands for purity in pregnancy generally focus on chemical or alcohol contamination but are linked conceptually to the problem of maternal sexuality. I argue in *Viral Mothers* (Hausman 2011) that idealizations of pure motherhood are based on fantasies of a sacred motherhood that is separate from the earth, its impurities, and the sexual basis of maternity (114–129).

Chapter 18

MORE BODY
A Performance for Five (or More) Bodies
GRETCHEN A. CASE

P LEASE perform the following text. You do not need any special acting skills, only a willingness to try something different from reading words on a page. First, think about what performing means for *your* particular body. Any perceived limitations might actually be assets. Embarrassed? Shy? Dubious? Reluctant? Include those feelings as part of your performance. Next, consider how your body will perform alongside the other bodies. Every body does not have to translate the text in the same way. Your body can't or won't do something called for in this script? Do something else. You can't make an incorrect choice because there are no correct choices; this performance is simply your interpretation of these words.

This performance, like every performance, won't go the same way twice. The most important thing is that you use your body to think about the *idea* of the body.

In this performance, there are six short scenes of increasing complexity to be performed by five people. At the beginning of each scene, *italicized*, are directions for the performers, followed by lines for each performer to speak. Try this performance without rehearsing or reading ahead, trusting the ideas that come to you in the moment. The directions assume you are in a classroom—you may, of course, improvise if you are in a very different sort of space.

SCENE 1

Spread yourselves out along the walls of the classroom so that you are as far away from each other as possible. If you have an audience (people who are watching but not performing), they should be in the center of the room. Face the center of the room and put your body in a posture that expresses some level of reluctance. Then speak in turn:

ALPHA This is ridiculous.
BRAVO Impossible.
CHARLIE Not impossible.
DELTA Possibly ridiculous.
ECHO I won't do it.

SCENE 2

Take several steps toward the center of the room, considering each step a sign of your willingness to engage in asking questions that might not have clear answers. Look to the other four performers and note your relative distances to each other and to the center. Facing the center, speak in turn:

ALPHA   What can a body do?

BRAVO   How do we describe a body?

CHARLIE   Who controls a body?

DELTA   Where does a body begin and end?

ECHO   What is a body?

SCENE 3

Turn to face one of the other performers; it's fine if more than one person is facing the same performer. Pretend that he or she is the only other person in the room, the only one who can hear you. Then speak in turn:

ALPHA   Is your body at full attention? Can your body stand? Can your body sit? Can your body roll back its shoulders? Can your body lift its chin? Can your body come to attention without moving at all?

BRAVO   Are you speaking out loud? Are you speaking loudly? Are you listening for your cue? Are you watching the next move?

CHARLIE   You assume a lot. You assume I can read these words. You assume I can speak them. You assume that reading and speaking will answer the question.

DELTA   I cannot translate from body to body. This body does not do what that body does. That body does not end like this one. This body fights for control with that one.

ECHO   More body! We need more body, not more bodies.

SCENE 4

Get ready to move and take up as much space in the room as feels appropriate. Listen to the words as you speak them. At the end of your line, use your body to demonstrate what you have just said. Go with your first instinct. Ready? Then speak in turn:

ALPHA   To ask, What is *a* body? is different than asking, What is *the* body? A singular body or a template for all bodies? In what spaces? To ask what a body can do is to ask how a body moves in its world. What is it doing? Asking goes like this. [*Alpha demonstrates.*]

BRAVO   To ask for a description of a body is to ask for words, ask for gestures, ask for concepts, which is to ask the brain to think the thoughts, to ask the lips, the hands, the eyes to describe a body by being a body. Asking about a body is impossible without a body. Asking goes like this. [*Bravo demonstrates.*]

CHARLIE   To ask who controls a body is not as simple as it seems. To begin with, "who" might be the wrong question, but you'll never know, so you have to ask.

You also have to ask why and when control matters and if it ever doesn't matter, and still you have to wonder if you would recognize control if it looked you in the eyes or had you by the nape of the neck or kept you off the grass. Asking goes like this. [*Charlie demonstrates.*]

DELTA To ask where a body begins and ends is to ask about another body and another and another. Is a body greater or lesser than another, closer or further away from a center, connected or disconnected or both, and in which directions? You can try to ask about a body, but you are always asking about bodies. Asking goes like this. [*Delta demonstrates.*]

ECHO To ask for more body is to ask for less. I can dance if you tell me how to dance, but I can also dance if you do not. The less you tell me about dancing the more I can dance because I won't know where to end or when to begin. Dancing goes like this. [*Echo demonstrates.*]

SCENE 5

The performers playing Alpha, Bravo, Charlie, and Delta should get ready to use gestures, movements, sounds, and words to express the adjective given below. You may choose whether or not to actually say the word. Echo, moving to face each of the other performers in turn, will respond to each performance with his or her own gestures, movements, sounds, and words. Again, relying on your first instinct, speak in turn:

ALPHA [*awkward*]

    [*Echo responds.*]

BRAVO [*inappropriate*]

    [*Echo responds.*]

CHARLIE [*excessive*]

    [*Echo responds.*]

DELTA [*grotesque*]

    [*Echo responds.*]

SCENE 6

Drop your body to the lowest comfortable level you can reach: this might mean lying on the floor, crouching down, or simply dropping your head or shoulders. Facing the center, speak in turn:

ECHO What did we do here?
DELTA What can a body do?
CHARLIE A body can describe a body.
BRAVO All bodies cannot describe all bodies.
ALPHA We didn't.

    [*The end.*]

You can take time now to discuss your performance, or you could try it again immediately, perhaps with different performers, to see what changes occur. Both performers and audience members might think about what was surprising or confusing or provocative. Consider the difference between reading a text silently and being part of a text as it is performed. How does your body matter?

Many authors write about what "the body" is and does. A recent article by Barbara Browning (2010) particularly inspired this text and reminded me to look again at some of the practitioners and scholars who have challenged my own thinking about the body: Judith Butler (1993, 2006), Jacques Derrida (1998), Mary Douglas (2002), Michel Foucault (1994, 1995), Donna Haraway (1990), and Mary Russo (1994).

Part VI

GENDER AND SEXUALITY

Chapter 19

ADULT INTAKE FORM

ALLAN PETERKIN

W HILE doing research for the textbook, *Caring for Lesbian and Gay People: A Clinical Guide* (Peterkin and Risdon 2003), I asked patients what made them feel welcome or unwelcome in clinical settings. The number one complaint was the "one size fits all" intake forms. Queer people of all stripes found them to be limiting and heterosexist if not downright homophobic. They showed me how almost every question, starting with gender as binary, through marital status (assuming heterosexual marriage when gay marriage is still not a legal option for most), through questions (or a lack thereof) on specific health concerns made them feel invisible, excluded, or shunned. With those many voices in mind—some political, others angry, many funny—I decided to riff off a standardized demographic form. Here are the results.

What's wrong with this form?

ADULT INTAKE FORM

Date: _____ Male/Female ◄─ *That's it?*

Drag name/Porn Name/Name you would choose?

(Birth) Name: _____

Now Ask about My Identity: G LB T T Q Q Not Sure / *Circle one (or several!)* /

Ask if I'm afraid to come out here ☐ In general ☐

Address: _____

Street   City   State   / *Do I have to?* / *Is a state of mind*

Zip Code: _____ Date of Birth: _____ Age: _____

Telephone: _____ (*Don't leave any messages at home—check with me first*)

Home / Work e-mail: _____

You don't let me get married in this state! Give me options → single/ polyamorous/co-habiting/in a domestic partnership/searching!

Marital Status: _____   No. of Children: _____   No. of Pregnancies: _____

Age and Sex of Children: _____

Blood Type: (if known) _____   ← *Red*   *Would like to*

Who referred you: _____

Occupation: _____   *Ask me about work:*

I'm out / not out

Workplace is cool / hostile

Your medical doctor: _____

Doctor's Phone # _____

Is your MD aware you are seeing a specialist? If so, would he/she like a report from us? _____

Emergency contact name and telephone number and relationship: ◄

Will you let my same sex partner make decisions for me in hospital if I'm really sick?

_____

Do you have insurance coverage for our services?

   Yes ☐   No ☐ ◄ *Why am I not covered under my partner's plan?*

Other health care providers: *Now ask me if I trust them!*

1. _____   2. _____   3. _____

Have you received the following:

Naturopathic medicine ☐   Acupuncture ☐   Chiropractic ☐

What are your health concerns, in order of importance to you, and when did you first notice symptoms?

Fear of being bashed on the street

1. _____

Fear of being bullied at school

2. _____

HIV concerns—had a close call

3. _____

Breast cancer

4. _____

5. _Stopping smoking_ _____

p.s. Body Image stuff, too _____

Have you been given a diagnosis for the problem? If so, by whom?

My birth family thinks I'm crazy/sick/sinful _____

If you are female, are your currently pregnant?

Yes ☐   No ☐ ◄—— _Can only females get pregnant? What about FTM?_

Medical History

Today? Assess your general state of health?

Excellent ☐   Good ☐   Fair ☐   Poor ☐

Please indicate any serious conditions, illnesses, or injuries and any hospitalizations, along with approximate dates:

Partner beat me up (didn't report it) = broken arm/heart

_____   _____

_____   _____

All cheap perfume, doctors with an attitude

Do you have any allergies (medicines, environment, etc.)? ◄

_____   _____

_____   _____

Please list current medications (prescription, over-the-counter, vitamins, herbs, homeopathics, etc.): ◄———— _Far too many!_

OTC diet pills, Black market hormones

_____   _____

_____   _____

_____   _____

_____   _____

How many times have you been treated with antibiotics? _____

Do you use any of the following?

Aspirin ☐   Laxatives ☐   Antacids ☐   Diet Pills ☐   _I wish_

Birth control pills ☐   Implants ☐   Injections ☐

2 or 20 (The bar is the only place for us to meet in my own town)

Alcohol—how much per day or week _____

Tobacco—form and amount per day _____

Caffeine—form and amount per day _____

$\left\{\begin{array}{l}\textit{Ask me why: To forget/relax/enjoy sex} \\ \textit{Coke/E/special K/Tina/MJ/other: medical marijuana (not all drugs are fun)}\end{array}\right\}$

Recreational drugs—what and how often _____

Please indicate what immunizations have you had:

☐ DPT (diphtheria, pertussis, tetanus)   ☐ Haemophilus influenza B

☐ Hepatitis A ☐ Hepatitis B   ☐ MMR (measles, mumps, rubella)

☐ Tetanus booster; when? _____   ☐ "Flu" ☐ Smallpox

☐ HPV │ *Why can't guys get the vaccine?* │   ☐ Polio

Other:

   Please indicate if any caused adverse reactions:

_____

│ *HIV/VDRL every year (just in case)* │

   Do you get regular screening tests done by another doctor (*Pap*, blood tests, etc.)

Yes ☐   No ☐   │ *Do lesbians need a Pap? Do FTM?* │

Please list the latest blood work taken: (provide a copy if possible)

_____

│ *How confidential is my file?* │

Have you ever had any dental work done? When? Please describe:

◁ *Just switched—Dentist wouldn't treat my HIV+ roommate*

_____

Diet

Do you have any food allergies or intolerances? Please list. ◁ *Anything fattening* ◁

_____   _____

_____   _____

_____   _____

Do you have any dietary restrictions (religious, vegetarian/vegan, etc.)

│ *Do you binge/purge/restrict/over exercise?* │ ▷   │ *Body fascist* │ ◁

Chapter 20

WHAT IS SEX FOR? OR, THE MANY USES OF THE VAG

ALICE DREGER

T HIS meditation begins at Oprah's feet, for it was there that I found myself sitting when I finally caught up with pop culture's relationship with the vulva.
Or was it with the vagina?

At this point in American culture, lady parts have become so messed up—
verbally, at least—that I should probably start with some definitions. *Vulva* is the
term that describes the typical female external genitalia, which includes the clitoris, the labia minora, the labia majora, and the introitus (i.e., the opening) of the
vagina. Or, as one friend puts it, the vulva is "the little man in the rowboat, with the
big pontoon boat sailing right behind." Although in this case, the pontoon boat has
a biggish hole in the middle, leading to the deep.

At least *vulva* is the term *I* use for the external package because it is the *right
term*, dang it. *Vagina* is the wrong term for a female's external genitalia. *Vagina* is
supposed to refer to one specific organ, what *WebMD* (2011) describes as "an elastic, muscular canal with a soft, flexible lining that provides lubrication and sensation. The vagina connects the uterus to the outside world." (Because, you know,
without the vagina, the uterus wouldn't get out much.)

So I'm sitting at Oprah's feet, and I'm sporting seven layers of eye makeup, four
coats of lipstick, and enough hairspray to keep a flower arrangement fresh for a
year. All because I've been called in as a "medical expert" on intersex. I am actually
a historian of medicine, not a medical doctor, but the producers couldn't find a
clinician who could speak English about sex anomalies, so they tapped me. The
occasion is the *Oprah* "Book Club" meeting on Jeffrey Eugenides's novel *Middlesex* (2001), whose main character, Cal, is born with a sex anomaly, namely 5-alpha
reductase deficiency. Cal appears to be a girl at birth and is raised as such, but
because of the 5-AR deficiency, Cal undergoes a masculinizing puberty, ending up
as a man. Pardon me for skipping the biochemistry lesson here; take my word,
it's rare, but it can happen. In the novel, Cal belongs to the nonfictional Intersex
Society of North America, which at the time of the book's publication was legally
registered to my Michigan address although it was mostly operating out of the California home of Bo Laurent, founder of the group.

Happily, the producers of the show have also invited actual, living, breathing
people born with various disorders of sex development, so they can talk about

what real life is like with sex anomalies and show the world that these folks are—when all is said and done—uh, human. Thoughtful, funny, sympathetic . . . even boring sometimes. Because I am not an affected individual but rather just a professor to whom Oprah only need turn for authoritative-sounding clarity, I'm not on stage but positioned in the audience's second row.

Up on the stage with Oprah is Katie Baratz, then a medical student (now an M.D.), and her mother Arlene, a physician. Yes, it's rather silly to have me as a "medical expert" when there are a highly educated medical student and a physician on stage, but such are the rules of daytime television: medically affected individuals can never be medical experts, or else the audience wouldn't *feel* the critical difference between patients and doctors. In order to maintain the fiction of the dichotomy in this case, the doctors are playing the patients, and the historian is playing the doctor.

Thus, Katie and Arlene are there not for their medical knowledge—which exceeds mine—but because Katie has complete androgen insensitivity syndrome, or cAIS. What this means is that Katie has XY chromosomes and was born with testosterone-producing testes. Pre- and post-natally, her testes put out the usual male-typical hormonal mix, but because her cells lack the receptors to respond to the masculinizing hormones, her body—including her brain—developed before birth mostly along the typical female pathway. With cAIS, there are no ovaries, no uterus, and so no cervix, but girls born with cAIS do have vaginas. Medical texts describe cAIS vaginas as "ending in a blind pouch" on the internal end, wording that always makes me imagine such a vagina as Diogenes, swinging a lamp in search of an honest man, but I think I have Diogenes—who swung the lamp seeking honesty—confused with Tiresias—the blind prophet—and the vagina's needs confused with my own search for an honest man where intersex treatment is concerned. (More on the honesty problem later.)

Meanwhile, development of the external genitalia depends largely on functional levels of androgens (how much the cells perceive). In cAIS, the external genitalia develop as pretty much female-typical: clitoris, labia minora and majora, that is, the little man in boat, and so forth—pretty much the same marina as most girls.

Even though I thought I'd been pretty clear in my descriptions of sex development, Oprah still hadn't grasped the finer points of cAIS. She wanted to ask Katie about her privates—what she had or didn't have—but couldn't quite bring herself to do it. Finally, after a bunch of hemming and hawing, Oprah did it: she asked Katie whether or not she had a "vajayjay."

Okay, so back in 2008, *you* might have known what a "vajayjay" was, but *I* had literally never before heard the term. When Katie laughed and answered, yes, she had a vajayjay, and the audience sort of breathed a big happy sigh of relief (was it relief that Katie had one of these? or relief that no one was going to mention *actual parts?*), my heart began pounding. I was terrified that Oprah would turn to me for an explanation of how Katie could have XY chromosomes and a vajayjay, at which point I would have to confess that *I had no idea what we were talking about.* Sweating profusely, I suddenly became grateful for the hairspray.

Many people think that being on *Oprah* changes your life. But being on *Oprah* changed my life in only two ways:

1 I spent the next six months with a neighborhood dad at the school bus stop telling me, every morning at 8:30 A.M., "You sure don't look as good as you looked on *Oprah*!"
2 After hearing of the "vajayjay," and having my little adrenaline reaction, I became obsessed with people who say "vajayjay" when maybe they mean "vagina" and especially with people who say "vagina" when they probably mean "vulva."

Frankly, it is very messed up not to know the difference between the vulva and the vagina, and even more messed up to use a term that acts like there isn't really a difference. I mean, call me square for not having met the vajayjay at the clubs before Oprah's bouncer ushered me into her green room, but I at least know exactly which organ my baby came out, you know? We in the humanities are supposed to be fascinated and generally cool with language shifts like this—language reveals and shapes human realities; we humanists just watch and provide color commentary—but this was just one language shift I could not abide.

I am not exaggerating when I say I become downright obsessed with this trinity of tragic confusion—vajayjay, vagina, vulva. I became like one of those crazy old people carrying around empty tin cans and newspaper clippings in a ratty bag and yelling at street lights. Only I would wander around yelling at people, "IT'S A VULVA, NOT A VAGINA! STOP CALLING IT A VAGINA!"

Well, not always yelling. I tried to be calm and polite when I had to tell a friend who is not only a sex researcher but also a certified Lothario that he was using the word *vagina* in his professional writing and in his six-hundred student human sexuality class when he actually meant *vulva*.

"Oh, right," he answered. "Well, you know what I mean."

I believe I was equally calm and polite when, as an aside to a history of an anthropological controversy I was working on, I discovered that the well-known anthropologist Napoleon Chagnon had translated a Yanomamö folktale about a man's admiration of a woman's beautiful vagina. I wrote to Chagnon, with whom I had an active correspondence by then: Didn't he mean to translate that as *vulva*? Surely this tribe in South America wasn't actually looking into women's vaginas, something you could only do with a speculum-like tool? He responded that, of course, I was right and that he'd correct the translation to *vulva* in the next edition of his book. (He added that, for once, a feminist had taught him something useful.)

I distinctly remember that I positively strained to remain calm and polite when a medical student of mine who was presenting on African female genital mutilation said something like "For cultural and religious reasons, they cut the vagina."

"Wait, wait, wait," I said, "they cut the *vagina*?"

"Oh, I guess I mean the labia," she answered.

And I think I was sort of calm and polite when I wrote to my friend Dan Savage, the sex advice columnist, complaining about how he let one of his readers talk about her inability to reach orgasm from stimulation of her "vag" without asking her what the heck she meant by *vag*—did she mean her vagina or her clitoris?

Because here's the thing: there are important differences among the various members of the female flotilla, *especially if you want to reach orgasm.*

No matter what Hollywood would have you believe, science shows that the great majority of women cannot reach orgasm through mere vaginal intercourse. Somebody has to engage directly the external part of the clitoris if happy climax is to be reached. Freud attempted to convince the world that clitoral orgasm is immature while vaginal orgasm marks the grown-up lady (Gerhard 2000), a psycho-physiological theory that feminist humanities scholars have reasonably noted is awfully handy for any guy who doesn't want to be bothered with a woman's satisfaction beyond simple penile-vaginal intercourse. ("Wham, bam, thank you, ma'am, and if you didn't enjoy it, *grow up!*") But the truth is that stimulation of a woman's vagina—while often quite satisfying—will not move the earth for the average woman.

In the mid-1990s, as a historian and philosopher of science and medicine encountering modern-day versions of Freud's kind of lame, patriarchal approach to women's sexuality, I became driven to produce extensive criticisms of the contemporary treatment of young girls with sex anomalies (Dreger 1998a). Until recently—until we made progress through the Intersex Society with help from artistic works like Eugenides's—the standard of care within medicine was to shorten girls' "big" clitorises "for social reasons," even though doing so necessarily risked their sexual sensation and potentially also their ability to orgasm. In fact, clinicians historically didn't worry that much about this, wanting merely to stop the clitoris from looking "cosmetically offensive" (Dreger 1998b).

In the early 1990s, when a surgeon from Johns Hopkins was asked, "How do you define successful intercourse [in the population of girls subjected to genitoplasties for 'social reasons']? How many of these girls actually have an orgasm, for example?", the surgeon responded: "Adequate intercourse was defined as successful vaginal penetration" (quoted in Dreger 1998a, 256n32). It's true: in the history of the treatment of girls with atypical genitals, vaginas have been treated simply as lazy receptacles for hard-working penises, and clitoral tissue has been treated as downright disposable. (Bo Laurent's clitoris had been completely excised in the late 1950s, when she was eighteen months old, so offensive was it to her specialist pediatricians [Weil 2006a, 24].) Pediatric surgeons long had a saying that the reason you should make genitally ambiguous children into girls is because, surgically speaking, "you can poke a hole, but you can't build a pole." That's all a vagina is in this scheme—a hole. Here's one group putting it officiously in the medical literature but with the same import: "It is much easier [when a boy is born with a micropenis] to create a vagina as a passive organ than an erectile phallus with sufficient dimension. Therefore the authors suggest that most such infants be reared as females" (quoted in Dreger 1998a, 256n32).

But really? To my mind—and *WebMD* has apparently got my back on this one—the vagina is not just there to entertain the visiting penis any more than the clitoris is at the table merely to be polite or to offend. The vagina is *more* than "what connects the uterus to the outside world"—more than the Verrazano Narrows

Bridge to the uterus's Staten Island. Remember, it's also "an elastic, muscular canal with a soft, flexible lining that provides lubrication and sensation."

So now's probably a good time to confess—although I can hear my husband's voice saying there is never a good time to confess this—that I was thirty years old when I realized I had a vagina. And it wasn't because I didn't know the right names for my parts, and it wasn't because I hadn't used them all.

The year was 1996, the year after I had finished my Ph.D. on the history of the treatment of people labeled *hermaphrodites* in France and Britain in the late nineteenth and early twentieth centuries, and I was busily turning my dissertation into a book. In other words, I'd actually been studying sex anatomy for *years*—four years at that point—at the *doctoral level*. I'd also just married a medical student. (Not coincidentally, he was not a disciple of Freud.)

I was at the University of Minnesota, hired as a one-year sabbatical replacement, and I was hanging out in their medical school's rare book library and looking at texts that I hadn't yet consulted. One day, I took a look at the Johns Hopkins surgeon Hugh Hampton Young's 1937 tome, *Genital Abnormalities, Hermaphroditism, and Related Adrenal Diseases*. And there, on page 64, in figure 43, I came upon it: a sketch of a vagina that had been removed from a man. The accompanying report explained:

P.O., aged 34 years, who was admitted June 19, 1924, had been reared as a boy. At birth the absence of urethra and the presence of a vagina were noted, but there was no doubt that the patient was male. Erections commenced at the age of 12, and since then sexual desire had been normal, although intercourse was never attempted, because of the marked curvature of the penis which was accentuated on erection. The patient desired to marry and came for operative correction of his deformity. His general health and psychology were normal. (Young 1937, 60)

The doctors decided that the patient's request—trying to correct the curvature of his penis and remove his vagina—was perfectly reasonable, and so they obliged. Lots of surgeries and lots of complications (and so more surgeries) later, "The patient married, and on October 23 came here with his bride of a week. They reported that sexual intercourse was satisfactory" (Young 1937, 71).

None of the wording surprised me. By then, I'd met (textually speaking) plenty of men born with vaginas, and I was familiar with the story of the treatment of intersex as a story of heterosexual triumph. That was, after all, why girls needed holes and boys needed poles. What stunned me was the "photo of specimen removed"—a drawing, really, of the excised vagina. Because it was a big, strong organ. *Not an absence of a thing at all, but a real thing in and of itself.* Beefy, strong, substantial—looking rather like a typical penis that way.

I flashed back at the moment to another penis-like vagina, namely the one drawn by the revolutionary anatomist, Vesalius, in the sixteenth century. It, too, looked rather like a penis. In his 1990 book, *Making Sex: Body and Gender from the Greeks to Freud*, Thomas Laqueur claims Vesalius's penis-like vagina as proof that anatomists of his time had a "one sex" model, in which women were just variations on the theme of man. Supposedly by the early twentieth century, we would have been well into the "two sex" model, in which vaginas were no longer viewed like penises, females no longer viewed like males. So why did Hugh Hampton Young's 1937 vagina look so substantial, like a penis? Maybe because both Vesalius and Young saw the vagina as really *something* (a pole), rather than *nothing* (a hole)?

And maybe they were right?

I suddenly realized that, like the contemporary doctors whose work I was sharply criticizing, I had also been thinking of vaginas as holes. I had thought of my own vagina basically as a hole, and I was stunned to see that it could really be so much more than that. Don't get me wrong; I had seen plenty of those neat cutaways of the female anatomy in gynecology offices and biology textbooks, but because they always showed the vagina cut away, what I saw in those pictures was the tunnel going through the vagina—not the *amazing walls.*

I called my husband who was still back in Indiana, finishing his fourth year of medical school.

"Honey!" I exclaimed excitedly, "I have a vagina!"

"Yes, dear," he answered. "I know. I've been there."

"But seriously!" I responded, and I went on to tell him about how exciting the vagina really is, and how interesting it was that, for me—for Johns Hopkins University!—to really see the vagina as a something and not as a nothing, the vagina had to show up in a man.

"I think," I said to him, confusing us both, "in the medical management of intersex, only men have vaginas. Women have holes in which to put penises. But when a man has a vagina, it's a *real organ*—albeit one that has to come out."

And so, at age thirty, just short of halfway into my sexual life, I began to really appreciate my vagina and to insist that all my girlfriends realize that they, too, *had vaginas.* Muscular, innervated, fleshy, self-lubricating objects of wonder! I mean, I didn't describe them that way, I just said, "We have vaginas!"

Which, of course, now makes me wonder if they thought I was talking about vulvas.

Maybe now you can understand why it is that I have never seen a production of Eve Ensler's (2001) *The Vagina Monologues.* I am truly afraid that, were I to see it, and a woman were to read the monologue called "Hair"—"He made me shave my vagina" (2001, 9)—or someone were to mention "a huge vagina cake" that has a clitoris (2001, xxix)—well, I'm just afraid that I would stand up and scream, "IT'S A VULVA! STOP CALLING IT A VAGINA!" I might actually scream, "EVE ENSLER, HANDS OFF MY VAG!"

But really. It's disturbing that so many putative feminists—like the medical student in my class—blithely refer to the *vag* or even the *vagina* when what they really mean is the clitoris, or the clitoris with the labia, or what have you. Why on earth would you go and lump them all together in one vague word that indicates you don't really care about each part? Why would you not be as disturbed as I am when you come upon a current-day advertisement from the Pediatric Urology Clinics of Weill Cornell Medical College (2011), whose website claims (without any evidence) that "female patients are able to undergo a more natural psychological and sexual development when they have a more normal appearing vagina [*sic*]"?

Shouldn't we care that a surgical clinic is going to mess with a little girl's clitoris while calling it her vagina?

Listen, I get what Ensler is trying to achieve in *The Vagina Monologues*. I admire her efforts (see also Bell and Reverby 2005). I realize *vag* and all the other supposedly cute nicknames for our packages are supposed to function like terms of endearment. But I hear them as terms of estrangement.

The standard of care emerging after 1950 in the United States held that it was best not to tell people who were born with sex anomalies and had had childhood genital surgery for social reasons about their real diagnoses, about their real medical histories. As late as 1995, the Canadian Medical Association handed out a cash prize to a medical student who argued that it was more ethical to lie to a woman born with a Y chromosome than to tell her the truth (Dreger 1998a). It is impossible for me not to feel as if a cultural system in which we cannot speak clearly about the clitoris, the vagina, the vulva, and the labia minora and majora—but must instead only voice them all as "vagina" or, worse, as the drunken howl "vajayjay"— is a system in which people who are born just a little too different will continue being changed, deceived, and hidden for our sake.

I presume that, by this point, I don't have to explain to you why I am completely creeped out by labiaplasties and vaginoplasties advertised to perfectly typical women who are sold on the idea that they need to look prettier down there. Rather than backing off on "normalizing" children with benign genital variation, we're headed in the other direction, convincing ordinary men and women that they're freakishly in need of surgery, making everyone intersex—not in the good way, but in the way that demands correction.

Many approaches in the medical/health humanities make what appears clear, fuzzier—what seems real, more tentative. But I think that the medical/health humanities also hold the potential to do something even more interesting—to suggest that, in medicine, we've missed some key realities. To point to roads not taken. I think about looking anew at Vesalius's vagina and matching it up with Young's vagina as I work on using the history of medicine to show physicians the shocking paucity of data to support their assumption that ambiguous genitalia left alone cause psychosocial problems, I'm struck by a beautiful possibility: that maybe one of the things the humanities can do is to give us back our biology in medicine.

I went on *Oprah* when our son was eight, which means that he has spent the last three years listening to me complain about people saying *vagina* when they mean *vulva*. A few months ago, when my son was still ten, he asked me, within earshot of my husband, "What does a vulva look like?" I thought about how to find a picture to show him. Porn was out, obviously, as were all of the modern medical texts that sliced the woman in half, as if she were an architectural model meant to allow you to appreciate how her staircase sweeps up from her living room. My son didn't want a cross-section view; he wanted to know what the vulva looked like straight on. I was stumped.

Finally, my mate suggested something helpful: "How about Dickinson's *Atlas of Human Sex Anatomy*?" (Dickinson 1949).

I went to our living room, to our own collection of old medical books, and pulled out that big volume of medical drawings of the naughty bits from 1949. I first showed my son one of the coolest things about Dickinson, the thing that had made Bo Laurent gift this book to me: he has tracings showing the various sizes and shapes of penises and clitorises he has come across. Marvelous variation, visually presented as if the variation is perfectly normal.

Then we turned to Dickinson's drawings of vulvas. These are highly naturalistic sketches, showing rather typical vulvas—hairy here and there, asymmetrical, complex. Dickinson shows what a grown-up, furry vulva looks like both ordinarily (usually not much to see with the labia touching) and then when one pulls the lips apart. I pointed out to my son the various parts of the vulva, naming them specifically, reminding my son that the clitoris is the same organ developmentally as the penis, and the labia majora are the homologue to the scrotum.

All of this got me thinking about what sex education is for. I had already decided, before I pulled out Dickinson, that the education I gave my son about sex would not be for me—not to satisfy me in an attempt to prevent his making the same stupid sexual mistakes as his mother, not to result in his making grandchildren for me, not even to make me proud of him as a sexually progressive, well-educated person. And the sex education he got from me would certainly not be for the heterosexual order; there would be no implicit lessons about how sex must be about monogamous, opposite-sex, long-term bonding. The sex ed he got from me would be whatever he needed it to be to feel comfortable with himself. I wasn't going to leave him baffled as I was by having a childhood sex education that consisted mostly of Mr. Rogers singing, "Boys are fancy on the outside, girls are fancy on the inside." (Besides, I don't think Mr. Rogers could have been a very good lover if he believed that song.)

This, then, got me thinking about a question I'd been mulling since long before our son came across my Verrazano Narrows Bridge: what is sex for? I don't mean sexual intercourse. I mean sex—as in the parts that make us male or female or specifically in between. Our sex parts have been used for so much: to prove power, to derive pleasure, to reproduce, to secure kinship, to glorify God, sexism, heterosexism, women's liberation, feminism, nationhood—even innate white moral supremacy.

Inevitably, this got me to the question I never know how to answer, the question that I think is at the center of the medical/health humanities: What is medicine for?

And what should medicine do with sex?

If medicine got up anew to dance with sex, and sex knew the names of its parts and could even draw them from memory—correctly—what might be conceived instead?

Chapter 21

"I ALWAYS PREFER THE SCISSORS"
Isaac Baker Brown and Feminist Histories of Medicine

MARJORIE LEVINE-CLARK

I N his now infamous text, *On the Curability of Certain Forms of Insanity, Epilepsy, Catalepsy, and Hysteria in Females* (1866), the Victorian gynecologist Isaac Baker Brown detailed the removal of the clitoris as his preferred method of treatment for the female "nervous diseases" specified in the title. In the introduction, weaving between scientific "objectivity" and his own subjectivity, Baker Brown expounds on his method: "When I have decided that my patient is a fit subject for surgical treatment, I at once proceed to operate. . . . The patient having been placed *completely* under the influence of chloroform, the clitoris is freely excised either by scissors or knife—I always prefer the scissors" (Baker Brown [hereafter BB] 1866, 17; emphasis in original).

Isaac Baker Brown used the scissors on at least forty-eight female patients in the 1850s and 1860s. His *Curability* and the medical community's reaction to it have provided an opportunity for scholars to explore questions concerning medical ethics, professionalization, and, especially, ideas about women's bodies and female sexuality in Victorian Britain. The very outrageousness of the text to late twentieth- and twenty-first-century sensibilities has made it an object of medical fascination and feminist anger. While we cannot help being astonished by the connections Baker Brown drew between female sexual organs and diseases like epilepsy, the astonishment is not enough: we need to understand why and in what context he came up with his ideas and practices.

Feminist histories of medicine emerged at the intersection of the women's liberation movement and a broadening of the discipline of history in the last third of the twentieth century. While "traditional" history in general and the history of medicine in particular tended to focus on powerful people, prominent institutions, big events, and groundbreaking processes, the development of social and cultural history expanded the purview of what we consider historically important, inquiring into everyday lives, social inequalities, and cultural assumptions. Historians of medicine long celebrated a progress narrative where great individuals and significant discoveries brought us out of the Dark Ages and into the modern world of scientific medicine. Social and cultural historians of medicine began to ask different questions: about patients' perspectives, the meanings of symptoms in their cultural contexts, patient-practitioner encounters, the role of medicine in understandings of social differences, and medical contributions to our sociocultural expectations and norms (Porter and Porter 1988; A. Wear 1992; see also Porter and Bynum 1993).

A central argument in this regard is that categories like gender and sexuality indeed *have* histories. Rather than seeing gender and sexuality as fixed elements of a static nature, scholars investigate their changeability and the ways that different historical contexts have constructed different practices, beliefs, and meanings surrounding gender and sex (Clark 2008; Porter and Hall 1995). Feminist histories of medicine uncover the ways in which medical systems have informed ideologies of sexuality and gender, ideologies that often privilege men, masculinity, and heterosexuality (Russett 1989; Schiebinger 1989; Showalter 1985). While historians are prominent in this literature, a wide variety of scholars and activists have used historical approaches as a means to emphasize the constructed nature of gender and sexuality and the possibility of change.

In this chapter, Baker Brown's text provides a window through which we can look at relationships among medicine, gender, sexuality, and history. I explore the context that produced a gynecological surgeon who so nonchalantly articulated his preference for scissors in performing a useless operation on numerous female patients. I then offer a critical reading of Baker Brown's *Curability* itself. Finally, I examine scholarship relative to Baker Brown, which highlights the centrality of medical understandings of gender and sexuality to feminist histories and politics.

THE CONTEXT

As scholars such as Londa Schiebinger and Thomas Laqueur argue, when in the eighteenth century liberal political theory opened up possibilities to challenge inequalities based on custom, men of science drew on the evidence of the body to elaborate new gendered and racial boundaries that would reinforce old hierarchies (Laqueur 1990, 151–153; Schiebinger 1989, 214–216). Medical ideas lent crucial support for what historians have labeled the ideology of separate spheres and the related ideology of domesticity. This belief system held that men and women were complementary beings: men were strong, active, rational, productive, and suited to the public sphere of politics, commerce, and education; women were weak, passive, emotional, reproductive, and suited to childbearing and rearing in the domestic sphere of hearth and home (Schiebinger 1989, 215–227; Steinbach 2004, 11–12, 42–43). Beliefs about female sexual desire were also tied to these social expectations: respectable women of the middle classes were not supposed to reveal sexual desire independent of motherhood, but it was assumed that less-respectable women, like libertine aristocrats, working-class women, and prostitutes, had an aggressive sexuality (Clark 2008; Nead 1988). Of course, large gaps existed between ideology and practice, especially for the masses of women who could not afford to obey the supposed constraints of their bodies and who had to work for survival (Levine-Clark 2004). Identifying these gaps between prescriptive discourses and the realities of people's practices has been an important project undertaken by historians of gender and sexuality.

The same historical moment in which domestic ideology was taking hold also saw the emergence of obstetrics and gynecology as a respectable medical field. The medical historian Ornella Moscucci argues that the professionalization of gynecology "crystallized deeply-held beliefs about the instinctual, pathological, and primitive nature of femininity" (1993, 60). This "hystericization of women's bodies," as Michel Foucault describes it in *History of Sexuality*, made women into patients who needed medical practitioners (Foucault 1980, 104). Nineteenth-century medical texts emphasized that their reproductive and sexual organs determined women's physical and mental well-being, compelling women to walk an egregiously thin line between health and illness, sanity and insanity (Digby 1989; Moscucci 1993; Poovey 1986; Showalter 1985).

Isaac Baker Brown practiced obstetrics and gynecology at a time when increasing numbers of women were bristling against the expectations of these domestic and sexual ideologies. Movements to improve opportunities for women's education and employment, challenge marriage laws, and demand the suffrage for women grew from the 1850s (Steinbach 2004, 245–285). Opponents of women's expanded rights and roles used medical evidence to assert their cases, and doctors themselves participated actively in debates on the "woman question" (Rowold 1996, xviii–xix). For example, prominent psychiatrist Henry Maudsley argued that women who devoted energy to educating themselves damaged their reproductive responsibilities by diverting that energy away from their reproductive functions to their brains (Russett 1989, 116–125; Showalter 1985, 125). Claiming that women "unsexed" themselves by challenging their "natural" domestic roles (Showalter 1985, 123), doctors used women's very lack of education to justify female dependence on medical practitioners while arguing that women's bodies unfitted them for serious knowledge (Rowold 1996; Russett 1989).

Feminist scholars and medical practitioners alike have been drawn to Isaac Baker Brown as an extreme example of Victorian medical ideas about women's health. Baker Brown's story has been recounted many times: he was a well-known, respected obstetrician and gynecologist in Victorian Britain. As both a co-founder of St. Mary's Hospital and later as founder of his own London Surgical Home for Women, Baker Brown developed significant gynecological surgery procedures and in 1854 published an important study, *Surgical Diseases of Women*. In 1865, he was elected president of the Medical Society of London (Black 1997, 403; Dally 1991; Sheehan 1981, 10).

Clearly feeling comfortable in his professional position, Baker Brown published *Curability* in 1866, revealing the clitoridectomies he had been performing since 1858 to cure a variety of women's "nervous diseases," which he believed were caused by masturbation. As a result of these revelations, however, he was barraged with hostile responses from his profession, most particularly from the powerful *British Medical Journal*. His colleagues accused him of failing to obtain patient consent and of lacking evidence that his "results" could actually be attributed to the removal of the clitoris (Black 1997, 404–405). Many were distressed that Baker Brown called too much attention to masturbation, inciting "non-medical persons to ponder indelicate questions" (Porter and Hall 1995, 147). In April 1867, Baker

Brown was called before the Obstetrical Society of London in order to convince colleagues of the efficacy of his operation. He failed. The society expelled him, and, eventually disgraced, Baker Brown was forced to rely on charity for his survival. He died shortly after his professional downfall (Sheehan 1981, 13–15).

In recounting this story, scholars have emphasized that professional jealousy, as much as issues surrounding medicine itself, was at the heart of the attacks on Baker Brown. Indeed, other British gynecologists practiced clitoridectomy, and even more practiced ovariotomy. Elizabeth Sheehan has observed that, "while condemning Brown's operation, few doctors disputed his contention that female emotional disorder was based on genital disfunction. Brown's particular methods were slurred at the same time that accepted medical theory of the period supported the widespread practice of ovariotomy as a cure for hysteria" (1981, 13). Such operations were even more prevalent in the United States (Barker-Benfield 1978). Thus, while Baker Brown may have been extreme in his approaches to women's health, he was certainly on a continuum with his colleagues. The context that emphasized the centrality of reproductive and sexual processes to women's health made clitoridectomy as a treatment for systemic diseases plausible.

THE TEXT

To analyze primary sources—materials from the era under study—historians rely both on related primary sources and secondary sources—the existing scholarly literature on the subject. The goal is to develop a relationship between text and context, to situate a document (written, visual, oral) in its historical moment. My interpretation of Baker Brown's text draws on the Victorian medical and social understandings of gender that I have just described, a context in which medical authority was growing, in which expertise in women's health was rooted in claims about the reproductive body, and in which women were recognized as patients but not as practitioners.

The very title of his work, *On the Curability of Certain Forms of Insanity, Epilepsy, Catalepsy, and Hysteria in Females*, points to Baker Brown's assumptions about the gendered nature of mental and nervous illness. The ailments he discusses in the book were only a small group of those to which women were considered susceptible. As he states in his introduction: "I do not intend to occupy the attention of my readers with all the numerous varieties of insanity and other nervous disorders to which females are liable, but only those which I believe to be curable by surgical means" (BB, 3). That Baker Brown, a gynecological surgeon, published a book about female nervous diseases immediately suggests the taken-for-granted links between female sexual and reproductive processes and women's mental health. Women, as women, were "liable" to "numerous" nervous troubles that gynecologists, as experts on women's bodies, had the potential to cure through sometimes invasive procedures targeting reproductive and sexual organs.

Baker Brown appeals to his experience of observing women's bodies to support his claim that "a large number of affections peculiar to females, depended on loss of nerve power, and that this was produced by peripheral irritation, arising originally in some branches of the pudic nerve, more particularly the incident nerve supplying the clitoris" (BB, 7). With this, Baker Brown presents his central hypothesis: masturbation—the "irritation" of the clitoris—causes hysteria, epilepsy, catalepsy, and eventually mania and death. To prove the seriousness of his argument, Baker Brown cites one of his cases in which a nineteen-year-old under treatment "was found dead, with every evidence of having expired during a paroxysm of abnormal excitement" (BB, 8). In this instance, orgasm most plainly equals death.

In order to contain the tide of disease brought on by "irritation" of the clitoris, Baker Brown presents the seemingly logical solution: eliminate the offending organ. He counters objections that clitoridectomy results in "unsexing the female, preventing the normal excitement consequent on marital intercourse, or actually, as some most absurdly and unphilosophically assert, causing sterility" (BB, 9–10). Rather, clitoridectomy was a means to transform masturbators into "happy and useful members of the community," to enhance "the well-being of the whole human race" (BB, 13).

Victorian medical men were rather obsessed with masturbation, connecting it to a wide variety of ailments (Porter and Hall 1995, 138–152). For men, doctors railed against the loss of vital energy through the wasteful spilling of semen. For women, masturbation connoted a range of behaviors that challenged expectations regarding feminine character and behavior. It indicated an active, solitary sexuality, calling into question dominant theories about women's sexuality or at least middle-class, white women's sexuality, which envisioned female desire solely connected to motherhood and dependent upon marital union.

Baker Brown uses the connections between gendered social roles and female sexuality throughout his text. While it does not appear that patients came to his clinic worried about masturbatory habits, Baker Brown was quick to diagnose "peripheral irritation" as the source of their troubles. He points to social behaviors and physical signs to identify patients whose problems would be solved by clitoridectomy. For example, Baker Brown indicates his ability to recognize a girl or young woman made nervous through chronic masturbation, as she would be "listless and indifferent to the social influences of domestic life" (BB, 14). She would show "a great disposition for novelties" and a desire "to escape from home" (BB, 15). He lists a variety of physical "affections" to go along with these social transgressions, focusing particularly on menstrual irregularities (BB, 15). Married women additionally suffered from "a distaste for marital intercourse and very frequently, either sterility or a tendency to abort in the early months of pregnancy" (BB, 16). Social and behavioral symptoms were confirmed by examination of the genitalia, which would reveal signs of "peripheral irritation" obvious to Baker Brown. These included "peculiar straight and hirsute growth [of the pubic hair]; the depression in the centre of the perinaeum; the peculiar follicular secretion; the alteration of structure of the parts, mucous membrane taking on the character of skin; and muscle having become hypertrophied and generally tending towards a fibrous or cartilaginous degeneration" (BB, 16). Any or all of these signs led Baker Brown to recommend clitoridectomy.

Once he performed his "usual operation," Baker Brown expected a full recovery in about a month. He gloated that "the rapid improvement of the patient immediately after the removal of the source of the irritation is most marked; first, in the countenance, and soon afterwards by improved digestion and other evidences of healthy assimilation" (BB, 18). Assimilation here clearly had both social and physiological meanings, as his cases reveal. Post-surgery, patients no longer exhibited symptoms of hysteria, paralysis, tumors, spinal irritation, fits, or whatever ailment had existed when they were presented to Baker Brown. Not only were bodily processes restored to their proper working order but so, too, were social functions—Baker Brown reported that his post-operative patients got married, got pregnant, resumed relations with their husbands, and other behaviors that assured readers of the significant role clitoridectomy could play in maintaining proper gender and sexual relations.

For Baker Brown, evidence of cure was specific to a woman's "station and opportunities" (BB, 15). The success of the operation on married women relied on whether the patient could adapt to her wifely role. In Case III, Baker Brown relates the situation of a thirty-three-year-old patient who, although she had been married for three years, "has had no children" and "has always had distaste for marital intercourse" (BB, 22). Whether it was the patient or her husband who related this information is unclear. Post-operatively, the patient became pregnant, and Baker Brown commented: "This was the first case of this nature under my care, in which the patient, formerly sterile, became pregnant after removal of the cause of her illness" (BB, 23). A case from 1862 described a woman on the verge of insanity. She, too, was married—for twelve years—without pregnancy. Her husband told Baker Brown that his wife would become violent during her menstrual periods: "she would fly at him and rend his skin, like a tigress." Yet after the operation, she "became in every respect a good wife" (BB, 30). While it may be obvious to twenty-first-century readers to question whether these women were in unhappy marriages or unprepared for sexual experiences, Baker Brown and other practitioners of his era looked to gynecological explanations to find a "cure" for these women's "diseases."

A particularly interesting case from 1863 concerns a married woman who, according to Baker Brown, suffered from mental disturbances that "caus[ed] her to have [such] a great distaste for her husband" that she refused to live with him (BB, 84). The operation was a "success"—the woman "returned to her husband, resumed cohabitation, and stated that all her distaste had disappeared; soon became pregnant, resumed her place at the head of her table, and became a happy and healthy wife and mother" (BB, 84). Baker Brown was so impressed by this result that he wrote: "From observations of this case, one feels compelled to say, may it not be typical of many others where there is a judicial separation of husband and wife, with all the attendant domestic miseries, and where, if medical and surgical treatment were brought to bear, all such unhappy measures would be obviated?" (BB, 84). This seems the most glaring evidence of medicalization in Baker Brown's text: the social problem of women seeking separation and maintenance from their husbands could be solved through surgical intervention. It was the clitoris, not the circumstances, that led a woman to leave her husband.

Baker Brown considered married women cured if they adapted to their domestic and reproductive roles. Single women's cures were measured by a consequent post-operative marriage or, if working-class, an ability to return to work. Baker Brown saw a servant in 1860 who had fits during her menstrual periods and could not keep a job. He proceeded to cut the clitoris "down to the base," and within six months she returned to service (BB, 43). In 1863, Baker Brown treated a "young lady" of twenty who exhibited symptoms including "almost constant menorrhagia, during which time she had suffered great irritability of temper, been disobedient to her mother's wishes, and had sleepless nights, restless desire for society, and was constantly seeking admiration . . . culminating in a monomania that every gentleman she admired was in love with her" (BB, 37). Having determined that the woman suffered from "no organic disease," Baker Brown "quickly discovered that all these symptoms arose from peripheral excitement," which led to "the usual plan of treatment." Shortly thereafter, the patient made plain her cure by getting married and becoming pregnant (BB, 37).

How did Baker Brown's patients react to their diagnoses and treatments? One of the challenges historians face is uncovering patient perspectives in sources like case histories in which patient experiences are translated by the practitioner or assistant taking the case (see Levine-Clark 2004, 77–83; Risse and Warner 1992). When Baker Brown does give his patients a voice, it is mostly to confirm his own representation of their "problems" and to affirm how much better their lives are after the operation. He recorded that one woman, for example, said "she feels a different being, and is quite astonished at her own improvement" (BB, 31). Another "expressed herself as not having been so well for many years" (BB, 25). Baker Brown reported that seven months after an operation in 1861, "I received a letter from this lady, stating that she now suffered no pain and was perfectly well . . . better in every respect than she had been for the last twelve years" (BB, 36). It is difficult to know what to make of this material. On the one hand, we can be skeptical of the opinions of the women still in the clinic; Baker Brown might have asked them how they were feeling, and they gave expected answers. On the other, the letter writing suggests some reflection. In a rare glimpse of a patient's perspective, one case indicates that, after the operation, the patient complained to Baker Brown's son (also a doctor) that his father "had unsexed her." Her husband was pleased, however, as Baker Brown reported that the husband returned to the clinic "many weeks later to express his gratitude for the complete restoration of his wife to health" (BB, 70).

Baker Brown also mentions when patients "admitted" to their masturbatory practices: "acknowledges great and constant irritation of pudic nerve" (BB, 62) and "acknowledges to frequent injurious habits, but is unconscious of their being the cause of her illness" (BB, 64). One married woman was "anxious to be cured of her attacks, of the cause of which she is fully conscious," while another "confirmed my opinion of the cause of her attacks" (BB, 46). In a case obviously written by a third person, the transcriber noted that "Mr. Baker Brown ascertained both from [the patient's] mother and herself, that she had long indulged in self-excitation of the clitoris, having first been taught by a school-fellow" (BB, 52). Here, too, some patients may have felt compelled to provide Baker Brown with the information he wanted; alternatively, some may simply not have understood what he was asking.

MEDICINE, FEMINISM, AND HISTORY

Feminist scholars have been drawn to texts like Baker Brown's to demonstrate the patriarchal nature of Western medicine, to highlight the victimization of women by male physicians and surgeons, and to challenge biological explanations of the differences between men and women that emphasize women's natural inferiority. The women's history that first emerged with the women's liberation movement of the 1960s and 1970s was closely interwoven with histories of medicine. Feminists in Europe and the United States pointed directly to the impact of a male-dominated medical profession on women's private and professional lives and made the women's health movement a central part of women's liberation. Self-help books such as *Our Bodies, Our Selves* aimed to aid women in reclaiming their bodies from what was seen as a hostile takeover by male practitioners, who, from the eighteenth century, usurped women's roles as midwives and healthcare givers and convinced the well-to-do that reproductive processes needed medical intervention (Schiebinger 1989, 102–112).[1]

Feminist authors marshaled history to argue that this process was dangerous for women's health. As Barbara Ehrenreich and Deirdre English write in a well-known 1973 pamphlet: "It is no accident that the women's liberation movement today puts so much emphasis on health and 'body' issues. Women are dependent on the medical system for the most basic control over their own reproductivity. At the same time, women's encounters with the medical system bring them face to face with sexism in its most unmistakably crude and insulting forms" (7). Ehrenreich and English additionally argue that the medical profession benefited financially from the Victorian "myth of female frailty," which was in its interest to maintain (23). This construction of women's health supported both a male-dominated medical profession as well as a male-dominated society.

Sexual surgery has a central role in feminist critiques of medicine's past and present. As Ehrenreich and English write, "If a woman's entire personality was dominated by her reproductive organs, then gynecological surgery was the most logical approach to any female psychological problem . . . and was undoubtedly effective at keeping certain women . . . in their place" (1973, 34–36). In a study originally published in 1976, G. J. Barker-Benfield makes a very similar point: "Excision of the clitoris (clitoridectomy) and extirpation of the ovaries (female castration; also called oophorectomy and normal ovariotomy) were two out of an array of new gynecological operations. Gynecologists' case histories are suffused with male anxieties over, and attempts to deal with, women out of their place" (1978, 21). These early feminist interpretations argue that, through practices like clitoridectomy, Victorian medicine as a profession was complicit in maintaining separate spheres and women's inferiority.

Isaac Baker Brown himself features in several analyses examining the medical profession's role in defining gender and sexuality. In line with the general feminist critique of medicine, one strand of interpretation stresses the control of women through control of their sexuality as the key to understanding Baker Brown. Literary critic Elaine Showalter's *Female Malady* (1985) is a major text in this regard. According to Showalter,

clitoridectomy has a symbolic meaning that makes it central to our understanding of sexual difference in the Victorian treatment of insanity. Clitoridectomy is the surgical enforcement of an ideology that restricts female sexuality to reproduction. The removal of the clitoris eliminates the woman's sexual pleasure, and it is indeed this autonomous sexual pleasure that Baker Brown defined as the symptom, perhaps the essence, of female insanity. . . . With their sexuality excised, his patients gave up their independent desires and protests, and become docile child-bearers. (76–77)

Of the women on whom Baker Brown operated, Showalter writes: "His patients seem to have been unusually sensitive to the hypocrisy and repressiveness of Victorian social codes. . . . The mutilation, sedation, and psychological intimidation of . . . deviant and unladylike women seems to have been an efficient, if brutal, form of reprogramming" (1985, 76). In Ann Dally's 1991 *Women under the Knife: A History of Surgery*, Baker Brown appears in a chapter tellingly titled "Mutilation." Identifying herself as a "practising doctor and psychiatrist," Dally writes: "The clitoris symbolized the aspect of women that men could arouse but not control. Uncontrollable, unconforming women seemed to threaten men and aroused intense anxiety in many, as they still do today" (ix, 163). Both Showalter and Dally see Baker Brown's patients as social resistors whose masturbatory practices stood for a wide range of nonconformist impulses; sexual surgery controlled women by excising their rebellion.[2]

The historian of medicine Moscucci has argued strenuously against feminist interpretations of clitoridectomy that stress Baker Brown's and other doctors' fear of female sexuality and their efforts to repress it. According to Moscucci, Baker Brown was not attempting to erase female sexual desire; rather he was channeling it toward marital heterosexuality, an argument my reading of Baker Brown's text supports. By examining gender and sexuality together with race and class, Moscucci offers a more nuanced feminist reading of Baker Brown's theories and practices. She argues that a prominent or enlarged clitoris had become a common marker to the Victorian medical community of blackness and criminality—observed in African "Hottentot" women as well as British prostitutes—and was, therefore, dangerous. It was not female sexuality per se that was problematic: "Sexual pleasure in women was pathological and socially problematic if it was the result of solitary, homosexual, or promiscuous sexual activity, healthy and socially constructive if it was pursued within the context of the marital relationship" (1993, 71). In this way, systems of gender and sexuality were linked: marital heterosexuality dictated a woman's social and sexual roles.

In another strand of interpretation, several scholars have used Baker Brown's history to complicate contemporary European and American thinking about female genital mutilation (FGM). Like veiling and child marriage, FGM has been a flashpoint in feminist debates about the role of Western women in the gender and sexual politics of non-Western nations. More often than not, FGM is held up as one "proof" of the primitiveness of certain parts of the world and the need for Western intervention to "rescue" victimized women. Anthropologists and physicians of the "West" alike have looked at Baker Brown as a way to challenge the "barbarism" of African traditions, noting, in the words of the physician John Black, that "we should reflect that it is not long since our attitudes to female sexuality and mental and physical disease in women gave rise, mainly in Britain and USA, to the subjection of ill or mentally disturbed women to clitoridectomy as a cure for their symptoms" (1997, 402). In an article in *Medical Anthropology Quarterly*, the well-known anthropologist Nancy Scheper-Hughes mentions that while "male clitoriphobia . . . is found in Africa, it is *also* found on London's Harley Street [known for its concentration of medical offices]" (1991, 26). Similarly, the anthropologist Elizabeth Sheehan notes that while Victorians used the supposed "primitiveness" of places like India and Africa to define their own sense of civilized superiority, "British gynecological medicine of the mid-nineteenth century was engaging in practices equally strange, certainly at least as 'unscientific,' and clearly ritual in nature" (1981, 10).

These are points well taken and certainly call into question the steady progress narrative that had dominated histories of medicine for so long. Yet I would also like to highlight a significant difference in the above analyses. Black relies on Baker Brown's case histories to determine women's status as "ill" or "mentally disturbed," and later in his paper he refers to the patients as "clearly hysterical" (1997, 404). These categories themselves, however, have been called into question by feminist scholars, who, pointing to texts like *Curability*, argue that the nineteenth-century nervous diseases themselves are culturally constructed. Hysteria, for example, from the physician's perspective, seemed to show up "in young women who were especially rebellious" (Showalter 1985, 145). Illness and the defiance of gender and sexual norms, as we have seen in Baker Brown's text, could be conveniently and persuasively conflated. Showalter and Carroll Smith-Rosenberg have explored whether, from the patient's perspective, hysteria was an expression of women's dissatisfaction with domestic ideology, "a mode of protest for women deprived of other social or intellectual outlets or expressive options" (Showalter 1985, 147; Smith-Rosenberg 1986, 207–211). To reproduce uncritically the illness categories used by late nineteenth-century doctors runs the risk of accepting diagnostic frameworks that were weighted with their historically situated cultural baggage of sex and gender.

CONCLUSION

Because Isaac Baker Brown's use of clitoridectomy seems so shocking to us now, analysis of his text makes it easy to highlight the ways his cultural assumptions about gender and sexuality influenced his ideas. Sometimes, however, these assumptions are not so obvious either historically or in current medical systems. Feminist histories of medicine have worked to uncover these assumptions with the hope of creating more humane and inclusive institutions and practices. Asking how cultural norms regarding gender and sexuality inform our medical models,

feminist histories of medicine, such as the ones I have examined, provide important evidence for opening the medical profession to women practitioners, for
questioning historical understandings of women's health "problems," and for articulating more general dissatisfaction with male-dominated institutions from which
women were excluded.

While the feminist medical histories of the 2000s are perhaps less overtly politicized than those of the 1970s, the work they do analyzing structures of power surrounding gender, sexuality, race, and class in medical theory and practice continues
to be significant. Feminist studies have been at the forefront of challenging notions
of objectivity in science and medicine, carefully detailing the ways that cultural
assumptions about gender have not only affected women's and men's experiences
but also the ways that the professions of science and medicine have developed.
Although it is a commonplace now to call attention to the manner in which science
and medicine are embedded in and not outside of culture, studies of the medical
construction of women's health and the medical treatment of women were some of
the early historical works to make this point particularly clear.

NOTES

1   First published in 1973 by the Boston Women's Health Book Collective, the ninth edition
of *Our Bodies, Our Selves* was published in 2011.
2   In 2006, a leading gynecologist gave a lecture to the London Medical Society comparing
historical and contemporary views of female sexuality very much in the tradition of these
interpretations, drawing on Baker Brown's story and using phrases like "horror of female
sexuality" and "assaults on the female genitalia" (Studd 2007, 674).

Chapter 22

COMICS IN THE
HEALTH HUMANITIES

A New Approach to Sex and Gender Education

SUSAN M. SQUIER

It's important to remember that these first editions [of *Our Bodies, Our Selves*] were not a book but course material to be used in a group for discussion. They were never considered a finished product. . . . It was very open and forward looking. There was a sense of "there's always another way to look at it."

KATHY DAVIS (2008, 23)

IN 2006, about forty years after the Boston Women's Health Book Collective published *Our Bodies, Our Selves* (1973) a "Think Tank on Emergent Paradigms in Women's Health" took place at the University of Toronto Medical Center. Organized by neuroscientist Gillian Einstein and philosopher Margret Shildrick, the meeting addressed the fact that "the practice of women's health [had] become a jumble of biomedical expectations, reproductive health politics, and surveillance of conditions more common in women" (2009, 294).

Einstein and Shildrick hoped the meeting would encourage the development of a more complex understanding of health and illness and a fuller account of the way that biomedical technologies were shaping our embodied experiences. They urged the physicians and scholars present to draw on feminist theory and philosophy to move the field of women's health beyond "medicine as usual": as institutionalized, as taught, and as practiced. Participants shared analyses of the current state of women's health care, described emerging techniques in tissue engineering, discussed new findings in immunology, and debated contemporary reinterpretations of scientific data. Despite the diversity of the participants—clinicians, biologists, feminist theorists, and science studies scholars—a consensus statement was reached at the end of the meeting: "Anyone who seeks to focus on the wellbeing of the body—bioscientist, clinician, theoretician—must do so from a more integrated interpretive stance that involves *contingency, complexity, collaboration, and conversation*" (2009, 299). This consensus statement and the core principles it affirms provide the context for the phenomenon this essay addresses: the emergence of comics as a medium for sex education.[1]

Consider how medical students and residents were once taught about sexuality.

In 1968, the first elective evening lecture series in human sexuality was offered at Indiana University in response to a request from the entire second-year class of medical students to the dean (Tyler 1970). The focus of this series of four two-hour lectures was normative, indeed masculine and heteronormative: in addition to lectures conveying information about human sexual behavior, the program explored sexual problems in the female, homosexuality, and marital and parental counseling. The course was sufficiently appealing (more than four hundred medical students apparently participated) that it led to the addition of a follow-up course in the curriculum. "Human Sexuality" was then listed as one of the organ systems covered in the twenty-six-credit required "Introduction to Clinical Medicine" course. Designed by an interdisciplinary planning committee that included the director of the Kinsey Institute for Sex Research, the resulting course in human sexuality was offered for five mornings from 8 A.M. to noon.[2] The course objectives included the goal of increasing "the student's awareness that: (a) a wide variety of sexual problems exist; (b) many of these problems are presented to physicians; (c) a physician needs more than his personal experiences and private opinions to help these patients; and (d) a physician's judgment is frequently handicapped by his own personal taboos, biases, and over-reactions to sexual information and stimuli" (Tyler 1970, 1026). Moreover, the course was intended to "make the students more tolerant of the wide spectrum of 'normal' human sexual responses (including their own sexuality)." Exposing the students to controversial points of view, desensitizing them to sexual stimuli, retraining them in a humanistically oriented approach to patients' sexuality, and introducing them to therapeutic techniques, diagnostic tools, and the curiously termed "preventive procedures and materials"—all were part of the course mission (Tyler 1970, 1026).

In addition, the course included lectures by a psychiatrist on "The Sexually Provocative Patient," by a family physician on "Sex Problems as they present to the GP," by a male-female team of sex therapists on "Therapy of Impotence, Premature Ejaculation, and Frigidity," and by an educator and a pediatrician on "Sex Education for Children" (Tyler 1970, 1027). Films drawn from the "scientific and stag collections" at the Kinsey Institute for Sex Research were shown for their "desensitization value," while an "actress" offered "three short vignettes of a physician interacting with a female patient who is subtly sexually provocative" in order to demonstrate "how the physician is exposed to sexual stimulation in his daily practice" (Tyler 1970, 1028). Desensitization included "an illustrated lecture on homosexuality, transvestite-transexuality, fetishism, and sadomasochism." Although the lecturer "emphasized the physician's need to be as tolerant of his patients' variations in their sexual behaviors as he is of their biochemistry," the explanation that "a homosexual individual seeking therapy for influenza should be treated only for the complaints he presents and not those that happen to offend the physician" suggests the limits of tolerance as either a curricular item or an institutional posture (Tyler 1970, 1029).

By 1972, a survey under way by the Center for the Study of Sex Education in Medicine indicated that "at least 29 U.S. medical schools . . . [offered] formal courses and 17 others incorporate[d] sex education into other areas in their curriculum"

(Golden and Liston 1972, 761). Yet if sex education was taking root in the medical school curriculum, it had yet to flourish. The year earlier, the Sex Knowledge and Attitude Test (SKAT) had been administered to second-year students at the University of California, Los Angeles, School of Medicine enrolled in the required course on human sexuality. The hope was "to determine some of the characteristics of the students and to . . . evaluate the extent to which this course increased their sexual sophistication" (Golden and Liston 1972, 764). Rather than revealing the sweeping changes in attitudes toward and knowledge of sexuality that the course's designers must have expected, the SKAT results revealed that the course failed to have any measurable effect.[3] Instead, the test, designed to gauge "knowledge and attitudes concerning sexual behavior," revealed that "the students were no better informed about sex than is the general population whose problems they will be expected to address—even after receiving specific instruction in this area" (Golden and Liston 1972, 770). Worse still, "a number of questions . . . produced rather startling responses, some even pointing to the absence of learning." For example, when presented with the sentence, "There are two kinds of physiological orgastic response in women, one clitoral and the other vaginal," 44 percent of the students pre-test and a disappointing 36 percent of the students post-test held that the statement was "True." The assertion that masturbation caused mental instability was affirmed by 14 percent pre-test and 10 percent students post-test. And perhaps most disturbing from the perspective of women's health, when exposed to the assertion that women could not respond to further sexual stimulation after orgasm, 24 percent pre-test and a remarkable 28 percent post-test marked the statement "True" (Golden and Liston 1972, 765). Psychiatrists Joshua S. Golden and Edward H. Liston argued that a new way was needed to carry out sex education in the medical school context: "Research is needed to determine whether clinical teaching . . . is better than traditional passive participation—listening to facts and then reproducing them for examinations" (1972, 770).

During that same period Justin Green published *Binky Brown Meets the Holy Virgin Mary*, a remarkably explicit and powerful underground comic detailing the protagonist's obsessive compulsive disorder, characterized by elaborate sexual negotiations around masturbation (Green 1972). This "hugely influential text . . . inaugurated comics as a medium of self-expression" (Chute 2010, 14). And what was expressed, more often than not, was the complex panorama of human sexuality in all of its varieties, anxieties, and desires. From Robert Crumb's *Zap Comics* in the late 1960s and Justin Green's *Binky Brown Meets the Holy Virgin Mary* in 1972, to the work of Aline Kominsky-Crumb and the feminist Wimmen's Comix Collective, the late 1960s and 1970s saw an explosion in underground comics that, to the willing reader, offered a different kind of sex and gender education. Sexually graphic, these comics challenged the silencing effects of enforced normativity by defiantly imaging and voicing previously taboo personal experiences from defecation, condom use, and the use of sanitary napkins to fornication, masturbation, sodomy, and cunnilingus (Chute 2010). Phoebe Gloeckner, whose own *A Child's Life and Other Stories* (1998) is a landmark work in this genre, recalls getting her own informal sex education from those underground comics.[4]

Gloeckner's experience suggests that comics—underground or not—may already have been providing sex education from the margins before the medical profession began to teach formal sex education classes. Rather than either the lecture/text method ("traditional passive participation") or clinical teaching, even in the 1960s and 1970s comics was providing value as a medium for sex education. But what exactly is that value? I argue that comics offers the "perspective by incongruity"—rhetorician Kenneth Burke's term for the way that "taking the vocabulary of one discipline to study the subject matter of another produces ideas that expose the limitations of the prior discipline as well as reveal novel insights into the nature of the subject" (Chambers 1990, 152). Disciplinarily far from the positivist realm of science and drawing on both words and images, comics as a medium encourages a broader, more accepting, and distinctly non-normative understanding of human sexuality, one reflecting the qualities valorized by Einstein and Shildrick: "1) an understanding of bodies in context, 2) an epistemology of ignorance, and 3) an openness to the risk of the unknown" (2009, 293).[5]

Yet the turn to comics may still seem a startling one for medicine, even though comics are deeply interwoven in our history, culture, and society and may even be personally significant for those of us who recall being belly down on the living room floor reading the brightly colored funny pages. For those for whom comics were the fare of children and teenagers, the very concept of using comics in medicine may seem counterintuitive. "What can possibly be *funny* about medicine?" a neurologist acquaintance asked me when I told him about the "Comics and Medicine" conference where I'd presented an early version of this research (Squier 2011b). As his response suggests, we are facing two issues here: not only may we resist supplementing existing modes of medical education (despite the evidence of surveys like the SKAT that some supplementation is needed), but we are also unfamiliar with comics as a medium.

More than a decade ago, a group of physicians and public health researchers proposed in the journal *Nature Medicine* that comics were more powerful at conveying information than even refereed journals:

As kids most of us read comic books. Many of us have gone back to our parents' home, and opened a comic book not read in 30 years. Amazingly, upon seeing the first page, the story and images spill forth from memory. We know what happened to Superman, where the Kryptonite brings Superman to his knees, and what Jimmy Olson and Lois Lane will say. Why is the recall over 3 decades of our comic books so good, yet we barely recall the contents of *Nature Medicine, BMJ, Lancet,* or *Science* from 3 months ago? What can comic books tell us about improving journals? . . . One may think that it is rather absurd to consider publishing journals in a comic book format. But is it? (Aaron et al. 1998)

As members of the Global Health Network dedicated to expanding the accessibility of medical information, Aaron et al. argue that comics are better at conveying information than medical journals because comics weave narrative and pictures together in a mode we are physiologically primed to remember: "Our perceptions and memories are sensory grounded and organized through our senses so that what can been seen, heard, felt, tasted and smelt are best remembered. Scientifically, in terms of cognitive theory, Pavio has described this as Iconic Memory"

(Aaron et al. 1998). Comics scholar Scott McCloud defines the icon—"any image used to represent a person, place, thing or idea"—as the most important part of the comic vocabulary (1994, 27). Icons convey information by simplifying, according to McCloud, and they *provoke identification.*

If we explore the essential aspects of the comics medium, we can see some of the reasons it offers a better approach to sex education both for medical students and everyone else. Comics combines gesture with words, thus providing the opportunity to draw on and integrate our multiple modes of learning: the spatial and the verbal, the right brain and the left brain, the embodied and tactile, the rational and linear. Consider additional reasons that comics might be ideal in expressing an experience as complex, layered, and context dependent as sexuality and gender. Comics present time through space, thus inviting the reader/viewer to integrate each moment in time with a new moment in space. The reader thus always experiences the temporal body as a spatial body as well. Moreover, the reader is constantly called on to attend to context—to the relationship between subject or event and the situations in which it is embedded or, to put it in other words, to contingency. Additionally, with its unique formal feature of panels in sequence separated by a gutter, comics produces a collaborative mode of engagement between reader, text, and images by requiring the reader to fill in information between panels. As a result, a reader cannot simply be a passive participant while reading a comic: a reader must collaborate with the cartoonist and his or her creation. Finally, comics as a medium has traditionally been the voice of those who are marginalized, whether by race, class, sex/gender, sexual preference, age, ability, and so forth. As David Hajdu observes in his history of American comics, "Comic books, even more so than newspaper strips before them, attracted a high quotient of creative people who thought of more established modes of publishing as foreclosed to them: immigrants and children of immigrants, women, Jews, Italians, Negroes, Latinos, Asians, and myriad social outcasts" (2008, 25). Even comics whose heteronormativity may seem to shut out marginalized groups, such as superhero comics in particular, have long nurtured a fan culture in which gender queering has been an active response to comics characters from Batman and Robin to Wonder Woman.

Yet this is not to portray comics as a free zone of self-expression in the twentieth and early twenty-first centuries. Although a vibrant culture of queer counterreadings has continued right up to present-day comics, the social and cultural access to mainstream culture that marginalized groups found in comics was abruptly blocked in the early 1950s. Responding to the moral panic produced by Fredric Wertham's muckraking 1954 book, *The Seduction of the Innocent: The Influence of Comic Books on Today's Youth,* the Comics Magazine Association of America (CMAA) created a forty-one-point Comics Code to be followed voluntarily by all members so that "violations of standards of good taste, which might tend toward corruption of the comic book as an instructive and wholesome form of entertainment, will be eliminated" (Senate Committee on the Judiciary 1995). This code governed both editorial matter (general standards, dialogue, costume, religion, marriage, and sex) and advertising matter, leading to a number of internal contradictions. For example, the code affirmed "the development of comic books as a unique and effective tool for instruction and education" even as it banned "advertisement of sex or sex instruction books."[6]

With the voluntary adoption of the Comics Code by a preponderance of comics publishers, the dissenting voice so characteristic of comics—and so essential to a broader, post-conventional view of sexuality—was softened, if not entirely silenced, by a raft of regulations, among them:

- "Nudity in any form is prohibited, as is indecent or undue exposure."
- "Suggestive and salacious illustration or suggestive posture is unacceptable."
- "All characters shall be depicted in dress reasonably acceptable to society."
- "Females shall be drawn realistically without exaggeration of any physical qualities."
- "The treatment of live-romance stories shall emphasize the value of the home and the sanctity of marriage."
- "Passion or romantic interest shall never be treated in such a way as to stimulate the lower and baser emotions."
- "Seduction and rape shall never be shown or suggested."
- "Sex perversion or any inference to same is strictly forbidden." (Senate Committee on the Judiciary 1955)

Much has been written about the negative effect of these strictures on the comics industry and particularly on their role in consolidating the enforcement of sex and gender normativity. Yet by the early 1960s and 1970s, the very same qualities that the CMAA code declared off-limits had returned in the form of self-published, informally distributed underground comics. And this was happening precisely at the same time that medical schools were beginning, slowly, to consider adding sex education to their curricula. We know what the result of those additions was, and we also know that underground comics like *Binky Brown* were simultaneously making it possible for authors and readers to explore sexual experiences, desires, and anxieties about sexual issues. That very tradition of attention to sexuality would make comics useful for sex education, moving through a gradual development from careful normativity to brave autobiographical frankness.

The Cartoon Guide to Sex, published in 1999 by Larry Gonick and Christine DeVault, was one of the first full-length sex ed comics published by a mainstream press. Although composed of images and words in panels separated by gutters rather than words in lecture format, it shares the expert knowledge format of those early medical school sex ed classes: information still flows one way only— from authors to readers. Yet this is expert knowledge with a twist, as a sample of the chapter titles from the table of contents makes clear: "Sex Is Paradoxical," "Reproduction Causes Sex," "Doing It," "Sexual Health and the Alternative," and "Uninvited Sex." In their drawings and word bubbles, Gonick and DeVault take a critical perspective that operates at a provocative remove from their deadpan text. Although the text refers in a factual tone to the tradition of gender stereotyping,

232 SUSAN M. SQUIER

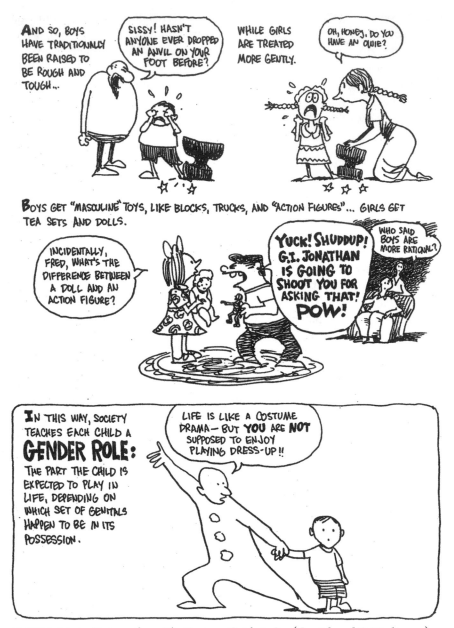

FIGURE 22.1 Cartoon from *The Cartoon Guide to Sex* (Gonick and DeVault 1999).

the exaggerated images convey that stereotyping hurts—physically as well as emotionally. The parent's clown suit undermines the sagacity of his advice, "Life is like a costume drama, but you are NOT supposed to enjoy playing dress-up!" (Gonick and DeVault 1999, 61).

Gonick and DeVault still register the chilling effects of the CMA Comics Code in their preface: "In a graphic medium, we wondered, exactly how graphic should we make it? Should we use sensitive line drawings? Bawdy cartoons? Fig leaves?"

Perhaps in jest, they offer a warning: "THIS BOOK CONTAINS EXPLICIT MATE-RIAL" (1999). Yet they also rely on the contemporary comics world to send up such caution. In a nod to Chris Ware's (1998) *Jimmy Corrigan: The Smartest Kid on Earth*, which includes instructions for an origami project using the jacket for its hardcover edition, they counsel: "In case you're easily embarrassed, you can make your own dust jacket by cutting out a rectangle from a brown paper bag and folding it along the dotted lines as shown" (Gonick and DeVault 1999, front matter).

Web-based publication brought the potential for interactivity to sex education comic books not only through the incorporation of hypertext but also through links to discussion boards, reader groups, and group projects (McCloud 2000, 166). The work of Martina Fugazzotto exemplifies this. An award-winning comics artist and illustration graduate of Pratt Institute in New York City, Fugazzotto contributes to "gURLcomix," a growing online library of over one hundred and fifty multi-panel web comics exclusively available on gURL.com.[7] This website intends to offer "a different approach to the experience of being a teenage girl. gURL.com is intended for girls age thirteen and up and is built on the principle that information is a positive thing."[8] Like *The Cartoon Guide to Sex*, gURL is careful to set out its perspective explicitly in a tone aimed at a teenage audience so readers who may be uncomfortable have the option to read no further: "Through honest writing, visuals and liberal use of humor, we try to give girls a new way of looking at subjects that are crucial to their lives. We hope to provide connection and identification in a way that is not possible in other media. Our content deals frankly with sexuality, emotions, body image, etc. *If this is a problem for you, you might not like it here. Please see our note to parents about that.*"[9]

Fugazzotto's contributions to gURL include "I ♥ Orgasms" and "I ♥ Fantasies." These lively and irreverent comics introduce women to a sex-positive perspective, debunking myths that position women as passive victims, such as the one described in Emily Martin's now classic essay, "The Egg and the Sperm": "Sperm . . . have a 'mission,' which is to 'move through the female genital tract in quest of the ovum.' . . . Sperm carry out a 'perilous journey' into the 'warm darkness,' where some 'fall away exhausted.' 'Survivors' 'assault' the egg, the successful candidates 'surrounding the prize'" (1991, 490). The approach to sex ed in Fugazzotto's "hero's tale" is distinctly post-conventional. Deconstructing the narrative of macho spermatic competition, the comic reveals that sexual activity need not be tied to reproduction.

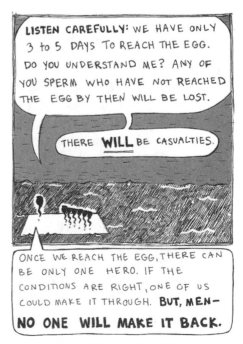

FIGURE 22.2 Cartoon from "Sea Men, a Hero's Tale" (Fugazzotto n.d.)

Instead, in the last panel drawn from the woman's perspective, we realize who is really in control of the sexual narrative.[10] Combining visual punch with feminist perspective, Fugazzotto's beautifully crafted comics explore the physiology of sex, correct cultural distortions, calculate the real—and asymmetrical—costs of sex (for women), and offer women important information about little known contraceptive technologies.

One final example of a sex ed comic focuses not on instructional push but what might be called educational pull: the illuminating knowledge gained when people share their experiences as a community. *Not Your Mother's Meatloaf* (2011a; *NYMM*) is a series of sex ed comics drawing on personal experiences to offer an intentionally non-expert perspective on sexuality. (Indeed, *NYMM* embraces the *amateur*, in all senses of the word.) After its inaugural issue, five issues of *NYMM* have appeared to date with themes of "Firsts," "Bodies," "Health," and "Age" (the first issue had no theme). When Liza Bley began compiling the first issue of *NYMM* in 2008, she wasn't interested in being "the authoritative voice on sexual health." With her co-editor Saiya Miller, she aspired to "offer a different kind of tool that has the ability to communicate something lacking between the pages of anatomic books and STD brochures." They also felt the power of personal stories would "humanize and offer a different kind of access to our questions on sex and sexuality than the sterilized, clinical speak of most sex ed curricula" (Squier 2011a; also see *Not Your Mother's Meatloaf* 2011a). They felt that while some issues related to sex can be explained relatively easily, like the function of the reproductive systems or how to use a condom, there are other questions "not as easily answered, but [that] desperately need to be discussed. Often there are multiple issues and dynamics occurring in these situations, which can be difficult to process, often confusing, and alienating" (Squier 2011a).

Just as *Not Your Mother's Meatloaf* deliberately emphasizes the personal over the expert narrative, the graphic standards for submissions are pluralistic. Miller and Bley have no specific criteria for the comics they accept, affirming the ability of anyone to create a comic except that the submissions must be on 8½ × 11 "paper and in black ink." They explain: "Our primary focus is educating youth and each other about important issues surrounding sexuality, safer sex, consent, gender, etc. Also: Submissions are anonymous unless you put your name on the comic itself."[11]

In its democratic and non-expert approach to sex education, *Not Your Mother's Meatloaf* reflects "one of the most important functions of the women's health movement" according to Einstein and Shildrick: "to lay ignorance bare" (2009, 294). In an aptly titled essay, "The Speculum of Ignorance," feminist philosopher Nancy Tuana explains how "epistemologies of ignorance" function in feminist praxis: "There is no better system of the epistemological practices of the women's health movement than the speculum" (2006, 2). While it is first of all a material and instrumental object that has given access to a previously unavailable perspective on our own bodies, the speculum is also a powerful metaphor for the new perspectives that are possible via a feminist analysis of the different ways that women's ignorance is produced and experienced. As Tuana taxonomizes it, ignorance comes in a variety of modes:

Knowing that we do not know, but not caring to know.
We do not even know that we do not know.
They do not want us to know.
Willful ignorance.
Ignorance produced by the construction of epistemologically disadvantaged identities.
Loving ignorance: accepting what we do not know. (Tuana 2006; my paraphrase)

Tuana's essay argues that the systematic study of ignorance is an essential part of any feminist theory of knowledge, which must make us aware not only of what we do not know but also of how that ignorance comes into being, whether systematically produced, haphazard, or merely part of the nature of life.

While all five issues of *NYMM* include many comics exploring forms of ignorance about sexuality, two comics treating two diametrically opposed forms of ignorance featured in Tuana's taxonomy can give a good sense of the series as a whole. Tuana's categories are "Ignorance produced by the construction of epistemologically disadvantaged identities" and the countervailing position, "Loving ignorance: accepting what we do not know." The former mode, positionally produced ignorance about sexuality, clearly has a strongly negative effect, while the latter mode, accepting ignorance and being constrained by normative expectations, can actually have a positive effect.

"The Appointment," Nik M. Sonfield and Jessica Ryan's three-page, five-panel-per-page autobiographical comic, illustrates the first category (Sonfield and Ryan 2008). The protagonist, a first-time gynecology patient and only eighteen years old, goes to her physician in order to obtain birth control. She is epistemically disadvantaged by her novice status and her age, and she is also positionally disadvantaged as young woman alone in a male physician's office. The comic begins with a telling interaction that emphasizes those disadvantaged identities: "In the examination room Dr. Plant told me I'd put my robe on backwards. 'Sorry,' I said. 'I've never done this before'" (Sonfield and Ryan 2008).[12]

The physician takes advantage of her ignorance of the gynecological situation, persuading her to give him her e-mail address in the pretense of putting her in contact with a patient who shares her genetic defect, *gastroschisis*. We learn in succeeding panels that not only has he acted inappropriately in the office (failing to leave the exam room for her to dress in private, asking her inappropriate questions, and badgering her for her address) but that he also continues his abusive behavior after she leaves, e-mailing her repeatedly.

Her disadvantaged positions (and identities) as a patient with a genetic defect, as a patient subject to the power of the physician, and as an individual without a community, all converge to create the ignorance that harms her. Yet the comic does not end with harm, isolation, and grief. A concluding panel shows her sitting at her computer, sharing the news about this physician with an online community, generating not only social support and empowerment but also the knowledge she needs to escape such mistreatment in the future.

THE APPOINTMENT

Drawn By Nik M. Sonfield
Original Story By Jessica Ryan

I had my first appointment with a gynecologist when I was 18. He was an attractive, young doctor. On the desk in his office was a framed picture of his beautiful family. I was really nervous but pretending not to be.

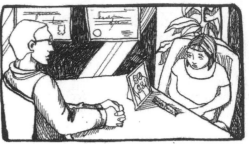

I told Dr. Mark Plant that I was in my first real relationship and that I wanted to go on birth control.

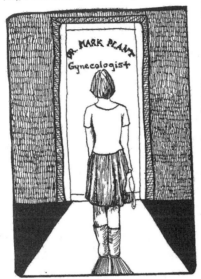

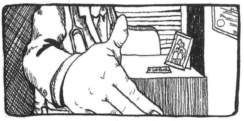

In the examination room Dr. Plant told me I'd put my robe on backwards. "Sorry," I said, "I've never done this before." During the breast exam Dr. Plant asked about the scar on my stomach. "I was born with gastroschisis," I told him. "My intestines were on the outside at first and they had to sew them back in.

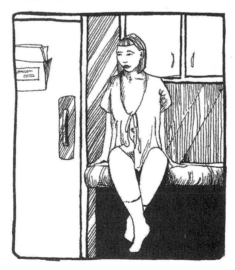

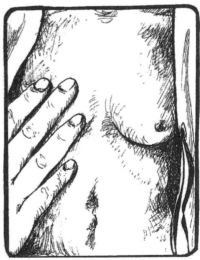

FIGURE 22.4 Cartoon panel from "The Appointment" in *Not Your Mother's Meatloaf* (Sonfield and Ryan 2008).

He told me he had a pregnant patient with a child with the same defect. He asked if I'd leave my contact information in case the mother had any questions.

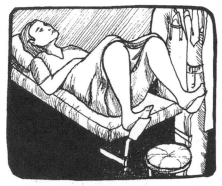

Dr. Plant began the pelvic exam. I winced. It was painful. "That hurts you doesn't it? I can tell by the look on your face," he said. While I got dressed Dr. Plant stayed in the room with me. He asked how long I had been with my boyfriend...

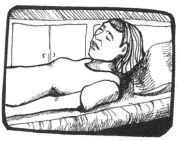

And reminded me again to leave my contact information.

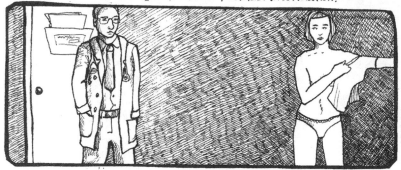

I left my e-mail address with his receptionist.

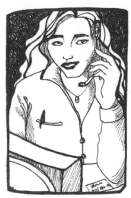

Back in my dorm room I had two new e-mails. They were both from Dr. Plant.

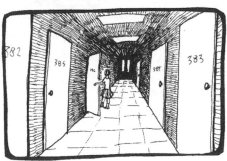

FIGURE 22.5 Cartoon panel from "The Appointment" in *Not Your Mother's Meatloaf* (Sonfield and Ryan 2008).

The first e-mail read...

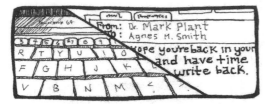

And the second...

It was great meeting today.
I hope we can stay in touch.

The next day there was another e-mail. It said...

What's your phone number?

I felt sick. There was no pregnant patient. He had lied to me to get my e-mail address. He had watched me change when he should have left the room. He had physically hurt me on purpose. I cried in my room. I felt completely alone.

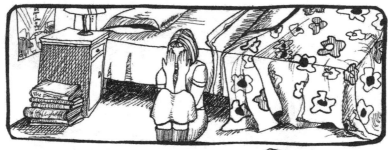

Later I started doing some research. I found sites like Ucomparehealth.com and wrote about my experience so other people would know about Dr. Mark Plant, and so other people could learn from what I had gone through.

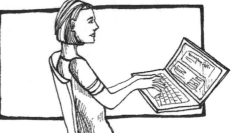

FIGURE 22.6 Cartoon panel from "The Appointment" in *Not Your Mother's Meatloaf* (Sonfield and Ryan 2008).

While "The Appointment" demonstrates the profoundly disempowering effect of ignorance, Liza Bley's one-page comic, "Defining Sex and Virginity" (2008), takes the delightfully counterintuitive position of what Tuana (2006) calls "loving ignorance"—accepting ignorance as an inevitable part of embodied experience. In contrast to experts' claims to authoritative definitions of sex and virginity, this comic lightheartedly refuses such closure. Instead, it offers a range of different definitions of sex and virginity, affirming the fact that conversation and context lend multiple possible meanings to any experience, including the sexual.

Fundamental to sex education and a cardinal tenet of the women's health movement since its origins in the Boston Women's Health Book Collective's (1973) *Our Bodies, Our Selves* is the fact that gender, like sex, is also complex, negotiable, and a product of the interaction of biology and society. A final panel, from Sparky Taylor's "My Body, Myself," illustrates how sex education can introduce the broader issue of gender identity, reinvigorating that iconic intervention of the women's health movement. Surveying how being "5/2, stocky, boyish, 26, punk" has taught her "a lot of things about body image," this comic explores the insecurities associated with affirming a particular and individual gender identity, from the discomforts of working out in public or being told that her frame is "stocky," to a stinging interaction with a friend. "My friend Jon said: "don't worry, the frat boys aren't looking at you," and even though I don't want to be objectified, it still really hurt my feelings" (Taylor 2010). The final three panels provide an alternate vision of a healthy attitude toward sexuality and gender identity. And they do so not by denying our uncertainties but by accepting them, by affirming not only the uncertainty associated with sexuality but the ambiguity of gender role identity as well.

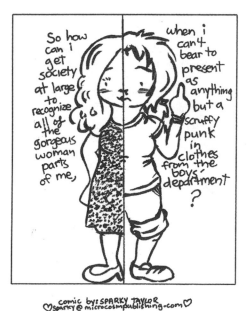

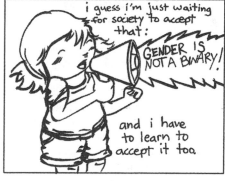

FIGURE 22.8 Cartoon from "My Body, Myself" in *Not Your Mother's Meatloaf* (Taylor 2010).

In its consensus statement, the Think Tank on Women's Health concluded that physicians, healthcare workers, philosophers, and feminist scholars must collaborate to generate new energy, and a new direction, for the women's health movement by incorporating an interpretive stance based on *"contingency, complexity, collaboration, and conversation"* (Einstein and Shildrick 2009, 299). The history of comics in the twentieth and twenty-first centuries reveals that the medium incorporates each of these aspects of a new post-conventional interpretive stance, serving as outlets for immigrants and other socially marginal voices, as sites of state power and social and biomedical regulation, as alternative zones of resistance to that surveillance culture, and finally as spaces of productive collaboration and negotiation between the dominant cultures and the many, and increasingly various, perspectives and positions of subcultures and countercultures. As comics as a medium nurtures these new attitudes toward gender and sexuality, it continues the project of the original *Our Bodies, Our Selves*: to develop the awareness of "economic and social systems that make women sick or influence the kind of health care available to them." The introduction of comics to medical education can return the embodied experiences of sexuality and gender to the social, interpersonal, historical, and cultural realms by enabling conversation, collaborative learning, continual change, and openness to alternative and innovative perspectives.

NOTES

1 Although the post-conventional exploration of both sexuality and gender expression/identity are integral, interconnected features of the comics I survey in this chapter, I use the shorthand term *sex ed* for ease and familiarity. To distinguish between gender expression, gender role, gender identity, and biological sex and sexuality, see "Talking the Talk" (Gay, Lesbian, and Straight Educational Network 2002). As to the term *comics*, the field of comics studies is still standardizing its terms and usages. When I am discussing comics as a medium, I use the singular verb, but when I am discussing comics as an aggregate of individual examples of the medium, I use the plural.

2 According to Edward A. Tyler, M.D., the interdepartmental planning committee included "Paul Gebhard, anthropologist and director of the Kinsey Institute for Sex Research; Eugene Levitt, clinical psychologist; John Melin, obstetrician; Irving Rosenbaum, pediatrician; and the author, psychiatrist" (Tyler 1970, 1026).

3 This test was the creation of Harold Lief and David Reed of the Center for the Study of Sex Education in Medicine, Department of Psychiatry, University of Pennsylvania School of Medicine (Golden and Liston 1972, 771n15).

4 See Gloeckner (2011).

5 I am arguing that comics as a medium nurtures these new attitudes, just as it illustrates the four theoretical postures essential to further the well-being of the body in general, and women's health in particular, according to Einstein and Shildrick: contingency, complexity, collaboration, and conversation (Einstein and Shildrick 2009, 299).

6 Senate Committee on the Judiciary (1995). See also McCloud (2000), 87.

7 Fugazzotto won the Kim Yale award for best new talent at the Friends of Lulu Awards. See her biography (Fugazzotto, n.d.).

8 Fugazzotto (n.d.)

9 Fugazzotto has also contributed a multi-part comic, "The Sex Mission," to "*Sex, Etc. . . .*

part of the Teen-to-Teen Sexuality Education Project developed by Answer" (Fugazzotto, n.d.)

10 Fugazzotto (n.d.). A final panel reads, "your little sperms don't know I'm a virgin. The semen might get on my hands but it stays far away from my eggs!"

11 *Not Your Mother's Meatloaf* (2011b).

12 Two other aspects of the epistemology of ignorance explored by *NYMM* comics from the first issue are

   ○ *Knowing that we do not know, but not caring to know*: a comic explores the difficult process of acknowledging that a love relationship had become abusive and had to be ended. ("I'll Be Your Mirror," 2008)

   ○ *Willful ignorance*: "Holes," by Cynthia Ann Schemmer, tells the story of her "first serious sexual relationship [that] spawned the relationship [that revealed] that our society lacks decent sex ed. A huge factor in this personal story is that my first boyfriend was raised as a born again Christian. . . . So, imagine my reaction when he revealed to me that females only have ONE HOLE to perform our many bodily functions!!!" (Schemmer 2008)

Chapter 23

I AM GULA, HEAR ME ROAR
On Gender and Medicine

RAFAEL CAMPO

"I've got a great riddle for everyone," Latvi says, mischievously. We're hosting a dinner party for a group of medical friends, polishing off a bottle of Chianti while we start to clear the dishes. Latvi is a Turkish optometrist with an ebullient personality who is doing research on some kind of retinal implant that promises to restore sight in blind diabetics; his grin is as big as his ambition. He continues, "A young boy and his father are driving home from a football game, and they are involved in a terrible head-on collision. Both are severely injured and rushed to the nearest hospital. They are wheeled into separate operating rooms, and two surgeons are called in to perform emergency surgery, one doctor for each patient. The surgeon operating on the father gets started right away, but the surgeon assigned to the young boy stares at him in surprise. 'I can´t operate on this child!' the surgeon exclaims to the exasperated nurses. 'He is my son!'" Latvi pauses for dramatic effect, pleased by the baffled looks on our friends' faces. "How can that be?" After he asks the question, he drains the wine from his glass and sets it in front of him with a self-satisfied flourish.

I wait for a few moments, letting the unconscious bias the riddle depends on cast its spell. I hate this riddle, or maybe I hate what it reveals about gender-based stereotypes, especially in medicine. "The surgeon is the boy's mother," I proclaim, a little too gleefully, and immediately everyone at the table recognizes with a collective incredulous groan the sexist supposition preventing them from arriving at such an obvious answer. Clearly, even among this enlightened group of Harvard-affiliated physicians in politically progressive Boston, we have difficulty imagining that a trauma surgeon could be a woman *and* a mother—or at least our automatic assumption is that it must be a man under that surgical mask, charging into the OR in the middle of the night to save the accident victim's life. I wonder whether we would do much better even if the scenario were changed and it's an obstetrician rushing in to the delivery room to perform an emergency C-section on a pregnant young woman after the head-on collision who turns out to be her daughter. Though women physicians probably now outnumber men in the medical specialty of obstetrics and gynecology, I suspect we might persist in unconsciously assigning a man to the role of imaginary savior.

Such bias against women in the role of physician perhaps is not so shocking when we consider the representations of women in relation to healing that predominate in American culture—or the lack thereof. Almost all of the best-known physician characters from literary works in English are men, from Mr. Hyde's kinder and compassionate Dr. Jekyll, to Sherlock Holmes's best friend Dr. Watson, to (more recently) Captain Jack Aubrey's sidekick Dr. Stephen Maturin. Even the great female novelist George Eliot's idealistic Dr. Lydgate from *Middlemarch* is male. The renowned physician-writers of the past are all men—John Keats, Anton Chekhov, William Somerset Maugham, Walker Percy, William Carlos Williams— which might be explained by the demographics of both professions during the times in which they lived; however, even the most recognized and lauded (or most actively promoted) contemporary physician writers are also all male—Ethan Canin, Atul Gawande, Jerome Groopman, Oliver Sacks, Richard Selzer, Abraham Verghese—despite the existence of many outstanding and prolific women physician writers such as Pauline Chen, Perri Klass, Susan Love, Danielle Ofri, and Rachel Naomi Remen.

On the small screen at the moment, we have only the frequently petty and vindictive character, Nurse Jackie (notably an RN, not an MD; *Nurse Jackie* 2009–) to compare against a long line of male physicians from the graciously white-haired Marcus Welby (*Marcus Welby, M.D.* 1969–1976) to the deceptively bumbling Quincy (*Quincy, M.E.* 1976–1983) to the unshaven and surly House (*House, M.D.* 2004–2012), all generally much more heroic main characters who have lent their names to their own television shows. Perhaps needless to say, all the other "real" TV doctors currently, from CNN's Dr. Sanjay Gupta to *Oprah's* Dr. Oz, are—you guessed it—most definitely not female. A couple of women have achieved some past notoriety as radio and TV personalities such as the irrepressible sex therapist Dr. Ruth Westheimer and the impeccable psychologist Dr. Joyce Brothers, but neither are, in fact, MDs. Arguably, one of the most famous female physicians is a fictional character from the later *Star Trek: The Next Generation* TV series (1987– 1994), the unfortunately but tellingly named Dr. Beverly Crusher—but alas, she seems very much an afterthought, considering her much more memorable and beloved predecessor on the original show, Dr. Leonard "Bones" McCoy (*Star Trek* 1966–1969). Runners-up to Dr. Crusher, while not quite as well known, are also both fictional characters. The first, Dr. Quinn, from the long-running show *Dr. Quinn, Medicine Woman* (1993–1998), improbably played by the willowy Jane Seymour, depicted frontier medicine as if contemporary social issues were tackled in the late 1800s as matter-of-factly as rattlesnake bites; Seymour's character, though hardly masculine, is often referred to as "Dr. Mike." The other, portrayed by Lorraine Bracco on the celebrated HBO series *The Sopranos* (1999–2007) is psychiatrist Dr. Jennifer Melfi; intelligent, insightful, but just a bit too sexy, she seems to pay for the vulnerability she exposes in the mafioso lead character she treats by being brutally raped upon leaving her office in one episode, and the perpetrator of the crime is never brought to justice. None of the female physician characters in more recent medically themed shows featuring ensemble casts such as *E.R.* or *Grey's Anatomy* particularly stand out, and in fact all seem to be overshadowed by their male counterparts.

Even what little we teach of the history of medicine in medical school typically omits the contributions of women. All medical students solemnly recite the Hippocratic Oath on entering the profession, which comes to us from the Greek physician Hippocrates, roundly credited as the father of Western medicine; most are already familiar with his Roman successor, Galen, and his perpetuation of the long-discredited but somehow still appealing theory of the four bodily humors. And perhaps just as many have marveled at Vesalius's anatomical drawings made during the 1500s (probably by artists training with Titian and not Vesalius himself). Little did I know, making my way through my own medical training at Harvard, that the powerful Babylonian goddess Gula (or Bau, as she called in the earliest Mesopotamian inscriptions), known as "The Great Physician," actually predated by several thousand years the Greek god of physicians, Aesculapius, after whom our medical humanities club was named. I was also left blissfully unaware that the first recorded female physician, Peseshet, practiced in ancient Egypt around 2400 B.C., a millennium or two before Hippocrates' name appears in the historical record, nor did I learn of his female contemporaries, whom we know through classical scholarship were widespread and, in a number of well-documented cases, received the same kinds of honor and social standing as male physicians of the time. Their names, such as Antiochis and Auguste, were also recorded by the ancient Greeks for posterity. Roman civilization benefited as well from the care of female physicians who similarly were established throughout the empire and participated actively in the scholarship and debate around the same medical controversies concerning Galen. One such female physician, Metrodora, sometime around the third century A.D., produced a tome devoted to gynecological pathology and treatment, making her particularly renowned; this remarkable text is the earliest surviving written work by a woman doctor.

Contrary to the unchallenged assumptions I had during medical school, women are also known to have practiced medicine during the Middle Ages—and not only as midwives or witches. Hildegard of Bingen, perhaps the best known of these, was a mystic who is said to have healed through incantation. In 1276, Virdimura, a Jew and the wife of a doctor, was publicly licensed to treat the poor of Sicily. During the early Renaissance in Naples, just before Vesalius's time, one Costanza Calenda became the first woman known to receive a doctorate in medicine from a university. In fact, the only woman to receive any significant attention during this impressionable time in my own training was Florence Nightingale, whom everyone knows was not a physician but who founded the modern profession of nursing in the mid-nineteenth century. While she certainly made tremendous contributions to the development of medicine, looking back I wonder why I never heard anything about the life and career of her nearly exact contemporary, Dr. Elizabeth Blackwell, the first woman to graduate from medical school in the United States. While Florence Nightingale famously cared for soldiers during the Crimean War, advancing our understanding of the importance of hygienic practices in reducing wound infections, Elizabeth Blackwell was struggling just as courageously to establish a medical practice in New York City, even after contracting "purulent ophthalmia" from a patient, which led to the loss of sight in one eye and which forced her to give up her dream of becoming a surgeon; facing intense discrimination that effectively banned her from practicing her vocation, she eventually went on to found her own infirmary, one of the first medical institutions to train women physicians. Of course, though Nightingale more than merited the passing mention she was given, she received nothing like the kind of reverent attention lavished on another great healer of her time who happened to be a male doctor, the demigod Dr. William Osler.

Growing up in an immigrant family in New Jersey, I had already observed that gender seemed to matter profoundly in healing. The only doctor in the family was my Uncle "Doc," a bespectacled psychiatrist from Cuba who married my grandmother's sister, Isabella, his office manager; another sister, my sturdy and indefatigable Aunt Teresa, was a nurse. At an early age, I saw how very differently these two medical professionals were regarded and how they used their skills both within the family and in the larger world. On the one hand, I was always encouraged to be like my Uncle "Doc," who drove a sporty red Mercedes convertible to family gatherings with his beautiful wife (who, according to family lore, almost became a Broadway star) and spoke very little to any of us children; I should excel in my studies so I could attend the most competitive college, which in turn would help me to gain admittance to medical school. On the other hand, what my Aunt Teresa did (who was homelier than her sister but acknowledged to be smarter) was considered women's work, like helping my ailing great-grandmother to the toilet or patiently feeding her a bowl of *pasta e fagioli*; I cringed when she would take me forcibly by the hand to give the decrepit old woman a peck on the cheek. My uncle was cool and detached, emitting quiet, polished, almost disdainful competence that seemed poised to solve any complex problem, while my aunt seemed more like a servant, willing and able to approach the awfulness of illness up close and without flinching. My uncle represented the manly ideal of stoicism in the face of suffering, meeting the cries of the afflicted with rational equanimity, for the trouble of which he was rewarded handsomely; my aunt, in contrast, offered the well-worn hand of compassion dutifully, as if it was a kind of privilege to be soiled in the act of ministering, and for whom recompense was more importantly in the spiritual or moral realm, not in a paycheck.

So for me, to become a physician was to live up to my masculine potential of what might be called a kind of benign heartlessness, while, for my female cousins, the alternative of nursing, which promised a more emotional and unequivocally virtuous self-sacrifice more suited to girls and ladies, was held out instead. I found myself in an unusual and awkward bind: I wanted to be a doctor, like a good little immigrant boy should, but I also wanted to be compassionate and caring, in the way little girls in my family were more explicitly expected to be. At one fateful family gathering, my cousin Denise, who was a year older than I was and considered a tomboy—she was certainly tougher than I ever was and would in our later adolescent years introduce me to such vices as tattoos, piercings, and smoking—proclaimed she wanted to be a doctor. She then proceeded to demonstrate her aptitude by devising a technique for tooth extraction that involved tying one end of a long string around my younger brother's loose incisor and the other to a doorknob, and then slamming the door shut. I remember the collective harsh scolding she got; while my brother shrieked and bled more profusely than either of us had anticipated, I hid in the bathroom, her cowardly and furtive assistant, listening to the adults remind her that girls could become nurses but never doctors. The terrible consequences of defying these gender roles were now obvious! Meanwhile, it was my Aunt Teresa who carefully tended to the wound left behind by that lost tooth, not to mention all of the high drama of subsequent temper tantrums, while my Uncle "Doc" urbanely smoked cigarettes with the other men somewhere outside on the back lawn. As I watched her stop my brother's bleeding with fascination, mixing her technical proficiency with kindly consolation, it seemed to me she was far better at doctoring than my uncle was.

Denise, all these years later, is not a physician, while I did go on to earn an MD. One of the many ironies of this personal history is that, according to the growing scientific literature on gender differences in the care of patients, of the two of us she would probably have been the better doctor, just as I imagined Aunt Teresa might have outshone Uncle "Doc"—at least in many of the terms I personally value so greatly as an internist providing primary care. A recent review of this literature reports that female primary care physicians spend more time with their patients, allow them more time to speak, and in general engage in more patient-centered communication and active partnership behaviors. Perhaps not surprisingly, such patient-centeredness, in turn, is associated with higher levels of patient satisfaction, improved patient adherence to treatment recommendations, and ultimately better health outcomes. While the data clearly support that the presence of women in medicine benefits patients, we continue to fail as a culture not only in recognizing their contributions but also by depicting them in our collective imagination as somehow lesser than male physicians. Studies also reveal that we pay women less for the same medical jobs, that they are much more likely to work part-time in medicine, and that they go into low-paying fields such as pediatrics and primary care more often than their male counterparts. At best, women can be nurses and midwives, safely in keeping with how we perceive them in their most common and culturally acceptable nurturing role as mothers; at worse, women who dare to interrogate the body's mysteries or to claim any kind of power over it risk being associated with the threatening likes of sorceresses, temptresses, and witches.

It seems obvious that the olden duality in our thinking about women as healers, which arose sometime during the Middle Ages (perhaps to erase the memory of compelling heathen figures like Gula and Metrodora)—that they are either fertile, nurturing, primitive earth goddesses at one extreme or evil, spell-casting, potion-brewing succubi at the other—has long colored how we regard them as physicians. Since we also associate power and competence with ruthlessness and detachment rather than with kindness and compassion, it becomes obvious why it may be so difficult for us to lionize female physicians the way we do Hippocrates, Galen, Vesalius, Osler, and the other giants of medicine. No wonder, then, why we must substitute nurses like the lovely Florence Nightingale (who was described in a popular account of the time as "a 'ministering angel' without any exaggeration . . . and as her slender form glides quietly along each corridor, every poor fellow's face softens with gratitude at the sight of her. . . . When all the medical officers have retired for the night and silence and darkness have settled down upon those miles of prostrate sick, she may be observed alone, with a little lamp in her hand, making her solitary rounds") for the likes of the brainy but unbeautiful Elizabeth Blackwell. We wish to romanticize and sexualize the female healer, disempower her as the innocuous, naked, big-breasted idol from the Stone Age or the modern-day subservient nurse in relation to the male order-giving physician. And if she has any intelligence at all, we must recast her as the callous and bitchy Nurse Jackie, or as the infinitely worse Mel Brooks caricature, Nurse Diesel, with her screechy German accent and exaggerated, sharply pointed breasts (Brooks 1977), or as the sadistic, more banally heartless Nurse Ratched from the well-known film *One Flew over the Cuckoo's Nest* (Forman 1975).

"Nurse Diesel" was one of the childhood taunts aimed by me and my other male cousins and brothers against another female cousin of mine, Elsie, this one on my father's side. Bookish and introspective, she also dreamed of becoming a doctor someday. A born diagnostician, she could immediately discern when an adult relative had enjoyed one too many Cuba libres and when the moment was right to ask for some outlandish privilege, like baking cookies (she was equally skilled in the arts of weights and measures) or staying up late to watch *The Tonight Show* (1962–1992; Elsie even did a passable impersonation of Johnny Carson and, to our astonishment and suspicion, actually seemed to understand some of his jokes). However, when she wasn't serving our needs, we could be cruel. We ceaselessly mocked her interest in medicine, not only calling her Nurse Diesel but also a number of other creative and insulting names ranging from "Doctor Dickless" (an unimaginatively obvious reference to her scary, lesser gender) to "Wilhelmina Shakespeare" (to be associated with any kind of sophisticated culture, especially from effete England, was felt to be especially damning), not to mention the more generic characterization of "Bruja" (Spanish for "witch," which took on the connotation of extra evil since it was pronounced in our forbidden and therefore quasimystical tongue). Perhaps it was all just harmless child's play, but I still wonder these several decades later if the reason Elsie is a nurse today has something to do with our blatant rejection of a notion that seemed at the time worthy only of our most hurtful scorn and derision.

Because of such deeply ingrained unconscious bias, it seems, my female colleagues continue to struggle to be taken as seriously as my fellow male colleagues, forever caught between these two archetypes. Those silly enough to try to embody the power of empathy and compassion are usually dismissed as emotional or subsumed into the stereotype of "the good nurse"; those who make claim to power and dare to challenge male authority are often viewed as her antithesis—criticized as manlike, discredited as unfeeling, never to be accepted as "one of the boys." The irony of this position is all the more palpable for me, as a gay man in medicine, who can more easily "pass" in a profession that remains such a bastion of male advantage. The conscious decision I make every day to be open about this aspect of my identity I imagine in some way approximates what women doctors must experience; I worry whether my colleagues will treat me differently, assume I am less competent, belittle me behind my back, expect me to behave less aggressively or more passively, while I wonder whether my patients will manifest the same homophobic and heterocentric biases.

At the same time, the optimist in me imagines whether my female colleagues might feel something that has always seemed a benefit to being regarded as an outsider in the medical profession. Though empathy in our postmodern moment continues to be viewed with suspicion, not only but especially in medicine, those of us who have directly felt its absence paradoxically can perhaps speak most persuasively about its power. I wonder if we can all take heart in looking back across the millennia to our origins as a civilized creature, back to the dawn of recorded history, to our very first stories passed down by the warring Sumerians and Babylonians, whose kings built massive ziggurats to commemorate themselves and their worldly power and yet who elevated a woman, Gula, to the greatest position of healing they could conceive. We will likely never know the reasons for her mythical ascendance—whether it was a profound recognition of the extraordinary life-giving capacity of femininity itself, or perhaps even something deeper and more astonishing, a collective admission that this awesome power, housed in a physically less powerful body, created a kind of vulnerability that should be cherished, that itself was an even greater kind of potency. So I pray to you now, Gula, Woman, Great Healer, Physician-Goddess: were you revered simply for your ability to cure illness or instead, for your wise, womanly insight into the human condition itself? May we continue to ponder this abiding mystery, through honoring your modern-day counterparts, the inspiring women physicians whom we must recognize as indispensable healers in their own right.

Part VII

RACE AND CLASS

Chapter 24

LISTENING AS FREEDOM
Narrative, Health, and Social Justice

SAYANTANI DASGUPTA

WHOSE STORY IS IT? THE CASE FOR MUTUALITY IN STORYTELLING

I begin this essay on storytelling and listening with a story, an Indian folktale that undoubtedly makes the case for mutuality in narrative more elegantly than I will thereafter:

A long, long time ago, before there were things like mirrors in homes, a wandering story-teller was traveling from village to village, telling stories, when he happened upon a magi-cal mirror propped up in the woods. Not knowing what the image he saw was, he assumed he was looking upon the face of his long dead father who had passed away at about the age that the storyteller was at that moment. He became overjoyed. "Baba! Baba!" he cried.

As this was happening, a wandering minstrel came by, on his way traveling from village to village singing his stories. And *he* looked in the mirror, and became convinced that he saw *his* long dead father, whom he had last seen when the father was the age that *he* was at that moment. And he too was beside himself. "Father! Father!" he cried.

This, as you can imagine, caused a good deal of consternation, and the two men began to fight. "It's *my* father," said the storyteller to the minstrel. "No, it's *my* father," argued the minstrel with the storyteller. As the men began to scuffle, yelling "My father!" "My father!" "My father!," it so happened that they both ended up looking in the mirror together. And as they now gazed at not one but *two* familiar faces in the glass, the storyteller turned to the minstrel and said, "Oh, that's just *you!*" And the minstrel turned to the storyteller and said, "Oh, that's just *you!*" So it was that only when they looked in the mirror *together* could they each see the truth about themselves.

This seemingly simple story is about the nature of intersubjectivity, and the state of mutuality that facilitates the intersubjective encounter. Even as the Other is allowing one to more fully access the Self, the reciprocal relationship is taking place as well. This also gestures to the dyadic nature of the teller-listener relation-ship, whereby listeners inevitably co-author stories with their questions, their responses, and their sheer embodied and relational presence. In a slightly differ-ent formulation, as memoirist Anatole Broyard (1992) wrote in his posthumously published *Intoxicated by My Illness*, even as the doctor diagnoses the patient, the patient is diagnosing the doctor. And we can imagine them, the minstrel and the storyteller, the clinician and the patient, gazing together into the mirror—or to borrow a phrase from Salman Rushdie (1991), into the *stream of stories*—that is their medical relationship.

Oral historian Alessandro Portelli notes: "An inter/view is an exchange between *two* subjects: literally a mutual sighting. One party cannot really *see* the other unless the other can see him or her in turn. The two interacting subjects cannot act together unless some kind of mutuality can be established. The field researcher therefore, has an objective stake in equality, as a condition for a less distorted communication and a less biased collection of data" (2001, 31). This formulation regarding oral history can be extended to clinicians and teachers working at the intersection of humanities and health care. Healing and teaching are fundamentally intersubjective inter/views and as so, experiments in equality. Equality here does not imply that physicians, nurses, or scholars give up their knowledge and authority; rather, it implies putting ourselves in a place of mutuality and transparency in order to promote a better care of our students, clients, and patients and a more satisfactory professional relationship for ourselves.

Whether in the classroom or clinic, work at the intersection of humanities and health care is necessarily storied. Indeed, stories are the way that we human beings make sense of the world around us and in situations of crisis, including illness, draw what Arthur Frank (1995) calls a "new destination and map" to our permanently altered lives. However, stories are also about power. They demand that practitioners and teachers ask questions regarding stories, including Whose story counts? Who owns the story? What voices or stories go unheard? Because certain stories can also silence other stories—the less "neat," socially acceptable stories, stories from marginalized communities, stories that challenge the social power structures as they stand.

Moreover, examinations of interpersonal and sociopolitical power are integral to approaching mutuality and equality in the intersubjective encounter. We must ask additional questions: What is the role of the witness in eliciting and co-constructing the illness story? What is our responsibility to it? What do we as witnesses expect from illness stories? What do such stories do to us? These are compelling in regard to any illness story, but they are particularly so in regard to vulnerable stories—narratives whose tellers are traditionally marginalized or silenced owing to their cultural, social, sexual, or economic identities. It not enough, then, to think about the listener/teller dyad and all the narrative nuance of a story—like plot, or frame, or genre—without contextualizing that listener and teller in broader social contexts. At the same time, it is not enough to draw broad conclusions based on sociopolitics without examining the way that these issues are manifested in particular, unique individuals and their stories because, of course, any group is composed of heterogeneous people with heterogeneous, idiosyncratic stories. The key is simultaneously listening to multiple levels of narratives—the individual and the social, the personal and the institutional—if we are to engage with the political underpinnings of narrative acts and to think about our responsibilities in witnessing narratives from the margins.

This approach to stories can be the first step in not just a shared consciousness but also in activism. We only have to remember that social movements from the civil rights movement to the 1970s feminist movement were rooted in the personal to political connection that enacted stories can make. If disease, violence, terror, war, poverty and oppression manifest themselves narratively, then resistance, justice, healing, activism, and collectivity can equally be products of a narrative-based approach to ourselves and the world.

This essay explores the connections between narrative, health, and social justice through a discussion of three texts I have used in teaching health and humanities students: Anne Fadiman's nonfiction book *The Spirit Catches You and You Fall Down* (1997), Zana Briski and Ross Kauffman's documentary film *Born into Brothels* (2004), and Logan Smalley's documentary film *Darius Goes West* (2007). These texts are used to explore issues of mutuality—as well as the sociocultural challenges to such mutuality. My discussion focuses on race, ethnicity, and nationality but through an intersectional lens, recognizing that we cannot talk about race, class, gender, ability, nationhood, and the like as isolated identities (or, similarly, about racism, classism, or sexism as isolated phenomenon). Ultimately, I hope this essay broadens the mandate of health and humanities fields by challenging us to bring a critical, self-reflective eye to our scholarship, teaching, practice, and organizing. How are the stories we tell, and the stories we are told, manifestations of social injustice? How can we transform such stories into narratives of justice, health, and change?

STORIES CATCH US AND WE FALL DOWN; OR, WHOSE GENRE IS IT?

As an interdisciplinary field, humanities and healthcare studies have historically grappled with issues of genre. In the teaching of future clinicians, what sorts of narratives "count"? Traditionally, written short stories, novels, and poems about illness or medicine told by canonical authors such as Anton Chekhov, Fyodor Dostoyevsky, Henry James, and Raymond Chandler were common fare, sometimes joined by stories written by physicians such as Oliver Sacks or Richard Selzer. Naturally, such curricula suffered from a distinct lack of diversity—of content, aesthetic sensibility, and authorship. However, expanding the health and humanities "canon" to include fiction by Chimamanda Adiche, essays by Nancy Mairs, or poetry by Eduardo Galeano is only part of the answer. The incorporation of other genres—including memoir, film, television, visual arts, oral history, and spoken testimony—in health and humanities classrooms allows not only for other modes of narration but a greater diversity of experiences and voices. For instance, I often begin my course in "Illness and Disability Memoirs" by playing spoken word poetry, including "Tamara's Opus" by Joshua Bennett (2009) and "My Body Is My Temple" by Emiliano Bourgois-Chacón (2004). These readily accessible works, performed by young male poets of color, are not only a compelling way to begin a semester; they also signal to students that the course itself will honor genres, authors, and experiences often silenced in our classrooms. Vital, of course, is the willingness to approach all such genres and authors with a critical eye, not to assume that inclusion of diverse stories or voices *necessarily* equates to a more socially just curriculum.

Over the last decade or more, the classic text with which to teach clinical trainees about culture has been anthropologist-journalist Anne Fadiman's *The Spirit Catches You and You Fall Down: A Hmong Child, Her American Doctors, and the Collision of Two Cultures* (1997), a nonfiction account of a Hmong child's epilepsy and the family's cultural experience of her condition in Merced, California. The text elegantly describes the dire consequences of cultural conflict, what physician anthropologist Arthur Kleinman (1998) would call different "explanatory models" of illness. In the Lee family's explanatory model, seizures are a manifestation of "the spirit catching you and you falling down," signaling difference/illness as well as a desirable spiritual marking. They, like families from many immigrant communities, seek a healing at the intersection of cultures, including both trips to the hospital emergency room and visits from a community shaman. For their daughter Lia's physicians, whose understanding of epilepsy is solely neurobiological, the Lees' language, behavior, and expectations are all incomprehensible. They are, at best, a "noncompliant" family and, at worst, neglectful/abusive parents. Stuck in the middle is Lia Lee, a young girl with a horrible disease whose management is only made worse through these conflicts.

While the nonfiction narrative has many strengths, including a structure that alternates accounts of Hmong immigration history with Lia's illness story, it also functions in certain ways that reinforce racialized hierarchies in humanities curricula and privilege certain sorts of stories about subjects of color. Medical anthropologist Janelle Taylor's (2003) essay "The Story Catches You and You Fall Down" discusses the ways that the story and its racialized representations function at odds to one another. According to Taylor, the compelling narrative drive of Fadiman's book creates a particular kind of love story between the text and the reader who is caught up by the story despite, or perhaps because of, its ethical vexations. In her words, the story itself catches the reader so that he or she falls down, such that the emotional pull of the narrative drive convinces the reader to overlook the book's problematic treatment of, among other things, Hmong culture as exotic, monolithic, fixed, and static. In answer then, to the question, Whose story is it? one might posit that Fadiman's text exists first and foremost for its non-Hmong, American reader who is unwittingly placed by the text in a position of voyeurism and simplistic understandings of both the Other and cultural conflict in general.

After being taught in so many institutions for so many years, *The Spirit Catches You* risks being interpreted by health and humanities students as an authoritative text, something that speaks the last word on something called "culture." This sort of uncritical reading replicates the totalizing formats of "cultural competency" courses of yesteryear whereby students were handed lists of cultural "traits" to memorize as pertaining to various ethnic communities (e.g., when a Dominican says *susto* this is what he means, or when you see round marks on a South East Asian's back, it is undoubtedly due to the practice of cupping). However, teaching Fadiman's book alongside a critique like Taylor's allows students to deepen their reading of this text while making them more comfortable with the inherent complexities of narratives in general—the idea that stories can be learned from and simultaneously critiqued.

KIDS WITH CAMERAS; OR, WHOSE GAZE IS IT?

Fundamental to the teaching of health and humanities are questions of representation. Who speaks? Who is heard? Who is spoken for and about? These questions inevitably break down along lines of race, class, gender, and power. The following comments of cultural critic Trinh T. Min-ha in regard to the anthropological project are perhaps equally applicable to the health professions. She writes that anthropology is "mainly a conversation of 'us' with 'us' about 'them,' of the white man with the white man about the primitive-nature man ... in which 'them' is silenced. 'Them' always stands on the other side of the hill, naked and speechless ... 'them' is only admitted among 'us,' the discussing subjects, when accompanied or introduced by an 'us'" (quoted in Alcoff 1991–1992, 6).

Consider the "rescue narrative" omnipresent in the writing of New York Times correspondent and two-time Pulitzer Prize–winner Nicholas Kristof. Indeed, Kristof has responded to critiques that he often portrays "black Africans as victims" and "white foreigners as their saviors" by saying that he believes "readers" need a foreigner as a "bridge character," someone they can "identify with" in order for them to care about the problems of "distant countries" (2010). The implicit assumption here is that all of Kristof's readers (acting subjects) are white, privileged, and situated in the Global North. Anyone else, whether reading the New York Times or not, is not an actor but someone to be acted upon.

In her essay "The Problem of Speaking for Others," feminist philosopher Linda Alcoff suggests, "Where one speaks from affects the meaning and truth of what one says ... The practice of privileged persons speaking for or on behalf of less privileged persons has actually resulted ... in increasing or reinforcing the oppression of the group spoken for" (1991–1992, 6–7). Yet she simultaneously problematizes the stance of not speaking up against injustice, instead suggesting, as does literary critic Gayatri Chakrovorty Spivak (1988) in her classic essay, "Can the Subaltern Speak?" that it is the more powerful Self's responsibility to create a space where dialogue with the Other becomes possible.

Zana Briski and Ross Kauffman's Oscar-winning 2004 documentary Born into Brothels seems, at first glance, to address these problems of "speaking for" head on. Briski, a photographer, documents her own journey seeking to photograph the lives of the sex workers living and working in Kolkata's (formerly Calcutta) red-light district, Sonagachi. Unable to get permission from the women themselves to photograph them, Briski gives cameras to the children of the brothels and lessons in how to use them. Not only are the children's lives and communities documented through their own eyes, but money is also raised for their education through public showings and sales of their photographic work arranged by Briski. Some children with particular talents in photography end up achieving goals that would otherwise have been impossible, including travel abroad and higher education. Indeed, it was Briski's experiences in Kolkata that led her and Kauffman to form their organization Kids with Cameras,[1] which works in impoverished communities in several other developing countries.

With *Born into Brothels* in mind, one can propose a corollary of the "Who speaks?" / "Who is spoken for?" dichotomy, that is, "Who sees?" / "Who is seen?" Indeed, one might suggest that Briski's work indicates an acknowledgment of her own status as foreigner and outsider, putting the power of gaze into the hands of her subjects. And yet Briski's film itself undermines the project of self-representation she seemingly undertakes with "her" children. In the words of one Indian reviewer:

In the end, the film seems more about Briski's journey and less about the hard reality of prostitution and the effects of her interference in young lives. . . . Intentionally or not, Briski is the noble soul in the film, faced with the mountain of Indian bureaucracy, teaching the children photography, trying to move them to good schools, getting them tested for aids [*sic*] and taking them to the zoo. The film's self-congratulatory tone thickens as it progresses through "Zana Aunty's" triumphs and travails, making us wonder who the real subject is. (Sirohi 2005)

Like Kristof's newspaper stories, *Brothels* places the white, foreign savior firmly at the center of the plot, suggesting that Briski herself is the only adult who cares for these children. This is done in particular through a placement of "Zana Auntie" (as she is called by the children), if not in direct opposition, then in cinematic opposition to the mothers of Sonagachi. Mothers are overwhelmingly absent from the film, and, when shown, they are portrayed, at best, as naive and neglectful and, at worst, as foul mouthed and abusive. Yet, when the voices of the Sonagachi mothers are listened for, they tell a very different story. In my graduate seminar on narrative health and social justice, I teach *Born into Brothels* alongside a book based on hundreds of interviews giving voice to the very women Briski silences: Sinha and Das Dasgupta's *Mothers for Sale: The Women of Kolkata's Red Light District* (2009). By teaching this interview-based text alongside Briski's film, I seek not only to complicate our reception of *Brothels* but also to problematize the "rescue" narrative itself, which is most often based on foreign (read: white) protagonists in relation to "innocent victims" (read: children, non-sex-worker women) who are in turn made acontextual—taken *out of relation* to their families, communities, local activist groups, and the like. In the words of Swapna Gayen, secretary of the Durbar Mahila Samanwaya Committee in Kolkata:

The film is a one-sided portrayal of the life of sex workers in Sonagachi. It shows sex workers as unconcerned about the future of their children. This is not true. Being a sex worker and a mother, I can say that we are more protective as mothers than can be imagined. . . . In this age, when it is the norm to respect ethical considerations while making documentaries, the film used hidden cameras to shoot intimate moments in the lives of sex-workers and their work zones. . . . We fear the global recognition of such a film, giving a one-sided view of the lives of sex workers in a third world country, may do a lot of harm to the global movement of sex workers for their rights and dignity. It can even have an impact on their hard-won victories for rights, un-stigmatized healthcare and access to resources. (Gayen 2005)

What impact, if any, do such classroom-based discussions of authorial power, representation, gaze, and subjecthood have on the healthcare enterprise? Of course, power sharing is of critical import in health care: is a patient *spoken of* and *about* or *spoken with*? Is a clinician made the hero, rather than the partner, of the patient's story? Are vulnerable patients, such as children, "saved" by good-intentioned healthcare workers who place themselves in opposition to "bad"/"irresponsible" families and communities?

Teaching for social justice in the health and humanities classroom helps students place their individual encounters with patients and clients within greater global forces of history, culture, and sociopolitical environments while broadening the mandate of our work itself beyond the dyadic patient-provider encounter.

GO WEST, YOUNG MAN; OR, WHOSE BODY? WHOSE NARRATIVE?

Although less well known than Fadiman's book and Briski's film, the narrative drive of Logan Smalley's 2007 documentary *Darius Goes West* is similarly irresistible: an amateur documentary film crew of eleven white young men from Georgia decide to take a fifteen-year-old African American boy with Duchenne Muscular Dystrophy (DMD) on the RV road trip of a lifetime.[2] They are heading from Georgia to Los Angeles in order to get Darius's wheelchair souped up on MTV's hit show *Pimp My Ride* (2004–2007). At the time of the film, Darius Weems had been in what he describes as a "raggedy old" electric wheelchair for six years and had never crossed the county line beyond his home in the housing projects of Athens, Georgia. On the three-and-a-half-week midsummer journey from Athens to Los Angeles, Darius and his boisterous crew experience an odyssey of American experiences: seeing alligators on a Florida swamp ride; collecting beads and female attention on Bourbon Street; wondering awestruck at the rim of the Grand Canyon; and dipping their toes in the Pacific Ocean. Along the way, the film includes elements of the conventional "buddy" trip, while providing snapshots of America's accessibility and the day-to-day realities of caregiving. The crew's first rest stop is at a gas station with no curb cuts, and Darius is forced to use the bathroom in the RV. The group celebrates the fifteenth anniversary of the Americans with Disability Act (ADA) with the rangers at the wheelchair-accessible Carlsbad Caverns but later are terribly frustrated at the inaccessible St. Louis Gateway Arch. Even more poignant are the scenes in which the young men of the crew roll heavyset Darius over in bed, adjust his swimming trunks, and cover his immobile legs with sunscreen and in which six or more fit, able-bodied young men drag Darius, on a blanket, to the edge of the lapping Pacific Ocean.

However, it is Darius himself who becomes "customized" by visual media rather than his wheelchair. Despite its good intentions, *Darius Goes West* ultimately robs its titular character of his subjecthood; instead, he becomes the vehicle for his crew members' and the viewing public's enlightenment regarding disability and access. This is a film about eleven young men who are transformed by their journey alongside Darius, rather than a film about any journey that Darius himself takes. In the words of one sobbing crew member: "Everything we do we have to do through Darius and none of us will be as good a person as Darius is." The emotional mark of the journey on all these young men is quite moving and genuine. Several get tattoos ("Darius Went West" and "DGW") as remembrances of journey and weep as they imagine a near-future world without Darius in it. In the words of Logan Smalley, the film's director, "We took this trip to celebrate Darius' life not to save it, and I realized Darius knows that. And that shook me—it shook me to action. The cure he's looking for isn't for him, it's for the next generation. He's saying look out for my brother when I'm gone. He is the vehicle. And that doesn't make me want to cry, it makes me want to fight" (2007).

As moving as this sentiment may be, it ultimately reduces Darius to the position of, at best, teacher, and at worst, a moral lesson. This is made particularly complex by the films nontreatment of race and ethnicity. Not once does anyone in the film comment that the crew consists of eleven able-bodied, white young men from Georgia (many of whom are college students) who are the caretakers of one wheelchair-using African American teen from the housing projects. When it is mentioned, race is referred to obliquely (and class almost never); it is the elephant in the RV. This is ironic in light, particularly, of laws of segregation in the American South that not so long ago prohibited African American and white people from traveling together, even using the same rest stops. Referring perhaps to the American South's legacies of racism, one of the crew says, "In the past it's been an issue of race, but now it's an issue of practicality." In this comment, race is relegated to a (resolved?) oppression of the past; disability access is the modern, "practical" (apolitical?) problem of the times. Similarly, Mark Johnson, one of the few other disabled individuals in the film (who is himself white), calls disability a "civil rights issue" without actually discussing the civil rights movement itself.

Director Spike Lee has roundly critiqued the trope of the "Magical Negro" in mainstream film[3]–a character who is purely a vehicle for the growth of the white protagonist (Gonzalez 2001). If *The Spirit Catches You* simplifies and exoticizes an immigrant community's "culture," and *Born into Brothels* reinforces the trope of the white savior who saves the vulnerable in distant lands, then *Darius Goes West* is a film whose imperialist discourse is profoundly American. Set in an imagined, postracial American frontier, the body and subjectivity of the disabled African American person becomes the vehicle for the growth of the white protagonists. This formulation is perhaps not dissimilar to well-intentioned healthcare students and practitioners who become deeply moved by their encounters with patients of differing economic or ethnic backgrounds but ultimately do not recognize the rhetorical violence they potentially commit on their patients themselves.

AN INWARD ORIENTATION: NARRATIVE HUMILITY

What are the implications of such critiques on the health and humanities classroom? This essay does not suggest that health and humanities educators *not* teach the above texts; rather, it suggests that teaching around race, class, ability, gender, or power opens up our understandings of the way we approach narratives themselves by situating them firmly within broader political contexts. By learning from, as well as critiquing, their assumptions, students of health and humanities integrate their classroom narratives into the real-life work of anti-oppression advocacy and social justice.

Simultaneously, teaching social justice in the health and humanities classroom cannot be a solely outward exercise—teaching about "them" while ignoring the internal workings of "us"—one's own personal, cultural, and institutional assumptions about race, class, ability, or gender. In a 1998 essay, Melanie Tervalon and Jann Murray-García suggested the term *cultural humility*, as opposed to *cultural competency* or *cultural sensitivity*, to guide clinicians in serving the needs of diverse populations. *Cultural competency* as a term suggests it is somehow possible to become entirely competent about another's culture. Tervalon and Murray-García suggest *cultural humility*, a practice committed to a lifelong process of self-evaluation and self-critique, as a more socially just alternative.

Building off of Tervalon and Murray-García's cultural humility, *narrative humility* (DasGupta 2008) can be a guiding force in the work of narrative, health, and social justice. Narrative humility is in many ways a response to Rita Charon's (2006) term *narrative competence*—the important idea that health and humanities teachers can train people to be competent in eliciting and interpreting patient stories. In contrast, the practice of narrative humility suggests an engagement with stories that acknowledges that stories are not objects that we can comprehend or ever become entirely competent regarding, particularly when those stories are oral interchanges with real live people on the other end. A position of narrative humility understands that stories are relationships that we can approach and engage with, while simultaneously remaining open to their ambiguity and contradiction and engaging in constant self-evaluation and self-critique about issues such as our own role in the story, our expectations of the story, our responsibilities to the story, and our ownership of the story. Also by thinking about it as narrative humility, we recognize that this is a perspective we take with *all* the stories we engage with (not just something we do when one of "those *other* people" walks into our office, whatever that may mean to us), while simultaneously not losing the idea that there are larger sociopolitical power structures that marginalize certain sorts of stories and privilege others.

A PEDAGOGY, AND HEALTH CARE, OF FREEDOM

A stance of narrative humility is a way to approach mutuality, what physician-anthropologist Paul Farmer has called *partnership in health* (2005) and a position of *accompaniment* ("Paul Farmer" 2011). In Farmer's words:

To accompany someone . . . is to go somewhere with him or her, to break bread together, to be present on a journey with a beginning and an end. . . . There's an element of mystery and openness. . . . I'll share your fate for awhile, and by "awhile" I don't mean "a little while." . . . [True accompaniment] does not privilege technical expertise above solidarity or compassion or a willingness to tackle what may seem to be insuperable challenges. . . . It requires cooperation, openness, and teamwork. ("Paul Farmer" 2011)

Educator and activist bell hooks suggests that education can also be a process of enacting justice and promoting freedom, a process of *accompaniment* (hooks

1994). This is not the model of education that is about facts being poured into learner's heads—what Brazilian educator Paolo Freire called the *banking model of education* (Freire 2000). Rather, it is a model of education that values what learners bring to the classroom, that co-constructs knowledge between teacher and student, that poses problems rather than ready solutions. If teaching is a parallel process—in other words, if the way we teach our clinical students (hierarchically, non-hierarchically, what have you) will then translate into the way that they treat their patients—then these approaches to power in the classroom can affect the clinic room as well.

Health and humanities faculty are ideally working toward a sort of health care, a sort of listening, that values the knowledge and experience of the sufferer; a health care that co-constructs meaning between clinician and patients, as well as teachers and learners; a health care dedicated to exploration and shared knowledge rather than a one-way flow of information. This sort of a narratively rendered and socially just approach can facilitate what might be called an "engaged health care." Here, I borrow again from hooks, who calls the kind of education she is interested in an *engaged pedagogy*. She draws from the work of Buddhist monk Thich Nhat Hanh, who says that "the practice of a healer, therapist, teacher or any helping professional should be directed toward his or herself first, because if the helper is unhappy, he or she cannot help many people" (quoted in hooks, 1994, 14). Such a stance of self-critique, transparency, and inward looking is what enables that state of engaged mutuality in which the storyteller and the minstrel of our opening folktale first found themselves.

Narratively humble, engaged, and socially just approaches to health and humanities will ideally facilitate the classroom or the clinic room to become, as hooks urges, a "location of possibility." In her words: "In that field of possibility, we have the opportunity to labor for freedom, to demand of ourselves and our comrades, an openness of mind and heart that allows us to face reality even as we collectively imagine ways to move beyond boundaries, to transgress" (hooks 1994, 207). This would indeed be a health care, and a health and humanities education, that could be "a practice of freedom."

NOTES

1 Learn more about Kids with Cameras, now called Kids with Destiny, at www.kids-with-cameras.org/home.
2 Duchenne Muscular Dystrophy is an X-linked degenerative neuromuscular condition that often takes the lives of its young sufferers by their twenties. The film is now part of a broader advocacy campaign (located at www.dariusgoeswest.org).
3 For example, *The Legend of Bagger Vance* (Redford 2000), in which an African American character in the 1930s seems less concerned with lynchings and prevalent racism than improving Matt Damon's golf swing, or *The Green Mile* (Darabont 1999) in which an imprisoned African American character seems to exist solely to heal the white protagonists—body and soul.

Chapter 25

RACE AND MENTAL HEALTH

JONATHAN M. METZL

Race and insanity share a long and complicated past (see Metzl 2010). In the 1850s, American psychiatrists believed that African American slaves who ran away from their white masters did so because of a mental illness called *drapetomania*. Medical journals of the era also described a condition called *dysaesthesia aethiopis*, a form of madness marked by "rascality" and "disrespect for the master's property" that was believed to be "cured" by extensive whipping. Even at the turn of the twentieth century, leading academic psychiatrists shamefully claimed that "Negroes" were "psychologically unfit" for freedom (Cartwright 1851; Evarts 1914; Lind 1914).

American medicine has undoubtedly progressed since that time; terms such as *drapetomania* fill the dustbin of history, and rightly so. Yet instances arise in the present-day suggesting that seemingly hermetic clinical encounters between psychiatrists and patients unconsciously mirror larger conversations about the politics of race. For instance, a prominent story appeared on the front page of the *Washington Post* on June 28, 2005. "Racial Disparities Found in Pinpointing Mental Illness" read the headline, above an article that detailed how researchers had examined the largest American registry of psychiatric patient records looking for "ethnic trends" in the ways in which doctors diagnosed schizophrenia. As the *Post* described it, schizophrenia, "a disorder that often portends years of powerful brain-altering drugs, social ostracism and forced hospitalizations . . . has been shown to affect all ethnic groups at the same rate." And yet, the large government study uncovered striking categorical differences in its analysis of 134,523 case files: doctors diagnosed schizophrenia in African American patients, and particularly African American men, *four times* as often as in white patients. The *Post* cited the study's lead author John Zeber, who explained that doctors overdiagnosed schizophrenia in African American men even though the research team uncovered no evidence that "black patients were any sicker than whites" or that patients in either group were more likely to suffer from drug addiction, poverty, depression, or a host of other variables. According to Zeber, "The only factor that was truly important was race" (Blow et al. 2004; Vedantam 2005, A1).

Paradoxically, we live in an era when the opposite is supposed to be the case: race should be entirely unimportant to psychiatric diagnosis. Present-day psychiatry believes that mental illness results from disordered brain biology at levels that are presumably the same in people of all races and ethnic backgrounds.

And psychiatrists consider schizophrenia to be the most biologically based of the mental illnesses. Leading journals routinely attribute symptoms of the illness— officially defined as delusions, hallucinations, disorganized speech, disorganized or catatonic behavior, or so-called negative symptoms such as affective flattening— to defects in specific brain structures, peptides, or neurotransmitters. Articles that describe research into the causes of the illness thus carry titles such as "Conserved Regional Patterns of GABA-Related Transcript Expression in the Neocortex of Subjects with Schizophrenia" or, incredibly, "Smaller Nasal Volumes as Stigmata of Aberrant Neurodevelopment in Schizophrenia." Meanwhile, textbooks routinely claim that, as a biological disorder, schizophrenia is an illness that should occur in *one percent* of any given population, or one out of every hundred persons regardless of where they live, how they dress, who they know, or what type of music they happen to prefer (*DSM-IV-TR* 2000; Regier et al. 1993).

Yet stories such as the *Post* article persist over time. In the 1960s, National Institute of Mental Health studies found that "blacks have a 65% higher rate of schizophrenia than whites." In 1973, a series of studies in the *Archives of General Psychiatry* discovered that African American patients were "significantly more likely" than white patients to receive schizophrenia diagnoses and "significantly less likely" than white patients to receive diagnoses for other mental illnesses such as depression or bipolar disorder. Throughout the 1980s and 1990s, a host of articles from leading psychiatric and medical journals showed that doctors diagnosed the paranoid subtype of schizophrenia in African American men five to seven times more often than in white men and also more frequently than in other ethnic minority groups (Delahanty 2001; Mukherjee et al. 1983).

The persistence of these findings suggest that, though we might wish otherwise, medical training does not entirely free certain clinicians from preexisting racial beliefs, assumptions, or blind spots. While medicine has made significant progress toward addressing multicultural issues in clinical practice, some individual doctors surely continue to harbor negative opinions about particular patients based on stereotyped cultural assumptions. As University of California at San Francisco psychiatrist Francis Lu explains it, "Physician bias is a very real issue. . . . We don't talk about it—it's upsetting. We see ourselves as unbiased and rational and scientific" (Vedantam 2005, A1; see also Sack 2008, D1; Sequist et al. 2008).

Recent work in the humanities and social sciences suggests that broader forces are at play as well. Vital texts such as John Hoberman's *Black and Blue* (2012), Harriet Washington's *Medical Apartheid* (2006), and Keith Wailoo's *Dying in the City of the Blues* (2001) show how, from a historical perspective, race affects medical communication because racial tensions are structured into clinical interactions long before doctors or patients enter examination rooms. This scholarship suggests that, to a remarkable extent, anxieties about racial difference shape diagnostic criteria, healthcare policies, medical and popular attitudes about mentally ill persons, the structures of treatment facilities, and, ultimately, the conversations that take place there within.

Stokely Carmichael, the civil rights activist, once described such a process as institutional racism, by which he meant forms of bias embedded, not in actions or beliefs of individuals, but in the functions of social structures and institutions. "I don't deal with the individual," he said. "I think it's a cop out when people talk about the individual." Instead, Carmichael protested the silent racism of "established and respected forces in the society" that functioned above the level of individual perceptions or intentions and that worked to maintain the status quo through such structures as zoning laws, economics, schools, and courts. Institutionalized racism, he argued, "is less overt, far more subtle, less identifiable in terms of specific individuals committing the acts, but is no less destructive of human life" (1968, 151).

In a perfect world, interactions between doctors and patients should be immune from any process deemed destructive to health. The Hippocratic Oath decrees that the primary aim of medical encounters is to restore, not to harm. Most physicians enter the practice of medicine out of a desire to help people. And most patients seek the aid of physicians in times when they require palliation and care. However, evidence increasingly suggests that structural forces supersede even the best individual intentions when race and insanity are the topics of diagnostic interaction.

SCHIZOPHRENIA

Schizophrenia is an example of a disease whose material realities have been profoundly influenced by the politics of race. American medical and popular understandings of the illness shifted radically during the civil rights era of the 1960s and 1970s. Over this vital period, new clinical ways of defining mental illness unintentionally combined with growing cultural anxieties about social change. Meanwhile, reports about new "psychochemical" technologies of control merged with concerns about the "uncontrolled" nature of urban unrest.

From the 1920s to the 1950s, American medical and popular opinion often assumed that patients with schizophrenia were largely white and generally harmless to society. Psychiatric textbooks depicted schizophrenia as an exceedingly broad, general condition, manifest by "emotional disharmony" that negatively affected white people's abilities to "think and feel." Authors of research articles in leading psychiatric journals, many of whom were psychoanalysts, described patients with schizophrenia and, all too often, their "schizophrenogenic mothers," as "native-born Americans" or immigrants of "white European ancestry." Psychiatric authors frequently assumed that such patients were nonthreatening and were therefore to be psychotherapeutically nurtured by their doctors, as if unruly children, but certainly not feared (Noyes 1927, 127–128).

Leading mainstream American newspapers in the 1920s–1950s similarly described schizophrenia as an illness that occurred "in the seclusive, sensitive person with few friends who has been the model of behavior in childhood" or that afflicted white women or intellectuals. In 1935, for instance, the *New York Times* described how many white poets and novelists demonstrated a symptom called "grandiloquence," a propensity toward flowery prose believed to be "one of the telltale phrases of schizophrenia, the mild form of insanity known as split personality" ("Psychiatrists Are Told of 'Literary Artists' Who Evidence Schizophrenia: Grandiloquence Is Sign" 1935, 17). Meanwhile, popular magazines such as *Ladies'*

Home Journal (Marsden and Adams 1949) and *Better Homes and Gardens* (Cooley 1947) wrote of unhappily married, middle-class white women whose schizophrenic mood swings were suggestive of "Doctor Jekyll and Mrs. Hyde," a theme that also appeared in Olivia de Havilland's infamous depiction of a "schizophrenic housewife" named Virginia Stuart Cunningham in the 1948 Anatole Litvak film *The Snake Pit*.

Of course, it was far from the case that all persons who suffered from a disease called *schizophrenia* during the first half of the twentieth century were members of a category called *white*. Rather, American culture marked schizophrenia as a disease of the mainstream in ways that encouraged identification with certain groups of persons while rendering other groups invisible. For example, popular magazines in the 1920s through 1950s incorrectly assumed that schizophrenia was a psychoanalytic condition connected to neurosis and, as a result, affixed the term to middle-class housewives. Meanwhile, researchers conducted most published clinical studies in white-only wards. Such strategies occluded recognition of the countless men and women diagnosed with schizophrenia who resided in so-called Negro Hospitals and suffered well outside most realms of public awareness ("Insanity: Mental Illness among Negroes Exceeds Whites, Overcrowds Already-Jammed 'Snake Pits,'" 1949).

American assumptions about the race, gender, and temperament of schizophrenia changed beginning in the 1960s. Many leading medical and popular sources suddenly described schizophrenia as an illness marked not by docility but by rage. Growing numbers of research articles from leading psychiatric journals asserted that schizophrenia was a condition that also afflicted "Negro men," and that black forms of the illness were more hostile and aggressive than were white ones. In the worst cases, psychiatric authors conflated the schizophrenic symptoms of African American patients with the perceived schizophrenia of civil rights protests, particularly those organized by Black Power, Black Panthers, Nation of Islam, or other activist groups.

As but one example, in a 1968 article that appeared in the *Archives of General Psychiatry*, psychiatrists Walter Bromberg and Frank Simon described schizophrenia as a *Protest Psychosis*, whereby black men developed "hostile and aggressive feelings" and "delusional anti-whiteness" after listening to the words of Malcolm X, joining the Black Muslims, or aligning with groups that preached militant resistance to white society. According to the authors, the men required psychiatric treatment because their symptoms threatened not only their own sanity but also the social order of white America. Bromberg and Simon argued that black men who "espoused African or Islamic" ideologies and adopted "Islamic names" that were changed in such a way so as to deny "the previous Anglicization of their names" in fact demonstrated a "delusional anti-whiteness" that manifest as "paranoid projections of the Negroes to the Caucasian group" (1968, 55–60).

Meanwhile, mainstream newspapers in the 1960s and 1970s described schizophrenia as a condition of angry black masculinity or warned of crazed, black, schizophrenic killers on the loose. "FBI Adds Negro Mental Patient to '10 Most Wanted' List" warned a *Chicago Tribune* headline in July 1966, above an article that advised readers to remain clear of "Leroy Ambrosia Frazier, an extremely danger-ous and mentally unbalanced schizophrenic escapee from a mental institution, who has a lengthy criminal record and history of violent assaults" ("FBI Adds Negro Mental Patient to '10 Most Wanted' List," 1966). Hollywood films such as Samuel Fuller's 1963 B-movie classic, *Shock Corridor*, similarly cast the illness as arising in black men, and particularly men who participated in civil rights protests (Crowther 1963, 32).

Schizophrenia's rhetorical transformation from an illness of white docility to one of black hostility resulted from a confluence of social and medical forces. Some of these forces were obvious, such as the biased actions of individual doc-tors or researchers. Other forces were less apparent, such as the shifting language associated with the official psychiatric definition of schizophrenia. Prior to the 1960s, psychiatry often posited that schizophrenia was a psychological "reaction" to a splitting of the basic functions of personality. Official descriptors emphasized the generally calm nature of such persons in ways that encouraged associations with middle-class housewives. But the frame changed in the 1960s. In 1968, in the midst of a political climate marked by profound protest and social unrest, psychia-try published the second edition of the *Diagnostic and Statistical Manual*. That text recast the paranoid subtype of schizophrenia as a disorder of masculinized bel-ligerence. "The patient's attitude is frequently hostile and aggressive," the *DSM-II* (1968, 33–35) claimed, "and his behavior tends to be consistent with his delusions."

Growing numbers of research articles from the 1960s and 1970s used this lan-guage to assert that schizophrenia was a condition that also afflicted "Negro men" and that black forms of the illness were more hostile and aggressive than were white ones (*Mental Disorders* 1952, 26–27; *DSM-II* 1968, 33–35). Some African American patients *became* schizophrenic because of changes in diagnostic criteria rather than in their clinical symptoms. Emerging understandings of the illness shaped Ameri-can cultural fears about mental illness more broadly, particularly regarding cultural stereotypes of persons with schizophrenia as being unduly hostile or violent.

THE RELEVANCE OF HISTORY

In no way is this type of analysis meant to suggest that schizophrenia is a socially fabricated disease or, worse, that people's suffering is somehow inauthentic. As the clinician and activist E. Fuller Torrey writes, "The lives of those affected [by schizophrenia] are often chronicles of constricted experiences, muted emotions, missed opportunities, unfulfilled expectations. . . . The fate of these patients has been worsened by our propensity to misunderstand" (Torrey 2001, xxi–xxii).

At the same time, humanities scholarship helps illuminate the mechanisms whereby the material reality of schizophrenia is shaped by social, political, and, ultimately, institutional factors in addition to chemical or biological ones. As the *Washington Post* article demonstrates, this history continues to affect the lives of African American men who receive higher dosages of antipsychotic medications than do white male psychiatric patients and are more likely to be described by healthcare professionals as being hostile or violent (Segal et al. 1996). History also lives on in instances where associations between schizophrenia and race suggest a loosening of associations, to use historian Keith Wailoo's insightful description of the ways assumptions about the virulence of particular racial groups expand to affect all sufferers of a particular disease. For instance, negative perceptions of persons with schizophrenia as being unduly hostile or violent thrive in American society, even though these persons are exponentially more likely to be the victims than the perpetrators of violent acts (Delahanty 2001; Mukherjee et al. 1983; Segal et al. 1996).

As such, humanities scholarship helps us take aim at the belief that the stigma of psychiatric illness cannot be changed because stigmatizing attitudes against the mentally ill are timeless, eternal, and, ultimately, immutable. Beliefs about the volatility of madmen are as old as time itself, this logic implies. As the eminent historian Roy Porter (2002) aptly describes it, narratives of insane violence "may be as old as mankind" and course through disparate religious texts and object lessons. Yet arguments about the timeless nature of schizophrenia as stigmatized often fail to address the impact of relatively recent events on present-day attitudes and beliefs. Schizophrenia was a European term invented in the early twentieth century and imported to the United States around 1915. For decades, schizophrenia connoted white, American neurosis. Only during the civil rights era did emerging scientific understandings of schizophrenia become enmeshed in a set of historical currents that marked particular bodies and particular psyches as crazy in particular ways. The tensions of that era then changed the associations that many Americans made about persons with schizophrenia in ways that altered, not just the stigma attached to the illness, but the definition of the illness itself.

CONCLUSION

It has been argued that we inhabit a current cultural moment in which American racial systems, ideas, and social relations promise improvement. The election of an African American president, this logic goes, suggests a transformation, not just in governance but in long-held attitudes, beliefs, and everyday practices. Change is here, the moment tells us, and change will come. Yet the ongoing tension between race and mental health provides a cautionary tale about the complex ways in which moments of change, and particularly moments that portend changed race or gender relations, produce anxieties about the stability of the status quo. The battles that follow—when the idea of change produces actual change—appear for all the world to play out on the public stage: in an election, for instance, or in the White House, or in other highly visible sites, where newfound leaders, freedoms, or rights become markers of progress for some people and symbols of inquietude for others.

History teaches us, however, that the brunt of the pushback against change is borne most by persons who, for various reasons, are least able to defend themselves. These persons then become doubly or triply stigmatized based on unfounded generalizations about deviance, or perceived volatility, or abnormality that remain acceptable modes of discrimination. Public concern about the actions or proclivities of these persons then grows, even as the persons themselves are rendered less-than-full citizens or are progressively removed from public life. As we know all too well from plagues past, the rhetorics of health and illness become effective ways of policing the boundaries of civil society and of keeping these persons always outside.

In this sense, humanities scholarship that studies the connections between race and mental health is faced with a complex task. Such scholarship frequently respects attempts to uncover the ontology of illness. But it also recognizes that the search for ontology is an ongoing process and that the frames aggregating certain symptoms into particular psychiatric diagnoses exist in an ongoing state of flux. Such flux can be a positive force, to be sure: it allows psychiatry to redefine illnesses in ways that are more scientifically precise. But flux can also have abjectifying or stigmatizing consequences if its mechanisms are not closely monitored.

In other words, for better and for worse, humanities scholarship helps uncover how the frames aggregating certain symptoms into particular psychiatric diagnoses exist in an ongoing state of flux. Recognizing such a process does not mean that psychiatrists should vote about whether a particular diagnosis is either socially constructed or real. Indeed, the polarizing dichotomy serves no one and makes it harder to see how mental illness is always already both. Rather, psychiatry should remain continually aware of how social contexts, historical moments, and violent structures shape perceptions of psychiatric reality. Psychiatry, in other words, must persist in its pursuit of the ontology of mental illness. But history suggests that it must also persist in developing methods for recognizing who its ontologies, categories, and provider networks leave out.

Chapter 26

LAW'S HAND IN RACE, CLASS, AND HEALTH INEQUITIES

On the Humanities and the Social Determinants of Health

DANIEL GOLDBERG

To understand law's power in shaping health along social strata like race and class, it is important to first say something, however brief, about law's capacity to change society and culture. The extent of this power is evident in the fact that law is one of the crucibles for the humanities; Socrates's words and acts in the *Apology* are forged against the anvil of prosecution, trial, and punishment. But antiquity was mediated in ways critical for the contemporary humanities by the medieval and Renaissance humanists who bequeathed to moderns the educational program known as the *studia humanitatis*. And as practiced by the Renaissance humanists, the humanities had as their raison d'etre practical engagement with the world, a task for which mastery of rhetoric was critical. Charles Nauert observes that "humanistic education claimed to provide rhetorical skills that would help . . . young men participate effectively in political life. It also claimed to provide an emphasis on moral training and moral obligation that seemed directly relevant to a ruling elite" (2006, 15).

Contrary to the contemporary tendency to see rhetoric as empty sophistry, for the humanists rhetoric was deeply practical and necessary to live not just an engaged political and social life but a virtuous one. Discussing Coluccio Salutati, Nauert explains that "his success as the [Florentine] republic's principal civil servant, which made him a central figure in Italian diplomacy, rested on his skill at applying the humanistic art of rhetoric (persuasive speech and writing) to the task of making the hard moral (that is, political) choices required by the politics of the day. His humanistic learning was not just an ornament. It was essential to his success" (2006, 28).

The key here is that, for the humanists, rhetoric was inextricably connected to the cultivation of virtue. This is not because the practice of rhetoric is inherently virtuous. The humanists well understood that *res* and *verba* were not necessarily linked; Gorgias admits that Socrates is correct that "rhetoric apparently is a creator of a conviction that is persuasive but not instructive about right and wrong" (*Gorgias* 455e; see Plato 1989). Yet effective rhetoric "alone could speak to the hearts of men, quicken faith, and transform lives," much more so than the disputations of the Scholastics (Nauert 2006, 28). Directed for virtuous ends, no skill was more useful in facilitating virtuous practice than rhetoric.

Accordingly, it is no coincidence that many of the humanists trained in law. William Bouwsma notes that "the culture of Renaissance humanism, especially in its earlier stages, was largely a creation of lawyers and notaries" (1973, 308). Their influence reached well beyond the Renaissance itself: "Lawyers played a large part in public support for the scientific movement of the seventeenth century in both France and England . . . and the so-called Scottish Renaissance of the eighteenth century was dominated by lawyers" (Bouwsma 1973, 308). Indeed, figures like Hugo Grotius and Jeremy Bentham, who hoped to reform the social order, "devoted themselves primarily to juridical thought" (Bouwsma 1973, 308).

From this brief excursion into the history of the humanities, several points follow. First, the humanists who crafted the educational program that forms the core of the contemporary humanities saw law as a critical tool for practical engagement with the world. The humanists' emphasis on practice and pragmatism was a direct response to the high Scholasticism of the monasteries and universities, from whence the term "cloistered" as a pejorative for academics originated. Second, insofar as a central objective of this engagement was the use of erudition and learning in the service of virtue, law has moral content. Like rhetoric, law can be used for good or for ill, but the humanists understood it as an extraordinarily powerful tool in shaping society, in answering the Aristotelian question: What kind of people do we wish to be?

Thus, law is in many ways a crucible of the humanities and of the essence in cultivating or, sadly, diminishing civic virtue. There are few better examples for analyzing these capacities than that which occupies the remainder of this essay: the extent to which law mediates the distribution of health along lines of race and class.

LAW AS A SOCIAL DETERMINANT OF HEALTH

One of the salutary effects of the recent terminological shift away from the "medical humanities" and toward the "health humanities" or "health and the humanities" is that it underscores the critical distinction between health and medicine. This distinction is so important precisely because robust historical and contemporary epidemiologic evidence suggests quite strongly that medical care is only a minor determinant of health and its distribution in human populations (Goldberg 2011; Lantz et al. 2007). Rather, the evidence shows that a number of social and economic factors are primary determinants of health, disease, and the distribution of each (Commission on Social Determinants of Health 2009; Link and Phelan 1995; Phelan et al. 2010). Such factors include but are not limited to income, class, education, housing, transportation, occupation, environment, violence, race, and stigma and discrimination.

Collectively, these factors are referred to as the social determinants of health. While medicine and medical care are unquestionably social determinants of health in their own right, strong evidence suggests that myriad other social determinants exert comparatively larger and more enduring effects on health and its distribution than medical care (Goldberg 2009, 2011; Lantz et al. 2007; Woolf et al. 2007). I have developed and defended these claims in detail elsewhere; the key point for this essay is understanding law itself as a critical social determinant of health (Burris 2011; Burris et al. 2002). What this means is that law is one of the central pathways through which social and economic factors shape health. There are many examples of such processes: (1) public transit laws and policies mediate the number of automobile fatalities; (2) laws regarding occupational conditions mediate both injury and chronic stress, the latter of which is robustly correlated with poor health outcomes (Brunner and Marmot 2006); and (3) laws and policies governing the allocation of resources to early childhood development programs have a pronounced effect on health given the compelling evidence linking socioeconomic conditions of early childhood to health over the lifespan (Anderson et al. 2003; Irwin et al. 2007; Raphael 2011). Other examples are not difficult to find, but the point for now is to perceive that laws and policies that go far beyond health insurance schemes have a pronounced effect on health and its inequitable distribution in human populations in both the global North and the global South. In fact, the epidemiologic evidence strongly suggests that many domains of law *other than* healthcare and health insurance law are by a fair margin more important in determining health and the lived experiences of illness.

The next part of this essay is devoted to exploring the interplay between law and two of the most powerful social determinants of health: race and class. Before proceeding, it is important to understand that health status and health outcomes are shaped by long causal pathways consisting of a large number of causes, determinants, and exposures. Thus it is not sufficient simply to state that social and economic conditions are the prime determinants of health outcomes—although they are—but rather that such conditions also shape the causal factors along the pathways that result in those health outcomes. As such, it is not just health that is distributed unequally across the globe but exposures to risks and deleterious social and economic conditions that are distributed unequally. As social epidemiologist Hilary Graham puts it, "Unequal social positions carry with them unequal probabilities of being exposed to health hazards along the environment/risk factors/illness pathway" (2004, 113).

Moreover, disadvantage tends to cluster (Commission on Social Determinants of Health 2009; Powers and Faden 2006; Wolff 2009). This well-documented phenomenon demonstrates that persons of lower socioeconomic status do not just suffer the impact on health from that determinant by itself but also face higher risks of having lower educational achievement, greater exposures to environmental hazards, poor working conditions with high stress, low job autonomy and little leisure time, poor access to public transit and/or long commutes, greater exposures to violence, an so on. Of course, such clustering is a population-level phenomenon; there is no guarantee that any individual will experience all or even most of these disadvantages. But across a population of disadvantaged persons it is much more likely that a person who experiences any single social disadvantage will experience others, and the clustering of these disadvantages has an enormous and deleterious impact on health. The clustering of social disadvantages and their effects on health signifies that both the social and economic conditions that determine health and health outcomes themselves—disease, suffering, and death—are distributed highly unequally. This fact has profound ethical ramifications, especially considered from the vantage point of social justice (Powers and Faden 2006). Although full exploration of these implications is beyond the scope of this essay, the intensely normative aspects of the humanities require confrontation with the fundamental Aristotelian question: What kind of people do we wish to be? It is imperative to keep this question in mind as the discussion proceeds on race, class, and health inequities.[1]

RACE AND CLASS INTERSECTIONALITY

The race-health and class-health relationships are tight and extremely well documented. Indeed, some of the foundations of the modern history of public health and social medicine are predicated on the class-health connection in particular (Engels [1845] 2005; Goldberg 2011; Waitzkin 2006). Before detailing some of this evidence and law's hand in shaping their health effects, two points are significant.

First, it is essential to understand that race and class are *social* rather than *intrinsic* determinants of health. Especially as to race, this matters a great deal because American histories of public health and medicine are saturated with the pernicious belief that race is an inherent cause of all manner of diseases and susceptibilities. For example, American Progressive public health reformers widely believed that groups like African Americans and Native Americans were more susceptible to infectious disease because of inherent racial degeneracy and deficiency (Chowkwanyun 2011; Jones 2004; McMillen 2008; Molina 2006). African Americans and other socially marginalized groups were frequently denied access to anesthesia in the latter half of the nineteenth century because of beliefs that they could endure much higher levels of pain and suffering than socially privileged white persons (Pernick 1985). One of the progenitors of obstetrics, J. Marion Sims, adopted a similar justification for his use of slave women as opposed to his well-heeled white patients as subjects in his experiments on vesicovaginal fistula (Pernick 1985).

The point is that understanding why race is so strongly correlated with health and inequities must not devolve into an essentialist, racialized discourse that posits inherent connections between race and health. Rather, the evidence shows that social, economic, and political structures that shape the lived experiences of race in the United States are the primary determinants and pathways by which race is linked with health and its inequitable distribution. Where race is a social category, so, too, are the pathways between race and health fundamentally social.

Second, while race and class are not identical phenomena, for purposes of assessing their health effects, they are nevertheless not independent variables. Trying to abstract the health effects of race from those of class is inadvisable because race and class shape and affect each other on multiple levels. Indeed, the pathways between social conditions and health are best conceptualized as complex adaptive systems in which myriad variables, attractors, and outcomes repeatedly interact with and shape each other in feedback loops (Jayasinghe 2011). Thus, classical scientific models that proceed by abstracting each system variable from all the others fundamentally distort the causal pathways between the variables and overall system behavior. As pioneering social epidemiologist Nancy Krieger puts it, it is the "interrelationships between—and accountability for—diverse forms of social inequality, including racism, class, and gender" that are most important to discussion of health (2010, 107). While the effects of race and class on health are therefore not identical, they are coextensive, and the ensuing discussion examines them in concert.

RACE, CLASS, AND HEALTH INEQUITIES

Race and class, individually and collectively, exert enormous influence in shaping health and its distribution in human populations. In the United States, racial health inequities exist in a number of indicia, including infant mortality, heart disease, and cancer (Gee and Ford 2011). As Gilbert Gee and Chandra Ford put it, "Health inequities among racial minorities are pronounced, persistent and pervasive" (2011, 115). Although there is no shortage of research on the race-health relationship, much of the early twentieth-century research on the subject suffered from the aforementioned sin of positing an intrinsic connection between race and health. More responsible research has focused on race as a social category and attempted to account for the socioeconomic conditions to which marginalized racial communities are inequitably exposed. Social epidemiologists have more recently attended to the relationship between racism and health, noting that stigmatization alone is a significant determinant of health and that "persons who self-report exposures to racism have greater risk for mental and physical ailments" (Gee and Ford 2011, 116; Krieger 2003). Even after controlling for almost every conceivable confounding variable, there is significant evidence that persons exposed to persistent racism suffer more illness and die sooner than similarly situated persons not so exposed (Krieger 2003; Krieger and Sidney 1996).

As Nancy Krieger and George Davey Smith (2004) explain, humans are embodied creatures, and social disadvantages become embedded in our bodies over time, with profound health effects. The daily psychosocial burden of living with stigmatization and discrimination in the form of racism is only one such disadvantage, although the weight of the evidence suggests it may be a particularly powerful determinant.

While the effect size of racism on health remains a relatively open question, the effect size of class on health is less so. Social position is one of the preeminent determinants of health in human populations. There is little better demonstration of this than the Whitehall studies, an enormously influential and significant series of longitudinal studies of the health of British civil servants.[2] Drawing on a rich and high-quality data set, Sir Michael Marmot and colleagues produced a number of startling and significant findings (Marmot 2003). For purposes of the discussion here, among the most relevant is the fact that all of the subjects had access to healthcare services through the National Health Service, which implies that significant differences in health among the subjects cannot be explained by access to medical care. The existence of such differences constitutes the other highly relevant finding: Marmot and colleagues demonstrated an almost linear correlation between health and occupational status, the latter of which is a powerful marker of class. The results from Whitehall have been substantially reproduced at local, state, regional, national, and international levels across the globe, thereby establishing that health typically follows a social gradient, with class being one of the primary determinants of the distribution of health in a given society (Goldberg 2011).

LEGAL PATHWAYS TO RACE AND CLASS-BASED HEALTH INEQUITIES

Law can of course impact race-based and class-based health inequities at the micro level. An obvious example is a law barring members of a certain race or class from accessing social services that are connected to health (using racial criteria to determine eligibility for public housing, denying enfranchisement to non-landed persons, etc.). However, such overt and blatant forms of discrimination are, while certainly not extinct in the United States, less common than race-based and class-based structural and institutional discrimination. In terms of race, Gee and Ford clarify the distinction between racism on the individual and the structural level through the iceberg metaphor: "The tip of the iceberg represents acts of racism, such as cross-burnings, that are easily seen and individually mediated. The portion of the iceberg that lies below the water represents structural racism; it is more dangerous and harder to eliminate. Policies and interventions that change the iceberg's tip may do little to change its base, resulting in structural inequalities that remain intact, though less detectable" (2011, 116).

Moreover, a focus on structural aspects of race and class powerfully demonstrates law's hand in health. Gee and Ford (2011) point out that immigration is a highly significant social determinant of health, and immigration in the United States is shaped at a deep level by U.S. laws and policies regarding immigration. For example, U.S. immigration law for many years essentially treated Haitian Americans as a deviant underclass (Simon 1998), in all likelihood playing a role in the intense stigmatization directed at Haitians and Haitian Americans during the early years of the HIV/AIDS epidemic (Galarneau 2010). More generally, Gee and Ford argue that

the exclusion of non-Whites from citizenship has been a defining characteristic of U.S. immigration policy.... Immigration control today retains many of the actions (e.g., the use of quotas, screening for undesirable traits, exclusion of those likely to be public charges) developed during one of America's most xenophobic and racist periods.... Immigration policy is a form of structural racism: exclusionary policies provide the most permanent and broad-scale type of segregation by prohibiting groups from entering the country, deporting those already here, and limiting the rights of those deemed to be threats. (2011, 119, 122)

Thus, insofar as immigration and social segregation exert significant effects on health, laws and policies that institutionalize racial inequities determine health inequities as well.

Other examples also show law's influence in shaping health along strata of race and class. Consider transportation policy. Over the past two decades in the United States, "traffic fatalities have averaged approximately 43,000 annually, with approximately 2.5 million people injured on our roads every year" (American Public Health Association 2008, 3). To put these numbers in some perspective, annual approximate mortality statistics in the United States include 18,000 deaths from HIV/AIDS and 23,000 deaths from diabetes. There is no dispute that transportation laws and policies have ample power to improve or worsen these statistics: a 2003 meta-analysis noted that laws targeted against drunk driving are one of the most effective transport interventions in improving health (Morrison et al. 2003), and legislation enhancing the availability of public transit also has a salutary effect on health (American Public Health Association 2008). Moreover, transportation policy mediates health equities along strata of race (Ross and Leigh 2000) and class. As to the latter, a 2008 report of the American Public Health Association notes that many families of lower socioeconomic status "have been forced to live outside city centers where housing is more affordable and access to public transportation is limited. These families often spend more on driving than healthcare, education, or food. The poorest fifth of U.S. families, earning less than $13,060 per year, pay 42% of their income to own and drive a vehicle. Those families earning $20,000 to $50,000 spend as much as 30% of their budget on transportation" (American Public Health Association 2008, 5). Transportation laws and policies relating to, for example, the availability of public transit, road conditions, and traffic safety have a tremendous capacity to alleviate or exacerbate these trends, which demonstrates how law mediates health inequities along lines of race and class.

This essay has already noted that racism is a powerful social determinant of health. Racism is fundamentally related to stigmatization and discrimination, which exert significant effects on population health and its distribution (Burris 2002; Link and Phelan 2006). One of the most obvious examples of this is HIV/AIDS stigma, which not only can cause devastating psychosocial harm and worsen disease outcomes but also in historical terms has disproportionately targeted marginalized social groups such as intravenous drug users, African and Caribbean immigrants, and gay men (Burris 2002). There is solid evidence that changes in U.S. law and policy regarding HIV/AIDS dramatically ameliorated the hitherto crushing levels of stigma directed at those marginalized social groups (Herek et al. 2002). Examples of such changes included enactments in privacy, disability, and antidiscrimination laws and policies (Brimlow et al. 2003). Because diminution of disease stigma improves both the psychosocial impact of illness and clinical outcomes of disease itself, these public policy changes had ethical significance.

Although time and space preclude further examples, those offered suggest that law mediates health and its distribution along lines of race and class in myriad domains, from immigration and transportation to housing and environment. Law may therefore be a powerful tool for ameliorating or intensifying the relationships between race, class, and health.

CONCLUSION

The Renaissance humanists laid the groundwork for the modern humanities. The possibility that, like rhetoric, law is less an institution of intrinsic worth than one that may possess significant instrumental value would not have troubled them. As Nauert puts it, for the humanists, "the ultimate goal is not knowledge of truth . . . the purpose of human life is to make sound moral decisions in the course of daily living" (Nauert 2006, 15). The humanists were thus profoundly interested in the question, What kind of people do we wish to be? but for them, the study of moral philosophy "involved not primarily a body of knowledge to be understood but rather a set of values to be internalized and applied in making the moral choices that arise in every human's life" (Nauert 2006, 201).

Rhetoric and law were so crucial for the humanists because they were critical tools for encouraging virtuous practice in the everyday world. Different stakeholders are responsive to different rhetoric, which is itself an element of classical oratory. Tailoring the communication to suit the audience is the notion of *decorum*, which was instrumental in, for example, Erasmus's mode of humanist toleration (Remer 1996). There is in this suggestion the barest beginning of an account of the potential use of the health humanities in public health policy. If health policy requires practical engagement, and if the model of the Renaissance humanists encourages the marriage of such engagement with virtue, then there is reason to believe that this model may have particular insight for weighing issues of social justice as to race, class, health, and policy. Michel de Montaigne, who was both a lawyer and a judge, was deeply concerned with questions of justice, but he was dubious of the value of formal codes in ensuring virtue. In "Of Vanity," he remarks that "the sentence I pass upon myself is sharper and stiffer than that of judges, who only consider me with respect to common obligation; the grip of my conscience is tighter and more severe" (Montaigne [1588] 2003, 897). Many scholars have taken this as a rejection of the significance of justice, but Andre Tournon suggests a more plausible alternative: "In fact the point is to stake out a space of freedom in which the *virtue* of justice can be practiced, the mere obeying of laws being its worthless *Ersatz*" (Tournon 2005, 111).

Ultimately, law understood as a crucible of the humanities, as a critical tool in the cultivation of virtuous practice, can hardly be more suited to analyses of race, class, and health. The evidence is compelling that race and class are significant social determinants of health. Members of racial and ethnic minorities and lower-class communities are much more likely to experience the accumulation of risk factors and social disadvantages that result in material deprivation, increased suffering and burdens of disease, and premature death. And while law is not the root cause of race and class-based health inequities, it is a powerful determinant of the lived experiences of race, class, sickness, and health.

NOTES

1 This essay utilizes the term *inequities* rather than *inequalities* or *disparities* because the first term conveys a normative valence (Evans et al. 2001). Disparities are merely differences, and inequalities can at least in theory be natural. But the term *inequity* implies some notion of unfairness or injustice, which, especially as to issues of race, class, and health, is critical. That is, those disparities or inequalities that matter most in terms of race and class are those that are unfair or unjust.
2 The Whitehall studies have produced a large number of papers and works devoted to documenting the findings and explaining their significance. A short bibliography of some of these works is available; see Michael Marmot (n.d.).

Chapter 27

THE ROOMS OF OUR SOULS

MAREN GRAINGER-MONSEN

No form of art goes beyond ordinary consciousness as film does, straight to our emotions, deep into the twilight room of the soul.

INGMAR BERGMAN (1987)

DOCUMENTARY film gives us a chance to walk in someone else's shoes for a time. If the narrative is compelling, it can indeed "go straight to our emotions, deep into the soul," as Bergman says, and it is capable of altering an audience's cultural perspective and personal opinion of the world. As a physician filmmaker, I make character-driven documentary films in an effort to trigger discussions about important issues in contemporary health care. My goal is for individuals to develop empathy and make connections that extend across cultural, racial, and economic divides, and my hope is that this new cultural perspective and awakened compassion leads to improvements in the delivery of health care and the reduction of disparities on multiple levels.

I have always felt that character-driven stories are more compelling than listening to a series of interviews on a certain issue, so for me as a filmmaker the selection of the story and characters are of the utmost importance. There are three major components that I consider when selecting a story for a documentary. First, the story must address crucial and substantive issues in contemporary health care and must not be held hostage to the sensationalism that often drives television shows and news coverage. Second, while sensationalism is the enemy, drama and suspense are the goals. The characters must embark upon a journey or a quest, giving the audience a reason to engage and to experience a new perspective. Third, the story needs to show the complexity of issues, depicting shades of gray and expanding an audience's understanding of the issues rather than creating or reinforcing stereotypes. This process requires developing profound trust with the subjects in the film.

In this essay, I describe how these three objectives play out in my body of work as a documentary filmmaker.

During my residency in emergency medicine, I found that the medical staff would leave the room after a resuscitation, saying: "I'd never want that done to me." Yet the public generally had very little understanding of what resuscitations were like and what was at stake. This clearly fit the first goal of story selection—an

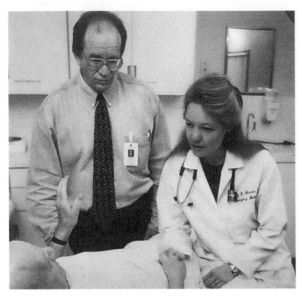

FIGURE 27.1 Still image from the documentary *The Vanishing Line* (Grainger-Monsen 1998).

intriguing and substantive issue that deserved being explored in its complexity. The film that resulted was *The Vanishing Line* (copyright 1998, Monsen), a personal documentary exploring the art and issues of dying, which was broadcast on *POV*, the Emmy Award–winning national public television series. The film follows my personal journey as a physician-in-training, struggling to understand how to care for patients at the end of their lives and learning from a remarkable hospice social worker, Jim Brigham, who takes us to visit patients in their own homes. Brigham is remarkable in his ability to communicate skillfully and compassionately with patients. For instance, we visit one patient who appears to be moments from the end of his life, and instead of a dramatic resuscitation, Brigham reaches out, takes the man's hand, and asks if he is afraid. With this simple act, we see the man's face relax, and Brigham is able to comfort him. It is my hope that *The Vanishing Line* allows viewers to experience a different and more compassionate way of interacting with dying patients, which they can carry with them in their own lives and work.

In my next film, *Worlds Apart*, which I co-directed with Julia Haslett (copyright 2004, Grainger-Monsen), we followed four patients from different racial and ethnic backgrounds for several years as they navigated the healthcare system in the United States. Our goal was to understand and thus better address disparities. However, the challenge was to dramatically illustrate the issues and allow their complexity to emerge yet avoid the sensationalism that can lead to stereotypes and perpetuate the problems. We realized that the key would be the selection of the characters.

As in most documentary films, particularly cinema verité, character selection makes a huge impact on the film. We searched for patients who were actively engaged in their health care as well as physicians who were making a sincere effort to care for their patients. With a graduate degree in public health and in his starched, button-down shirt and cufflinks, Robert Phillips shattered widely held stereotypes of African Americans who suffer because of healthcare disparities. In the film, Robert confronts the perception "that an African American male with hypertension and diabetes is just going to ruin [a kidney] anyway, so why give him a kidney, when all these other folks who are more deserving, should get it. . . . Most of the white patients here, either have had transplants, or are going to have transplants . . . most of the African American men here, aren't."

The film allows viewers to experience the challenges of Robert's life, as he juggles his professional responsibilities, his dialysis requirements, and his strenuous efforts to obtain a transplant. His story is personal, giving viewers a chance to see into the healthcare system and witness the racial and ethnic disparities that exist, I hope moving them toward change. Fortunately, since the completion of the film, Robert has had a kidney transplant and completed his doctorate at Harvard.

The quest or journey of a film's subjects is another critical element of storytelling that can foster empathy for their situations. In *Rare*, a recent film I co-directed with Nicole Newnham (copyright 2012, Grainger-Monsen and Newnham), we document the story of Donna Appell, an extraordinary mother, racing against time to fill a clinical trial for her daughter's rare genetic disease. Donna is relentless in her search for patients, using every possible means—from surfing the Internet to handing out flyers on the streets of Brooklyn. The film highlights the isolation of people with rare diseases, especially in economically and culturally marginalized communities. Donna literally takes viewers along with her on a journey full

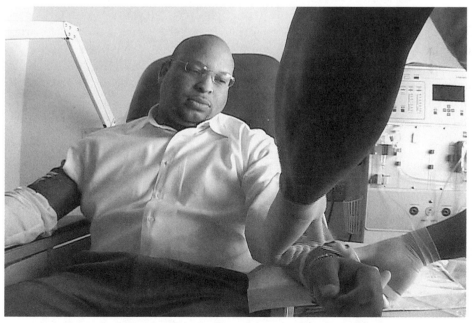

FIGURE 27.2 Still image from the documentary *Worlds Apart* (Grainger-Monsen and Haslett 2004).

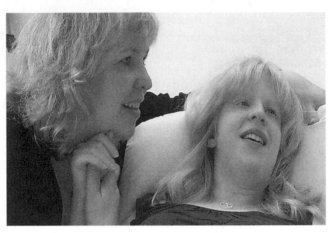

FIGURE 27.3 Still image from the documentary *Rare* (Grainger-Monsen and Newnham 2012).

of twists and turns, while the clock ticks for her daughter, Ashley. A unique element of the film is how it opens a window onto the world of clinical trials, both a patient's and her family's experience as well as a medical researcher's. We not only see the human side of illness but also the scientific pursuit of information that could lead to treatment and cure. The dramatic tension of Donna's search to fill the trial draws viewers into the story and creates a space for them to consider deeply what is at stake.

In *The Revolutionary Optimists*, co-directed with Nicole Newnham and theatrically released as well as broadcast on national PBS on the Emmy Award–winning Independent Lens Series in 2013 (copyright 2013, Newnham and Grainger-Monsen),we felt that there was an urgent need to tell the stories of those visionaries in global health who are striving to improve the situation of their own country in a way that is replicable. Our research led us to Amlan Ganguly, a lawyer turned social entrepreneur in Kolkata, India, working to improve the public health of some of his city's worst slums by empowering and training children to become activists and peer educators. The film follows Amlan and several of the children over three years as they use street theater, dance, and data as their weapons.

Our vision of the film was both as a window into the Kolkata slum where the children live and as an image of the children's own experience. For us, this is where the complexity and texture of the film resides. But in order to achieve this, we needed to build trust with the community, the children, and their parents to have the access necessary to make this kind of film. Consequently, we put significant energy into building relationships with the community for more than five years, making multiple trips to India to work with Amlan and the children. The first challenge was gaining Amlan's trust. Working in the community for fourteen years, he has developed the kind of relationships in these marginalized, often exploited neighborhoods that are rarely achieved by outsiders or non-governmental organizations. When we began the project, there was already great resistance to what the community saw as "poverty porn," the style of many recent films made about Indian slums. We had to prove both to Amlan and to the community that we wanted to create a film that represented the children with respect as well as the neighborhood from the residents' own point of view. This involved establishing a relationship with Amlan that moved well beyond that of filmmaker and "subject." He has not only become a real partner in our plans for the outreach and distribution of the film but also a trusting stakeholder in the film's ultimate mission and purpose.

The children and their families also needed to be persuaded, and we discovered that by releasing short educational films about their work, such as one on polio prevention for TEDxChange (an event convened by Melinda Gates, in partnership with the TEDx program, which had livestream events in eighty-two different sites throughout forty countries around the world in September 2010), we could go a long way toward demonstrating how and why we were interested in their endeavors. We needed a director of photography who could build trust with the children and their families, and we were fortunate to work with two Bengalis, Ranjan Pallit and Ranu Gosh. Ranu did a photography workshop with the children, and afterward, whenever we would ask permission to film something, people would say, "Is that with Ranu, who did the workshop? Then of course!" Through sustained dedication and commitment to our subjects, we have been able to gain their trust in order to be allowed into their lives and to tell a more true and complex story of the actual situation in Kolkata.

As my development as a physician filmmaker continues, I remain excited to explore the ways in which I can create meaningful stories that will trigger discussion, shift perspectives, and change the course of contemporary health care. Not only do I feel compelled to tell stories that address substantive issues, but I

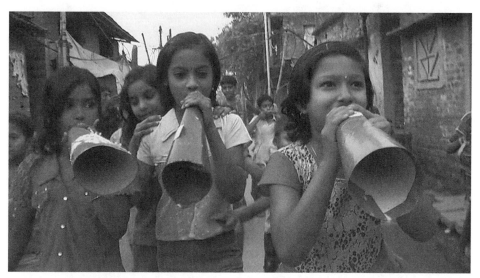

FIGURE 27.4 Still image from the documentary *The Revolutionary Optimists* (Grainger-Monsen and Newnham, 2013).

also realize how fully engaging the storytelling process must be. By dramatically representing the journey of another, I can draw the viewer in and form a trusting relationship, one built upon the honesty and integrity of the story. It is that trust that brings filmmakers, viewers, and film subjects together into a space where real change can actually happen.

Part VIII

AGING

Chapter 28

"OLD AGE ISN'T A BATTLE, IT'S A MASSACRE"

Reading Philip Roth's *Everyman*

THOMAS R. COLE AND BENJAMIN SAXTON

I N the late twentieth and early twenty-first centuries, Philip Roth's fiction has been populated by a certain kind of Dirty Old Man. Like Roth himself during this period, these characters are in their sixties or seventies, struggling with bodies that can no longer be counted on. They are obsessed with younger women, sex, and death; they flout conventional morality; they are dogmatically antireligious. The most conspicuous of these Dirty Old Men—perhaps because he is a nondescript, ordinary guy—is the nameless protagonist of *Everyman* (2006), Roth's harrowing portrait of late-life deterioration and demise. This essay places Roth's *Everyman* in the context of his other (anti)heroes and also against the background of Western attitudes toward aging—from Plato's "wise old man," Cephalus, to the medieval Everyman to the old man surrounded by the prejudice of ageism and the pressures of "healthy aging" in contemporary society. We read *Everyman* as a kind of postreligious morality tale that is grounded in secular Jewish restoration rather than Christian resurrection.[1]

Roth's old men are far from an isolated or temporary instance in his late fiction. Indeed, some of them also appear in his earlier fiction and, as a result, stand in tension with previous, healthier versions of themselves. David Kepesh, for example, is a self-proclaimed "rake among scholars, a scholar among rakes," who first appears as a professor of literature in *The Breast* (1972) and then in *The Professor of Desire* (1977). *The Dying Animal* (2001) follows Kepesh, now in his sixties, and his pursuit of Consuela Castillo, a gorgeous undergraduate whom he seduces at an end-of-semester party. Kepesh's desire for Consuela develops from a fascination into an obsession: he fears that, as his body and sexual prowess decline, she will abandon him for a younger man. "I was all weakness and worry," he explains, because, while Consuela "hundreds of times said to me, 'I adore you,'" she never, even insincerely, could bring herself to whisper, 'I desire you, I want you so—I cannot live without your cock'" (Roth 2001, 23).

Nathan Zuckerman is an even more prominent figure in Roth's fiction, narrating nine of his novels.[2] In *Exit Ghost* (2007), Zuckerman, seventy-one, lives a reclusive life in upstate New York until recurring health problems of impotence and incontinence force him to visit New York City for treatment. While in the city, he becomes enamored with Jamie, a thirty-one-year-old aspiring writer. In spite of infirmities that would rule out a sexual encounter—not to mention Jamie's husband, Billy—Zuckerman fantasizes about seducing her, but his deteriorating body will not keep pace with his libido. Zuckerman wonders where this leaves him: "What could I, an exhausted 'no-longer' with neither the confidence for the seduction nor the capacity for the performance, say to make her waver? All I had left were the instincts: to want, to crave, to have" (Roth 2007, 276). After Jamie refuses his final, desperate proposition, Zuckerman leaves the city (and probably Roth's fiction) for good.

Mickey Sabbath, the sixty-four-year-old failed puppeteer in *Sabbath's Theater* (1995), may be the most memorable of Roth's Dirty Old Men. Part of Sabbath's distinctiveness comes from his quest to make sex the absolute priority of his life. "Most men," the narrator tells us, "have to fit fucking in around the edges of what they define as more pressing concerns: the pursuit of money, power, politics, fashion, Christ knows what it might be—skiing. But Sabbath had simplified his life and fit the other concerns in around fucking" (Roth 1995, 60). The novel, which is one of Roth's most ambitious and outrageous, details Sabbath's sexual exploits with Drenka, an Eastern European woman who is an incredibly prolific and inventive lover; a phone-sex episode with one of his twenty-year-old students, which gets him fired from a university teaching post; his fond reminiscences of trysts with Spanish and Italian prostitutes; and, while in the bedroom of his friend's teenage daughter, Sabbath's seduction of a Mexican cleaning lady.

The Humbling (2009) features Simon Axler, a sixty-two-year-old stage actor who inexplicably loses the ability to perform. In an effort to combat loneliness, thoughts of suicide, and an increasing sense of failure, Axler begins seeing Pegeen, an intriguing ex-lesbian whom Axler hopes will provide physical and professional rejuvenation. Axler tells Pegeen that he's been alone "long enough to be lonelier than I ever thought I could be. It's sometimes astonishing, sitting here month after month, season after season, to think that it's all going on without you. Just as it will when you die" (Roth 2009, 54). But, just as Axler considers committing to Pegeen and even having a child with her, she abruptly ends the relationship, plunging Axler into an even deeper depression and, ultimately, suicide.

Roth's Everyman, then, joins the ranks of Kepesh, Zuckerman, Sabbath, and Axler—all self-proclaimed Dirty Old Men who deal in the raw truths of sex and death, reveling in the unending and unwinnable struggle against "the cold friction of expiring sense," as T. S. Eliot memorably put it in the *Four Quartets* (1968, 54). Like them, he has no use for refined discussions of meaning and metaphor. He is unconvinced about the virtues of sublimation—that is, he sees no reason to renounce or restrain sexual desire in order to live within conventional sexual morality. And, like their author, all these protagonists categorically reject the possibility of religious truth.[3]

However, before we condemn Roth for his depressing, nihilistic, loveless picture of the aging American male, let us take a more sympathetic or—if we can manage it—empathic look at the nameless protagonist in *Everyman*, an unexceptional character whom we might prefer to ignore because of our moral repugnance or because he comes to an end that is possible for any man (or woman).[4] Roth challenges us on all counts: he questions our sense of moral superiority and reminds us that, for all our individuality, we *are* also ordinary mortals. Roth is in the business of puncturing illusions about morality and mortality. Conventional morality, he suggests, is filled with hypocrisy and false piety. Furthermore, popular faith in medicine's power cannot save us from the terrors of death. But before we can fully appreciate Roth's *Everyman*, we need to understand what it is that he is rejecting, for Roth brings a wrecking ball to traditional Western philosophical and religious views on aging.

AGING AMONG THE ANCIENTS: THE WISE OLD MAN

By and large, classical male Western philosophical and literary authors advise transcendence of the individual body.[5] Whether they are optimistic or pessimistic about the outcome, these writers believe that the fruit of living a good life should be a good old age. They counsel discipline, character, willpower, and spiritual and religious commitment—in short, forms of sublimation that transform waning physical desires into moral and spiritual strength and wellbeing.

In Plato's *Republic*, for example, Cephalus notes that many of his friends lament the loss of their youth, "reminiscing about sex, drinking bouts, and feasts" (1968, 5). Cephalus, however, prefers Socrates' view of old age. When asked whether he is still capable of having sex, Socrates responds: "Most joyfully did I escape it, as though I had run away from a sort of frenzied and savage master." Old age, he adds, "brings great peace and freedom from such things" (1968, 5). Likewise, in Cicero's *De Senectute*, Cato declares that "pleasure hinders thought, is a foe to reason, and, so to speak, blinds the eyes of the mind. It is, moreover, entirely alien to virtue. . . . I quit life as I would an inn, not as I would a home. For nature has given us a place of entertainment, not of residence." Hence, he concludes, "my old age sits lightly on me, and is not only not oppressive but even delightful" (Cicero 1909–1914, 27, 52).

This view, of course, is addressed to an elite male audience without so much as a nod toward women or to the lower strata of the social order. It also fails to do justice to the very real losses of physical capacity that accompany aging. And, as Simone de Beauvoir points out in *La Vieillesse* (Beauvoir 1970), it amounts to a coercive idealization of the old in which "they are required to be a standing example of all the virtues" (quoted in Small 2007, 11). Nevertheless, Plato's and Cicero's writings on aging are characteristic of the dominant Western, premodern cultural narrative in which physical decline is offset by knowledge and virtue. Even Aristotle, who is pessimistic about our capacity to flourish past the prime of life, holds old men to the same standards of virtue as those in mid-life.

When Christian writers take up themes of aging, they graft theology onto their classical inheritance. For example, when describing the journey through the stages of life, Cicero writes: "Life's racecourse is fixed. Nature has only a single path and that path is run but once and to each stage of existence is allotted its appropriate quality" (quoted in Cole 1991, xxxii). Christianity transformed nature's racecourse into a sacred pilgrimage to God. Perhaps because Christ was crucified in the prime of his life, there is no classical Christian focus on longevity, no Christian equivalent of *De Senectute*. Augustine articulates the authoritative view that aging, along with death, is punishment for original sin and hence the fate of all human beings after expulsion from the Garden. The Christian answer is to transform finite, mortal life into a pilgrimage to God. Through repentance and good deeds, each one must embark on a harrowing journey through the sorrows and temptations of this life toward salvation and eternity in the next life.[6] This is the essential message of the medieval *Everyman*, which Roth chooses as the implicit counterpart to his own morality tale.

EVERYMAN FOR THE MIDDLE AGES

Everyman (ca. 1495) is one of five extant fifteenth-century English morality plays,[7] all of them written and performed for nonliterate audiences, offering moral instruction through dramatic action and allegory (King 1994, 235). The play has no temporal setting, suggesting that its message is timeless, and it centers on the life of an individual male human being who, as his name suggests, is meant to stand for all of us. The other characters are personifications who stand for virtues, vices, and, of course, Death. While other fifteenth-century morality plays are essentially optimistic, comic, and move toward a resolution, *Everyman* emphasizes transience and loss as the permanent human condition. In the opening scene, Death, God's "myghty messengere" (Davidson 2007, 21), explains to Everyman that his time is running out. Everyman, of course, is not ready: "O Deth, thou cummest whan I had thee leest in mynde" (Davidson 2007, 23). He offers Death a thousand pounds in order to delay the date of his departure. Death, of course, will have none of it.

Seeking companionship for his journey, Everyman calls together those friends whom he hopes will accompany him: Discretion, Strength, Five-wits, and Beauty. It is not long before everyone deserts Everyman, and he realizes that he has been forsaken by everything that he loved most. Abandoned, Everyman turns to Good Deeds, whose help he desperately needs to set his affairs in order. Good Deeds agrees to accompany him, suggesting that only Everyman's deeds will outlive him on earth. It is also worth noting that, in many modern stage performances of the play, Good Deeds appears as an attractive young woman. The medieval Everyman's relationship with Good Deeds thus implicitly acknowledges sexual desire and transforms it into sacred love. While there is no ambiguity over her chastity, some productions of the play even feature Good Deeds lying down with Everyman in the coffin (Davidson, 2007, 13). Good Deeds, then, can be interpreted as a proxy for imagining the relationship between Sex and Death.[8] In any case, Good Deeds accompanies him into the grave, through death, and into the next life, where Everyman's soul is received as the "excellent electe spouse" to Christ (Davidson 2007, 77). The final message is clear: sin and death are inevitable, but repentance and salvation are possible.

ROTH'S *EVERYMAN*

Between the medieval *Everyman* and Roth's *Everyman*, Western ideas about aging undergo a fundamental transformation. Spurred by the development of modern society, ancient and medieval understandings of aging as a mysterious part of the eternal order of things gradually give way to the secular, scientific, and individualist tendencies of modernity. Old age is removed from its place as a way station along life's spiritual journey and redefined as a problem to be solved by science and medicine. By the second half of the twentieth century, the central goal of the modern scientific enterprise—the conquest of premature death from acute disease and the prolongation of healthy, vigorous life—has become a realistic expectation for most people in Western, urbanized societies. And by the turn of the new millennium, Americans in particular have increasingly come to view aging not as a fated aspect of existence but as one of life's problems to be solved through willpower, aided by science, technology, and expertise.

In the novel, Roth demolishes both the medieval and the modern views of aging. Rather than accepting American culture's relentless hostility to physical decline, he forces the reader to address it head on. Moreover, like its medieval counterpart, Roth's *Everyman* treats the inevitable transience and finitude of our lives with a directness that is rarely encountered today. Indeed, Roth treats his eponymous forbear with great seriousness—and for good reason. Roth, who began work on his own *Everyman* in the shock and grief following the death of his friend, Saul Bellow, described his appreciation for the medieval text in a recent interview: "It was hair-raising . . . All the terror that's in it. It's told from the Christian perspective, which I don't share; it's an allegory, a genre I find unpalatable; it's didactic in tone, which I can't stand. Nonetheless, there's a simplicity of approach and directness of language that is very powerful" (McGrath 2006). Almost in spite of himself, Roth admires the direct, didactic message of *Everyman* and appreciates its universal claims about the meaning and purpose of human life—claims that he is eager to demolish and replace with his own counternarrative.

We first meet Everyman at his funeral in a broken-down Jewish cemetery in northern New Jersey. A small group of family and friends are gathered around his coffin: Randy and Lonny, two estranged sons from his first marriage; his brother, Howie, and Howie's wife; his daughter, Nancy, and her mother, one of Everyman's three ex-wives; his private-duty nurse, Maureen, with whom he has had an affair; some former advertising colleagues from New York; and friends from a retirement community at the Jersey Shore. There is nothing even vaguely religious about the ceremony. Everyman, who had not stepped foot in a synagogue since his bar mitzvah, has long concluded that "religion was a lie . . . he found all religions offensive. . . . No hocus-pocus about death and God or obsolete fantasies of heaven for him. There was only our bodies, born to live and die on terms decided by the bodies that had lived and died before us. . . . Should he ever write an autobiography, he'd call it *The Life and Death of a Male Body*" (Roth 2006, 51–52).

After family and friends depart, Everyman alone is left at the cemetery. The story shifts to his childhood and gradually moves forward, revealing the simple truth that Everyman's life will end in the grave. In fact, the narrative is built around the medical history of his body, woven into the checkered history of his intimate — or at least sexually intimate—relationships.[9] Everyman's life is punctuated by four major episodes of illness that in medieval, medical, and theological parlance would be known as the Four Ages of Life (Covey 1985). Chronologically, his life is also divided into periods marked by a succession of three wives—Cecilia, Phoebe, and Merete—followed by a final period of isolation and loneliness. In other words, the story of Everyman's body, like the story of his relationships, is a tale of gradual and repeated breakdown.

As a young teenager in the fall of 1942, Everyman's mother takes him on a bus for a hernia repair in the hospital where he had been born. Everyman is haunted by the death of the other boy in a shared hospital room where he spends four nights recovering from the operation. One evening his father, who owns a jewelry store in Elizabeth, New Jersey, arrives to comfort and strengthen him: "You can do it, son. . . . It's like when I give you an errand to run on the bus or a job to do at the stores. Whatever it is, you never let me down" (Roth 2006, 23). For reasons never made clear in the novel, Everyman's reliability never extends past the period of his childhood and adolescence; moreover, his only consistent, unbroken relationships are with his parents, the moral anchors in his life.

Fifteen or so years later, Everyman has abandoned his first wife, Cecilia, and their two children for Phoebe, a young copywriter. Despite a pleasant summer vacation at Martha's Vineyard and bouts of passionate lovemaking, Everyman experiences terror and anxiety as they walk along the beach together: "The dark sea rolling in with its momentous thud and the sky lavish with stars made Phoebe rapturous but frightened him. The profusion of stars told him unambiguously that he was doomed to die, and the thunder of the sea only yards away . . . made him want to run from the menace of oblivion to their cozy, lighted, underfurnished house" (Roth 2006, 30). Concealing his thoughts from Phoebe, Everyman wonders why he is so haunted by the fear of death in the prime of life.

Back in Manhattan, Everyman falls ill. He cannot concentrate on his work, gives up his morning swim, and cannot even look at food. Almost overnight he is transformed "from someone who was bursting with health into someone inexplicably losing his health" (Roth 2007, 34). Everyman's doctors (who are also nameless) can find nothing wrong with him, but he is actually close to death, suffering a burst appendix and severe peritonitis, a hereditary problem that killed his younger brother, Sammy, at age eleven. He survives the surgery and leaves the hospital after a month of recovery.

For the next two decades, Everyman is in excellent health, enjoying the "boundless self-assurance that flows from being fit" (Roth 2006, 41). He never smokes, rarely drinks, and swims a mile every day at the City Athletic Club. Although Everyman seems to live an amoral life focused around personal freedom and sexual pleasure, he actually embodies the unstated moral calculus embedded in the religion of health (Katz 2005, 161). In the medieval morality tale, he would be condemned to the despair and sense of failure inherent in worshiping a false God, but in the novel, he eventually finds consolation, connection, and blessing in relationships with his parents that extend beyond the grave.

We follow Everyman into retirement, another divorce, Social Security and Medicare, and then into a relentless cascade of physical ailments that culminate in his death on the surgeon's table. After he moves from Manhattan into a New Jersey retirement community, Everyman suffers an obstruction in his left carotid artery which is relieved by insertion of a stent. But operations and hospitalizations accelerate on a yearly basis, and the absence of stable, loving relationships leaves him alone with his body and his memories: "He'd married three times, had mistresses and children and an interesting job where he'd been a success, but now eluding death seemed to have become the central business of his life and bodily decay his entire story" (Roth 2006, 71).

Once Everyman realizes that he will never regain his health, he begins some moral accounting of his own. Looking back, he thinks about his estranged sons, Randy and Lonny, whom he had abandoned as young children. His sons call him a "cunthound," referring to his infidelities, and a "happy cobbler," mocking his recent interest in art (Roth 2006, 96). Sadness, followed by anger, descends upon Everyman as he recalls their insults: "You wicked bastards! You sulky fuckers! You condemning little shits!" he thinks (97).

To ease his loneliness, Everyman has taken up amateur painting, giving lessons to fellow retirees. His class includes a woman named Millicent who has recently lost her husband and suffers from depression and severe back pain. Perhaps she stands for Everywoman, a rare and brief female perspective in Roth's male-dominated fiction. Millicent, however, has internalized the traditional male standard of self-reliance. Her pain not only removes her from the land of the upright, but it is also a source of shame and suffering for her. Everyman tries to console her by pointing out that pain is not shameful. "You're wrong. You don't know," she responds. "The dependency, the helplessness, the isolation, the dread—it's all so ghastly and shameful. The pain makes you frightened of yourself. The utter otherness of it is awful" (Roth 2006, 91).Ten days later, Millicent Kramer kills herself with an overdose of sleeping pills, and Everyman cancels the painting class.

One morning on his daily trek along the boardwalk, Everyman spots an attractive young jogger and awkwardly propositions her. "How game are you?" he asks. "What did you have in mind?" she replies (Roth 2006, 133). Concealing his fear of humiliating rejection, he writes his phone number on a piece of paper. She stuffs it into her bra. "'You know where I am,' he said, feeling himself growing hard in his pants unbelievably, magically, quickly as though he were fifteen. And feeling, too, that sharp sense of individualization, of sublime singularity, that marks a fresh sexual encounter or love affair and that is the opposite of the deadening depersonalization of serious illness" (133–134). Here and throughout the novel, there is an uncanny connection between the medieval and the Rothian depictions of aging Everyman and beautiful young women. Doesn't every old man want a young woman to sleep with him and save him? As he has with so much of conventional sexual morality, Roth also challenges the image of the Dirty Old Man. Everyman acts out this urge unconstrained by fear of being seen as an over-the-hill lecher; he is only constrained by fear of failure and humiliation.

Everyman's last sexual assault on mortality is, of course, futile. The young woman takes off down the boardwalk, never to be seen or heard from again. So where does Everyman turn when he can no longer find sexual satisfaction and his body refuses to cooperate? "Would everything be different . . . if I'd been different and done things differently?" he asks himself rhetorically. "Would it all be less lonely than it is now? Of course it would! But this is what I did! I'm seventy-one. This is the man I have made. This is what I did to get here, and there's nothing more to be said!" (Roth 2006, 98). Like Tolstoy's reluctant invalid, Ivan Ilyich, Everyman questions the foundations on which he has lived his life.[10] Unlike Ivan, however, there is no last-minute conversion. Hospitalized for the seventh year in a row, Everyman goes into cardiac arrest and dies on the surgeon's table. As Roth notes in *Everyman*, "Old age isn't a battle, it's a massacre" (156).

ROTH, RELIGION, AND RESTORATION

What is the core message of Roth's postreligious *Everyman?* To some degree, the novel can be read as a cautionary tale against our culture's dominant ideal: the biomedical management of aging, which implicitly regards health as a form of secular salvation. The approach to aging as a problem to be managed rather than a mystery to be experienced has come at a high spiritual and ethical price. It disguises American culture's relentless hostility to physical decline and to those who are dependent. It appears to be optimistic but only by denying the harsh realities of decline and death—hence, the frantic, futile search for youth and the undiminished negativity of ageism and devaluation of older people.

Everyman's only weapon in this losing battle is the desire for sexual pleasure divorced from love or intimacy, and to be fair, one might argue that he (along with Kepesh, Sabbath, Zuckerman, and Axler) has internalized our culture's ageism—Everyman hates himself for his failing health. The only narrative available to him is one of decline (Gullette 1997). Old men in Western culture have traditionally faced a dehumanizing dichotomy: either embrace sex and be mocked as a Dirty Old Man or behave with the dignity accorded to a Wise Old Man. Roth's Everyman refuses either choice, an apparently liberating move, but one that leaves him less in the position of a rebel and more as subject to a new form of cultural coercion. Like the rest of us, Everyman lives in an eroticized commercial culture that hawks products guaranteeing hot sex and long-lasting erections, where "sexual inadequacy is more unseemly than indecorous lust" (Fiedler 1986, 40). Rather than banish old men from sex, contemporary American culture pressures them to retain sexual vitality and functioning or risk being perceived as or feeling like failures. There are no commercial interests that incentivize intimacy.

Everyman also appears to epitomize the antireligious message of our secular age: religion is fiction; the soul does not exist; there is no life after death; aging has no meaning; and the material world is all there is. In a way, then, Roth's (anti)morality tale seems to invert the message of its medieval Christian counterpart, which holds that living a moral life before God softens the sting of Death. But (and this is the point, even for Roth), Everyman cannot escape the weight of the moral and philosophical questions that religion thrives on. And, as with the medieval *Everyman*, this weight arrives in the form of a package from Death that cannot be returned to sender.

At the end of the novel, we return to the rundown cemetery off the New Jersey Turnpike where we first met Everyman at his own funeral. This time, Everyman's father is being buried next to his mother's grave in a traditional Jewish ceremony in which the mourners bury the dead. The taste of dirt lingers on the inside of his mouth long after he leaves the cemetery. In a poignant conversation with his dead parents at the cemetery—shortly before his own death—Everyman is overcome by "the kind of sobbing that overpowers babies and leaves them limp." (Roth 2006, 169). Despite himself, Everyman turns to the realm of the spirit, getting as close as he can to the bones of his parents, "as though the proximity might link him up with them and mitigate the isolation born of losing his future and reconnect him with all that had gone" (170).

The passage is reminiscent of Ezekiel 37, in which the Israelites cry out over the loss of their ancestors: "Our bones are dried up, and our hope is lost; we are cut off completely" (37:11). For the Israelites—and for Everyman—the dry bones offer the possibility of continuity and restoration. Like the Israelites, Everyman is strengthened by the presence of his parents' bones, enduring long past the flesh they once sustained. But his spiritual sustenance rests not on divine deliverance but in symbolic, generational immortality.[11] "The bones," the narrator tells us, "were the only solace there was to one who put no stock in an afterlife and knew without a doubt that God was a fiction and this was the only life he'd ever have" (Roth 2006, 170).

Everyman spends an hour and a half at his parents' graves, musing and conversing in ways far more meaningful than his conversations with living friends and relatives. In a spare dialogue filled with tenderness and longing, he finds meaning beyond sex and death, beyond resignation: "I'm seventy-one," he tells his parents. "Your boy is seventy-one." "Good," his mother replies. "You lived." His father answers: "Look back and atone for what you can atone for, and make the best of what you have left" (Roth 2006, 171). Everyman, then, has received forgiveness and a final blessing from parents who still carry the moral authority of a residual ancestral Judaism. In the end, he is not spared the losses incurred in the battle—or massacre—of old age. He accepts the consequences of a life largely squandered but finds solace in the knowledge that he will be laid to rest beside the bones of his ancestors.

NOTES

1 Our opinion has been shaped by Stephen Hazan Arnoff's fascinating essay on *Everyman*. He writes that Roth creates a "transcendent, iconoclastic, post-religious tale—a morality play for a time when inherited views, practices, and narratives of traditional

religions appear either threatening or obsolete" (Arnoff 2006, 4). For two other illuminating discussions of the novel's (post)religious dimensions, see Bernard Rodgers and Derek Parker Royal (2007) and Victoria Aarons (2007).

2 Zuckerman, who shares many biographical parallels with Roth, especially his profession as a novelist, first appears in *The Ghost Writer* (1979) and narrates *American Pastoral* (1997), *I Married a Communist* (1998), and *The Human Stain* (2000).

3 In a 2005 interview with the *Guardian*, the interviewer asked him if he was religious. "I'm exactly the opposite of religious," Roth replied. "I'm anti-religious. I find religious people hideous. I hate the religious lies. It's all a big lie" (Krasnik 2005).

4 As wife Linda says in *Death of a Salesman*: "I don't say he's a great man. Willie Loman never made a lot of money. His name was never in the paper. He's not the finest character that ever lived. But he's a human being, and a terrible thing is happening to him. So attention must be paid. He's not to be allowed to fall into his grave like an old dog. Attention, attention must finally be paid to such a person" (Miller 1998, 40).

5 See Thomas Cole (1991), esp. chap. 1; and Helen Small's (2007) *The Long Life*.

6 See Cole (1991), 3–31.

7 While its precise date of origin is unknown, most scholars consider *Everyman* to be adapted from the Dutch original *Elckerlijc* (Davidson 2007, 1).

8 I am indebted to my dear friend Marc Kaminsky for pointing out the sexuality of Good Deeds and linking it to the psychoanalytic theme of family reunion.

9 Before settling on its current title, Roth called his novel *The Medical History*. "As people advance in age," he explained in a 2006 interview with the *Independent*, "their biography narrows down to their medical biography. They spend time in the care of doctors and hospitals and pharmacies and eventually, as happens here, they become almost identical with their medical biography" (Freeman 2006).

10 Before his conversion, Ivan goes through a similar process of introspection and denial: "'Can it be I have not lived as one ought?' suddenly came into his head. 'But how now so, when I've done everything as it should be done?' he said, and at once dismissed this only solution of all the enigma of life and death as something utterly out of the question" (Tolstoy 137). For a discussion of Roth's debt to Tolstoy, see Ivanova (2011).

11 As Victoria Aarons has noted, "the imagined presence of those buried bones suggests a link to a historical continuity that depends upon and finds meaning in a past not entirely of one's own making. [Everyman's] very proximity to those bones suggests a connection with others, a link to those with a shared history. . . . Such a desire to be connected to something in the past larger and more sustaining than oneself is a very ethnically inflected, very Jewish expression, an expression of a collective ethos, an obligatory ethic to bear witness to the past and, in this way, to secure a future" (Aarons 2007, 123). See also Rodgers and Royal (2007), esp. 10–15.

Chapter 29

"DO YOU REMEMBER ME?"

Constructions of Alzheimer's Disease in Literature and Film

E. ANN KAPLAN

As we are told repeatedly in a growing mountain of articles and books, Alzheimer's is perhaps the cruelest disease of all: in robbing the victim of her memories, Alzheimer's robs her of herself. But what concept of self is involved in such statements? And is there only one kind of "self"? In this chapter, I explore such questions through two case studies: a memoir by Judith Levine, aptly titled *Do You Remember Me? A Father, a Daughter, and a Search for Self* (2004) and Sarah Polley's film, *Away from Her* (2006), adapted from the Alice Munro story "The Bear Came over the Mountain" (Munro 2001, 2007). Fictional works like these show the elderly suffering from dementia in a far more complex, empathic, and sensitive way than medical models can transmit. Each text brilliantly reveals how the protagonist suffering from dementia changes with his or her condition but is still not necessarily "deviant" or needing institutional care.

However, I am not questioning the clear scientific data on Alzheimer's disease (AD). In its full-fledged form, AD involves the brain's inability to deal efficiently with the protein beta amyloid, which normal brains produce and flush out each day. As the brain ages, it continues to produce the same amount of beta amyloid. As Rebecca Frey writes in a summary of the science research: "Neurofibrillary tangles (i.e. what's not flushed away) are the accumulation of twisted protein fragments found inside the nerve cells in the brains of Alzheimer's patients" (2003, 36). Thus plaques and neurofibrillary tangles form on the neurotransmitters, not only clogging up the mechanism and hindering efficient memory recall and processing of language but also causing disorientation, breakdown of personality, and eventually preventing the body's ability to perform its many routine functions.

One of the problems in this research, however, is defining when symptoms indicate AD and when something else (such as drug-induced confusion) might be the cause of phenomena that appear similar (Harding and Palfrey 1997). Scientists are still exploring the differences between AD as a specific disease and ordinary confusions, which are more pervasive among the elderly but are seen also in other people. This state is often called *dementia*, and for the purposes of this chapter, that is the term I adopt when talking in general terms. When I discuss two case studies in which the more specific diagnosis of Alzheimer's is used by an author, I refer to AD.

What I do want to challenge through my case studies is the medical lens through which United States and Canadian societies view people with dementia. This lens contributes to how they are stigmatized and considered "deviant," resulting in exclusion from functioning in their families and communities. Judith Levine's memoir itself is more than just an account of her father's illness; it also takes up a position vis-à-vis AD. As Nancy Harding and Colin Palfrey argue, we need "alternative conceptual frameworks in order to explore the phenomenon of dementia" (1997, 2; see also Brody 2011, D7). Through analysis of book and film, I argue that the "demented" (as Levine calls them) may develop new subjectivities: just because they are new, perhaps causing pain to loved ones, does not mean that these people should not be recognized as subjects with their own ways of being.

But first some statistics on the increased number of North Americans being diagnosed with Alzheimer's, especially in the context of media attention to the disease.

MEDIA AND THE MEDICAL MODEL

Articles on dementia have proliferated during the last decade, matching the increasing number of people now being diagnosed. Before 1982, AD was barely in the news, but in 1986, an editorial in the *New England Journal of Medicine* by Robert Katzman labeled AD as the fourth leading cause of death in the United States—a statistic that became widely reported by 1992 (Ewbank 2004, 63). However, Douglas Ewbank cites data from 1991 showing that 14,112 deaths in the United States were attributed to AD, making it the eleventh, not the fourth, leading cause of death among those over sixty-five years of age. In any event, scientists agree that "between 1979 and 1991, the reported age-adjusted death rate for Alzheimer's disease increased twelve-fold" (Ewbank 2004, 64).

There are two possible reasons for the increased reporting of AD: the obvious one is the ever growing number of people living longer—often by a significant number of years—making them susceptible to the illness. Centenarians are increasingly featured in the news, and obituaries show people dying at 105 or more. As the baby boomers advance in age, with their well-known attention to health and exercise, the numbers of the extreme elderly are likely to rise. Everyone over sixty-five is liable to get dementia over a twenty-year period, so the math is not complicated as to numbers. Moreover, genetic inheritance is only a small part of the story, with the environment increasingly being targeted as a contributing factor, in addition to the normal shrinkage of the brain.

However, if the media are a lodestone, it is not clear that the sheer numbers of people being diagnosed is the real reason for such anxiety about the disease. Arguably, the kind of subject (or self) that dementia produces is anathema to the Western celebration of "Rational Man"—following Descartes's long-revered concept, "Cogito, ergo sum"—at the expense of other kinds of humans or other aspects of being human. Wilhelm Reich (1983) and later followers such as R. D. Laing and Aaron Esterson ([1964] 1990) attempted to validate illnesses like schizophrenia by theorizing their emergence as a result not only of dysfunctional families but also of pressures that capitalist societies, insisting on rationality, put on people. More recently, neuroscientists such as Antonio Damasio have demonstrated how wrong Descartes was. In a review of Damasio's (2004) book, *Descartes' Error: Emotion, Reason, and the Human Brain*, Daniel Dennett writes: "Even among those of us who have battled Descartes' vision, there has been a powerful tendency to treat the mind (that is to say, the brain) as the body's boss, the pilot of the ship." Dennett continues:

Falling in with this standard way of thinking, we ignore an important alternative: viewing the brain (and hence the mind) as one organ among many, a relatively recent usurper of control, whose functions cannot properly be understood until we see it not as the boss, but as just one more somewhat fractious servant, working to further the interests of the body that shelters and fuels it, and gives its activities meaning. (1995, 3)

According to Damasio, "Nature appears to have built the apparatus of rationality not just on top of the apparatus of biological regulation, but also *from* it and *with* it" (1994, 128; emphasis in original). The failure to see this was, according to Damasio, Descartes's error.[1] Dennett notes that "far from there being a separation, sharp or ragged, between mind and body, mind cannot exist or operate at all without body" (1995, 3).

In their provocative volume *Social Construction of Dementia* (1997), Harding and Palfrey argue strongly for recognizing a cultural angle to dealing with people with dementia.[2] The media and the larger culture, they believe, have adopted the medical model in regard to the elderly who suffer mental confusion—a model that encourages situating them perhaps unnecessarily in institutional care. Harding and Palfrey cite research that argues for both a "core" self and an "adapted" self—for example, the self that functions according to social norms and prohibitions rather than according to "core" desires and feelings. Perhaps, in dementia, the adapted self wanes, but the core self remains, expressing itself in ways that those of us using adapted social selves find "deviant." Emotions, in particular, are not as well controlled once the adapted self wanes. While some scientific studies have tried to study emotions in people with dementia, these have not been able to say more than that subjects with dementia are as able as the control group to suppress emotions when told to but not as able to amplify emotions as the control group (Henry et al. 2009). All this really tells us is that we know very little about the way the core or emotional self functions. After all, most experiments (if we accept this theory) study the adapted self.

Especially important for understanding dementia is to understand the sometimes drastic changes in how subjects relate to their spouses and/or children. While such changes can be difficult for family members, they do not mean that the subjects are "mad" or "bad," as often labeled in cultural discourse (Harding and Palfrey 1997, 3–8). In this regard, art can inform us much more than science about subjectivity, relationships, and especially about emotions and values in people with dementia. The two texts studied here are different: Levine's is an autobiographical piece detailing her father's dementia as it related to changes in him and thus to their relationship. *Away from Her* is a fictional work detailing a husband's attempt to stay close to his wife, whose dementia seems to pull her away from him—to change her into someone else. However, the nonfiction/fiction difference is less important than the surprising affinities in the way the persons with dementia change in each work. While one way of describing the change is to think in terms of a core self (relying on emotion) that remains while the adapted self (social/cognitive) gets lost, another is to see the difference as analogous to what Brian Massumi, following Gilles Deleuze, distinguishes as affect versus emotion (Massumi 2002). Discussions of people with dementia focus on their loss of coherent speech and their apparently strange affective ways of being, which we see in the works discussed below. For Massumi (1995), emotion is a cognitive experience—a feeling consciously known; affect is rather a nebulous sensation that works beneath regular linguistic, narrative, and teleological levels. Both descriptions are pertinent to changes in the protagonists in the two works I turn to now.

TWO CASE STUDIES

Judith Levine's (2004) memoir begins with two brilliant pieces of writing. The "Prelude," an account of her parents' fiftieth anniversary party, not only establishes the character of Stan, Levine's father, who shows early signs of some mental confusion, but also tells us something about the daughter's relationship to her father up to this point in their lives. It is clearly a conflicted relationship, if not as unhappy as Stan's relationship with Judith's brother, James. For James, Levine says, Stan's senility "is just the final straw. Indeed, James's theory seems to be that Dad has managed to mangle his brain just to bug his son." Judith concedes that "Dad might yet deploy his dementia in some nefarious way," but she tells James "that Dad can't help what's happening to him" (8). Judith's sympathy, she tells us, is still tentative, but in making sure Stan manages the party we see some tenderness for him developing in her manner. The chapter ends with the diagnosis from a psychiatrist, handing Stan what Levine calls a "sentence" (in applying the medical model), namely "that he will lose his self."

But Levine is too smart to take this at face value; indeed, her memoir is far more than just about her family and a demented father. She explores the social construction of dementia, and perhaps, most tellingly, she quotes research on the normative discourses at work in support groups for those caring for AD patients.[3] Groups, we learn, "enforced a 'ruling narrative' that brooked little divergence" (Levine 2004, 117). Further, the disease classification of Alzheimer's, Levine notes, gives people both a sense of fellowship and an illusion that they can learn what to expect. For Levine, one of the main characteristics of AD or dementia is the unpredictability of the illness: nothing remains the same for long, and sometimes people's memories can return. A permanent feature of the disease is that short-term memory goes quickly while long-term memory can function quite well. However, in general, memory in dementia is never stable, seemingly returning or leaving without any particular pattern. I should note that this is only an exaggeration of how memory works for people without the illness—all of us suffer from unstable memory. In contemporary research, memory is almost by definition considered unreliable.[4]

On the personal side, meanwhile, Levine sees her father's diagnosis as an invitation. After spending her life fighting him, she is now determined to find her father at the very time when society thinks he is lost. But in the process, she discovers something about "this multifarious, elusive thing, the self." She learns that the self "cannot exist but in relationship," that "the self's demise cannot be accomplished by a brain disease alone," and that "like a father, a self is a hard thing to lose" (Levine 2004, 9). Her implication is that we have selves that are more than simply *rational*, as discussed in the critique of Descartes's view of humans. Levine suggests that, as she relates to her father in his new stage, a different self emerges. She theorizes a self-in-relation in the present, as against the usual concept of a self only being possible if one has memories and self-consciousness. Provocative as this might be, it is interesting to contemplate, and I explore it further in the later discussion of the two case studies.

In the film *Away from Her* (Polley 2006), the diagnosis is much longer in coming but paradoxically more rapidly results in the heroine, Fiona, being taken into institutional care. At first Fiona (Julie Christie) and her husband, Grant (Gordon Pinsent), mature adults who have retired to the relative calm of a Canadian suburb, seem happy in their relaxed and loving lifestyle. However, when Fiona puts the frying pan in the freezer, without noticing anything, Grant is disturbed. Soon after, she labels kitchen drawers with Post-its naming contents. When Fiona forgets what she has in her hand and why (she had intended to pour wine for her guests), she herself wonders if she is losing her mind. Her forgetfulness increases: during her habitual cross-country afternoon skiing trip, she forgets where she is going and how to get back home. As the camera follows her, we see her confusion and puzzlement about not finding her way. Concerned, Grant goes out to find her. Back at home, Fiona says that it's time to begin looking at places with people to take care of her. Fiona's awareness of her condition contrasts with Stan's complete lack of understanding about what's happening to him in Levine's memoir. It is Fiona who pushes her husband to place her in a home; Grant does not believe it's warranted yet, but she insists, and it is with grave misgivings that he takes her there.

Why might have Fiona insisted on leaving home as she begins to change, and what significance for her marriage lay in her retaining her long-term memory? When Grant questions Fiona about the need to label drawers with their contents when she could just open them to see inside, with an intense look at him she reminds him of a story she heard once at a dinner party about German soldiers. She heard it, she says, from Veronica, a Czech student of Grant's. "Don't be nervous," she says, looking at him significantly. "Each of the German dogs had a sign, 'Hund.' When asked why, they said 'because it is a Hund!'" She walks past Grant and pokes him as if to say "you naughty boy." Grant has a troubled, confused, and guilty look on his face, and with the remark about the student, we are given an image of a beautiful woman with long black hair at their dinner table, drinking. The memory of this story in close connection to Fiona's forgetting where objects are yet paradoxically remembering her husband's affair, suggests some kind of link between the two happenings. Fiona perhaps intended through the story to say, instead of lies, let's call an affair an affair! Let's label things as they are.

Also supporting an interpretation of some kind of unconscious mischief Fiona is making vis-à-vis Grant's affairs through her dementia is another moment just before she goes to Meadowlake, the facility for people with dementia; they are talking about it, and Fiona pretends to forget what place they are talking about. She has the puzzled look (now familiar) but then suddenly smiles and says, "Just kidding!" It suggests both her awareness of her confusion and her deliberate separation from Grant. Shortly afterward, we see them dancing closely, and we get a clear sense of Grant's now deep love for his wife, just at the moment that she is turning away perhaps to punish him belatedly for those painful years when she evidently even allowed the women into her house.

During the car ride to the institution, Grant is pleased that Fiona shows short-term memory in pointing to the forest where they recently enjoyed looking at plants. Fiona notes that she wishes she could not remember other things: "Things we don't talk about. . . . But you never left me; you still made love to me, despite disturbing demands elsewhere." Her next comments are almost taunting: "All those pretty girls, all those sandals and bare female toes! It didn't seem like any wanted to be left out!" She continues, "You did all right, not like others who left their wives." She also seems to justify her own tolerance: "And women who would not put up with it. People are too demanding. People want to be in love every single day! What a liability! That silly girl, silly girl Veronica; girls are always going around saying they are going to kill themselves. But that was that; we moved out here to start a new life. That is what you gave me; how long is it? Twenty years. So you see I am going but I am not gone."

During the car ride, the song to which they were dancing, "I Loved You with All My Heart," is playing on the radio. Images of Veronica and other students, presumably called up in Grant's mind as Fiona speaks, appear on screen. Since her last thoughts before going into the institution have to do with Grant's affairs and the pain they caused her, it is reasonable to see a connection between what happens once she is in Meadowlake and this conversation: Fiona is unconsciously motivated to hurt Grant or at least making him suffer as she has. Thus, her dementia brings on this new subjectivity of independence and distance—and also paradoxically an ego strength she lacked at the time.

Levine's memoir covers a greater span of time, and given the space available for development of details in a book, in contrast to the narrative drive that film must adhere to in a commercial production, we are given far more insight into the gradual changes in Levine's father, Stan, and into the rapidly deteriorating relationship to Levine's mother, Lillian (known as Lil). However, in both case studies, one spouse falls in love with someone else but in very different situations. In *Do You Remember Me?* Lil, made crazy by trying to deal with Stan, takes time away from caring for him and falls in love with an attractive, wealthy man, Sid, who is about her age. The relationship provokes varied responses from the couple's children and friends, but Lil sticks to her guns and in the end marries Sid. In *Away from Her*, it is Fiona who, once in the institution, becomes infatuated with or responds to the advances of a man, Aubrey.[5] Grant is greatly disturbed by this. He comes to the institution daily, hoping Fiona will recognize him, but she never does. Grant feels that she is changing in basic ways. For instance, she always had great taste in clothes and dressed smartly, and now he finds her in what before she would have considered tasteless clothes, her hair and appearance disheveled. Could this be an example of a person letting the "adapted" self go? Grant simply cannot understand this new Fiona, on either the level of dress or of her dedication to caring for the crippled, usually grumpy Aubrey.

Stan's dementia, meanwhile, enables him to articulate thoughts that might not have been spoken by the "adapted" self. For example, at one point, the family is in Vermont and going to the lake. Stan needs to put on a swimsuit, and when he doesn't return, Lil asks if he needs help. Levine writes, "But he doesn't want her help, which itself seems to accuse him of helplessness. 'I can't do anything,' he yells at her. *I have no boat, I have no money....* 'Why am I living?'" (2004, 115; emphasis in original). She and her partner, Paul, realize that this is a good and serious question, but a question most likely that Stan would not ask of his ordinary "adapted" self. We usually shy away from such questions or distract ourselves through daily tasks and preoccupations, our adapted selves pushing such questions away. Stan finds a brilliant, touching way to get around his embarrassment of forgetting the names of people he knows—something the adapted self finds difficult to handle as well. He simply asks people he meets: "Do you remember me?"—a question that gets him out of the bind.

Levine realizes that what she calls "the Alzheimer's narrative" can cover over an already deteriorating relationship. With group encouragement, caregivers attempt to redefine the entire relationship through the new lens of dementia. "The Alzheimer's story," Levine notes, "is told from one point of view, that of the caregiver, who is also the hero" (2004, 119). Further, the "cause of all distress is the patient, barreling toward the edge of dementia's cliff. Yet there is no villain besides a conspiracy of chemicals: 'Something is happening to your brain, Stan. It's nobody's fault'" (119). Levine contrasts this to the story of her parents' marriage, in which both narrators are unreliable, the plot is tedious and confusing, and the resolution will never come. If everyone is innocent in the Alzheimer's story, in the marriage story, no one is, Levine concludes. And, of course, the same is true of Fiona and Grant, although here it would seem that Grant shares the larger burden of marital grief, given his affairs with the women in his classes. As we saw, Fiona's adapted self in her 1960s era in Canada, entailed "forgiving" Grant or at least not making a big fuss. Clearly this came at psychic cost. Dementia possibly enables her to get even. If this is more an interpretation than something the narrative explicitly states, the staff assistant in the institution, with whom Grant talks about his loss and confusion about Fiona's new relationship, does hint at this possibility.

A very interesting aspect of *Do You Remember Me?* is how her father's dementia not only changes him but also changes Levine's relationships to both him and her mother. Levine resists the Alzheimer's narrative, as we have seen, while her mother, newly in love, wants to believe in it to justify her moving away from Stan. As she puts it, neither she nor her mother believes that Stan is coming back: "But," Levine writes, her mother "has long been parting from him and is ready to say adieu, and I am just meeting my father. To me, he is still here" (Levine 2004, 183). These opposing views of the disease become increasingly polarized as Lillian becomes more and more infatuated with Sid and Judith gets closer and closer to her father. Their trips together are fun, as Judith is able to enjoy Stan's new "demented" subjectivity, his new ways of thinking, which is often poetic in unexpected ways. However, this new subjectivity meanwhile merely annoys and irritates Lillian.

We can see in both works how prior aspects of each marriage partly condition the new subjectivities that Stan and Fiona adopt. The anger that Stan's dementia brings out seems directed at Lillian for never really having doted enough on a man with a very large ego in need of constant reassurance and praise. And Fiona's dementia triggers her painful life as a college professor's wife expected to turn a blind eye to her husband's affairs with his students. She seems finally able to confront Grant with the infidelities she suffered through with her new subjectivity at Meadowlake as handmaid to Aubrey: she is available at his beck and call, picking up things for him, and pushing him around in his chair. She hardly recognizes Grant who sits daily in the room, watching the two play cards and touching each other. Grant tries to get her attention, to insist on her recognizing him, but each time she refuses and rushes away back to Aubrey.

However, one day, Aubrey's wife, unable to bear the cost of Meadowlake, takes him home. Fiona collapses into despair and mourning—crying, not eating, and finally refusing to leave her room. Although the film refuses a teleological narrative, jumping back and forth between time periods, we do see Grant's final gesture to Fiona: a request to Aubrey's wife (played beautifully by Olympia Dukakis) that Aubrey return to Meadowlake because Grant can't bear to see Fiona grieving for him. It seems this is the transformation in Grant that Fiona's dementia has produced—finally thinking more about Fiona than about himself. The nurse at Meadowlake plays her part in this transformation by suggesting that there's always a reason for the way patients behave and that Grant might have been disloyal in their earlier lives.

But before Aubrey's wife and Grant prepare to return Aubrey to Meadowlake, she makes a romantic overture to Grant, and since Grant has given up any hope of Fiona recognizing him, he goes along. The plan is to return Aubrey permanently to Meadowlake and, it seems, to have his wife move into Grant's house. But in a surprising turnaround—not only in narrative terms but also in dementia as an illness—on the day that Aubrey returns, Fiona finally recognizes Grant and recalls the books he has been reading to her. They embrace, and the camera swirls around them time and again, as the credits appear.

How are we to read the endings of both works? The ending of the memoir leaves Stan still in his own space with different caregivers coming in and with Judith enjoying his surprisingly upbeat subjectivity. "As he loses language," Levine tells us, "my father sings the world. Car alarm, tea kettle, crow: he matches the pitch, taps out the rhythm. Like John Cage, he makes no distinction between music and sound, between sound and noise" (2004, 299). Sitting with her father in the living room, Levine hears "a man who sings the world. In this demented moment of history, in his own vague and vivid here and now . . . my father is singing the song of himself" (300). We don't know what will happen next, but Judith has found her father. *Away from Her* (Polley 2006) also leaves us in suspense. We can't believe that Fiona is cured, but we do see that, even if only temporarily, she has partially recovered her memory, if not her old subjectivity. Her gesture of an affair of sorts puts her in a different position than before vis-à-vis Grant, who, as noted, has also had to change.

For those teaching medical/health humanities and those training in the health professions, both texts represent dementia as far more complex than medical models would have us believe. It is highly possible that the core self does not change and that the changes people observe have to do with the adapted self. While we hope that research will continue to develop new ways of treating dementia, American culture (as Levine persuasively shows) needs to be careful regarding what assumptions are made about people with the disease. Slotting them into a preordained narrative that constructs a predictable path for both victims and caregivers can only be unproductive at best and cruel at worst. New subjectivities that dementia produces may make the family nervous, but if changes are seen as opportunities for revitalizing relationships, the result might be interesting and positive.

NOTES

1   In an interview, Levine asks Damasio: "Is there a level below which a person is no longer a person?" He answers that in the case of the comatose subject he might give up, but "with Alzheimer's disease, I wouldn't. My feeling is that we should err on the side of thinking the person is there" (Levine 2004, 295).

2   I am grateful to Levine for pointing me to the work of Harding and Palfrey. In the book, Levine cites research that supports her view, such as several clinics that have had success in showing that "high-quality care for demented people even in the last stages of 'global deterioration' results in ameliorated emotional outlook and behavior and retarded cognitive decline" (Levine 2004, 182).

3   Despite the memoir genre she's writing within, Levine includes reference to the scholarly research underlying her book. There is an impressive bibliography of works Levine consulted at the end of the memoir.

4   See Paul Antze and Michael Lambek (1996); Richard Terdiman (1993); and, most recently, Susannah Radstone and Bill Schwarz (2010).

5   Readers will recall the much-discussed case of Supreme Court Justice Sandra O'Connor, who retired early to care for her husband, who was suffering from Alzheimer's disease. Once in an institution, he attached himself to another woman, very much as in the film.

Chapter 30

LOVE IN THE TIME OF DEMENTIA

JERALD WINAKUR

After bathing him, Fermina Daza helped him to dress: she sprinkled talcum powder between his legs, she smoothed cocoa butter on his rashes, she helped him put on his undershorts with as much love as if they had been a diaper. . . . Their conjugal dawns grew calm.

GABRIEL GARCIA MARQUEZ, *Love in the Time of Cholera* ([1985] 1988)

H IS father, a shopkeeper, dies when he himself is only seven. A sensitive boy, he has the ability to capture any image that catches his fancy. A high school teacher sends a note home to his mother urging her to send this son to the Art Institute. She tears it up, the pieces fluttering to the ground in front of his eyes. It is the Depression, and each of his brothers and sisters are taken out of school in turn to run the pitiful shop that kept the family alive. The boy's name is Leonard.

Since he is the youngest of six, his turn comes late—he is, at eighteen, just a few months shy of graduation, but it is his turn, and he goes out into the world with as much formal learning as he will ever have.

She is so young. A raven-haired girl of fifteen, she waitresses in the tiny luncheonette across the street from his shop. And he comes in for lunch each day, sits at one of the few tables, and she comes over to take his order. She has a sweet smile, and he makes her laugh. And then he begins to draw her: as she bends to serve, or at the register, or as she stands—in a rare idle moment—staring out the window onto West Baltimore Street. Her name is Frances, and she has been born and raised in the tiny apartment above the luncheonette. She dreams of falling in love forever, living happily ever after.

Then comes the war, and just like that he is gone overseas. The shop, of necessity, closes. Five years he is away, first to England, then France. The Army Air Corps trains him as a photographer: his eye—that artist's eye—is good, and someone notices. But the things he sees over there—the hollowed-eyed waifs in dark doorways, whole cities in ruin after the bombers make their runs, the broken soldiers on the fields of battle, the survivors wrapped in white on the hospital wards, the decimated companies of men at attention as the bugle plays taps—he cannot get out of his head.

He sends copies of the photos to her, and she neatly anchors each and every one by its four corners onto soft, thick, black paper and then into albums. Books of memories he then spends years trying to forget.

She writes him letters every day. Chatty, newsy letters, girlish stuff, about her life in the luncheonette. She is careful not to mention other beaus. She seals each letter with a red-lipstick smooch on the back of the envelope, sprays it with the perfume he sends her from Paris. He puts every one up to his face once they finally find their way to him. He falls in love with her scent, her innocence. What does either of them know of love?

He returns, counts himself lucky to be in one piece. At twenty-six, he is aching to get on with his life; she is twenty-one and still knows nothing of the world.

The wedding album: rented top hats and tuxes, the bride veiled in lace, the tiered cake, the kiss, the dance, all recorded in black and white, more memories pasted onto blank, black pages, then stowed away. To what end?

And yet, life is ongoing, relentless. More memories: those two boys growing up, the brick Cape Cod in a new neighborhood full of them, the shop reopened, the rose garden, the collie dog, birthdays and graduations, a fleeting trip here or there. He is a photographer, after all; she is the keeper of memories.

The arguments, the frustrations: oh, she wanted a father-provider, and, oh, he so wanted to be deeply and passionately loved. Memories laid down deep in the depths, the good with the bad, resurfacing instantly, furiously. The worries over money, the tears over dreams deferred, promises unfulfilled, the weeping over losses: parents, siblings, friends. Intimacies that should have occurred but did not, or should not have occurred but did. This is a life to be lived through to the end. A test of wills, of endurance. For the children if nothing else. Isn't every marriage like this? This is a life and the memories pile up, the albums overflow, the excess banished to shoe boxes. The black paper, soft as crepe, crumbles over the years.

Who has time to paint portraits when it is time to repaint the kitchen? There was nothing for art's sake.

Now the boys are grown, educated, married. He loses the shop, the business, and with it the last vestige of self-esteem. He takes to the bed. She goes to work.

And then, for a brief few years he rediscovers something lost along the way. The old wooden easel that gathered dust leaning in a corner of the garage stands on its own feet again, a welcoming stranger. He retreats into his garage-studio, plucks a picture from the boxes of memories: his mother dressed up in her Sunday best; his oldest brother, Frank—the one who was a father to him—in the bow of a rowboat fishing on the Severn River; his own wife—startlingly young and beautiful, cutting roses off the vines he planted so many years ago: the blossoms, her lips, the same shade of red. Watercolors and oils flow from his studio, cover the walls of his home.

In the act of painting he is transformed, resilient, overflows with feelings he has never known—or no longer remembers. They surge through him. When he is at his easel he cannot sleep. Mornings she finds him in the garage, alive, paint-spattered, a new image glowing on canvas under the lights. Fran, what do you think? It's nice, Len, she says. She encourages him; helps pick out the frames that will hang on her walls. You must come by and see your father's latest work, she says to her sons.

And now they are old. Where did the years go? A couple of heart attacks, cancer, radiation therapy. Neither is immune. They are in their eighties, after all. What can one expect?

Of course, the worst. He keeps getting lost. Even in the neighborhood. Turn right, not left, she says. Something in her voice—or is it his own deepest fear—enrages him. She refuses to go out at night to avoid the fights. Not long after, it is the front door: he stands on the stoop, studies his keys, does not know what to do. The sons sell the car. He can no longer be left alone. She retires from her job, but now she is at home with him all day, all night. Not what she expected, yet somehow what she has come to expect.

The years go by like this. Friends stop calling. They sleep in separate rooms just so she can get a little rest. At night, he wanders the house, turns on the lights, peeps in through her door just to make sure she is still there. Closes it again, shuffles back down the hall.

He cannot remember names. Faces are familiar: he thinks his son is his brother or some old friend he recognizes but cannot place. He refuses to go out, lives in his pajamas, sleeps more and more. Refuses his meals, pees on the couch, falls in a heap at the front door. He is trying to locate his army unit—that's what he says when she finds him there.

She is beside herself. Life has always been tough—the Depression, the loss of his meager business just when they were trying to educate their boys. Then his depression. How did it come to this? What might her life had been had she married the dentist who came courting during the war when she was writing those letters she sent overseas? Was that love, too?

He thinks she is cheating on him, accuses her of every sort of mean betrayal. I can't deal with this anymore, she cries to her sons. But she does.

And the nights are worse. He calls her "Mom" now, knocks on her door in the darkness, shuffles in with his walker.

Are you asleep, Mom?

What is it, Len? It's the middle of the night, for god's sake.

He is sobbing, his face is wet. Please tell me who I am, he pleads with her. I can't remember who I am.

She does not hesitate, pulls back the covers.

Come here, Len. Lie beside me, she says.

In some way he is reticent. Like a first-time lover. Are you sure? he asks.

Come, she says.

She moves over to one side. He pushes his walker up to the bed, turns and sits on the edge. Are you sure? he asks again.

She switches on the light, reaches for him, holds him while he falls back into the pillows, helps him straighten himself, cover himself. She cradles him into her arms.

She keeps the photo albums on her bedside table.

Your name is Leonard, she begins. You were born in Baltimore, Maryland. The year was 1919, and you have three older sisters and two older brothers. She turns the pages.

Soon every night is like this. She feels him relax into her body. Sometimes he asks if one or another of his siblings is still alive. Yes, she says, though all are long gone.

Frank is living in Florida. Hilda is retired from teaching now . . .

Good, good, he says.

The story of his life unfolds page by page. Her voice, his story, spills into the tangled interstices of his mind, every cobwebbed corner. Embraced, he recalls the scent of her perfume on the letters she wrote to him all those years ago. He listens closely, anticipates with subdued breath. Up against her chest her words purr through his body, pour into his emptiness, fill him up. He falls in love all over again.

Now his breathing is deep, regular. His body is still warm. Sixty years they have been together. He is asleep. For the moment, she can stop reciting his story, but she does not. She will see it through.

This is what love comes down to, she thinks. There is no happily ever after; but perhaps, in the end, this is what it is all about.

Part IX

MENTAL ILLNESS

Chapter 31

NARRATING OUR SADNESS, WITH A LITTLE HELP FROM THE HUMANITIES

BRAD LEWIS

THE World Health Organization estimates that depression affects 121 million people across the globe. It is the fourth leading contributor to the global disease burden, and by the year 2020, it will be the second leading contributor (World Health Organization 2011). Moreover, the experience of depression can be intensely painful and debilitating. In his memoir *The Noonday Demon: An Atlas of Depression*, Andrew Solomon compares his experience of depression to that of a strong and dignified oak tree, persistently and maliciously conquered by a parasitic vine (Solomon 2001). At its worst, this kind of agony can lead to suicide, killing approximately 850,000 persons every year, and beyond those directly affected, the morbidity and mortality of depression deeply affects friends, co-workers, children, parents, and loved ones.

Despite the extensive experience with depression, there remains remarkable uncertainty and controversy about how to understand it. In the cosmopolitan world, depression is increasingly understood through the frames of biomedicine. "Broken brains" and "chemical imbalances" have become popular but crude catch-alls for a vast and ever growing body of biomedical research linking depression and depressive episodes to our bodies, our neural synapses, and our brains. However, the biomedical model of depression is hardly the only model available for under-standing our sadness. Depression continues to be understood through a variety of other models, including psychoanalytic, cognitive-behavioral, existential/human-ist, family, political/feminist, creative, spiritual, and biopsychsosocial model.

Humanities work in narrative theory provides invaluable tools for navigating this diversity and for linking the many models of depression with the particular life choices people make in the face of it. Even so, narrative theory is vast and not easy to master. How can people take advantage of it for telling sadness? Clinicians who have taken a humanities turn have found that the narrative elements most essential for clinical work are *metaphor, plot, character*, and *point of view*. Following this lead, this chapter first explores these elements and their relevance for depression and then recent memoirs of depression as examples of how people use such models to tell the story of their sadness (Lewis 2011, 2012).

NARRATIVE THEORY

Narrative approaches to *metaphor* move beyond commonsense notions of metaphor as simple embellishment or ornamentation. Scholars George Lakoff and Mark Johnson explain it this way: "Metaphor is not just a matter of language, that is, of mere words. . . . On the contrary, human thought processes are largely metaphorical" (1980, 6). By shaping our concepts, metaphor structures the way we perceive the world, what we experience, how we relate to other people, and the choices we make. It even organizes diverse cultural and sub-cultural approaches to suffering and healing (Kirmayer 2004).

Metaphors are critical for understanding the many models of depression because metaphors and models work in similar ways. A model, in short, is a metaphor developed over time. In ordinary writing or conversation, people use metaphors to provide a quick glimpse: "This hotel is a palace." But, in a clinical model, research communities (e.g., biomedical, psychoanalytic, cognitive-behavioral) develop a metaphor into systematic models that frame their work and that explain the world through a metaphorical re-description (Hesse 2000, 353). Just as the metaphor "Joe is a pig" re-describes Joe in a new way and allows us to perceive something new about him, so, too, the disease model of depression—"depression is a disease"— re-describes sadness and allow us to perceive something new about it. Philosophical psychiatrists Bill Fulford and Tony Colombo use these insights to develop the following definition of psychiatric models: "[Psychiatric] *models*. . . are the conceptual frameworks, or sets of ideas, by which, in any given area, people structure and make sense of the world around them" (2004, 130; emphasis in original).

Like metaphor, *plot* also structures our experience and provides form to our narratives. Plot creates a narrative synthesis between multiple elements and events, bringing them together into a single story. In addition, plot configures the multiple elements of a story into a temporal order that is crucial for our experience of time. Philosopher Paul Ricoeur sees the relation between time and plot as a two-way phenomenon: time makes sense to us precisely because it is organized by plot, and conversely, plot is meaningful because it portrays the features of temporal experience (1984).

Character in narrative theory helps us understand human identity by drawing a comparison between identity in life and character in fiction. Narrative theory helps us see that we understand ourselves similarly to the way we understand fictional characters. Ricoeur calls this approach *narrative identity*: "Fiction, in particular narrative fiction, is an irreducible dimension of self-understanding . . . fiction is only completed in life and life can be understood only through the stories that we tell about it" (1991, 30). Self-understanding, on this account, is an interpretive event, and narrative is the privileged form for this interpretation: "A life story [is] a fictional history or, if one prefers, a historical fiction, interweaving the historiographic style of biographies with the novelistic style of imaginary autobiographies" (1992, 114).

Bringing metaphor, plot, and character together, we can say that when models of depression seep from the clinic into the culture, they become part of our cultural resources of self-experience. In times of trouble, we look through the metaphorical structures of mental models to perceive, select, and plot aspects of our lives that we believe to be important. These culturally located "self" stories and the priorities within those stories combine with other cultural stories to scaffold our narrative identity and provide us with a compass for living. They tell us where we have been and where we are now, and they provide us with a trajectory into the future.

The power of models and plots to shape our narrative identity brings us to *point of view.* If a person with depression sees a clinician who is working from a disease model, the clinician's point of view (organizing metaphors, treatment recommendations, and narrative identifications he or she prioritize) will be very different if the person sees a psychoanalyst or a family therapist or begins a creative writing class. A biological psychiatrist will see a broken brain and recommend some form of biological intervention; a psychoanalyst will see loss and unconscious psychic conflicts and recommend psychodynamic therapy; a family therapist will see dysfunctional family patterns and recommend family work; and a creative writing teacher will see an undeveloped but very sensitive muse that needs further discovery and expression.

The implication of narrative theory for depression is that there are many ways to tell the story of sadness—not just one right way and many other wrong ways. All the models of depression involve a process of storytelling and story retelling. No matter which model or combination of models one uses, the process of healing involves an initial set of problems that the person is unable to resolve. The client and therapist use one or more models of depression to bring additional perspectives to their problems, which allows the client to understand them in a new way. The perspectives vary greatly depending on which models of depression are used because each model tends to foreground and background a very different set of variables. From the vantage point of narrative theory, what these different perspectives all have in common is that they rework, or "re-author," the initial story of sadness into a new story, which allows new degrees of flexibility for understanding past and present troubles and provides new strategies for moving into the future.

A narrative understanding of depression models fits well with an ethical approach to clinical work which philosophers of psychiatry refer to as values-based practice (VBP). The first principle of VBP gets to the heart of the issue: "All [clinical] decisions stand on two feet, on values as well as on facts, including decisions about diagnosis (the 'two feet' principle)" (Fulford 2004, 208; Fulford et al. 2006, 498). The first principle of VBP means that data and evidence alone cannot determine clinical decisions or choices of diagnostic models. Even in cases where there are good data to support a clinical model and intervention, that alone does not determine the decision. The final decision depends on how the intervention lines up with the person's life choices, life goals, and narrative identity (who the person wants to be).

Fulford gives an example of an artist who ultimately decides against taking lithium for mood swings even though there were good outcome data to support the use of the medication and an initial trial helped calm her instability. The artist makes this decision because lithium reduced her capacity to visualize color. For her, the effect of lithium on her experience of color was more important than its effects on her moods. Using narrative theory, we can say that the artist preferred to prioritize creative variables over biomedical ones. Hers was not simply a medical decision with a right or wrong answer with outcome data determining the choice. The artist made a personal decision that combined both facts and values (2004).

STORIES OF SADNESS

Memoirs of depression provide a wealth of examples that help us see how people use the many models of depression and integrate them into their lived-experience and narrative identity. And these memoirs show how important depression can be in shaping our sense of ourselves. Hillary Clark, a literary scholar who studies depression memoirs, finds that significant depression often becomes central to people's sense of themselves and their identity formation: "One cannot feel well one day, numb and oppressed the next, suicidal after a few months have elapsed . . . without seeking a narrative explanation—the cycle of bipolar disorder, for instance, or the Christian narrative of sin, repentance, and redemption—in order to make sense of it all, to trace a single self through all these changes" (2008, 2). Clark finds that personal "narratives give voice to the ill, the traumatized, and the disabled" and restore the insights and wisdom they have achieved—wisdom that is often lost by medical research and clinical "case studies" that too often turns people into statistics and diagnostic labels (3). For examples of how people narrate depression, it helps to look at two particularly rich collections of depression memoirs: *Unholy Ghost: Writers on Depression* (Casey 2002) and *Poets on Prozac: Mental Illness, Treatment, and the Creative Process* (Berlin 2008).

In "Planet No" from *Unholy Ghost*, Lesley Dormen emphasizes themes of loss and depression through a model of unresolved grief common in psychoanalytic theory (see also Leader 2008; Pollock 1989). Dormen explains that she initially spiraled into depression by two losses in her life: "An architect I'd loved for under a year left me for a woman he met in a supermarket parking lot. And my best friend, Tessa, a woman as central to my understanding of myself as my brown eyes and small feet, disappeared into marriage and withdrew from our friendship completely" (2002, 229). Dormen used psychotherapy to explore these losses and came to realize that they were compounded by earlier losses and traumas from her childhood. She lost her father after her parents divorced when she was six years old, she was sexually abused by her stepfather, and she had a painful emotional relationship with her mother. Dormen felt so isolated and rejected by these experiences that when her therapist asked her, "if [you] were a girl in a story, how would [you] see yourself?" Dormen answered: "Like an orphan" (232). Building on this insight, she eventually came to understand that her many ungrieved losses amplified one another, and these unresolved feelings were repeated in the present life. As an adult, she relived her past experiences of solitary isolation and failure as an unmarried woman in New York, feeling the pressure to be coupled like "normal and successful" people.

Psychoanalytic therapy and self-reflection helped Dormen to understand that her stepfather's sexual abuse was the central "curve in [her] depression story. His touch had caused the spine of the story to veer off into a new direction, had reconfigured the terms of my loves and longings" (238). Most pernicious for her ongoing development, the abuse left her confused about her desires, and this confusion left her "frozen in a girlhood made curiously old" (239). The dense and painful emotional conflicts that grew up around the sexual abuse knotted together shame, illicit sexual pleasure, heartbreaking loss, pity, betrayal, guilt, duplicity, and an aching distance between her mother and herself. These emotional knots were so tight that she could not begin to open them or untie the feelings, but at the same time she could not forget them. She found herself constantly and repeatedly returning to them "with the vague uneasiness that was a familiar part of [her] internal landscape" (232).

Slowly and often painfully, therapy helped her move past these knots in her character that seemed to rope her into depression and despair. She was able to separate herself from this history: "Something happened—something that was separate from me. There was a me that existed before the something and a me that existed after. Before and after were separate, not the same" (238). No longer tied together in knots, "it was possible to stand outside those events, to observe them and draw a conclusion about them. It was possible not to just be them" (238). And, not only that, it became possible to move past the grief, to feel joy, and to make new connections: "I fell in love with New York, with the giddy green of the first spring after the worst of the depression lifted, with new friends, travel, and wonderful books. I looked around my apartment and saw that there was pleasure in things, in their colors and shapes, and that one did not actually need a marriage certificate to buy good pots" (240).

In contrast to Dormen's psychoanalytically inflected story, an excerpt from William Styron's memoir, *Darkness Visible*, is paradigmatic of the disease model as narrative template (Styron 2002). Styron describes himself as "laid low by the disease," a "major illness" of "horrible intensity," which came on him like a "brainstorm . . . a veritable howling tempest in the brain, which is indeed what clinical depression resembles like nothing else" (2002, 114–115). This connection between depression and bad weather perfectly captures the disease model of depression as lying outside the frame of human goals, desires, losses, and disappointments. Like the weather, depression comes from the material world of inhuman forces, from physical and chemical interactions. For a strong disease model advocate like Styron, it makes no more sense to give human meaning to depression than to tell an atheist that thunder is caused by God's anger towards us. Styron explains how he sees it: "I shall never learn what 'caused' my depression, as no one will ever learn about their own . . . so complex are the intermingling factors of abnormal chemistry, behavior and genetics" (115).

Styron's memoir was one of the first and most influential to adopt such a narrative frame. He relies on biological metaphors for depression that perfectly match the disease model in psychiatry as well as an avalanche of pharmaceutical marketing and ghost research devoted to promoting antidepressant medications (Angell 2005; Applbaum 2006, 2009; Healy 2004, 2006; Matheson 2008; Rose

2003; Sismondo 2007, 2008). Depression, Styron writes, "results from an aberration of biochemical process. [It] is chemically induced amid the neurotransmitters of the brain . . . a depletion of the chemicals norepinephrine and serotonin" (2002, 120). This "upheaval in the brain tissues" causes the mind "to feel aggrieved, stricken," and it creates "muddied thought processes" like the "distress of an organ in convulsion" (121).

Styron is far from alone in his approach, and the disease model runs through many of the other memoirs. Indeed, this model is arguably the most dominant in the collections just as it is in mainstream culture. In the *Unholy Ghost* collection alone, Virginia Hefferman laments the "substandard physiology," which creates her depression (2002, 20). Chase Twitchell moves past the phrase, "chemical imbalance" to chime in with a more updated disease model explanation: "What happens in depression, for reasons that are still unknown is that the limbic-diencephalic system malfunctions" (Twitchell 2002, 23). And, similarly, Russell Banks fears that his wife's "malfunctioning limbic diencephalic systems" may result in her suicide (31). The popularity and pharmaceutical hype of the biological model does not make it "bad" or "wrong" and certainly not a "myth." Many people are clearly able to integrate the model into their lives in a helpful way, but the hype exaggerates benefits, downplays side effects, and makes it hard for those who cannot use the biological model to access other models without extra effort (Martin 2006).

It is instructive to compare the disease model of depression with a psychoanalytic unresolved grief model in two similar memoirs: Dormen's (2002) memoir (discussed above) and Liza Porter's memoir, "Down the Tracks: Bruce Springsteen Sang to Me" (2008). The two memoirs have a lot in common, and many of the same themes arise in Porter's memoir that arise in Dormen's—loss of a best friend, a complicated childhood, sexual abuse, excruciating breakups, and psychotherapy. However, for Porter the primary narrative frame through which she comes to understand herself is the disease model, rather than the psychoanalytic model. In a comparison of the two memoirs, we can see how either model can be used to make sense of similar experiences of depression, but we can also see how the disease model does not lead to instant cures despite the hype of a pharmaceutical advertisement (think of the dancing Zoloft blob). The disease model, like other models, requires patience and persistence on the part of the person who adopts it (Karp 2006).

After years of psychotherapy to battle her depression, Porter sees a biological psychiatrist who convincingly asserts that "you've been clinically depressed most of your life and have never been properly treated for it" (2008, 157). The psychiatrist goes on to "explain brain chemistry, dopamine, serotonin reuptake inhibitors," and he says, "I'll be able to help you. You may not feel better right away, and we might have to try many different medications, but I'll help you" (157). Even before they try any medications, Porter is dramatically relieved by the psychiatrist's pronouncement of depressive disease:

I raise my head and stare at him. I weep. And I believe him . . . . Finally I admit powerlessness. This is the first time I ever truly realize that it is not my fault; there is nothing more I can possibly to fight the depression. . . . I have an actual physical disease . . . , and there is treatment for it. I quit trying to convince myself that I have to fix it, or even that I can fix it. I decide to trust this doctor to help me find the right medications. Hope is back. (Porter 2008, 157)

And hope sustains Porter though three long years of medication trials: "We go through Wellbutrin, Celexa, Effexor, Zoloft, Ritalin, Lamictal, Provigil, and Sero-quel. More drugs I can't remember the names of, but I do recall the side effects— Zoloft gave me the shits, Effexor had me jerking and twitching in the night, Lamictal constipated me. . . . Almost all the drugs steal my sex drive. But something starts happening in my brain, I feel better." But gradually, through a combination of drugs, Porter comes to the other side of depression: "The depression and its voices recede into the background. I become able to write poems about things other than my sordid past" (2008, 157). She finds that she becomes more mature and more focused though "changes in [her] brain chemistry." Her writing, something she had always enjoyed and used to cope with her feelings, begins to change as well: "After the antidepressants begin to work, my [writing] becomes more universal. Others besides me can relate to it. I have energy to submit poems to magazines. Editors begin accepting them. I learn—as a writer friend has told me several times—to turn the hardships of my life into beauty" (158).

In contrast to biopsychiatry or psychoanalysis, David Budbill's memoir, "The Uses of Depression: The Way Around Is Through" (2008), provides a good example of more alternative models. Budbill approaches painful periods of depression through the less common but still vital models of spirituality and creativity. Because of what he calls his "rebellious, contrary" personality, none of the mainstream approaches is suitable for him, and he decides to push past the mainstream to develop his "own way of dealing with and using depression" that he calls his "give in" method: "I discovered that the only way around my periods of depression is directly through them; in other words, the sooner I can resign myself to the Angel of Depression, the sooner she will be done with me and leave me alone" (2008, 83). Drawing insight from Zen Buddhist teachings and the process of creative writing, Budbill discovers that if he lets go of his critique of depression and allows himself to be with the intensity of the feelings, the episodes are not all negative. Indeed, depression can be generative (or positive) as well (Wilson 2008), and Budbill finds that one of its most important positive dimensions is that is slows him down. Depression forces him to enter a "negative space" where he can neither work nor produce; instead, he tunes into a very different experience—"empty, open, quiet, passive, receptive, dark" (89). These slothful, withdrawn periods function as a kind of dormancy where he can store up energy for times when the Angel of Depression lets him go. During such times, he can better hear his muse, and this "receptacle" period later emerges in his poetry.

Susanna Kaysen also takes a generative approach to depression. In "One Cheer for Melancholy," she explains, "I think melancholy is useful" (2002, 38). It tunes in people to the fundamental contradictions of life: "failure, disease, death" are all standard life events. "Is it any surprise," she asks, "if some of the time, some of us feel like hell?" Kaysen does not frame her generative melancholia through a spiritual or creative model but through an evolutionary one. She speculates that the reason there is so much depression in the world is that it provides balance: "I've learned this from my optimistic friends. I rely on them and their cheerful attitudes. Together, we make a complete picture. My doom and gloom may be more often right, but they aren't the whole story." From a population perspective, Kaysen suspects a species may benefit from having the "majority of can-do types mixed with a significant minority of worriers and brooders" (40).

Kaysen does acknowledge that those people who insist on drawing a bright line between clinical depression and depression more broadly will not be convinced, but she finds that for her the distinction is too blurry to be of much use. If one relies on this distinction too heavily, the result is a futile "competition" about who is "more depressed" and about whether some "things in life were truly sad and worth feeling depressed about" (2002, 42). In addition, the distinction feeds a "pathologizing" culture that raises extraordinary hopes for a cure of ailments that "have plagued people for millennia," and it leaves people with "unreasonable expectations for happiness" (41). Kaysen does not try to argue with those who find the "disease" model helpful (and she is aware that many people do), but for her depression is not a disease because it allows her to "perceive, and more important, to tolerate the fundamental ambiguities of life" (45). After all, "the transient nature of happiness, beauty, success, and health may come as a shock to the upbeat person but it's old hat to the depressive" (45).

Joshua Wolf Shenk gives a good sense in his memoir of how an awareness of the many models of depression can be a tool of coping (2002). Looking at the history of depression and the role of metaphor in shaping what we know about depression, Shenk suggests that "what we call 'depression,' like the mythical black bile, is a chimera. . . . It is cobbled together of so many different parts, causes, experiences, and affects as to render the word ineffectual and perhaps even noxious to a full, true narrative" (2002, 245). Even so, the pain and suffering of depression is anything but a chimera, and Shenk understands our inevitable need to "abbreviate and simplify" in trying to understand it (246). He finds "no way around words like 'depression' and 'melancholy' . . . but it is one thing to use shorthand while straining against the limits of language. It is quite another to mistake such brevities for the face of suffering" (246). For Shenk, simplified phrases like "biochemical malfunctions" and "biological brain diseases" favored by well-intentioned activists and pharmaceutical companies can mystify as much as they inform. "When we funnel a sea of human experience into the linguistic equivalent of a laboratory beaker, when we discuss suffering in simple terms of broken or fixed, mad and sane, depressed and 'treated successfully,' we choke the long streams of breath needed to tell of a life in whole" (247).

This awareness allowed Shenk to seek consciously an array of different approaches to his depression. He gave medications a try (although found none that were helpful) and sought solace and guidance in several hundred afternoons of psychotherapy. He worked through the pain of his parent's divorce when he was seven—"the slow leakage of affection and kindness from my parent's marriage, the grim entrance of resentment, confusion, and anger"—and overcame the automatic tendency from his family life that "forbade expressing these emotions" (2002, 255).

All of this work went into the larger task of creating a life story that put his depression in perspective: "to find my story by living it, following moments of emotional clarity through life's maze. I look for help in therapy, [but also] in relationships, and faith in its broadest sense—faith in the gardener, the faith of the lover, the faith of the writer. The faith that I can experience what is real about the world, that I can hurt plainly, love ravenously, feel purely, and be strong enough to go on" (254).

Narrative reading of depression memoirs like these also fit well with empirical research in how change actually happens in the mental health (Duncan et al. 2009; Lewis 2011). A good example of such research is that by Damien Ridge and Sue Ziebland, who interviewed thirty-eight men and women with previous experiences of depression in order to discover the strategies they used to revitalize their lives (2006). Ridge and Ziebland found that people did not use any single approach but selected a variety of "narrative tools," such as talking therapy, medication, yoga, and complimentary therapies to regain mastery of their situation. Ridge explains: a "key finding . . . was that recovery tools considered effective by patients go hand in hand with telling a good story about recovering from depression" (2009, 174). The very process of assembling a range of tools for recovery helped create the stories that were effective. The people interviewed also found that therapists were most helpful if they could function not as experts but as "recovery allies." A recovery ally of this type does not function in a "doctor knows best" capacity but is someone who helps the person select the narratives and the recovery tools that feel most true to him or her.

As in Ridge and Ziebland's study, the writers of depression memoirs often (though not always) use a combination of approaches and models as recovery tools. Shenk's memoir is the most conscious of the process, but many other writers combine approaches to depression. Dormen, for example, not only uses an unresolved grief model but also finds creative expression as well as medications invaluable for coping with depression (2002, 240). Styron, who has the most muscular biochemical model of the group, sees loss as a key element of his sadness (2002, 117, 125). And throughout the memoirs, there are writers who combine cognitive, humanistic, family, and political (particularly feminist) approaches. There are also writers who are adamant about a more single model approach. Porter, for example, discredits the other models she previously tried once she settles on a disease model (2008, 157), and Budbill argues strongly against a society that reduces the spiritual dimensions of depression to a pathology that should be treated or a disease that should be medicated (2008, 91).

CONCLUSION

The implications of narrative theory for clinical encounters involving depression are many. Mental health practitioners will do well to develop their awareness and competency with regard to multiple models. They must come to appreciate the many stories of biopsychiatry, psychoanalysis, cognitive therapy, family therapy, humanistic approaches, political approaches, spiritual approaches, and creative approaches to name a few. Furthermore, they must come to understand the value of biography, autobiography, literature, and narrative theory for developing a narrative repertoire. Clinical competency for depression means a tremendous familiarity with the many possible stories of sadness. The more stories clinicians know, the more likely they are to help their clients find a narrative frame that fits their situation. In addition, the more stories clinicians know, the easier it is for clinicians to take a values-based approach and appreciate that the person who should most decide which models to use and which stories to tell is the person whose life is at stake.

For people going through the experience of intense sadness, the multiple models of depression mean that there are a range of possible therapists and healing solutions that might be helpful. An approach that is right for one person may not be right for another. There must be a fit between the person and the approach, and people should feel empowered to take seriously their own intuitions and feelings. If the person getting help does not feel this fit, he or she may be right. There may well be another approach, or an additional combination of approaches, that would work better with the person's proclivities. Like everything else, however, therapeutic experiences of all kinds can be frustrating, slow, and uncertain. How does one know when an approach misses his or her needs and when it is something that will take time, patience, and perseverance to be helpful? There can be no gold standard or simple answers to these questions. Only judgment, wisdom, and trial and error can decide.

Chapter 32

TEACHING NARRATIVES
OF MENTAL ILLNESS

ANNE HUDSON JONES

I N the preface to his book *Minds That Came Back*, the physician Walter C. Alvarez speaks to the educational value for physicians of attending to autobiographical accounts of mental illnesses:

In the past fifty years I have gathered what I imagine is the world's largest collection of autobiographies of people who have been mentally upset, highly eccentric, alcoholic, or otherwise ill or handicapped. To me, most of these books have been fascinating and invaluable; . . . I do not know of any books more worthy of study by us physicians, and especially psychiatrists. Readers can find . . . much hope and encouragement. Why? Because most of the authors show that, when nervously ill, we can often fight our way back to health and a useful life again. (Alvarez 1961, 5)

Alvarez's comments may seem naïve today, given the scientific advances in brain imaging, genetic information, molecular biology, and pharmaceutical research in the intervening decades. Why read "anecdotal" autobiographical accounts when advanced technologies provide more scientific and reliable data and offer hope for more accurate diagnoses and efficacious treatments? Some answers come from A. R. Luria (1979) with his "Romantic Science" and Oliver Sacks (1986) with his "Clinical Tales," who are both onto something in their narrative explorations of the lived reality of individual human beings when confronted with devastating illnesses or injuries. Sir William Osler's famous aphorism, "It is much more important to know what sort of a patient has a disease than what sort of a disease a patient has" (1950), still seems apt when trying to understand the baffling differences in response to mental illnesses. Out of fashion for a while, patients' autobiographical narratives still have much to offer those who want to understand what the subjective experience of mental illness is like and how some minds have "come back" despite the odds.

During the past two decades, I have taught courses in narratives of mental illness for undergraduate honors students at a large state university, for third- and fourth-year medical students, and for graduate students in medical humanities. I have also led discussions of narratives of mental illness for reading groups of health-care professionals, including residents in psychiatry, and for groups of the general public, and I have organized a film series—"Mental Illness in the Movies"—to bring medical and local communities together in conversation. The courses have all been elective, rather than required, and the reading groups and film series have been entirely voluntary. Yet these activities have always attracted students and participants from a wide spectrum, including those who are mentally ill themselves and want to learn more about others who suffer from mental illness, those who have struggled to understand and help mentally ill family members or friends, and healthcare students and professionals who want to understand more about the subjective experiences of their patients. These groups have always overlapped a bit—that is, some of the students and healthcare professionals have also suffered from mental illness, a fact they had usually concealed from their respective colleagues but sometimes disclosed in class or group discussions or confidentially to me at the time or some years later. The remarkable mix of experience among the participants has sparked intense and lively interactions as we have all learned from each other in response to the texts.

Illness narratives of all kinds have proliferated during the past several decades, especially in the United States, and narratives of mental illness are no exception. Both the increased incidence of mental illness in these decades—whether real, a result of better diagnosis, or an artifact of new diagnostic categories (Angell 2011a; Angell 2011b; Oldham et al. 2011)—and, arguably, a concomitant lessening of stigma (Jones 1998) may have encouraged patients and their family members to go public with accounts of mental illness. There are now far more compelling narratives of mental illness than could ever be used in any one course or by any one reading group or in a single film series (Gabbard and Gabbard 1999; Hornstein 2002, 2011; Jones 1995). Selection is always difficult and depends upon many factors, including the intended audience (healthcare students or professionals versus general public); duration of the course or discussion group (several weeks or months versus a shorter opportunity); and special focus, such as the history of psychiatry, an overview of several different mental illnesses, a close look at a particular illness (e.g., depression, bipolar disorder, or schizophrenia), the efficacy of contemporary versus historical treatments, or the need for parity in health insurance and for reform in health policy for mental illness. Literary and aesthetic qualities of a narrative are important but do not always ensure its inclusion. A narrative by a highly esteemed writer, such as William Styron's *Darkness Visible: A Memoir of Madness* (1990), may not be as helpful for a particular group or purpose as a less literary but more accessible account, such as Martha Manning's *Undercurrents: A Therapist's Reckoning with Her Own Depression* (1994). It is important, whenever possible, to read (or view) several narratives rather than just one or two because diseases manifest themselves so differently in different people, and never more so than in major mental illnesses. Severity of disease, access to care, response to treatments, and social support vary immensely and can make the difference between suicide and recovery.

When constrained to choose only one narrative of mental illness to include in a course or discussion group, in recent years I have often turned to *The Quiet Room: A Journey out of the Torment of Madness*, by Lori Schiller and Amanda Bennett (1994), which has much to teach about many aspects of mental illness and does so in an engaging yet powerful way. It is both an easy and terrifying read. Schiller's contribution to the book comes from her experience with a devastating mental illness for which no treatment was efficacious for many long years. She promises no easy cure but offers hope of sustained remission through new medications, such as clozapine, and continuing psychotherapy. Bennett's contribution comes from her experience as a journalist and editor for the *Wall Street Journal*. Indeed, the idea for this book evolved from the responses to an article she had published two years earlier about Schiller's emergence "from the torments of schizophrenia" (Bennett 1992, A1). Schiller's first-person account of her illness is, of course, the sine qua non of *The Quiet Room*, but the book benefits greatly from Bennett's skills as an experienced investigative journalist, as well as from the cachet of the *Wall Street Journal*, which no doubt helped the authors gain access to the many documentary records and psychiatric experts they consulted. Most who write a first-person narrative of mental illness do not have ready access to such resources, although some do as a result of their own professional or celebrity status. Schiller is in some ways privileged—she is smart and well educated with a devoted family and good health insurance—but she was neither a professional writer nor a celebrity before her illness, which makes her experience more like that of other "ordinary" patients. The result of Schiller and Bennett's collaborative authorship is seamless, unlike an earlier collaborative work, *A Brilliant Madness: Living with Manic-Depressive Illness* (1992), in which chapters by the actress Patty Duke about her personal experience with the illness alternate with chapters by Gloria Hochman about the medical history of the disease and its treatments (Duke and Hochman 1992).

In his taxonomy of first-person narratives of illness in *The Wounded Storyteller*, Arthur W. Frank describes what he calls the *chaos narrative* as one that paradoxically "cannot be told" because "those who are truly *living* the chaos cannot tell [it] in words" (1995, 105, 98). Having once recovered enough to write a coherent account of the illness, the person is, in Frank's taxonomy, writing either a *restitution narrative* or a *quest narrative*, neither of which can adequately capture or represent the true chaos of the full-blown illness. To a certain extent, this paradox may occur in all serious illnesses, but the psychotic episodes of mental illness are excellent examples of living in chaos. If the purpose of a first-person narrative of illness is to present primarily the subjective experience of the patient, narrative reflection and coherence may not matter. The unmediated phenomenological experience of the patient may provide the greatest value. Yet a narrative of schizophrenia written while the author is psychotic, even when edited by friends and later published, can be tedious reading. What one learns, first and foremost, is that the author is severely mentally ill, in great pain, and suicidal (Burke 1995). Such a desperate cry for help makes "moral and clinical" claims on readers (listeners) to "honor" the chaos story and care for the sick person (Frank 1995, 109), but such an account offers little help or hope to others suffering from schizophrenia. It is not surprising that most published narratives of mental illness are by those who have achieved at least a temporary remission from the chaos of their illness and are able to reach out to help those who have not.

In the "Author's [*sic*] Note and Acknowledgments" that opens *The Quiet Room*, Schiller and Bennett deal explicitly and effectively with concerns about Schiller's unreliability as narrator by explaining their choice to supplement her flawed memory with accounts by her parents, two brothers, college roommate, and psychiatrist: "In writing this book Amanda Bennett and I have done the best job we could to make sure that we rendered events as accurately as possible. All the people, places and events . . . are real, and are portrayed exactly as I recall them. . . . In the interests of accuracy, we tried to interview as many people involved with my life, my illness and my treatment as possible. We tried to take their perspectives into account in the telling of this book" (Schiller and Bennett 1994, vii–viii). They also include, for external "objective" accuracy, brief excerpts from Schiller's medical records at the Payne Whitney Clinic of New York Hospital–Cornell Medical Center and from those at the Westchester Division of New York Hospital–Cornell Medical Center.

Yet it is not only as compensation for gaps in Schiller's memory, caused both by her illness and some of the treatments for it, that these other stories are needed. She has vivid false memories that only others can contest. In a shocking example, the second section of the book opens with Schiller's "memory of the afternoon of the dog." She graphically describes her brutal beating to death of a helpless dog and her remorse over the years for "having committed such a terrible sin against an innocent creature." But her parents and brothers assure her that "it never happened" (Schiller and Bennett 1994, 9). The violence and detail of this false memory get readers' attention early on, making them extremely well aware of how essential the stories of others are in helping both Schiller and the reader understand better the horrific extent—and limits—of her illness. In addition to this vital function, including the stories of her family members and friend has the benefit of showing how those close to Schiller were profoundly affected by her illness.

Another issue that comes up in many narratives of mental illness is that of protecting the confidentiality of other patients while including them in the story. Schiller explains her efforts to do so: "With a few minor exceptions all names in the book are real too. Because of their deep involvement with cocaine, however, I have changed the names and other identifying details of Raymond and Nicole. I also changed the names and descriptions of Robin, Carla and Claire to protect their privacy as fellow psychiatric patients" (Schiller and Bennett 1994, vii–viii).

As evident in the previous quotation, the "Author's Note and Acknowledgments" is written primarily in Schiller's individual voice—"this is my life story"—although it is signed by both coauthors. "Amanda and I" and "we" are used when thanking medical people who have helped with the details about Schiller's experience: psychiatric consultants at Long Island Jewish Medical Center, Duke University Medical Center, the National Institute of Mental Health, and the National Institutes of Health; several editors at the *Wall Street Journal*; their agent and editor; and their families. The copyright to the book is held jointly by Schiller and Bennett, yet when the *New York Times* reported shortly after the publication of *The Quiet Room* that the movie rights had been optioned, only Schiller was mentioned as being paid $800,000 by Touchstone Pictures (Lombardi 1994). And, in another *New York Times* article two days later, only Schiller is reported to have "become something of a public figure, appearing on 'Prime Time Live,' 'Larry King Live' and the 'Today' program and making appearances around the country" (Brozan 1994).

Immediately after the "Author's Note and Acknowledgments" comes a "Foreword" written by Jane Doller, MD, who was the staff psychiatrist in charge of 3 South, the special long-term-care unit for worst cases at New York Hospital–Cornell Medical Center, Westchester Division at White Plains, when Schiller was a patient there. Dr. Doller, Schiller's case administrator on 3 South and then her therapist after discharge, summarizes well and succinctly those aspects of Schiller's case that are typical of her illness: "The onset in late adolescence after an apparently normal childhood; the initial difficulty in finding a correct diagnosis; her own denial, and that of her parents, and their refusal at first to recognize her illness for what it was. The initial failure of treatment . . . [and] turn in the meantime to illicit drug use in an effort to manage the frightening symptoms" (Doller 1994, xii). She also speaks eloquently of the importance of Schiller's "personal determination, courage and hope" and her "connection with another person" as "a powerful tool for healing in a curing arsenal that also includes drugs" (Doller 1994, xiii).

Much of the value of Schiller's story is, as Doller points out, that her illness is typical in many ways. The first child and only daughter of Marvin and Nancy Schiller, she was a bright and happy child until August 1976, just before her senior year in high school, when she begins to hear the abusive Voices that have plagued her ever since. The Voices relentlessly repeat "You must die!" and castigate her with taunts such as "You whore bitch who isn't worth a piece of crap!" (Schiller and Bennett 1994, 6). She tries desperately to hide the Voices, her increasingly black moods, and her agitation from all those around her during her last year in high school. As a number of other young people report having done, she, too, diagnoses herself as mentally ill after reading Sylvia Plath's *The Bell Jar* (1978) for one of her English class assignments. She confides to her diary: "The symptoms of the crack-upped Sylvia Plath–Esther Greenwood are me. Of course not everything, but enough. . . . I didn't sleep for 23 nights. Esther G. only didn't for 21" (Schiller and Bennett 1994, 17). And, just as many other mental patients have reported, she believes that Walter Cronkite, when he reads the nightly news on CBS, is talking directly to her, expecting her to take responsibility for the world's problems.

Somehow Schiller manages to hold onto her secret and enough of her sanity to finish high school and, in September 1977, she enters Tufts University, where she rooms with two young women, one of whom is also named Lori. Schiller manages to get through a junior year abroad in Spain, where the Voices revile her in the language she is studying. When she returns to Tufts, she tells her parents she needs "to talk to someone" (Schiller and Bennett 1994, 24), and with their approval, she begins to see a counselor at Tufts and then a private psychiatrist to whom she does not talk at all about the Voices that torment her lest they make good on their threats to kill her. The psychiatrist prescribes Valium. Schiller takes it, graduates from Tufts in June 1981, and moves with Lori Winters to New York City, where they room together again and start their first jobs. The extent of Schiller's illness during her final college year and first year in New York, as well as the strength of her parents' denial that anything is wrong, are vividly related in Winters's one section of

The Quiet Room. Seeking help for Schiller, Winters calls Schiller's mother on several occasions, only to be reassured that Schiller "is just in one of her moods. It will pass" (Schiller and Bennett 1994, 33). But Schiller's moods do not pass. They get worse, and after pleading for help from her psychiatrist one night and receiving none, she takes all the pills in the bottles he has prescribed. Fortunately, Winters is there and promptly calls 911, Schiller's parents, and the psychiatrist. Schiller is taken to Bellevue Hospital.

In the next section, one of two from Marvin Schiller's point of view, readers begin to get an understanding of the depth of his denial of his daughter's illness. A clinical psychologist himself, Dr. Schiller's is concerned first of all that his daughter's attempted suicide does not get documented in a way that could label her as a psychiatric patient. Afraid of the stigma that entering a psychiatric ward would bring her, he negotiates her admission to a medical ward instead. His resistance is primarily that of a father protecting his child, but it is not unusual in narratives of mental illness to see mental health professionals themselves resist admitting a patient to a psychiatric ward or hospital. Styron (1990) reports in *Darkness Visible*, for example, that had he not been admitted to the hospital against his psychiatrist's advice, he would not have survived his deep depression. Both autobiographical and fictional accounts of abusive institutions have left enduring images in the minds of the public and health professionals alike. Mary Jane Ward's *The Snake Pit* (1946; film, Litvak 1948) and Ken Kesey's *One Flew over the Cuckoo's Nest* (1962; film, Forman 1975) are iconic examples. Both novels were made into award-winning films that retain their cultural influence into the twenty-first century. Despite the power of such anti-asylum works, many narratives of mental illness, including Ward's novel, endorse as does Styron the healing effects of time spent in an asylum, even when it is far less than ideal (Jones 1993).

Marvin Schiller's denial of his daughter's mental illness goes much deeper, however. For his generation, he says, "there was only one cause for all mental illnesses, even the most severe: a faulty upbringing. Everything was tied to the way you were raised" (Schiller and Bennett 1994, 45). Not wanting to believe that he could be responsible for his daughter's illness, he denies that she is ill. Even his profound denial fails, however, when Lori makes a second suicide attempt just three months after the first. More frightened than before, he is finally convinced that his daughter is seriously mentally ill when she undresses before him and her brother Steven and starts to walk out of the hospital naked and shoeless. This time, Dr. Schiller pleads with his daughter to sign herself in voluntarily to the Payne Whitney Clinic of New York Hospital–Cornell Medical Center, an acute-care psychiatric facility.

Unlike her husband, Nancy Schiller does not at first blame herself for her daughter's illness, but she recounts two moments of sudden recognition that force her to acknowledge what she has tried so hard to deny. In the first, she is walking to meet Lori in Manhattan one day and sees "a woman laden down with heavy shopping bags. Although it was late spring and very hot, she was wearing an overcoat, hat, and boots." With a shock, she realizes that the bag lady before her is her daughter (Schiller and Bennett 1994, 66). In the second such recognition, she suddenly realizes that she has seen the vacant look in her daughter's eyes before, in her own mother's eyes. Then she remembers others in her family, like her cousin Sylvia, who was referred to by everyone as "crazy as a loon" (Schiller and Bennett 1994, 83). With these reawakened memories, she must face the fact that her daughter's schizophrenia is genetic, comes from her side of the family, and may threaten her sons' futures as well. Implausible as it may seem, such moments of sudden recognition of other family members' "craziness" are not unusual in narratives of mental illness.

Just as the older generation had done before them, Marvin and Nancy Schiller try at first to hide their daughter's illness, not telling anyone what is wrong with her or where she is when she is hospitalized. Their sons know, of course. Steven, six and a half years younger than his sister, is sixteen when she is first committed. Although he is resentful that she gets so much attention, he is also angry that his parents have put her away and accuses them of just trying to get her out of sight to avoid embarrassment. His greatest fear, however, is that what has happened to his sister could happen to him as well, because her illness is genetic. Like his younger brother Steven, Mark also resents the attention his sister receives after her suicide attempts. Not until he learns that she has been "mutilating herself" (Schiller and Bennett 1994, 179) does Mark realize the severity of her illness and feel sympathy for her. Away at college, he is somewhat buffered from his sister's suffering, but he feels overwhelmed when he comes home for the holidays and encounters her in his parents' home. He repeatedly breaks up with his fiancée just before his trips home so that she will not meet his sister. Like Steven, Mark fears for his own future because of his sister's illness. Even if Schiller's brothers do not develop a serious mental illness, their lives are shaped in many ways by the effects of her illness on the entire family. In this aspect, as well, *The Quiet Room* represents the experiences of most families in which mental illness is present.

Accepting her father's advice, Schiller voluntarily commits herself in June 1982 to the Payne Whitney Clinic, an acute-care psychiatric wing of New York Hospital–Cornell Medical Center, and moves into a new stage of her illness odyssey. She and her parents hope for what Frank calls *restitution*—for accurate diagnosis, effective treatment, quick recovery, and return to normal—to the life she had before her illness. As the young medical students who try to care for her rotate in and out of the clinic every few weeks, they prescribe psychotropic drugs—lithium, Thorazine, and Haldol—in ever-higher doses, but to no avail. They then give her six electroconvulsive shock treatments, then six more, and then six more, until Schiller has received twenty in all and still shows no improvement. At this point, they tell her parents that she suffers from schizo-affective disorder, a combination of bipolar disorder and schizophrenia, that she needs to be transferred to a long-term-care facility, and that she may never recover.

With this dismal prognosis, Schiller is admitted in September 1982 to the Westchester Division of New York Hospital–Cornell Medical Center in White Plains. By April 1983, showing little improvement, she is released, against medical advice, to the care of her parents and spends the next year at their home in Scarsdale. She gets a job as a waitress and begins to self-medicate, gradually developing a $1,000-a-week cocaine habit. Even though she manages, at her father's insistence, to break her cocaine addiction, Schiller's illness repeatedly overwhelms her, and, in the next several years, she makes more suicide attempts, enters and leaves hospitals and halfway houses, takes and quits taking an array of psychiatric drugs, and resumes her cocaine habit. As Doller attests, these episodes, unfortunately, are all too typical in the course of an illness as severe as Schiller's.

What is not typical in Schiller's case is the special unit at Westchester Division reserved for worst cases, the ones that many consider lost causes. When Schiller is eventually accepted there, she finally makes the kind of personal connection with Dr. Doller that becomes a necessary but not sufficient component of her successful treatment. The trust that Schiller develops with Doller can hardly be overstated; it is the essential groundwork for Schiller's recovery. Such a personal connection shows up in many narratives of mental illness as a turning point for patients (Jones 1993). The connection is not always with a psychiatrist or psychotherapist, but it is arguably most effective when it is. Knowing that she has been given a very special last chance, Schiller becomes at last an active participant in the demanding psychotherapy she has resisted for so many years. At this point her story becomes a true *quest narrative* (Frank 1995). And over time, she makes progress—but not enough for recovery from an illness so severe as hers. Not until Schiller has the opportunity to enroll in a trial of clozapine, then a new antipsychotic drug with potentially life-threatening side effects that was available only for those whose schizophrenia had not responded to standard treatments, does her true recovery begin. Both she and her parents decide that the drug is worth the potential risk of death because they believe that Schiller will die of her illness if she does not find relief. In the same year that *The Quiet Room* was published, Diana Ross starred in an excellent made-for-TV movie based on another true story of a woman suffering from severe schizophrenia who also begins taking clozapine as her last hope and who has a remarkable recovery (*Out of Darkness*; Elikann 1994).

With the combination of intense psychotherapy and this powerful new drug, Schiller gradually gets better and is eventually able to leave the hospital and live on her own. The book makes clear, however, that Schiller's recovery is tenuous and depends upon her adherence to a regimen of twenty pills a day and continuing psychotherapy. She has entered what Frank (1995) calls *the remission society*, but she will never be restored to the life she had before. That Lori Schiller is gone forever. *The Quiet Room* and Schiller's efforts to teach others—health professionals as well as patients—about living with schizophrenia fulfill Frank's call for those who have emerged from severe illness to tell their stories and thereby share their wisdom with others.

Sadly, the special unit that helped Schiller and many others with worst-case mental illnesses was closed by 1996, the result of budget cutbacks in New York. And in early 2002, the remarkably gifted and dedicated psychiatrist Jane Doller died suddenly, at age forty-six, of an acute myocardial infarction. The stress of caring for severely ill mental patients was identified by one of her colleagues as a contributing factor in Doller's premature death (Kroplick 2003, 1). Other gifted therapists featured in well-known fictionalized accounts of mental illness have also died prematurely from diseases that may have been exacerbated by the stress of their work. Two prominent examples are William H. R. Rivers (1864–1922), as portrayed in the three well-researched historical novels of Pat Barker's *The Regeneration Trilogy* (1991–1995), and Frieda Fromm-Reichmann (1889–1957), portrayed in the autobiographical novel *I Never Promised You a Rose Garden* (1964) by Joanne Greenberg (published originally under the pseudonym Hannah Green). Although Rivers, at fifty-eight, and Fromm-Reichmann, at sixty-eight, were a decade or two older than Doller when they died (Hornstein 2000; Slobodin 1997), both are described in these narratives as working to exhaustion because of their deep sense of responsibility for their patients.

Greenberg's and Schiller's accounts of their long-standing remissions offer two more autobiographical narratives of "minds that came back" and stayed back, despite the occasional relapse described by Schiller. There are a number of other recent narratives by very successful people who have found ways to control their severe mental illnesses well enough to function in highly demanding careers. The physician Mark Vonnegut (1975, 2010), who has written the foreword to this volume; the highly acclaimed clinical psychologist Kay Redfield Jamison (1995); and the law professor Elyn R. Saks (2007) are among the best-known examples. Recently, however, the *New York Times* has run a series of articles about less well-known people who have learned how to live with major mental illnesses and maintain demanding and stressful careers (Parker-Pope 2011). There now seems again, as there was sixty years ago in Alvarez's time, a willingness among mental health professionals to recognize and learn from the special expertise of such people and their stories.

Worth noting as well is the surprising popular and commercial success of *next to normal* (Kitt and Yorkey 2010), a rock musical that won several 2009 Tony Awards and the Pulitzer Prize for drama in 2010. Most impressive is the play's realistic presentation of the experience of bipolar disorder, its effects on all family members, and the ongoing struggle of the protagonist, Diana, to enter and remain in the remission society. Despite her best hopes, she finds no magic pills, no miracle cure, just very hard work, every day, day after day. Her endurance and resilience are not glamorous, but they are life sustaining and potentially transcendent. As increasingly more patients risk coming out to add their voices and stories in blogs, published narratives, films, and plays, the possibility of early diagnosis, better treatments, and lessened stigma seems more realistic than ever before. We are fortunate to have their compelling stories.

Chapter 33

COMMUNITY PSYCHIATRY AND THE MEDICAL HUMANITIES

MICHAEL ROWE

S EVERAL years ago, a few colleagues and I set out to collect, in one volume, a set of "classic" texts in the field of community psychiatry. They were to span the period from 1954—the year that institutionalization in state psychiatric hospitals in the United States reached an apex from which it would steadily decline through a process called "deinstitutionalization"—to the latter 2000s. Texts would fall into one of four categories: government, legislative, and policy; first person and literary; clinical and systems theory, conceptual, and historical; and practice and research. Those that made the final cut would be worthy in their own right *and* have either broken new ground or elucidated important aspects of the field, or both.

To select as representative a group as possible, we adapted a research method called "snowball sampling" (Goodman 1961): first, identifying a core group of leading researchers, policy makers, advocates, and scholars in the field; next, asking these experts to choose classics and suggest other nominators; and then repeating this approach with the next group. If our method worked, we would, over a few iterations, have consensus on both the experts in the field and on a group of classics they had recommended. From these we would select a final set, including our own nominations.

It didn't work. We were offered a new set of prospective nominators and more suggested classics with each turn of the snowball, which got larger, heavier and finally, unmanageable, leaving us with lots of good suggestions and sole responsibility for choosing our texts (Rowe et al. 2011). It seemed to us that we had been given an object lesson in the contested nature of our discipline, with multiple parties offering, through titles and nominators, their arguments regarding the accomplishments and failures of community psychiatry. Thus, while I would like to offer a succinct statement on how the field of community psychiatry sees itself, in relation to which humanistic inquiries in medicine can make a contribution, such a statement would be misleading. Instead, community psychiatry is better described as a field of tensions between poles that, while not necessarily contradictory, often perform as though they are (Freeman and Rowe 2011).

Community psychiatry is composed of policies, people, (mainly) public and private nonprofit organizations, and technologies aimed at providing treatment and rehabilitation services for people who are poor and have mental illnesses.

"A life in the community" has been the standard for the "community" half of the term. However, the efforts associated with this goal have involved removing hundreds of thousands of people from the "total institutions" of state hospitals (Goffman 1961) to urban ghettos or nursing home institutions, in effect making available to them a life "in" the community but not "of" the community (Ware et al. 2007). The other half of the term, "psychiatry," is, of course, a branch of medicine, but its involvement with the mind and emotions more so than with the body—artificial as these distinctions now seem to us—has sometimes pushed it to the margins of medicine. In this chapter, I will suggest some ways that the medical/health humanities can contribute to community psychiatry. In doing so, given the breadth of the field, I will focus on only one main theme—the notion of recovery both from and outside of mental illness (Davidson 2003). First, a whirlwind historical tour is in order.

COMMUNITY PSYCHIATRY: A VERY BRIEF HISTORY

Pre–Community Psychiatry (1850–1953)

From roughly 1850 to the mid-1950s, mental health care in the United States was largely institutional care that offered "moral treatment" to its patients, removing them from stressful environments and placing them in one set apart—an asylum—where their mental health could be restored through social activities and empathic care (Bockoven 1956; Martin and Flanagan 2011). Moral therapy claimed high success rates during its early years (Bockoven 1956). In retrospect, that success, which is contested today, appears to have been related to the similar cultural and social background of patients—native born, upper or upper middle class—to that of asylum superintendents as well as the leisurely census of those institutions (Grob 1991). As non-native persons began to constitute a higher portion of the patient population in the latter part of the nineteenth century, well-to-do patients eschewed public asylums for private facilities (Morrissey and Goldman 1986). Asylums devolved into the warehousing of people with serious psychiatric disorders in large state psychiatric institutions by the end of the nineteenth and well into the twentieth century, and by 1954, 350 hospitals across the country housed 559,000 patients (Martin and Flanagan 2011). During and after the Second World War, exposés and fictionalized autobiography (Deutsch 1948; Ward 1946) contributed to the increasing disrepute of these facilities, and financially pressed states became increasingly unwilling to pay for them (Grob 1994).

Deinstitutionalization and the Community Mental Health Center Movement (1954–1976)

Beginning in the mid-1950s, thousands of state hospital patients were discharged, many with prescriptions for one of a new group of psychiatric medications—phenothiazines—that, it was hoped, would make it possible for them to lead stable lives in their home communities. In 1963, President John F. Kennedy proposed a national effort for this purpose, supported in part by development of community mental health centers (CMHCs). Implementation of the Community Mental Health Centers Construction Act was passed in 1963 under Lyndon B. Johnson (Miller et al. 2011). Between 1966 and 1975, over two hundred fifty thousand people left U.S. psychiatric institutions (Gronfein 1985). John Talbott (1979) has argued that the prime movers of "deinstitutionalization" were shifts in funding for Medicaid, Medicare, and federal Supplemental Security Income (SSI); the emergence of the community mental health philosophy; new medications; and a number of other legal, judicial, and legislative actions. Studying the relationship between mental illness and the economy, Harvey Brenner (1973) argued for the causal impact of unstable economies on increasing discharge rates from mental hospitals separately from the incidence of mental illness.

By the mid-1970s, most assessments of the deinstitutionalization process were highly critical. An effective and coordinated system of mental health care was never put into place, and funding for construction and staffing was limited. Psychiatrists and psychologists, trained and personally and economically inclined to provide psychotherapy to the so-called "worried well," declined to work in CMHCs or fled them for private practice. Services eroded or were not implemented, planning was haphazard, and the CMHC movement lacked a base of knowledge for providing community-based care (Geller 2000). Deinstitutionalization for people with mental illnesses became "transinstitutionalization" for many, with discharge from state hospitals to nursing homes—mini-institutions physically located in local communities but otherwise largely separate from them—or to families who lacked the supports to care for them, or to single-room occupancy buildings, for which they paid with their federal entitlement (SSI) income. The community mental health centers that were to provide their mental health treatment were reluctant to do so (Davidson and Ridgway 2011).

The Community Support Movement and Its Demise (1977–1997)

During this period, community psychiatry moved from the messianic reformist zeal of the community mental health movement to a more modest but still ambitious attempt to consolidate lessons learned from the troubled implementation of the CMHC vision. Predicated on the need for comprehensive and wide-ranging community support service systems for people with serious psychiatric disabilities, the Carter administration's Community Support Program System (CSP) was pulled and patched together from existing programs and funding mechanisms(U.S. General Accounting Office 1977). However, much of the optimism and focus associated with the early stages of the CSP as well as financial support for it dissipated during the early 1980s as the Reagan administration eliminated the CSP funding that President Jimmy Carter had requested, reduced funding for CMHCs, and largely gave back to the states, through block grants, responsibility for funding mental health services and systems. In addition, the Social Security Administration reviewed current SSI cases for eligibility. Thousands lost their benefits as a result, and rates for approval of new applications dropped. Urban renewal and gentrification as well as cuts in federal housing programs and low-income housing

development further widened gaps in the safety net for people with mental illnesses, contributing to the rise of homelessness during the 1980s (Davidson and
Ridgway 2011; Mechanic and Rochefort 1992).

States began to create managed systems of community-based care through strategies that included integrated local mental health authorities, case management
and assertive community treatment, and various financing strategies. All fell short
of making up for the deficiencies in overall systems of care. In spite of its failures,
though, the CSP movement initiated a reform agenda that helped to shape the next
(and still present) era of community psychiatry (Davidson and Ridgway 2011).

The Contemporary Era (1998–Present)

Several service approaches have reached prominence in the present era of
community psychiatry. One is "evidence-based practice," including illness self-
management, supported employment, integrated treatment for dual disorders of
mental illness and substance use, and other forms of treatment that have been
shown to be successful through successive randomized controlled trials (Drake
et al. 2001). Cultural competence in mental health care has also been recognized
at federal and state levels, in keeping with a trend in medicine at large in our
increasingly multicultural society (National Alliance of Multi-Ethnic Behavioral
Health Associations 2008), but the application of multicultural principles in practice has lagged (Delphin and Rowe 2008). Mental health parity legislation has
been passed, although issues of entry into insurance programs, cost of care, and
determination of parity at the level of individual care remain (Lawless and Rowe
2011; Satcher 1999). Recognition of the need for integration of mental health and
primary care has increased with the dissemination of findings that people with
mental illness, on average, have significantly shorter life spans than those without (National Association of State Mental Health Program Directors 2006). And
finally, before taking up the issue of mental health recovery, healthcare reform
looms as a major, but still uncertain, source of change for the field of public mental
health care (Levinson et al. 2010).

RECOVERY FROM AND "OUTSIDE OF" MENTAL ILLNESS

Until the early 1990s, recovery from serious mental illness chiefly meant improvement in the social functioning or psychiatric symptoms of persons diagnosed with
schizophrenia, as documented in research studies showing diverse outcomes,
including, variously, long-term remission, substantial improvement, or periods of
higher and lower functioning (Harding et al. 1987; Strauss et al. 1985). Over the
past two decades, however, another view of recovery, fueled initially by the psychiatric consumer/survivor movement, has emerged. This view, which I will call
new recovery, neither negates nor downplays *traditional recovery* but instead argues
that even if or when mental illness persists, it is only one part of the person's life
and need not overwhelm the others. Recovery, in this sense, is a process not an
outcome—a way of seeing one's self and living one's life. Recovery, in general,

essentially incorporating both definitions, has been endorsed at the federal level, most recently in the President's New Freedom Commission on Mental Health (2003) report.

Traditional recovery has an impressive evidence base supporting it, although it has not penetrated the discipline of psychiatry as deeply as one might hope. New recovery has received both widespread support among persons with mental illnesses and at federal, state, and service system levels (although often without making the distinction that I do here between old and new recovery) and been the object of much skepticism (Davidson et al. 2005). This support and skepticism stem, in part, from new recovery's fluidity: it is a personal journey, a rallying cry for advocates that is usually coupled with a harsh critique of psychiatry historically, and an approach to direct care involving the provision of "recovery-oriented treatment" (Davidson et al. 2009). In addition, because new recovery, also called *social recovery* in order to distinguish it from traditional, or clinical, recovery, is often discussed in terms that make it appear more subjective than social, there is recent interest in other, more pointedly social forms of recovery, including *capabilities*, derived from Amartya Sen's economic theories (Hopper 2007); *social inclusion*, derived from European Union social planning approaches (Thompson and Rowe 2010); and *citizenship*, derived from mental health outreach to people who are homeless (Rowe, Benedict, et al. 2009; Rowe, Kloos, et al. 2001).

With the suggestion that those who engage in new recovery are likely to have more fulfilling lives than they would otherwise, there will be more and more push to show evidence of its success. Demonstrating recovery outcomes is complicated; not only is personal fulfillment difficult to measure but also increased social connectedness and participation are less persuasive to funders and policy makers and, therefore, more challenging to pursue through rigorous research than reduced hospitalization, substance use, homelessness, and other measures of progress, which recovery, properly defined and measured, may or may not facilitate. It is likely there will be attempts in the near future to develop a unified theory of old and new recovery that integrates its clinical and social impacts in order to overcome what may be an overwrought distinction between the two.

Recovery in both senses is relevant to the question that, as I suggested at the outset, lies at the heart of community psychiatry: can people with serious mental illnesses live clinically stable lives in their home communities and thrive as participating and accepted members of those communities? What follows are two case vignettes, one demonstrating clinical and functional recovery, and the other, at least in potential, belonging in the domain of new recovery. The first involves a well-known and highly accomplished mental health professional who was featured in a *New York Times* article (Carey 2011), from which I draw material for the vignette. The second involves a pseudonymous person, unknown to the public but about whom I have written, and who is not distinguished by what we typically recognize as major personal accomplishments (Rowe 1999). This brief telling and discussion of their stories is, I hope, consistent with the beginning of a qualitative inquiry in mental health. I will then take up the question of the link of such inquiries to the medical humanities.

TWO VIGNETTES

At age seventeen, Marsha Linehan was admitted as an inpatient to the Institute for Living, a psychiatric hospital in Hartford, Connecticut. Ms. Linehan spent much of her two years there in a seclusion room because of suicidal behavior, including cutting her arms, legs, and midsection. Diagnosed with schizophrenia and given powerful psychiatric drugs and multiple electroshock treatments, she attempted suicide a few years after leaving the institute and was rehospitalized. During this time, Ms. Linehan's Catholic faith sustained her, culminating in a revelation—that she loved herself—which proved to be a turning point in her life: "She had accepted herself as she was. She had tried to kill herself so many times because the gulf between the person she wanted to be and the person she was left her desperate, hopeless, deeply homesick for a life she would never know. That gulf was real, and unbridgeable" (Carey 2011, A17). Now she had found a way to begin to build that bridge.

Ms. Linehan became Dr. Linehan, a psychologist who treats severely suicidal patients, including those diagnosed with borderline personality disorder. The principle of *radical acceptance* of oneself that first appeared to her in a revelation linked with the patient's commitment to change his or her life became what is now known and practiced worldwide as dialectical behavioral therapy. Dr. Linehan, who lives with her adopted daughter and her husband, describes herself as a happy person with the usual ups and downs we all have.

Robert Andrews was in his late thirties when I interviewed him on a medical unit at Yale–New Haven Hospital in New Haven, Connecticut. Robert had grown up as an orphan in the state foster care system. In addition to his severe psychiatric disorder and polysubstance use, he had HIV and end-stage renal and liver failure. During my interview with him, Robert spoke of an abandoned building that he had lived in for a few years: "There was nothing wrong with the shelter, but it was inconvenient for me to get up at 4 o'clock in the morning and walk all the way across the city to the labor agency. So I found this vacant building that was about a ten-minute walk. . . . I fixed up my quarters, cleaned it up. There was no heat but I had about fifteen blankets that I kept sanitized." He also told me of his volunteer work at the soup kitchen, which he took up after injuring his hand at a glass factory: "I'd wipe the tables down, wash the chairs, sweep and mop the floor, run the washing machine, work with pots and pans scrubbing and washing them. . . . The staff began to like me there. They told me I was like part of the family."

I interviewed Robert at an auspicious moment. He'd just received a complete blood transfusion and saw this event as an opportunity to turn his life around: "I had the same body but my blood and everything has been changed . . . the places I once was at, I can't go there. I'm forbidden. There's still a chair, still a window, still a bed, still a house, still a moon. The people still exist but I have no right to go there. . . . I'm farther away from them. I'm letting them go" (Rowe 1999, 22–23).

Robert hoped to get married again and buy a home for his children from his first marriage. (Based on information we were able to gather, we think it unlikely that Robert was ever married and had children although it was clear that he believed he did, or believed it at times.) He died in 2000 after moving into his own apartment, where he kept himself fit until near the end with daily push-ups and sit-ups. Staff from the local mental health center arranged a funeral service for Robert so that he would not have a pauper's burial.

Excepting their common experience of having a serious mental illness, Dr. Linehan and Mr. Andrews appear to have little in common and much to separate them. Dr. Linehan, a white female who grew up in a middle-class family in Oklahoma, overcame the turmoil and suicidality of her teen and young adult years to become a world-renowned mental health clinician and researcher. Mr. Andrews, an African American male, grew up in one after another foster family setting in Connecticut and seems to have been doomed by his poverty, illness, and mental illness. Yet without downplaying these radical differences, there are suggestions of commonalities or points of connection between these two people. While Dr. Linehan's story may seem to be a classic example of clinical and functional recovery from mental illness, she also drew on her faith, her connections with others (her patients) who had similarly suffered, and in finding strength in the midst of weakness to construct the path of her own recovery. All of these are elements that proponents of recovery as a way of life identify as tools in planning and living (Davidson et al. 2009).

Mr. Andrews, in contrast, is a person whose life I have used to illustrate what I call the *five Rs* of social recovery by way of *citizenship*: He demonstrated his *responsibility* in taking care of his living quarters and making the most of the *resources* (abandoned building, cast-off materials) that he found or took pains to gather. He successfully pursued the valued *roles* of paid and volunteer work (and, if he had had the time and opportunity, he might have pursued the role of poet, as evidenced by his description of the meaning of his blood transfusion). He valued and benefited from his *relationships* with his soup kitchen co-workers, and he believed he had the *right* to pursue his dream of having a home and family. Although enumerating the barriers he faced is not to say that Robert had no responsibility for shaping his life—an idea I am confident that Robert would have rejected utterly—I think it is fair to say that his inability to exercise his capacities on a broader canvas is Robert's tragedy in contrast to Dr. Linehan's triumph. Either of their stories, however, if regarded through the narrowest medical lens (for the sake of illustration, even if the lens used in practice is rarely this narrow) would read quite differently: Dr. Linehan's story might be one of intensive clinical treatment and potential misdiagnosis of schizophrenia—since her eventual success, some would say, is so extraordinary for a person who is said to "have" schizophrenia that she must not have "had" it—as well as her own native talents and abilities. Mr. Andrew's story might be that of a disadvantaged individual who was further incapacitated by mental illness, drug use, and other poor choices, which led to his fatal illnesses. A role of the medical humanities has been to advocate for wider lenses than are typically employed, to incorporate subjective and social elements in clinical training and practice.

COMMUNITY PSYCHIATRY AND THE MEDICAL/HEALTH HUMANITIES

What, if anything, can the medical humanities do for community psychiatry? I would first posit that community psychiatry already has its own form of medical humanities represented in clinical care that is directly connected to community living and thriving, as with centers, assertive community treatment, homeless outreach teams, and newer innovative programs. Moreover, one aim of the qualitative and ethnographic research in the discipline is to elucidate the texture and meaning of living with mental illness in one's community. Second, the enduring question of mental health treatment in the context of community living for persons with serious psychiatric disorders is, in fact, a humanistic-medical question. Against this backdrop, I would like to offer four points regarding the potential contributions of the medical humanities to community psychiatry.

Recovery and Chronic Illness

In community psychiatry, no theoretical approach to mental illness and "a life in the community" speaks more loudly for "wellness" and to treatment approaches that privilege the choices, preferences, and full involvement in planning of persons with mental illness than "new" recovery. Therefore, a link between recovery and living with chronic illness may seem far-fetched at first glance. The suggestion that there was one astonished me when my colleague, Larry Davidson, made it during a 2010 meeting with directors of the psychiatric residency training at our institution. *Limitation* seems to be embedded in the very four syllables of *chronic illness*, while recovery is about moving away from the determinism of limits that people carry, along with the mental illness itself, from the time they are diagnosed.

As we talked, though, the similarities became clearer. Both fields confront the issue of the person's full life in the context of, in spite and outside of, the illness. "New," or "social," recovery, for all its own limitations, including the fact that its individual aspect—the subjective sense of "being a person in recovery"—sometimes threatens to overwhelm its social aspect—a life of engagement and participation with others in social life—does not ignore illness. People with mental illnesses, when they are "in recovery," often contend with symptoms and functional constraints associated with their mental illness, as do people living with chronic "physical" illnesses. Persons in both groups learn to consider health in relation to their activities and interests, not just illness symptoms, and see these elements of their lives as part of who they are beyond being a person with schizophrenia or a brittle diabetic (Charmaz 2006).

Another area of similarity, in logic if not always in fact, is the patient-doctor relationship. (I should note that, in public mental health, "patient-clinician relationship" is the more accurate term, as the clinician generally is a psychiatric social worker or psychologist, although psychiatrists either prescribe or oversee prescription of psychiatric medications.) If ever there were a case to be made for the patient-doctor "partnership" in clinical care, it is in the field of chronic physical illness care and in recovery-oriented mental health treatment. In both, the locus of energy shifts from cure to ongoing care and illness management, and the illness is not an interruption in and aberration from normal life but instead *is part of* normal life. The question is no longer "Will I live or die?" or "Will my life be different in the future than it is now?"—life *is different* now, with the limitations and compensations and even the rising above of limitations that are the province of life with a chronic illness. This is a simplification, of course, as in chronic illness there may be significant periods of reduced symptoms and functional limitations as well as of acute illness. My point here is that chronic illness pushes the patient-doctor relationship toward the "whole life" of the person.

While the link between the medical humanities and chronic illness, as well as that between the medical humanities and living with mental illness in one's community, must be made, not assumed, there is a natural fit in both cases, and community psychiatry can benefit from the link. Robert Andrews's life, for example, becomes meaningful when placed in its social as well as its medical context, and the medical humanities have technologies, or methods, that can be useful in this regard.

Research Methods/Technologies

Narrative medicine, a subfield of the medical humanities, is a term rarely used in community psychiatry research and scholarship. More to the point, narrative research and theory as practiced by scholar-researchers such as Rita Charon (2006), Arthur Frank (2010), and others, with their emphases on comparative medical and narrative telling of patient stories, offer additional models for use in qualitative research in community mental health care. These methods can be used in teaching clinicians as well as in offering frameworks to patients (often called "clients" in public mental healthcare settings) with which to understand their medical as well as their illness experiences. In a 2001 article, Charon writes: "The human capacity to understand the meaning and significance of stories is being recognized as critical for effective medical practice.... Narrative conceptual frameworks have been advanced . . . for examining and understanding medical reasoning, clinical relationships, empathy, and medical ethics.... The rise of narrative medicine may signify fundamental changes in the experience of disease or of doctoring" (Charon 2001b, 83).

Regarding specific theoretical frameworks, Frank's categorization of restitution, chaos, and quest narratives, for example, is not necessarily superior to other frameworks of qualitative inquiry already in use among a few researchers in community mental health for delving into social and subjective issues behind the lives of people like Dr. Linehan and Mr. Andrews. However, it is a shame that the silo effect in community mental health and primary healthcare practice and research assures that such frameworks and tools are largely missing in these settings.

Ethical Considerations

While there is often some tension between the fields of medical humanities and bioethics, the two disciplines remain linked, and the medical humanities are important approaches to in exploring the inherent moral and ethical consider-ations of patient-doctor relationships. Such is the case in community psychiatry where it is likely that if one asks an assortment of twenty psychiatrists, other clinicians, and case managers to name the first ethical issue that comes to mind for them in the field, the majority would say "boundaries between patients (or clients) and professionals." A psychiatrist or two might also mention involun-tary treatment for people with serious mental illnesses who are unengaged in treatment. A case manager or two might mention poverty as an ethical issue for work with people with mental illnesses, and among researchers, institutional review boards that approve human subject research might also be identified as an issue. Ethical considerations come up regularly in community psychiatry in many contexts—psychiatrists' roles as agents of social control, the national shame of homelessness among people with mental illness, and high rates of incarceration for people with mental illness whose crimes, in many cases, are related to their mental illnesses and who often receive little mental health treatment while incar-cerated, among many others. Yet there is remarkably little discussion of ethics in the field of community psychiatry as compared to its disciplinary presence in medicine writ large. Practitioners and researchers do make moral claims regard-ing the needs and rights of persons with mental illness, but these authors rarely draw on explicit ethical frameworks available to them in non-psychiatric medical research. In particular, *street-level* bioethics (my term) as practiced by sociologist-ethnographers in such areas as intensive care (Zussman 1992), medical errors in surgery (Bosk 1979), and inpatient nursing care (Chambliss 1996), which in my view share both medical humanities and bioethical concerns, can and should inform ethical inquiries in community psychiatry.

Mental and Physical Health

The link between mental health and early mortality, and poor coordination and integration between mental and primary health care, are concerns for public health, for medicine as a whole, and for both of these medical disciplines (Thorni-croft and Tansella 2004). The medical humanities, though, with their implicit and explicit concerns for the whole person, not just the patient, and for the experience of illness, not just specific clinical treatments, have a role to play in current efforts to integrate the two and improve medical care for persons with mental illnesses. Their expertise involves the three areas discussed above—the link between chronic mental illness and chronic medical illness, including a recovery-oriented approach to care; research methods that can contribute to current community mental health research on these topics; and ethical considerations, including the still-pervasive stigma of mental illness that reinforces the separation of people with mental illness from others in terms of medical care as well as within their communities. Increasing attention to this split in care and in health outcomes may be both encouraged by medical humanistic inquiries and their companion inqui-ries in mental health and open up opportunities for increased border crossings between the two.

CONCLUSION

Community psychiatry is a venue for the medical humanities in the fullest sense, whether or not its potential ties to the medical humanities as practiced in non-mental health (primary) care are exploited. It makes sense to pursue these potential ties, though, more systematically. Both community mental health and the medical humanities may benefit from the effort.

Chapter 34

CULPABILITY

IAN WILLIAMS

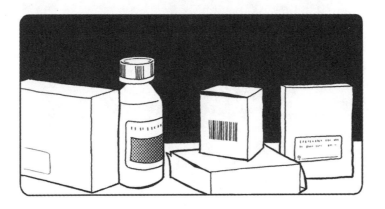

this is a fictional story in which any likeness to real events or similarity to real persons, living or dead, is entirely coincidental.

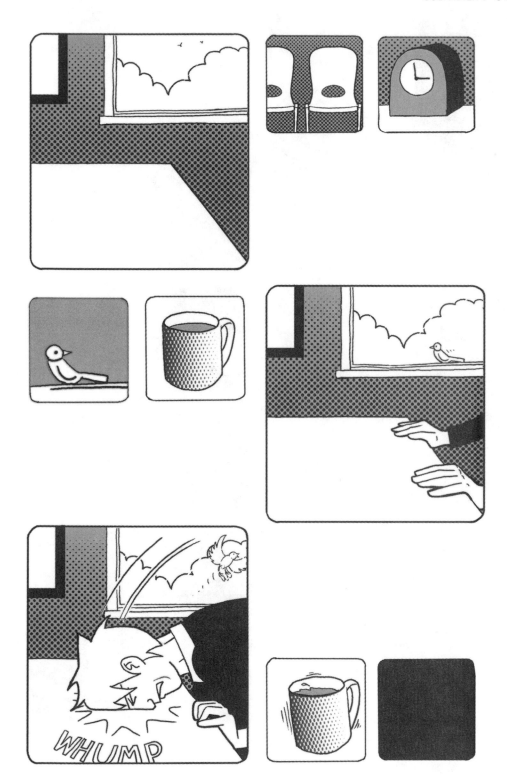

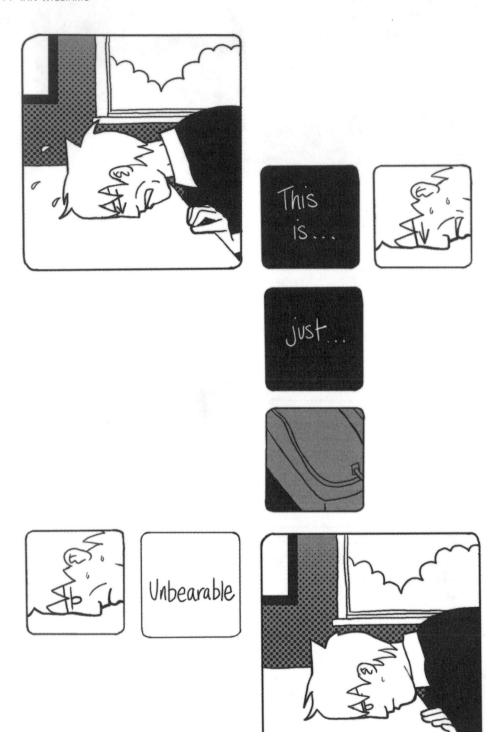

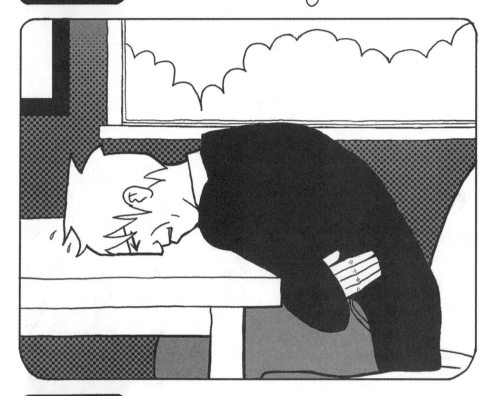

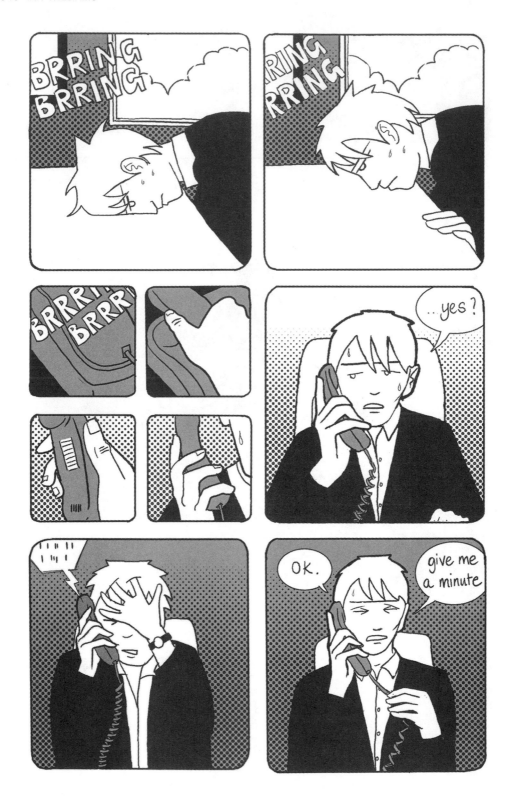

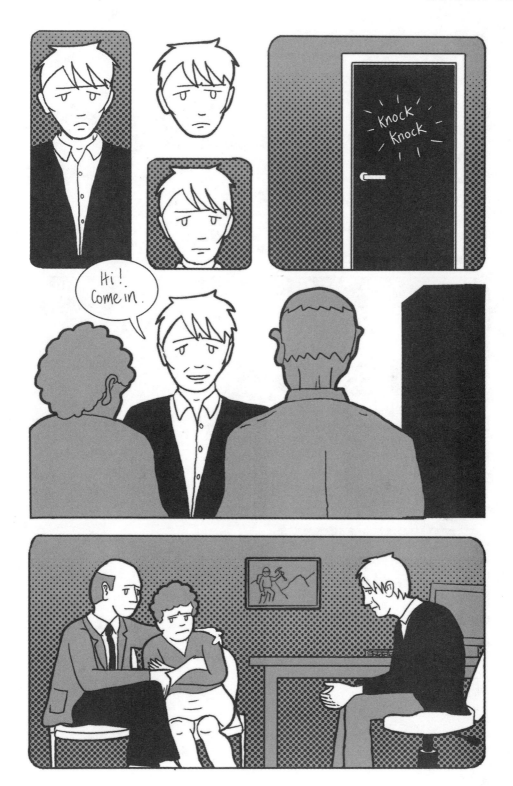

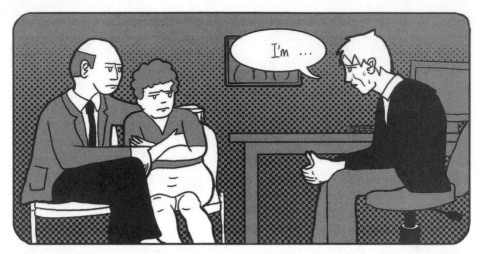

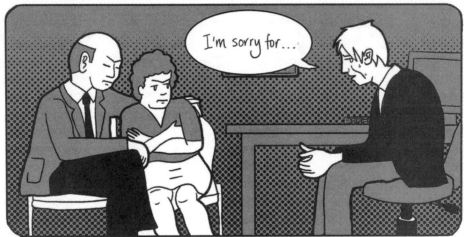

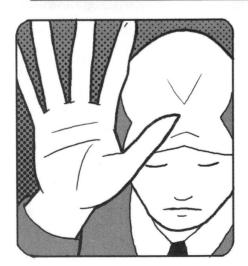

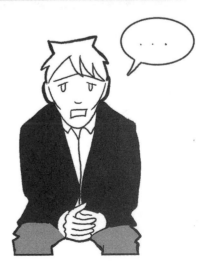

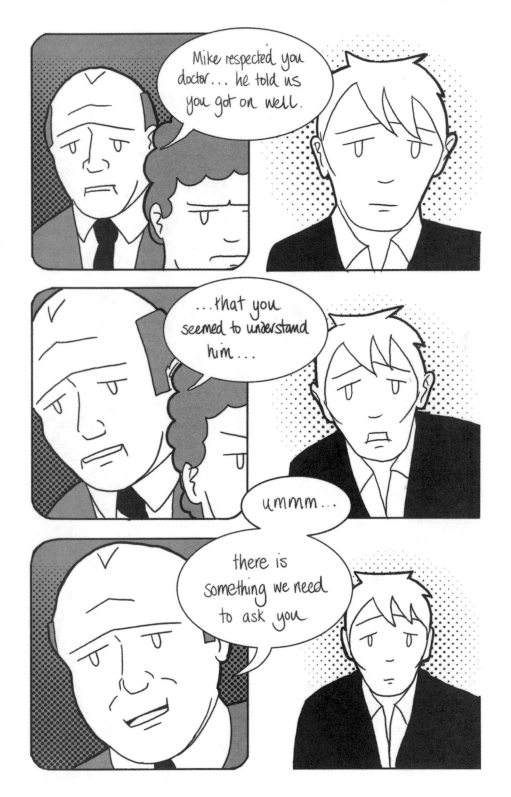

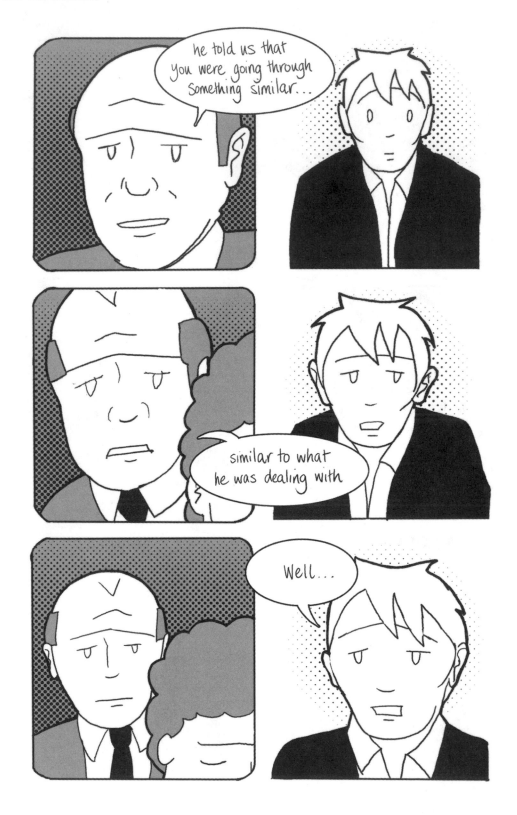

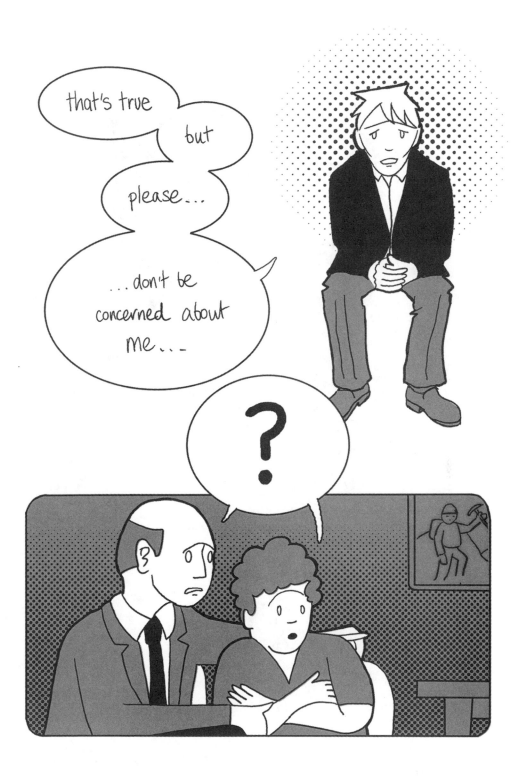

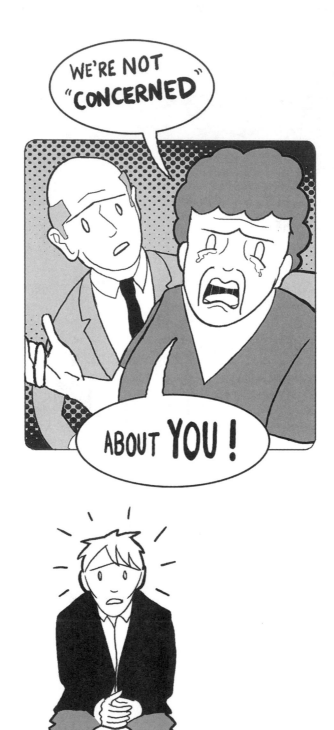

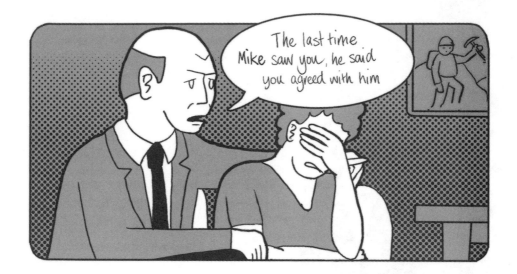

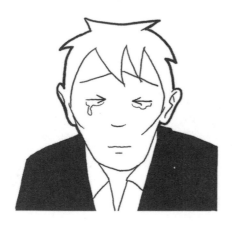

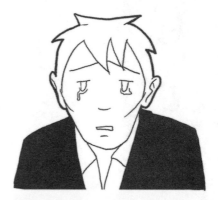

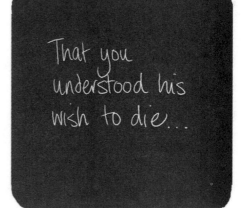

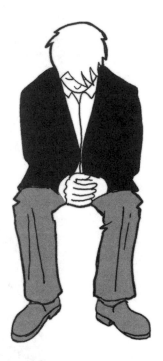

fuck

fuck

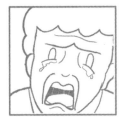

fuck

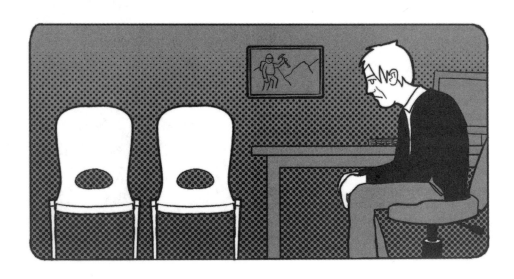

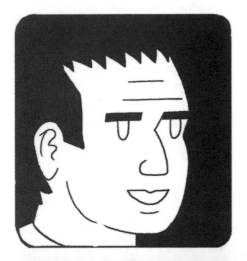

it's true...

Mike and I compared notes on the vicissitudes of life

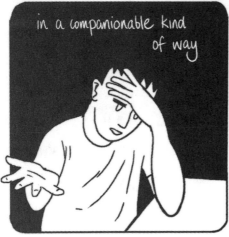

in a companionable kind of way

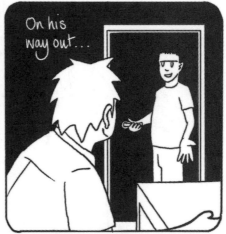

On his way out...

he asked me for sleeping tablets.

I gave him a prescription for twenty eight.

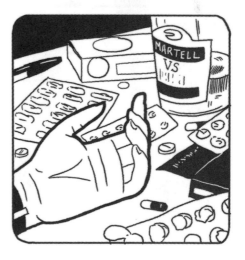

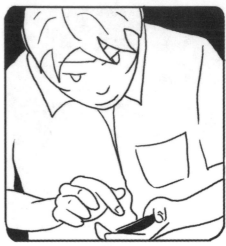

I knew what had happened the moment I heard that he had gone missing.

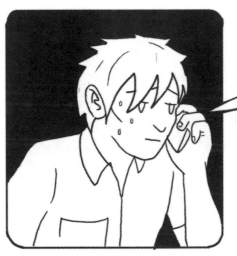

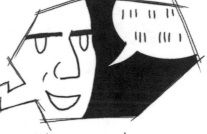

but his voicemail message sounded so **alive**

With fading hope, I left several messages

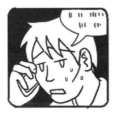
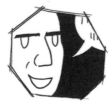
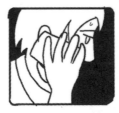
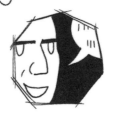

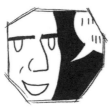
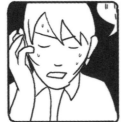
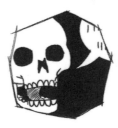
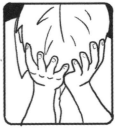

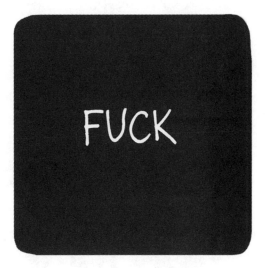

Oh God, I miss you

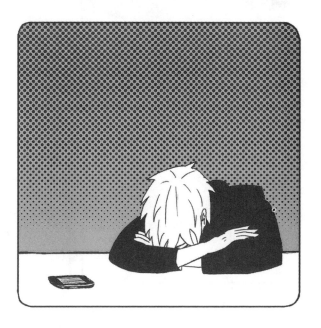

It might be easier
if YOU were dead...

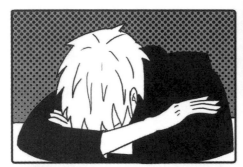

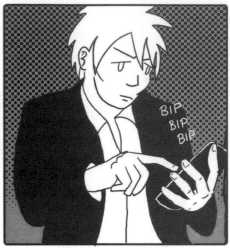

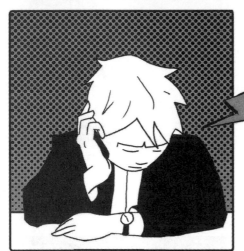

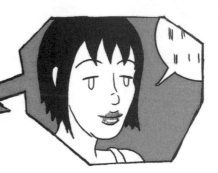

at least then I might not
have to bear the responsibility

for having screwed it all up.

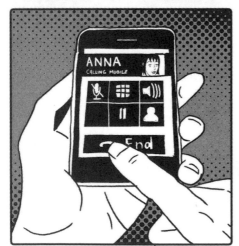

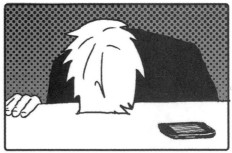

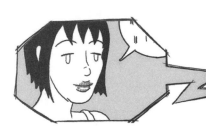

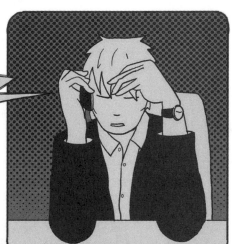

You are creating a
new life without me

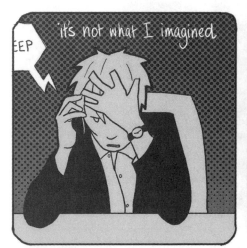

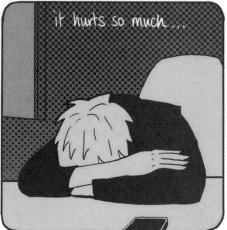

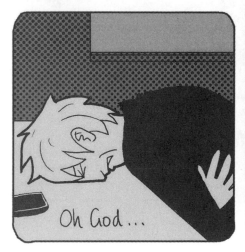

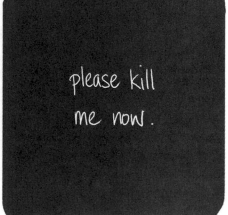

Ian Williams is a physician,
Comics artist and scholar
based in the U.K.
He has previously published
comics under the
nom de plume 'Thom Ferrier'
www.thomferrier.com

For more information about
Comics and Medicine visit
www.graphicmedicine.org

Part X

SPIRITUALITY AND RELIGION

Chapter 35

RITES OF BIOETHICS

TOD CHAMBERS

As a social animal, man is a ritual animal. If ritual is suppressed in one form it crops up in others, more strongly the more intense the social interaction. . . . It is not too much to say that ritual is more to society than words are to thought. For it is very possible to know something and then find words for it. But it is impossible to have social relations without symbolic acts.

MARY DOUGLAS (1996, 62)

ABOUT eighteen years ago, I attended my wife's medical school graduation, which concluded with the recitation of a moral code for physicians. The inclusion of a code—often some version of the Oath of Hippocrates—is a common part of many such ceremonies. As Alan Verhey notes, these ritual communal declarations were traditionally "a performative declaration rather than a descriptive one. It did not just describe reality; it altered it" (1987, 72). Yet at the ceremony I attended, the dean asked everyone to rise and recite the oath. I am not sure why anyone in some way related to a physician would wish to declare a duty to heal the sick (perhaps, the dean simply forgot to specify only physicians), but everyone in the audience did just that.

What occurred then may signify the degree by which this particular ritual action has lost some of its power to alter identity in the way that Verhey claims. I suspect that one reason for the loss of the oath's performative power lies in the rise of other rituals that have supplanted this virtue-based ceremony, for we now expect physicians to engage in a series of rituals that express a new ethic of medicine, one that primarily promotes patient autonomy. These new rituals include informed consent, ethics consultations, involuntary hospitalization hearings, advance directives, genetic counseling, do-not-resuscitate (DNR) discussions, surrogate decision making, competency evaluations, and ethics committee deliberations. Each of these social performances represents a distinct break from the ritual life of paternalism that characterized the traditional ethos of medicine in North America.

FROM TEXTS TO RITUALS

To refer to standard components of medical ethics as ritual performances is to reframe them in a way that is different from how ethicists and medical humanities scholars tend to see them. Outside of an interest in plays that portray medicine, the humanities rarely attend to the ritual and performative dimensions of clinical practice. One reason is that in the Geertzian blurring of genres (see Geertz 1983), the humanities has drawn primarily upon the text analogy to understand the medical world. However, as with all analogies (including the drama analogy), viewing clinical decision making through texts has distinct limitations. The anthropologist Michael Jackson observes that, "by fetishizing texts, [textualism] tends to ignore the flux of human relationships, the ways meaning are created intersubjectively as well as 'intertextually,' embodied in gestures as well as in words, and connected to political, moral, and aesthetic interests" (1989, 184). This bias toward textualism, for example, is evident in how "informed consent" has been traditionally conceived within bioethics and the medical humanities.

Informed consent is a central concept within the new ethic of medicine. Echoing Alfred North Whitehead's famous statement that all of European philosophy is but a series of footnotes to Plato, one ethicist states that all of contemporary medical ethics is but a footnote to informed consent (Kuczewski 1996). Informed consent represents the essential liberal political foundation of contemporary medical ethics with its basis in the promotion of patient autonomy; as Tristram Engelhardt summarizes this worldview, "Moral authority in secular health care policy is derived from permission and even in circumstances of complex collaborative undertakings is at its roots consensual or contractual. Moral controversies in biomedicine are public policy disputes to be resolved peaceably by agreeing to procedures for creating moral rules based on the principle that force cannot be used against the innocent without their consent" (1996, 73). In *The Principles of Biomedical Ethics*, Tom Beauchamp and James Childress define informed consent through a group of "analytical components": competence, disclosure, understanding, voluntariness, and consent (1994). And like most bioethicists, Beauchamp and Childress think of informed consent as a philosophical problem, not a social event. It is not surprising, therefore, that when surveyed, healthcare professionals state that they consider informed consent as the patient's signing of a legal document (Meisel and Kuczewski 1996).

To conceive of informed consent as a *ritual act* means viewing it in terms of a symbolic dramatization of social values; it means to *embody* the liberal moral ideal of contractual agreement, for ritual alters social relations by establishing particular kinds of interactions. Paul Wolpe has referred to informed consent as a "ritual of trust." Similar to Engelhardt, Wolpe notes that with the breakdown of a single shared community in which the notions of the Good are shared, the contemporary world entails that we are often being cared for by those who do not share our communal values—that is, strangers caring for strangers. Wolpe argues that "informed consent involves the physician trusting the patient with what used to be privileged professional information (risks, procedures to be used, the exact nature of the problem) and the patient returning the trust by allowing the physician to invade his or her bodily integrity despite the knowledge of risks. This formalistic ritual becomes increasingly necessary where informal bonds of trust have eroded" (1998, 50). Wolpe's inclusion of the modifier "formalistic" to ritual suggests a negative evaluation, which, akin to Engelhardt, indicates that he would prefer the notion of medicine as practiced in an arena where the "informal bonds of trust" have neither eroded nor corroded.

The devaluation of ritual aspects of informed consent can be found throughout bioethics literature. For example, in an article on informed consent, Charles Lidz, Paul Appelbaum, and Alan Meisel state: "Indeed, both empirical research and clinical observations indicate that informed consent often becomes an empty ritual in which patients are presented with complex information that they cannot understand and that has little impact on their decision making" (1988, 1385). Given this common concern among bioethicists that informed consent can become an "empty ritual," the authors propose two alternative models: "consent as event" and "consent as process." They argue that the superior model takes informed consent as a processual entity rather than a single event, and, in their conclusion, they make a second allusion to informed consent as ritual: "The resulting process is neither an arbitrary legal imposition on clinical care nor a ritual disclosure that the patient cannot understand" (1988, 1388). Terms such as *legal* and *ritual*—as well as *relativism* and *top-down*—are in bioethics what the rhetorician Richard Weaver refers to as *devil terms* or *terms of repulsion* within a particular community. Devil terms are usually paired with *god terms*, which are those expressions "about which all other expressions are ranked as subordinate" (1953, 212) Such a dislike of ritual has a long history in the West. Mary Douglas notes that, in our culture, "Ritual has become a bad word signifying empty conformity" (1996, 1) and that such prejudice has permitted social scientists to miss the importance that common symbols contained within ritual practice have for particular social structures. Thus, the attack on informed consent as ritual has its origin in the Protestant attack on any action that is not derived from an internal desire.

While the American worldview may be infected with an anti-ritual bias, the philosophical observations of the intimate association of ritual with moral behavior can be found in traditional Confucian philosophy. In this tradition, it is asserted that there is a profound need for ritual (*li*) to shape social ethics, regardless of the degree of familiarity between parties. Explicit rules and commands are thought to have only a limited influence on any true alteration in our moral life. Instead, by ritualizing our social interactions, the Confucian philosophers argue, one fashions the kind of actions and attitudes people take toward one another. In his analysis of the understanding of ritual by the Confucian philosopher Xunzi, T. C. Kline explains that "ethical theory may provide us with compelling visions of the good human life, but it is only through ritual participation that we are capable of living those lives and transforming ourselves into good human beings" (2004, 204). Correspondingly, rites of autonomy have the potential to enact and embody a new social ethic in the patient-physician relationship. However, I would argue that, at present, the ritual act of informed consent transforms the patient-physician interaction into a legal relationship rather than a therapeutic one. One study reveals that 80 percent of patients viewed informed consent as something that is done for the protection (and thus benefit) of the healthcare professional (Cassileth et al. 1980). A survey request by the President's Commission for the Study of Ethical Problems in Medicine and Biomedical and Behavioral Research shows that, of physicians polled, only 26 percent thought informed consent was related to the patient's giving consent to medical interventions (Faden and Beauchamp 1986, 99). To reframe informed consent as ritual performance stresses the way such cultural events are fluid, processual encounters between social actors.

RITUAL AS PERFORMANCE

One key feature of performance behavior is its transformation of the social world. Richard Schechner argues that performance is possible because it brings about distinct transformations of the self as the play frame puts social actors in a subjunctive mood (1985). During performance, I am no longer myself, but I also am not not myself either: "It isn't that a performer stops being himself or herself when he or she becomes another—multiple selves coexist in an unresolved dialectical tension" (1985, 6). Schechner gives the example of Laurence Olivier acting the role of Hamlet. While on stage, Olivier is not himself, but he is also not Hamlet; he enters a liminal mode of between the two identities. In *ritual* performances, there is an inevitable degree of idealization in such subjunctive transformations. Moreover, Clifford Geertz points out that in ritual performances "the world as lived and the world as imagined, fused under the agency of a single set of symbolic forms, turn out to be the same world, producing thus that idiosyncratic transformation in one's sense of reality" (1973a, 112).

During my own research on Thai Buddhist rituals, I watched as men during their initiation into the monkhood played the role of the Prince Siddhartha abandoning the world. The majority of Thai men who become monks are not expecting to (or expected to) remain monks for their entire lives. Instead, the *temporary* ordination permits these men to transfer the good merit accumulated in giving up their earthly possessions to their parents: an exchange of monetary capital for spiritual capital. Traditionally, men were not considered mature until they had undergone a period of time as a monk, and the ritual performance itself is an idealized enactment of core Buddhist beliefs. As the Prince, the men are casting away all their wealth for the quest for enlightenment with the knowledge that they would, in three months' time, return to the world with greater social status.

If we view informed consent as a ritual performance, we begin to judge its success in terms of its effectiveness in transforming the patient-physician relationship. It is only through cultural performances, like rituals, that the new ethic of medicine can be brought about, for as Edward Bruner observes, "[a] ritual must be enacted, a myth recited, a narrative told, a novel read, a drama performed, for these enactments recitals, tellings, readings, and performances are what make the text transformative and enable us to reexperience our culture's heritage" (1986, 7). Many healthcare professionals have been highly critical of informed consent, and they contend that it represents an impractical chore for three reasons. First, few people outside of medicine can understand the procedures being recommended. Second, it is impossible to describe all of the risks of any procedure. Third, people in the midst of a serious illness do not have the emotional autonomy to make an informed decision about their own care. However, in his analysis of ritual behavior, Jonathan Z. Smith emphasizes the importance of the incongruity between the ideal and the real in ritual's effectiveness in our social life, arguing that "ritual is a means of performing the way things ought to be in conscious tension to the way things are in such a way that this ritualized perfection is recollected in the ordinary, uncontrolled course of things" (1986, 480). Thus, the ritual of informed consent is of vital importance to our healthcare practices primarily in its ability to construct a performed ideal in conscious tension with the impossibility of making a truly autonomous decision. During informed consent, the physician and the patient enter into the subjunctive mood and act as if patient and physician were of equal power. In an article on legal rituals, Peter Winn examines the imposition of the Miranda warning on police procedures, which in many ways provides an instructive parallel to the imposition of informed consent on medical practices. Winn points out that there is little or no indication that the introduction of Miranda warnings in actual practice has changed the number of confessions made by suspects. He contends, however, that we should see the warnings as constituting an important new legal ritual, for prior to Miranda there were no rituals that indicated a person had been transformed into someone under arrest; the stating of the warning created a distinct legal rite of passage. The warnings, Winn argues, have been "highly successful in disrupting prior patterns of behavior and attitudes between the police and the public" and symbolically tie the actions of local police to the U.S. Constitution (1996, 561). While informed consent, in whatever form it is practiced, may not change the number of patients who ultimately agree to particular medical procedures, it can disrupt the prior pattern of behavior and attitudes between physicians and patients. In the end, informed consent can transform the patient-physician relationship so that, in Geertz's words, "the world as lived and the world as imagined . . . turn out to be the same world" (1973b, 112).

RITUAL CRITICISM

Attention to the performative dimensions of such practices as informed consent encourage medical humanities scholars to engage in what Ronald Grimes refers to as *ritual criticism*, which he defines as "the interpretation of a rite or ritual system with a view to implicating its practice" (1990, 16). Such a criticism aims toward the evaluation and improvement of practice and thus has a particular moral feature to it. That is, it does not merely describe but also prescribes. Critical to such a step is recognizing the power of ritual to constitute distinctive social relations and to judge whether such relations are morally just, for ritual can just as easily be a force for ideological conservatism and oppression as it can be for the generation of morally just associations. One of the steps that Grimes recognizes as important to the development of such a style of criticism is the recognition of "the possibility of ritual failure." By drawing upon J. L. Austin's description of the ways speech acts can be "infelicitous," Grimes creates a typology of ritual failure. It is interesting to note that Austin, himself, saw a direct connection between ethics and ritual action: he notes that "a great many of the acts which fall within the province of Ethics are *not*, as philosophers are too prone to assume, simply in the last resort *physical movements*: very many of them have the general character, in whole or part, of conventional or ritual acts, and are therefore among other things, exposed to infelicity" (1990, 19; emphasis as in original). As an example of the way ritual criticism can assist in the discussion of the performance of the rituals of bioethics, I briefly examine some of the ways that informed consent can fail as a ritual (although in many ways it could be said to have, at the same time, fulfilled the standards created by bioethicists). If we accept that the goal of informed consent is to transform the patient-physician relationship in the same manner that the Miranda warning alters the relationship of police to the public, then the kind of failure that can occur in this ritual concerns the way it leads away from this transformation and instead simply reinforces paternalism or legalism.

There are three obvious ways in which informed consent as a ritual practice can fail: omission, misapplication, and opacity. Omission is the easiest failure to understand as it involves the failure to perform the ritual. Not to perform the ritual of informed consent is not merely in its legal constitution "touching someone without his or her permission"; it also represents a refusal to accept the new morality of the patient's right to self-determination. Perhaps one of the most common ways in which informed consent fails is in a form that is sometimes referred to by medical house staff as "consenting the patient." This odd verbal construct entails merely getting a patient to sign the consent form prior to the performance of a medical procedure. The fact that "consenting" can be done by almost anyone on the medical team (including often inexperienced third-year medical students) indicates that this is a clear example of a form of ritual failure. Grimes refers to "misapplication" as a form of ritual failure that would involve inappropriate persons or circumstances in the performance of a ritual act.

Another form of ritual failure is the opacity in which the ritual does not function because the rite "is experienced as meaningless; the act is unrecognizable or uninterpretable" (Grimes 1990, 202). Informed consent as a rite cannot take place if the medical information is not presented in a way that is understandable to the patient, and thus the rites's capacity to equalize the power relation between physician and patient becomes corrupted by the opacity.

The most serious forms of ritual failure in informed consent concern *breaches* and *insincerities*. In his study of intensive care units, Robert Zussman discusses a patient who was admitted to a unit where the intern "documented his refusal thoroughly in the chart, providing an almost textbook application of the principles of informed consent." Zussman states that the next day, the attending physicians on the unit "overruled" the agreement between the intern and the patient that he should not be intubated because of "both the possibility of an AIDS-related mental impairment and a higher responsibility." Zussman records one of the attendings stating: "In effect, lie to him. . . . We have to save his life." The patient was soon intubated (1992, 84). This is an example of a *breach*: ritual failures that "are abrogations of ceremonially made promises" (Grimes 1990, 200). If there is anything that causes critical injury to the rites of autonomy, it is this form of failure. When healthcare professionals create breaches in the rituals of informed consent, advance directives, and DNRs, they in turn sever the moral power of these cultural performances and transform them into farces.

Another form of ritual failures particularly serious for rites of autonomy are *insincerities*, in which one says and does things "without the requisite feelings, thoughts, or intentions" (Grimes 1990, 200). When acts of informed consent are carried out by healthcare professionals as if they were legal requirements, insincerity fails to allow the ritual to transform the patient's relationship to professionals. The Patient Self-Determination Act requires all healthcare institutions that receive federal funding to give patients the opportunity to discuss advance directions when they are admitted to that institution. Most institutions have simply made such a directive another form for patients to sign during their admission, which is a form of ritual insincerity.

Schechner observes that scholars of drama rarely attend to those aspects of a performance that occur outside of the show itself. He recommends that we consider such features as training, workshops, and rehearsals as integral to performance. Many rituals include just such preparatory events. The men preparing for Buddhist ordination often prepare and rehearse aspects of the ritual prior to the day of ordination. If we think of informed consent and other cultural practices surrounding the new ethic of autonomy as ritual performances, perhaps we should also begin to ask what the best way is to prepare healthcare professionals for their roles in these social dramas. When asked about preparing students to give informed consent, bioethicists tend to provide them only with what information needs to be conveyed, and these bare scripts provide little assistance in being able to carry out these complex cultural performances. Schechner sees two tasks involved in all rehearsals. First, rehearsals tend to select out and simplify the basic components of a performance. Second, they work toward having "each performer perform her/ his part with maximum clarity" (1985, 183). Unlike a lecture on informed consent, a workshop emphasizes the full performative aspects of the process, including attention to the space, the social rhythm of the action, and the construction of a social role. I would also like to note the importance of improvisation during ritual. While we may think of ritual as simply the repetition of social codes, cultural life is fluid and processual. Just as each ordination ritual is slightly different owing to the engagement of the present actors with scripted roles, healthcare professionals also need to learn to improvise in relation to the present context (see Watson 2011). One of the strengths of the drama analogy for understanding social interaction, including medicine, is that it underscores the seriousness of play.

POSTSCRIPT: THE RETURN OF RITUALS OF VIRTUE

I began this chapter by observing the relative ritual weakness of the oath-taking component of a commencement ceremony I attended. It is important to note, however, that a new rite of virtue has arisen in medical schools, the white coat ceremony. It represents, I believe, an attempt by the medical profession to counter the perceived amoral contractual nature of the rites of autonomy with an appeal to traditional professionalism, and ritual criticism has something important to say about this new ritual of medical education. Promoted by the Arnold P. Gold Foundation, the white coat ceremony was created in order to "establish a psychological contract for the practice of medicine" (Arnold P. Gold Foundation 2010). The ceremony, as planned by the foundation, includes a "recitation or discussion of an oath (such as the Hippocratic Oath or a student-written oath)." A number of critiques have been made of this ceremony, the most cited by Delese Wear (1998), in which she explicitly discusses it as a ritual and addresses the symbolism of the white coat itself.

The anthropologist Victor Turner has noted that one of the properties of a ritual symbol is its *multi-vocality*, that is, its capacity to express a number of cultural meanings ([1967] 1981, 50). While Wear acknowledges that the white coat does express positive values such as altruism, she contends that it also expresses a number of negative values, including the distinct power differential between physician and patient. Howard Brody's (1993) work, *The Healer's Power*, argues that one of the unacknowledged dimensions in medical ethics is the various ways in which physicians are given power over patients: culturally, economically, socially, educationally. For Wear, the subtext of the white coat ceremony includes these various messages about the power that physicians have over their patients, leading her to conclude:

To link a white coat to a mythologic, Welbyized image of a physician who is always decisive, who is "immune" to variations in economic and social status, race, ethnicity, national origins, and sexual desire; to differences in body type, size, appearance, and hygiene; and to variations in family structure, religion, occupation, political beliefs, and moral life, sets students up not just for failure but also for guilt, cynicism, and denial when the ideal fails to materialize. (Wear 1998, 736)

However, it is clear that Wear is not against the presence of ritual elements or symbols in medical education; rather, she is against the reinforcing of physician privilege that she sees expressed in the white coat ceremony. She suggests alternative rituals for medical students, such as routinized monthly visits to domestic violence shelters or hospice units, which she believes will foster compassion and social awareness of the needs of patients.

Robert Veatch also disparages the white coat ceremony, criticizing it on two counts. First, he argues that incoming medical students are not, in a manner, given "informed consent" prior to the ceremony. He believes that most students are not informed about the oath that they are about to take, and for those students who might be informed, they are nevertheless coerced by the ceremony to consent to a particular moral code with which they probably would disagree. While Veatch's attack is in many ways a natural extension of his general critique of professional codes (see Veatch 1981), it seems a relatively weak argument, for one could fully inform students prior to the ceremony as well as give them a professional code that is an expression of the ethics a medical student should follow at a particular institution. Moreover, if students disagree with such a code, they could seek to attend another medical school, one that would sanction, for example, breaching confidentiality, misrepresenting one's educational status to patients, and cheating on exams. Veatch's second critique, I think, is more interesting, for he argues that the ritual itself represents a symbolic "calling apart," in which students are asked to separate from the lay community and to bond with others of a "priestly" caste. He recognizes the dramaturgy of the white coat ceremony as a divorcement from one's prior identification with laypeople.

S. J. Huber has responded to critiques like that of Veatch and Wear, arguing that Veatch conflates bonding and separation and conceives of it as an either/or dichotomy. Huber points out that bonding with a profession does not necessarily mean isolating oneself from other communities. In response to Wear, he contends that the multiplicity of meanings is the reason that rituals like the white coat ceremony can be particularly effective. While Huber acknowledges that the white coat has traditionally expressed both virtue and the abuse of power, it is this very multi-vocality that the "ritual can seek to sort out" (2003, 365). In many ways, his response reflects Winn's contention: "Because ritual is formalized social action, not expression, different meanings can be attributed to a single ritual action. There can often be more than one—sometimes mutually inconsistent—interpretations of the ritual's meanings. This ambiguity can be understood as essential to the working of ritual; it is not a weakness but a strength of ritual, in that it permits group solidarity and action in the absence of actual consensus or agreement" (Winn 1996, 555). Ultimately, Huber praises the white coat ceremony as an important and "well-crafted" initiation ritual but stresses that it merely marks the beginning of professionalism, rather than the completion of it.

While I find Wear's critique valid in relation to the medical profession's past and present status within society, I would argue that the alternative rituals that she suggests lack an essential element of ritual—the very features of drama—that would make them an adequate substitute for the white coat ceremony or a powerful addition to the entrance rituals of medical students. It is not that I believe that the white coat ceremony has more potential to foster social consciousness than monthly visits to facilities that care for the least fortunate, but a visit is not a ritual. Wear uses "ceremony" and "ritual" interchangeably; Turner points out that ceremonies are cultural institutionalized performances of "normatively structured social reality, and [are] also both a model *of* and a model *for* social states and statuses," while rituals are transformations, taking a prior social status and transforming it into a new status (1982, 83). Wear's analysis suffers because of the mistake of conflating ritual and ceremony. Ritual follows dramatic plot, and in the white coat ceremony (which I hope it is clear that I do not see as a ceremony), it is intended to transform the layperson into a medical professional. Ceremonies present the world as it is; rituals transform the world as we wish it to be. Wear's alternatives are, I believe, ceremonial representations of the status of others and not a ritual transformation of a medical student's status. In many ways, her critique of such entities as the white coat event questions the need for this transformation at all; that is, it challenges the moral status of the notion of professional identity.

But, while Wear questions the very presence of the white coat ceremony in medical school, Huber as noted above sees it as an important rite of passage for students, a ritual transformation, and one that is "well crafted." I contend, however, that the white coat ceremony is missing some of the essential elements of a successful ritual transformation because it is so unskillfully crafted. While Wear pays inadequate attention to the dramatic structure of rituals, Huber does not attend to those symbolic elements of ritual structure that create the drama of transformation. The directions, cited below, from the Gold Foundation for the white coat ceremony are themselves odd in their singular focus on administrative details rather than the actual ritual itself:

1 White Coat Ceremonies where students are given clear instructions prior to the event are enjoyed most:
    Organize the students in alphabetical line for processional.
    Row should stand as a group when instructed by row organizer.
    Encourage participants to shake hands and move quickly.
2 Before introducing the students, announce to the audience to hold their applause until the last student is announced and to stay seated at the end of the ceremony until the students finish the recessional. (Some schools use the time between calling students' names to mention each student's undergraduate school and major.)
3 The oath should take place as soon as all students are cloaked. Following cloaking and oath, formally end the program. Prior to ceremony, Dean should instruct and perhaps practice with students, that after reciting the oath and on cue: "And now I present to you the Class of 2003," all students will turn together in the same direction and face the audience.
4 Arrange for class photo if desired. (Arnold P. Gold Foundation 2010)

I confess to being a bit perplexed as to why Huber believes that this is well crafted, for many of the features that make rites particularly meaningful are simply not present in the foundation's minimalist directions. In his classic study of rites of passage, Arnold van Gennep observes a common structure to the transformation: rites of separation, transition rites, and rites of incorporation (1960). This structure exists primarily to develop a process by which the prior identity of the initiand is deconstructed and a new identity is created. In the rite of separation, an individual is "separated" from the normal social structure. While it can be a physical separation, the key symbolic feature of this stage in the ritual process is that the individual is detached from his or her prior social identity. There is little sense of separation in the white coat ceremony. Furthermore, it is following the action of separation that some of the most powerful features of rite of passage arise, that is, during the liminal stage. At this point, the neophyte exists between categories, or one might say, it is a structured period of no structure. Turner explains that the symbols during this stage "give an outward and visible form to an inward and conceptual process. The structural 'invisibility' of liminal *personae* has a twofold character. They are at once no longer classified and not yet classified. In so far as they are no longer classified, the symbols that represent them are, in many societies drawn from the biology of death, decomposition, catabolism, and other physical processes that have a negative tinge" ([1967] 1981, 96).

As it is, the white coat ceremony lacks any such liminal features. Interestingly, the *short* white coat that most American medical students are assigned to wear during their training itself acts as a liminal symbol. While the white coat represents medicine, its attenuated length signifies that the wearer is, in some manner, not really a physician. Such lack of attention to the dramatic structure and symbolic features of the white coat ceremony makes it far less effective and, in doing so, stunts the power of the rite. Lacking any liminal stage in turn makes the putting on of the coat a somewhat trite activity. As Grimes notes: "To enact any kind of rite is to *per*form, but to enact a rite of passage is also to *trans*form" (2000, 7). Yet I must confess to seeing the white coat ceremony as more a ritual of nostalgia, a desire to recapture an image of the physician as healer, than one that truly expresses the contemporary image of the physician. It exists in structural opposition to the rites of autonomy developed over the past fifty years. The physician's identity has been so radically transformed and translated in the contemporary practice that it is the virtue of the technician that is as much valued today as that of the healer (cf. May 2000), and it is the rituals surrounding this image of the physician as technician that have dominated the contemporary practice of medicine.

This chapter has been primarily concerned with how understanding these rituals of autonomy are the essential expression of contemporary Western bioethics. While the bioethics community has been quite good at creating the theory for these practices, they have been largely inattentive to the manner in which these theories need to be performed through ritual. As the epigraph from Douglas that began this chapter notes, one cannot have social relations save through ritual acts—that is, symbolically loaded, multi-vocal, scripted physical exchanges. I have argued that ritual criticism furnishes bioethics with a vocabulary by which it can begin to construct dramaturgically rich scripts for the practice of the new ethic of medicine. Ritual criticism—as its older sibling literary criticism—carries with it both descriptive and normative features: it entails both understanding its basic grammar and judging particular rituals as successful or failed. I have attempted here to provide a typology of failures in the ritual practice of informed consent as well as a criticism of the white coat ceremony, and each criticism is done "with a view to implicating its practice." Bioethicists need to view ritual as the embodiment of their particular vision of moral medicine and, I believe, spend as much time on scripting this embodiment as they have providing a philosophical grounding for their particular vision. What Alasdair MacIntyre once said about depriving children of stories can be equally applied to not explicitly providing rituals to those training in medicine: deprive them of ritual and "you leave them unscripted, anxious stutterers in their actions as in their words" (1984, 216).

Chapter 36

HEALTH AND HUMANITIES
Spirituality and Religion

RAYMOND C. BARFIELD AND LUCY SELMAN

S PIRITUALITY, conceived as a multidimensional aspect of all human beings, consists of experiences, beliefs, and values that provide a compass in difficult decision making and constitute our grasp of what kind of universe we are in. Often, but not necessarily, spirituality is embedded in a particular set of religious practices and teachings through which human beings relate to something greater than themselves and, thus, transcend everyday reality. Spiritual perspectives in turn affect some of the most important parts of our lives: how we view our relationships and obligations to others, how we choose our life work, and how we relate to our own body in health, illness, and death.

Medicine provides a unique challenge to the way we live our spirituality, and the challenge arises, in part, because of the astonishing success modern medicine has had in understanding and affecting human disease. As technology has advanced, medicine has increasingly become sequestered within the walls of complex institutions where the primary language is that of biology and technology (Foucault 1973) and where the distribution of power is unique and heavily weighted toward the physician (Starr 1983). At precisely the moments when we are most acutely in crisis—facing loss of function, opportunity, or life because of disease or injury—we are thus removed from the context in which we navigate the remainder of our lives. We find ourselves outside the familiar, "homelike" state of health and in the foreign, "unhomelike" world of illness (Svenaeus 2010).

For the many people who find a fundamental source of orientation in spiritual beliefs and values, the institution of medicine can seem strangely deaf to such considerations. Observing medical practice reveals what seems a striking failure of imagination on the part of those within the institution of medicine, not because of some malignant intent, but rather because of a distortion in medical education that arises in a society that fears death. For we, who will one day become sick, suffer, and die, are complicit in an illusion regarding what medicine is or ought to be and how it relates to the rest of our lives. This illusion, coupled with our astounding ability to deny death, is a formula for profound damage.

In this chapter, we seek to address the distortion in our current medical model by reimagining medicine through a more human lens. Drawing on the humanities, we argue, enables the link between medicine and human nature to be reasserted in all its complexity. We demonstrate the way in which the humanities can play this role by exploring at the end of the chapter the profound lessons that are expressed in Kazuo Ishiguro's 2005 novel *Never Let Me Go*.

THE BIOMEDICAL TRADITION: TECHNOLOGY AND THE FEAR OF DEATH

Gerald McKenny argues that, with rise of modern technology, a "moral imperative" developed that is uniquely actualized in medicine: "The imperative is to eliminate suffering and to expand the realm of human choice—in short, to relieve the human condition of subjection to the whims of fortune or the bonds of natural necessity" (1997, 2). This technological attempt is what McKenny calls the *Baconian project*, as Francis Bacon famously urged that manipulation of nature for human ends was not only permissible but was, in fact, morally imperative. Four hundred years after Bacon's birth, the Byzantine complexity of modern hospitals and academic medical centers testifies to our contemporary devotion to the project of staving off death. There is much for which we can be grateful in this endeavor, and yet there is an increasing worry that, in the process of building edifices devoted to preventing death and eliminating suffering, we have transferred the suffering and the dying to an environment in which the meaning of illness is neglected and the sufferer as a person ignored.

It is increasingly recognized that patients and clinicians are subject to an unrelenting pressure to render the body, with all its uncertainties and vulnerabilities, to technological control (Gawande 2010). The wild popularity of technological control as a goal of health care may be due to the "hope" it seems to offer that vulnerability and death can be delayed or eliminated. In modern medical practice and science, technical intervention on physiological processes and the discovery of standard means to achieve this pre-specified end is pursued unwaveringly and with little regard for subjective patient outcomes, such as quality of life or spiritual well-being. Suffering humanity all too often embraces the Baconian approach to technological "advance" out of fear of loss and death; witness, for example, the shallow and harmful distortions in contemporary debates regarding so-called death panels during U.S. efforts to reform an unsustainable medical system (Rutenberg and Chalmes 2009). In the United States, an enormous proportion of Medicare expenditure pays for intensive care interventions in the last month of life in the context of biological processes that cannot be reversed (Wennberg et al. 2008). This causes a great deal of suffering, threatens financial crisis, and often interrupts the work that is rightly done at the end of life, such as reconciliation, expressions of gratitude, and mindful preparation for death (Byock 1997). Nor does such work belong only at the end of life: any illness that reminds us of our vulnerability and frailty can serve to motivate us to reimagine our lives, our priorities, and our relationships.

When medicine is reduced to the science and technology it uses, it is inevitably distorted. The so-called medical gaze risks dehumanization, separating the patient's body from his or her identity and losing sight of the patient as person (Foucault 1973). Medicine is a repository of potent technologies with profound potential not only to help but also to harm (Illich 1975), even when, by the criteria of biomedicine, a person has been "helped." This occurs from the operating room to the intensive care unit and the medical research units in which frightened patients sign on to phase I trials without understanding the nature of the trial, driven by fear of dying. If how we treat the weak and the vulnerable, including the dying, is the basis on which our society is judged, these are crucial concerns (John Paul II 2000; also attributed to Gandhi).

THE NEGLECT OF SPIRITUAL NEEDS

The negative impact of the technological focus of modern medicine is compounded by the marginalization of spiritual aspects of the experience of suffering and dying. Within clinical care, spiritual care is always subservient to the structure of modern biomedicine and hence often neglected (Kristeller et al. 1999; Kuuppelomaki 2001; Ross 2006). Such neglect occurs despite evidence that patients with serious illness wish to discuss spiritual beliefs with their physicians (Astrow et al. 2007; Ehman et al. 1999; MacLean et al. 2003) and need spiritual support (Astrow et al. 2007; Moadel et al. 1999; Wilson et al. 2007). A national survey representing 33 percent of all hospitals in the United States found that patient satisfaction with the emotional and spiritual aspects of care had one of the lowest ratings among all clinical care indicators and was one of the highest areas in need of quality improvement (Clark et al. 2003). Similar results have been reported in Canada (Heyland et al. 2010).

One of the reasons healthcare providers give for their neglect of patients' spiritual needs is a lack of confidence and competence in the provision of spiritual care (Belcham 2004; Ellis et al. 1999; Kristeller et al. 1999) and a lack of support from the organizations and structures in which they work (Carr 2010; McSherry and Jamieson 2011). In a survey of family physicians in the United States, Ellis et al. found the top five barriers to spiritual discussions to be related to staff members' personal comfort: lack of training; uncertainty about identifying responsive patients; concerns about proselytizing; and uncertainty about managing spiritual issues (1999). Findings from other U.S. studies support the idea that subtle issues such as clinicians' discomfort are more significant impediments to spiritual care in a clinical context than other factors such as time constraints (Chibnall and Brooks 2001; Koenig et al. 1989). The discomfort felt by clinicians intimately involved in people's journeys through ill health and facing death translates into patients' perceptions that physicians are too busy to attend to their spiritual concerns or are simply not interested in doing so (Hebert et al. 2001). This state of affairs points to the need for an urgent rethinking of medicine, education, and social attitudes to the practice of medicine.

REIMAGINING MEDICINE

No one experiences illness, suffering, or impending death in terms of biology. As important as biological disciplines are and as grateful as we are for meaningful advances in the effort to relieve suffering and prolong life, these advances are important only in relation to some concept of human flourishing, well-being, or "positive health" (Bowling 2005; Wilkin et al. 1992). If health is to be considered something more than the absence of disease and its negative consequences (World Health Organization 2010, 100), an understanding of health in its fullest sense is required. Such a definition is generally based on maximizing quality of life through developing human potential (Boorse 1997). The concept of human potential, of what it means to flourish and be truly "well," is related to philosophical and spiritual questions regarding why we are here and what our goals, or ends, might be. Answering these questions, we draw not only on physical notions of full functioning but also on spiritual values and beliefs, the perspectives provided by the major religions of the world (Myers 2008; Taylor and Dell'Oro 2006), and the insights into the human condition provided by the humanities.

Recognition that there is something fundamental missing from the biomedical view of the medical endeavor, which largely ignores the issue of defining human flourishing, has led to the principle of patient-centeredness in modern medical policy (U.S. Department of Health and Human Services 2010). As a principle of health care, patient-centeredness is derived from an individual, rather than population-based, perspective on illness, recognizing the importance of "understanding the patient as a unique human being" (Balint 1969, 269). Definitions of patient-centeredness thus incorporate the idea of entering into the perspective or "world" of the patient, "to see the illness through the patient's eyes" (McWhinney 1989, 34). These understandings of patient-centeredness underpin the definition of patient-centered care as care that is sensitive and responsive to the way patients and their caregivers view the treatment and care that they receive (NHS Executive 1998).

Patient-centeredness advocates treating the patient as a whole person and ensuring care is directed by the preferences and priorities of that person (Brown et al. 1986; Levenstein et al. 1986). Yet how we conceive of the person at the heart of patient-centered care is open to debate. Holistic models differ with respect to which "units" or domains of personhood are included with the physical domain (Engel 1977; Sulmasy 2002), as well as the explicit or implicit importance accorded to those domains (Field 2000). The psychological domain is always recognized along with the physical, but the place of the social and spiritual domains and how they are delineated are more contentious and fluid. The principle of patient-centeredness also says nothing to the prevailing negative social attitudes toward death and dying, which seem to favor technological bombardment over considerations of quality of life.

Being caught up in what technology makes possible rather than following a deeper understanding of what it means to flourish is fundamentally a product of losing regard for the stories we tell about our history and our hopes for the future, our present toils and joys, and the ways we see the world and value and respond to its mysteries. Orientation toward technique is fine when the development of technology is called for, but patients and clinicians are often left longing for something more, even in the midst of fear. However, with the truncated language of modern medicine, we do not have available categories to name this "something more"; the rhetoric of patient-centered care is insufficient in this regard.

The humanities represent a vast resource for the development of a more humane medical model by offering stories of the human condition and conveying areas of experience that exceed the limits of scientific and physiological vocabulary. The limitations of language, although inescapable, are tested and shifted in artistic, philosophical, and theological responses to health and illness, which provide a richer and potentially more fruitful imaginative landscape than one that arises out of medical science alone. Medicine, in meeting and "treating" the person, not simply the physical body, is already a practice fundamentally concerned with the spiritual dimensions of the lives of those it serves. When this is not acknowledged, the recipients and providers of care perceive a "lack," which is associated with dissatisfaction with care and impaired quality of life (Astrow et al. 2007).

Drawing on the humanities thus provides us with the imaginative resources to describe the person at the heart of patient-centered care in all his or her mystery, to flesh out the concept of flourishing that is fundamental to an understanding of health, and to begin to challenge the hegemony of the social denial of death (Becker 1973). If, in medicine, the use of scientific discoveries applied to human ends is linked to a debate about ideas of human flourishing and identity in which the humanities have a voice, advances may be possible not only in the planning of medical education but also in the perceptions of those of us who will need medical intervention at some point and who will most certainly die. To advocate that medicine be practiced in right relationship to the human experience so profoundly expressed in the range of the humanities is to challenge and reconfigure Karl Popper's conception of scientific, objective knowledge as "knowledge without a knower . . . knowledge without a knowing subject" (1985, 60). Indeed, the most important aspects of much of clinical practice depend upon the intuitive and subtle "human knowing" that is in the room.

Pursuing an approach to medicine that is prudent and incorporates a comprehensive understanding of our condition thus involves an attempt to reimagine medicine in the context of a productive relationship with the humanities. "Health and the humanities" can serve, not as a minor complementary effort, but as a defining approach to how we understand and express the variety of spiritual questions arising in our response to illness, vulnerability, and dying as patients and care providers. Insofar as medicine embraces the advances offered by science and the attempts to apply them to individuals who are in a "context," one often built from and expressed through stories, medicine is best conceived as a human activity in which the content and methods of both science and the humanities are deeply related. The former provides a set of tools; the latter a vision of human complexity that can help guide the wise application of those tools.

IMPLICATIONS

The proposed model of medicine drawing on the humanities has implications for clinical practice and medical enquiry. First, narrative becomes central to the medical endeavor, a discipline that begins and ends with interpretation of human experience. While medicine may well talk about biological generalities and epidemiological trends, when it comes down to day-to-day practice, it is a deeply personal discipline requiring considerably more than charts and measures. It requires knowledge of persons, attained by the listening to and telling of stories. As we tell our own stories and listen to the stories of others, we discover who we are and what it means to live lives of meaningful encounter in sickness and in health. This was recognized by Cicely Saunders, founder of the modern hospice movement, who was much influenced by "the individual stories of carefully observed people. Here we are not meeting 'the dying,' but people" (Doyle et al. 2004, vi).

Anthropologists and sociologists have illuminated the ways in which human beings use narrative to make sense of and find meaning in their experiences, particularly those of suffering. Research has explored the reconstructive power of narrative in serious illness (Luoma and Hakamies-Blomqvist 2004; van der Molen 2000; Williams 1984). Patients' telling and retelling of their illness experiences or stories become a way of reasserting control, reestablishing personal identity, and (re)discovering meaning when these have been brought into crisis by illness (Frank 2000; Good 1994). Psychotherapeutic approaches such as dignity therapy (Chochinov et al. 2005), meaning-centered therapy (Breitbart 2001), and life review or reminiscence (Butler 1963) have been developed around the idea that constructing a narrative or dialogue with another person can help bolster a patient's sense of meaning, purpose, and dignity.

One of the functions of literature, theology, history, and philosophy is to clarify and make accessible the narratives of others. Spiritual worldviews often occur in specific contexts such as faith communities, which may be opaque to those outside them. One function of the humanities in resisting the marginalization of spiritual dimensions of health and illness is to provide expression of such life-shaping influences in a form approachable by those not embedded in a particular tradition but open to imaginative growth in the effort to understand others' experience. This is particularly important for clinicians who have some responsibility for the course of another's experience.

A second implication of the proposed model is that medicine, if practiced with genuine curiosity about the human condition, must take seriously the significance of the "phenomenology of illness," that is, "what it is like" to be ill, from the patient's subjective perspective (Svenaeus 2000a, 2000b). This concept has much in common with "illness experience" in interpretative sociology and phenomenologically oriented anthropology. Arthur Kleinman, for example, observed that while clinicians typically focus on the disease itself, patients, their families, and folk practitioners address the disease as an experience, an illness, in its social and spiritual context (Kleinman 1978a; 1978b; Kleinman et al. 1978). More recently, Michael Bury has demonstrated how the impact of chronic illness cannot be adequately described in a biomedical model of disease, as the impact of illness on everyday life is multidimensional. Through an empirical examination of patients' experience of chronic illness, Bury shows how illness can constitute a major instance of "biographical disruption" in which the relations among body, mind, and everyday life are threatened (1991). One of the tasks of medicine is to heal the relationships disrupted by illness, and this requires respect for the phenomenological aspects of illness (Sulmasy 2002).

In a phenomenological understanding of illness, narrative, literature, art, and music are considered, not epiphenomenal to the patient experience (and hence to the healer's task), but actually fundamental to it. The humanities, in conjunction with the spiritual and cultural traditions in which they are embedded, provide a resource for finding meaning in illness and for understanding others' experiences of illness. By reasserting the subjective, experiential, and spiritual dimension of illness, subjects such as philosophy and literature provide a resource for a humanity that is essential to the way good medicine should be practiced.

NEVER LET ME GO, BY KAZUO ISHIGURO

When we are caring for each other in the context of illness, suffering, or death, as a clinician or family member, one of the most important gifts we can both give and receive is to reveal the meaning of our experience from the inside. From within this context of meaning, conversations about goals of care arise as a response to a new reality that is consonant with how we live our lives and perceive our future. Meaning reveals itself through listening, and it is only through this habit that we come to understand another's grasp of the event we call "illness." The humanities— including literature, theater, film, and other forms of the human expression of experience—have the potential to open up the worlds of characters in such a way that our own capacity to imagine and respond to the inner worlds of others is enhanced. Following Aristotle's discussion of tragedy in the *Nichomachean Ethics,* such forms of storytelling and expression give us the opportunity to consider ideas and perspectives—sometimes quite disturbing—outside of the real-time events of suffering. For Aristotle, this is a training ground for virtue, from which we can change our lives for the better, respond to others in a more virtuous manner, and, when suffering comes, respond to it as people who are better prepared for having already made imaginative responses to possible experiences that life can bring.

Fictional worlds compel us to reconsider meanings within our own lived worlds. Kazuo Ishiguro's *Never Let Me Go* (2005) is one such work, raising questions such as What is it to be person? What is it to love? and How are lives valued? Ishiguro takes that last question and expands it into the more provocative and disturbing question, How are lives valued differently, and why? In doing so, he creates a reimagined world close enough to our own to call into question the meanings and values by which our society lives. The novel is a beautiful example of the imaginative expansion that the humanities can bring to the medical understanding of vulnerability, suffering, and illness.

The first element of the work that is relevant to such an analysis is its very tone. It is not the language of literature but the factual language of everyday life. The narrator, Kathy H, a thirty-one-year-old "carer," tells the story somewhat blandly, using language that assumes we already know its context. Reared in a progressive boarding school called Hailsham, she has become the *carer*—a term initially unexplained to the reader—for two of her friends, Tommy and Ruth. The facts of their situation are doled out slowly through explication and conversation. For much of the first half of the novel, the characters are portrayed during their teenage years—concerned with school, sex, and, nebulously, the future. Although Ishiguro has earned readers' trust with previous work, it is sorely tested as he creates this mundane atmosphere. It is, in a sense, the very atmosphere and language of a dull and repetitive life that many turn to the arts to escape. However, this is a critical element of the novel's strategy because it is the familiarity and drudgery of the young people's very "human" lives that allow Ishiguro to build toward the central, disarming revelation at the center of the novel regarding the identity of Kathy, Tommy, and Ruth.

Related to the bland tone is an understated mystery that pervades the first part of the novel—namely, the requirement that students produce art at Hailsham. Initially, this seems like an expectation of any boarding school, but the subdued urgency of several teachers for the children to produce good art betrays an as-yet-unknown strangeness around the task. To underscore this strangeness, the children are aware of a mysterious visitor known as "Madame" who takes away the best of the children's art. These elements—mundane daily living, childish romance and jealousies, the experience of education, thoughts about the future, and creative expression—form the same backdrop against which we experience the disorientation of unexpected illness and the inevitable yet shocking approach of death. The odd thing about these children, however, is that their suffering, their loss of bodily function, and their deaths are not random events looming on an uncertain horizon, as are ours. Rather, their lives and their suffering are scheduled, for they are clones whose destiny has been determined before their birth: they are raised to provide vital organs for transplantation to extend the lives of people who do not appear in the novel but who reside in the wings in a dystopian, alternative England where the moral horror of their experience is permitted for the perceived good of others' longevity. Once they reach maturity, the young people's organs are harvested until they die, which is called, significantly, "completing," recalling teleological conceptions of life and its cycle in religious traditions.

Gradually, the reason that the children are encouraged to create art becomes clear. In the course of conversation, Tommy, who has not been terribly successful because he does not want to participate, tells Kathy about an odd statement made by one of the teachers: "[Miss Lucy] says, 'Listen Tommy, your art, it is important. And not just because it's evidence. But for your own sake. You'll get a lot from it, just for yourself.'" Kathy responds, "Hold on. What did she mean, 'evidence'?" (Ishiguro 2005, 108). Hailsham is an experiment. It takes them a while to understand, but when another of the boys asks a teacher about it, he tells Tommy what he learns. "What she told Roy, what she let slip, which she probably didn't mean to let slip, do you remember, Kath? She told Roy that things like pictures, poetry, and all that kind of stuff, she said *they revealed what you were like inside.* She said *they revealed your soul*" (175). The question driving Hailsham is more directly revealed late in the novel when the characters encounter Madame and a teacher, Miss Emily. Speaking to Tommy, she says, "Why did we take your artwork? Why did we do that? You said an interesting thing earlier, Tommy. . . . You said it was because your art would reveal what you were like inside. That's what you said, wasn't it? Well, you weren't far wrong about that. We took away your art because we thought it would reveal your souls. Or to put it more finely, we did it to *prove you had souls at all*" (260).

The clones encountering non-clones' questions of whether or not they have souls not only evokes deep and interesting questions about what constitutes a human being—the soul traditionally being the placeholder for the spiritual dimensions of human experience—but also about the value of a "soul" in this context, given the destiny of the children as organ donors and whether the non-clones' behavior displays evidence of "soul." That is to say, if art shows evidence of a presumably valuable soul, what is suggested about those who comply with a system in which sentient clones capable of love and art are used for organ harvests until they die?

Here Ishiguro uses the novel to turn the question back upon the reader. We are forced to ask questions not only about the nature of being human but also about the impact and meaning of our own lives in light of what we are willing to tolerate in exchange for purported benefit to ourselves or society. Miss Emily states the reality in this way:

After the war, in the early fifties, when the great breakthroughs in science followed one after the other so rapidly, there wasn't time to take stock, to ask the sensible questions. Suddenly there were all these new possibilities laid before us, all these ways to cure so many previously incurable conditions. This was what the world noticed the most, wanted the most. And for a long time, people preferred to believe that these organs appeared from nowhere, or at most that they grew in a kind of vacuum. Yes, there were arguments. But by the time people became concerned about . . . about students, by the time they came to consider just how you were reared, whether you should have been brought into existence at all, well by then it was too late. There was no way to reverse the process. . . . There was no going back. However uncomfortable people were about your existence, their overwhelming concern was that their own children, their spouses, their parents, their friends, did not die from cancer, motor neurone disease, heart disease. So for a long time you were kept in the shadows, and people did their best not to think about you. And if they did, they tried to convince themselves you weren't really like us. That you were less than human, so it didn't matter. And that was how things stood until our little movement came along. (Ishiguro 2005, 262–263)

Jeremy Bentham, responding to Kant's claim that while we must treat humans as ends, we may use non-humans as we wish, stated: "The question is not, 'Can they reason?' Nor, 'Can they talk?' But, 'Can they suffer?'" (Bentham 1823, chap. 17, note). The nature of our spiritual lives, how we perceive our place and purpose in the world and the structure of our values and priorities are cast in bold when we enter the cauldron of illness, suffering, and impending death. But we also come to know more deeply that we are not merely individuals but people in relation to each other, so that what happens to another matters to my own life. Listening for value and responding to it where we find it is enriching. Ignoring the suffering of others, however, also has an impact on our souls. We do well to listen and to let the domain of our concerns go beyond local priorities. Ishiguro's novel thus reaches out toward the practice of medicine, asking practitioners and recipients alike that we open ourselves to the suffering of others and question our social response to mortality.

CONCLUSIONS

Medicine is practiced on the threshold of vulnerability, risk, and the threat of death. There we are most inclined, if not compelled, to ask: Why am I here? This is true perhaps especially in the context of "near-misses" or in the face of inevitable death from an incurable disease. Existential truths are brought home in the experience of illness and in the experience of meeting ill patients in their suffering. The spiritual aspect of our relation to the world, whether expressed philosophically or in religious terms, seems to come into focus. In recognition of this, Kleinman writes: "The study of the experience of illness has something fundamental to teach each of us about the human condition" (1988, xiii).

It is therefore fair to suggest that our actual experiences and practices in medicine fall under the domain of the humanities at least as consistently as they do under the sciences. To be human is, at the very least, to struggle toward our end, to struggle in light of our end, where "end" is both our purpose and our death. When mere prolongation of a biological process is considered an "advance" without reference to some notion of human flourishing—some idea of our ends and goals and of what it means to be a person—we risk being entangled in a technology that actually substitutes for our ends, that is no longer tethered to questions of meaningful human existence.

The question, Why am I here? is very nearly a paraphrase of the question, What is it to be human? However the question is phrased, it is profoundly relevant that we ask it against the backdrop of our mortality and lack of control. Such concerns arise in illness not only because it is a window into our mortality but also because illness brings into stark relief life's backdrop of uncertainty. In the absence of certainty, and in the knowledge that life is short and death inevitable, further questions arise: What are we willing to risk in order to make sense of the universe? What are we willing to imagine and to what shall we commit in our search for meaning? To what, if anything, is our sense of mystery and awe a clue? In what sort of universe do we live, and what is our place in that universe? Our answers to these questions, however half-formed, constitute the spiritual substance of our lives.

Science alone and narrowly conceived is insufficient to navigate these deep waters. As our discussion of Ishiguro's work attempts to demonstrate, the humanities allow the kind of imaginative expansion necessary to consider our own lives as individuals who must make decisions in the face of illness and impending death and respond to vulnerability and suffering. The humanities open up the worlds of others whom we may serve as clinicians, helping us to know more fully the vision of flourishing that others' embrace so that we can offer support in light of that vision and help people to make decisions that are fitting.

ACKNOWLEDGMENTS

Portions of this chapter are indebted to vigorous conversation on related topics over the course of the 2010–2011 academic year between RCB and Warren Kinghorn, Richard Payne, Esther Acolatse, and Allen Verhey at Duke University and John Swinton at the University of Aberdeen. We would like to thank Cicely Saunders International and the Halley Stewart Trust for funding LS while this essay was written.

Chapter 37

SCIENTIA MORTIS AND THE ARS MORIENDI

To the Memory of Norman

JEFFREY P. BISHOP

The only thing we do not know is how to be ignorant of what we cannot know.
JEAN-JACQUES ROUSSEAU ([1762]1979, 268)[1]

THERE are a series of terms in the medical and health humanities that share certain family resemblances. For example, the term *humanities* shares similarities
with *humanity* and with *humanism*. Each term sounds very nice. For those of us
who rail against the harshness of medical science—that razor sharp edge that cuts
precisely but not necessarily accurately at the joint of nature—we seem to want
to give medical science a dose of the *humanities* so as to help medicine improve
on its accuracy in *humane* treatment. We want more than anything to increase
humanism in medicine or to promote a more *humane* medicine for the betterment
of *humanity*. The similitude of the names elides differences among the terms, differences that, when pointed out, make us feel uncomfortable.[2] After all, who could
be against *humanity* or against *humanism* or against the *humanities*? What should
be at the center of our moral universe, the North Star for navigating through the
moral Charybdis and the ethical Scylla, if not the shining star of *humanism*?

Yet, there are different kinds of humanisms (Engelhardt 1991). Which one do
we mean? Renaissance humanism is different from the humanism that animated
the Republican revolution in France, which is different yet again from the humanisms of the twentieth century. We sometimes forget that both National Socialism
and Soviet communism were both humanisms, philosophically speaking, even
though those claiming the mantle of medical/health humanities would never
acknowledge these as humanisms. Moreover, what counts as human, what traits or
properties we like to assign to the human, and what counts as humane treatment
are actually contested, even while some in the medical/health humanities would
rather pretend that we all agree and know what these terms mean.

Much that is done in the name of a more *humane* medicine pierces to the heart,
to the spiritual core of what it means to be human. We desire to be *humane* practitioners, and because humans are spiritual creatures, we insist that spirituality be

central to the care of our patients. The story goes that we will be more humane if we create spiritual assessments to make sure that patients, especially dying patients, have access to good spiritual care. And the best way to assure good spiritual care is to appeal to the procedures of the human sciences, now more often called the social sciences.

It is just such a wonderfully misguided sentiment that animates the rise of spirituality in medicine. However, with spirituality, we find a slightly different dynamic at work. On the one hand, the similitude of meanings of *humane, humanism, humanity,* and *humanities* elides difference under the banner of the same; on the other hand, with the terms *spirituality* and *religion* (terms whose etymological roots are different, but whose meanings have historically been intimately linked), we find them now set apart from one another. For the educated elite, we desperately desire that religion and spirituality be separated from one another, as when people say, "I am spiritual, but not religious." After all, we must be all things to all people; how can we care for the spiritual needs of the non-religious unless we have a universal category like *spirituality*?

Sometimes the claim that "I am spiritual, but not religious" means something like, "I speak a spiritual language, but no particular spiritual language," or when people say, "I am spiritual, but not religious," they mean something like, "I speak my own spiritual language but not the language of an organized religion."[3] The term *spirituality* is thought to be personal and private, whereas religion is organized, part of an elaborate "group think" bent on destroying the world. Of course, those who hold such a view seem ignorant of the fact that it was religion (not spirituality) that became a private matter in the eighteenth and nineteenth centuries at the peak of optimism in Enlightenment science. It is certainly true that religion is more of a social idea; after all, *religio* and *religare* mean, in Latin, to bind or to tie people together in a community. And for many who claim to be religious, it is the Spirit that binds them together; it is the *spiritus*—Latin for breath—that animates the community. It is in the Spirit—*in nomine Spiritus Sancti*—that their community, their common unity, exists. So for many religious people, it is the privatization of the spiritual, the claim that I breathe a different air than all those crazy religious people, that is the height of radical individualism and anti-communitarianism.

It is just here, at the intersection of the *humane* and the *spiritual*, that I shall begin this exploration. For it is the worthy desire to be *humane*, the desire to uphold the *humanity* of dying patients, that animates the elevation of the *spiritual* aspects of life for those who are dying. But I shall be focusing on what is lost, what goes unassessed, or rather I shall be gesturing toward that which does not conform itself to our *spiritual* assessments. In other words, it is that which slips past the *spiritual* assessment, that which slips through the cracks of our measures, that interests me. Or, put differently, I am more interested in that *object* we call spirituality or the spirit that does "not go into [its] concepts without leaving a remainder" (Adorno 1973, 5). Spirituality is not what is measured in our assessments; it is, instead, the very thing that resists—nay, exceeds—all measure.

In what follows, I shall critique the attempts to maintain *humanity* through the sciences of psychology and sociology. The hope is to create a kind of *scientia mortis,* a science that allows us to uphold the humanity of our patients in and through a spiritual medicine, and the creation of spiritual assessments appeals to a social scientific process that I shall describe. At moments, these assessments with their conceptual and operational definitions might capture something of the human spirit. However, in this critique, I will show that the process of spiritual assessment creation is an exercise in circular thinking, and I shall claim that the very thing that these spiritual assessments seek to capture recasts the spiritual and religious dimension of human life in order to fit with the values of those who create them. Moreover, the most important aspects of the spiritual life at the end of life slip through the cracks of the assessment. Thus, our *spiritual* assessments either become part of the totalizing tendency of the human sciences, or they are utterly irrelevant to those who are dying. As a point of contrast to the *scientia mortis*, I shall describe an *ars moriendi*, one that resists the instrumentation of spiritual experts. It is an art of dying grounded in an *ars vivendi*; it is highly particular and local—and particularly storied.

SCIENTIA MORTIS: ASSESSING THE SPIRIT AT THE END OF LIFE

In 2004, the National Consensus Project for Quality Palliative Care (NCP) published the first edition of the *Clinical Practice Guidelines for Quality Palliative Care*. With an overall goal of achieving "quality by systematic evaluation of care, criteria for outcome data, and the development of validated instruments," the NCP *Guidelines* offered a "national definition of palliative care" (National Consensus Project for Quality Palliative Care 2009, 2). The group stated that "palliative care is operationalized through effective management of pain and other distressing symptoms, while incorporating psychosocial and spiritual care with consideration of patient/family needs, preferences, values, beliefs, and culture"(2009, 6).

Following from the NCP *Guidelines*, the Improving the Quality of Spiritual Care as a Dimension of Palliative Care Consensus Conference produced a comprehensive document addressing the fifth domain in the *Guidelines*: the spiritual, religious, and existential aspects of palliative care (Puchalski et al. 2009). The consensus group defined spirituality as "the aspect of humanity that refers to the way individuals seek and express meaning and purpose and the way they experience their connectedness to the moment, to self, to others, to nature, and to the significant or sacred" (Puchalski et al. 2009, 887). Among the seven areas addressed by this group, three areas deal explicitly with the concept of spirituality: spiritual care models, spiritual assessment, and spiritual treatment/care plans.

In the first area—spiritual care models—the Improving the Quality of Spiritual Care as a Dimension of Palliative Care Consensus Conference concluded that, because an essential component of humanity is deeply based in relationship and because relationship is spirituality, "spiritual care models should be integral to any compassionate and patient-centered health care system model of care" (Puchalski et al. 2009, 891). They claimed that spiritual distress ought to be treated with the same intensity and urgency with which physical pain is treated: "Spirituality should be considered a patient vital sign" and should be routinely assessed in much the way that blood pressure, heart rate, respiratory rate, body temperature, and pain are assessed (Puchalski et al. 2009, 891).[4] The authors argue that every palliative care team must have a chaplain, one who has been trained in a Clinical Pastoral Education training program and is board certified. Clinical Pastoral Education is required for many Christian denominations, and pastors who seek full-time employment as hospital chaplains are not only required to do the training but also to complete a residency program. A patient's pastor can be involved at the request of the chaplain.

Chaplains will need to utilize and/or create tools of spiritual assessment, allowing their work to meet the demands of rigorous science: "Failure to assess spiritual needs may potentially neglect an important patient need; it also fails to consider patients as whole persons" (Puchalski et al. 2009, 891). Moreover, spiritual screening, or triage, of patients is a simple way to identify those in need of immediate spiritual care, and specialized training will be necessary in order to conduct a full spiritual history and a full spiritual assessment on the patient (Puchalski et al. 2009, 893). The purpose of the spiritual assessment is to learn the patient's beliefs and values, to assess for spiritual distress (hopelessness and meaninglessness) and spiritual sources of strength (hope, meaning, and purpose), to assist the patient in finding "inner sources of healing," and to find those who are in need of referral to a board-certified chaplain or "equivalently trained person" (Puchalski et al. 2009, 893).

Once a spiritual history has been taken, one might identify needs or distress that should be addressed by a more thorough assessment conducted by a board-certified chaplain who will use a "screening tool" that is "simple and time-efficient" (Puchalski et al. 2009, 893). This tool will also allow for the assessor to assess the success or failure of spiritual treatment plans (Puchalski et al. 2009, 893–895, 899–900).[5] In other words, tools not only assess patient spirituality but also reflexively serve to assist the chaplain in defining how well he or she has done in first assessing and then intervening to treat the patient's spiritual distress or other spiritual needs.

Of course, spiritual treatment plans must be created so that the team will be able to meet the needs diagnosed in the spiritual assessment. Once an accurate diagnosis has been made of the patient's overall spiritual condition, the board-certified chaplain will deliver and monitor a spiritual treatment/care plan. Thus, frequent reassessment of the patient's spiritual condition will be necessary, and the examining chaplain will decide when to appeal to the patient's pastor or spiritual adviser. Certainly, no board-certified chaplain would ever prohibit the visit of a patient's clergyperson (Engelhardt 1998); nevertheless, it seems odd that it is the board-certified chaplain who is designated to enlist the assistance of the patient's clergyperson, should he or she have one. The doctor, however, remains the captain of the team, determining how the spiritual plan works in conjunction with the overall care plan. As a member of the interprofessional team, "a board-certified chaplain, as the expert in spiritual care, provides the input and guidance as to the diagnosis and treatment plan with respect to spirituality" (Puchalski et al. 2009, 894). Treatment plans can include

- referral to chaplains, spiritual directors, pastoral counselors, and other spiritual-care professionals including clergy or faith community healers for spiritual counseling
- development of spiritual goals
- meaning-oriented therapy
- mind-body interventions
- rituals, spiritual practices
- contemplative interventions. (Puchalski et al. 2009, 895–896)

And, as in all medical treatment plans, "Treatment algorithms can be useful adjuncts to determine appropriate [spiritual] intervention" (Puchalski et al. 2009, 897).

FINDING THE RIGHT TOOL

But how to find the right tool of spiritual assessment when there are too many to enumerate here? In fact, Peter Hill and Ralph Hood (1999) documented 125 different measures of spirituality and religiosity several years ago. Several differ-ent models have been used in order to conceptualize spirituality. For instance, the discipline of psychology conceptualizes religiosity or spirituality according to its dominant theories of psyche and its attendant methods; sociologists conceptu-alize it according to various social theories with its attendant methods. In short, religion and/or spirituality are transformed into psychologies of religion/spiritu-ality or into sociologies of religion/spirituality. Some measures focus on attitudes toward religion (Francis and Stubbs 1987, 741–743), others on concepts of God (Benson and Spilka 1973). Some conceptualize faith as a mode of psychological development (Fowler 1995), religious commitment (Roof and Perkins 1975), and religious coping (Pargament 1997; Pargament et al. 2000). Secular measures for spirituality have also been developed along the lines of both existential well-being and religious well-being (Ellison 1983; Paloutzian and Ellison 1982). Thus, rather than allowing spirituality and religiosity to remain in the language of particular traditions, it must be transformed into the universalizing language of science.

In addition, spirituality as it plays out in medicine is most often subservient to other goals. For example, Tracy Balboni and colleagues set out to demonstrate that more and better spiritual care would lead to "better patient QoL [Quality of Life] and less aggressive care near death" (2010, 446). Using an assessment instrument that defines and operationalizes religiosity as a form of psychological coping, they were able to show that patients "whose spiritual needs are met by the medical team have more than three-fold greater odds of receiving hospice care at the EoL [End of Life] in comparison with those not supported" (2010, 448).

Another set of researchers began by hypothesizing that the more positive reli-gious coping a patient might have, the more likely a patient would be to reject aggressive end-of-life care. First, it should be noted that the purpose of doing the study was to demonstrate that other medical goals—the rejection of "ineffective (i.e., not curative), yet physically burdensome, medical procedures that still result in death" (Maciejewski et al. 2011)—correlated to religious coping. While noting that religious faith can be a major coping resource for patients, much to the surprise of these authors, the more positive patients' religious coping, the more aggressive they were with end-of-life care (Maciejewski et al. 2011; Phelps et al. 2009). High positive religious coping has been shown to increase the likelihood that patients will opt to receive more aggressive care at the end of life (Balboni et al. 2007; Phelps et al. 2009; True et al. 2005). So, of course, their conclusion was that more study was needed to better understand why high religious copers would embrace futile aggressive medical care.

I have elsewhere discussed the problematic nature of the instruments used by Balboni et al. and Maciejewski et al. specifically and the development of all spiritual and religious inventories more generally. The instrument used in both of the studies reduces spirituality and religiosity to a means of coping with psychological trauma or angst (Bishop 2009, 2011a). For our purposes, two important points emerge from these recent studies. First, religion must be converted to the language of psychological coping or to the language of one of the social/human sciences. Second, the usefulness of the knowledge about the patient's religiosity is directed toward some other good external to the spiritual/religious tradition, namely a medical good. In other words, religion is best understood and used as a coping mechanism rather than to achieve enlightenment or salvation.

OF CONCEPTUAL FUNNELS AND EPISTEMOLOGICAL CIRCUITS

While one can hope that board-certified chaplains, in creating instruments of assessment, will not reduce religion to one of the social sciences, there can be little doubt that scientific rigor will be the coin of the realm. Thus, while chaplains may not convert theological, religious, and spiritual concepts and practices into psychological or sociological terms, they will, nonetheless, submit themselves to the paradigmatic and epistemic methodologies of the social sciences.

It is hard enough to know and understand natural objects like the brain. It is even more difficult to know and understand social or psychological objects like intelligence, mystical experience, religiosity, or spirituality. There is a long and complicated story to tell about the development of the social sciences and their relationships to the development of the natural sciences, for the *méchanique céleste* and the *méchanique sociale* were thought to operate on similar mechanisms in the nineteenth century (Bishop 2011a, 77, 82). To get at rather fluid objects, such as religiosity or spirituality, social scientists engage in a process by which conceptual and operational definitions are articulated and tested, a process known as *conceptual funneling*. The first step in research is to create a definition of what it is that one wishes to know. There are myriad ways that one comes up with definitions: some are empirical—for example, grounded theory; others are more conceptual or theoretical/philosophical. Sophisticated practitioners of the human sciences realize that social and psychological objects are not "real" in quite the same way that a brain is real (Babbie 2004, 119). Thus, since their objects are not palpably real, research in the human sciences relies heavily on definition—nominal definitions. Mystical experience, religiosity, or religious coping are difficult to study scientifically, so robust definition is necessary. Indeed, establishing a conceptual definition is the first step in the process of studying such fluid phenomena.

Yet conceptual definitions must also set out a list of operations or indicators that will allow the researcher empirically to recognize and register when he or she happens upon an instance of the concept of say, mystical experience or religious coping. Thus, the human scientist creates an operational definition, one that allows the concept of *mystical experience* or *religious coping* to be seen in operation: "Conceptualization is the refinement and specification of abstract concepts, and operationalization is the development of specific research procedures (operations) that will result in empirical observations representing those concepts in the real world" (Babbie 2004, 132). The process is referred to as a *looping process* in which the conceptual definition is refined in the process of operationalization, which further leads to better conceptualization and operationalization (Babbie 2004, 131; Fisher 2004, 130–131). After carrying out the study in which people or communities respond to the inventory of operations, one can, with statistical operations, then further refine the concept and operation. As conceptual and operational definitions become better and better refined, a definition is produced, finally becoming standard, such as in the IQ test for intelligence. Those who create inventory tests and assessments are always hopeful that their measure attains the status of such a gold-standard definition.

It is just such a process that led to the development of the RCOPE (Religious Coping Method) and the Brief RCOPE (Pargament et al. 2000, 520). As I have shown elsewhere, the reason for the functional view of religion taken by the RCOPE is that it can be harnessed for other goals and purposes, such as clinical intervention and better research (Bishop 2009, 261). Rather than appealing to Moses, Jesus, Paul, or Mohammed, the developers of the RCOPE and Brief RCOPE appeal to Clifford Geertz, Eric Fromm, Sigmund Freud, and Émile Durkheim, as its roots are in the social sciences and not the wisdom traditions. In addition, the RCOPE and the Brief RCOPE both have an inventory of operations directed at function—meaning, control, comfort, intimacy, and life transformation—and directed at purposes other than those of religion and spirituality: "Thinking functionally [with the RCOPE] should lead to stronger predictions of outcomes, easier interpretation of significant and non-significant results, and advances in our understanding of the ways religion expresses itself in critical life situations"(Pargament et al. 2000, 521).

Pargament et al. define religion/spirituality as a psychological coping mechanism and create operational inventories that force patient responses into categories of coping. The conceptual funnel, then, is really an epistemological circuit in which the researcher or practitioner finds what the assessment test has been constructed to find (Bishop 2011a, 250). The "being" of religion or spirituality or the spiritual or the sacred is the product of what the research has constructed the assessment or inventory to find. Spirituality or religiosity becomes what the measures developed by the human sciences say it is.

Consequently, by joining spiritual assessments and spiritual interventions with a biopsychosocial medicine, we now have a biopsychosociospiritual medicine, one in which each domain of a person's life is evaluated by the disciplines of psychology, social work, and now chaplaincy, all at the service of the medical. Or, put differently, religion is disciplined such that it must conform to the values, theories, and methods of the social sciences. Each discipline subjects the whole patient to various tools of assessment in order to treat them holistically. No area of the person's life goes unevaluated by a discipline; no area of a person's life goes undisciplined by expert assessment and treatment. That which is thought to be holistic, treating the patient as a whole, comes to discipline the total patient, and as such she is totalized: "Whereas the care of the dying . . . was once a handmaiden to the theological virtue of hospitality, now spirituality becomes the professionalized domain of a totalizing medicine" (Bishop 2011a, 274). And this whole enterprise is ushered in by a humanistic appeal and a desire to treat the dying patient spiritually. It is perhaps that which exceeds all the capacity of the measures that makes life meaningful.

LIVING IN THE SPIRIT

May 12
It's all rather surreal, for so many reasons. The doctors gave him 2 weeks; Monday we hit 2 months. My father told me to my face a year ago (sitting in the living room chair I'm sitting in now) that he could never have a relationship with me "because of your choices," and yet here I am, helping to change his dirty diapers, helping him into his wheelchair to go outside, giving his medicine. . . . I'm tired and isolated (I'd paid for satellite internet my third week here, after having to arrange for someone to be here and drive 15 minutes to town to use McDonald's wireless or visit a cousin) and constantly biting my tongue (so many landmines to walk around with a family that doesn't want to acknowledge that a man named Bert even exists) and yet I'm also so glad I'm here.

Thus began an e-mail to me from an old college buddy. I have known Ed for twenty-five years now. Though we were much closer in college, we have kept up periodically. I contacted Ed several years ago, in order to ask him if I could reprint one of his poems in my book, and he graciously agreed. Then, in the spring of 2011, I contacted him again to let him know the book would be out in the fall. It explores the ways that the dead body has become normative in medicine and how this attitude toward the body shapes the way we care for the dying. I had not known that Ed's father was dying from pancreatic carcinoma.

Ed, reminded of my work, wrote the e-mail. His father, Norman, is a conservative, evangelical Christian. This and subsequent e-mail conversations in addition to a few new poems chart a kind of spiritual journey for Ed and his family. Ed's words and poems are flashes of light and clarity in what was a rather dark time. Try as we might to make death a part of life, there is something about living that always sees death as unnatural; it is as though we have to lie to ourselves repeatedly in order to believe death to be a part of life. The journey that Norman took, that Ed and his mother and brother traveled with Norman, is a very complex one that resists easy categorization and fast and easy constructs, yet it is a spiritual journey. Though we probably did not need the National Consensus Project for Quality Palliative Care or the Improving the Quality of Spiritual Care Consensus Conference to tell us, spirituality seems to be very important at the end of life.

Norman and Ed are sons of rural Arkansas. Like his father before him and like so many Arkansans, Ed grew up in a small town, surrounded by physical labor and hard work that bend the back, by the Arkansas dirt that insinuates itself into sinew and flesh. Yet Ed is really more the cerebral type with keen interests in reading, writing, and thinking critically. No son of rural Arkansas can avoid being shaped by faith, and Ed grew up a conservative, evangelical Protestant of the free-church stripe.

Fiercely independent and moralistic, such Christians are rarely without an opinion. In a way, they are the heirs of the Reformation, certain that they can interpret scripture for themselves without priests, bishops, pastors, or scholars. For hundreds of years, however, such independent interpretations have concretized and ossified, and what were once idiosyncratic interpretations of scripture offered by frontier Protestants in the South have now become the foundation for what is good, true, and beautiful for the Christian Right. They have, after generations, been shaped by and sculpted themselves into a highly particular brand of Christian. Despite the narrowness of mind in their interpretation of scripture, they still emphasize the intellectual content of belief over the embodied practices of liturgy. Right belief (ortho*doxy*) is emphasized over right practice (ortho*praxy*); a work of the mind—belief—is emphasized to the neglect of the body. The body, with its attendant pleasures and pains, is meant for labor, and it is usually dirty. This Protestant group tends toward the binaries of Manicheanism—light and darkness, black and white, flesh and spirit.

Anything or anyone who challenges these beliefs is usually dismissed outright. If a beloved son questions these beliefs, it can cut to the bone, causing deep pain and suffering. Ed, by his very being, challenged much of what his father held as sacred, a word often misunderstood, but which literally means set apart—set apart as inviolable; he could inflict no worse pain upon his father. Of course, Ed did not intend, did not consciously choose to inflict pain upon his father. Loved ones can inflict pain so easily without ever intending to do so, and Norman could cause no deeper pain to his son than to reject Ed and Bert, his partner of nearly twenty years. A poem in Ed's most recent collection of poems, *Prodigal: Variations*, captures that pain:

SACRIFICE

When my father bound me, I submitted,
closed my eyes to the lifted knife in his fist.
Even now, the cords still hold my wrists,
rough ropes of love. My chest is bare,
my heart lies open. He loves his god more
than me. I open my eyes, watch my father
raise his fist against a bright and bitter
sky, no angel there to stay his hand. (Madden 2011, 1)

To Ed, his father appears to have rejected him, to have rejected something sacred to him. To Norman, his son has rejected certain understandings and beliefs about the body that radically challenge Norman's deepest convictions.

Yet neither Ed nor Norman is independent of one another. Ed could not have been who he is without Norman, and Norman could never have begotten and reared Ed to be any other man than the man that he is. Norman can never not be the father of Ed. Even in rejecting him, Ed only becomes more central to Norman's identity. Given what Norman holds as good, true, and beautiful, he cannot but see himself as a failure as a father. And in rejecting Ed, Norman seems to be trying to reconcile something in his own heart, trying to protect something that he feels cannot be violated.

But let us not judge Norman. Given what Norman holds as true, given what he holds as sacred, it is not difficult to see that he is being faithful to that which has guided his life. In one sense, Norman is to be commended for adhering to his beliefs, hoping that Ed will not only be reconciled to him but also to God. While we may want a quick and clear reconciliation between Norman and Ed, and while every board-certified chaplain may want to move Norman's relationship to Ed to a place more consistent with certain theories of pastoral counseling, should we not also marvel that it is Norman's robust faith that was able to create a man like Ed, a poet and scholar? As easy as it would be to condemn Norman for choosing a set of beliefs over a relationship with his son, would this not be for us—the enlightened elite—to do violence against something good, true, and even beautiful held by Norman? And wouldn't it be for us to reject Ed born of Norman and the soil of Arkansas? Is Ed not shaped by the dogged faith of his father—as well as his rejection of it? Can those of us in medicine ever accept the complexity of the body and spirit, the soil and soul, without turning it into some sort of therapeutic journey to what I, at least, have found to be a false place, a no-man's-land, a nowhere of the *scientia mortis*?

I sent Ed the "Prelude" to my book when I wrote to let him know that it was coming out but did not know that Norman was ill. In it, I describe one of my patients, who had been diagnosed with pancreatic cancer, and describe her journey through the medical system, including the biopsychosociospiritual landscape of medicine. Later that day, Ed responded:

May 12
Dear Jeff:
Much to deal with this—rings both so true (we wondered why we had a chaplain—it was a pretty worthless visit, and we don't really want him back) and so false to me (we don't tell Norman he's dying—he's been told that—you are right that they want to move to acceptance—but his cranky insistence that he will get on a tractor—do we encourage that delusional thinking? we're torn—we don't want to be blunt, but we also don't want to be unrealistic?).

All I know is I'm glad when the hospice nurse visits, and was thrilled when the social worker convinced my mom that whatever we do is right, that there is no one right way to deal with funeral arrangements. (My brother and I convinced my mom that getting them taken care of now while we're rational was better than waiting till we're emotional after he dies—so we've done it, and it's all planned, and what a burden that is to be lifted—and the conversation with the hospice social worker is what started the process.)

Norman has been in and out of hospitals the past 4 years—heart bypasses, diverticulitis, colon surgery. . . . What they've been thinking was abdominal they diagnosed mid-March as cancer—pancreatic, but tumors on one kidney, prostate, his liver, and a large abdominal mass right behind his navel. My Aunt Elaine goes off when she visits: she's angry, thinks they should have caught it last year, thinks they should have let him have chemo. (Aunt Elaine, have you seen how fucking weak he is?! Have you changed 3 liquid bowel movements in a row?) He wouldn't have lasted thru chemo.

I don't know.

Ed

May 12

Hi Ed:

It is not uncommon for folks to live longer in the familiarity and comfort of home. I am sure that your father, at some level, realizes the gravity of his previous statements and appreciates the fact that you are there. The best that we can hope for when it is our time is to be surrounded by those who love us and those whom we love. The fact that you are there, despite the hard words delivered by your father, still says something about a father who could raise a son who would be there despite the harsh words. He is a fortunate man; you are a fortunate son.

Best to gently redirect people when they start with delusions. "Dad, you are not out in the field; you are at home in bed. You are sick, but we are taking care of you . . ." or some such. I have found that when you tell them where they are and that they are sick, they have moments of lucidity and can actually converse for a short period of time about what is going on. It is very disconcerting, though.

I hope all goes well; I am glad you are there . . . I hope it is not too painful for you.

Blessings, I will say prayers for you and your dad. Wish we could get together for a drink or two.

Jeff

A day later, Ed sent me a poem that he had written.

May 13

POEM FROM MY FATHER'S HOUSE

Sundays someone always stops by
with the travelling show of crackers
and magic juice, the shuffle of little cups
from a Ziploc bag—Lord's Supper
for the shut-ins, the sick and afflicted
as they say in the ministry lingo.
They left behind the empty cups.
Washed up, they nest on my dresser,
hold the moment when together
we had prayer over Norman's bed
about flesh and blood
and something I'm not sure
I still believe—but I believe
in this: five people around a bed,
something shared,
a broken body, bowed heads.

May 30

Weird weekend. Major pain Friday, and said, finally, "I think I'm dying." After 10 weeks, he's just admitted. Told my aunt "I'm dying" Friday. Told my mom "I'm ready to go" this morning. Told the nurse Friday evening, "I'm through fighting."

It's weird, but it feels like such a blessing, a grace—for all of us—for him to accept this and be at peace and not be angry or agitated or asking when he can get up and get on a tractor.

Ed

May 31

Hi Ed

It sounds like things are better then . . . if "better" is the right word.

Jeff

May 31

Hi Jeff

I think "better" is the right word—if only because of the sense of peace it seems to have given both him and my mother.

We have had spiritual work here. The hospice chaplain assigned to us has only come once—perhaps more of use to folks who don't have a church community or don't have ministers they know well. My parents' minister has come by about once as week, and many folks from church have asked to pray with Norman. (I do like that they all ask him if they can pray with him: no one assumes.) But because of my own relationship with my family and with the church I grew up in, even when I'm in the room, I feel weirdly alien. It's not that I don't believe, it's that I don't believe the way they do.

I don't know if you've seen my new book, *Prodigal: Variations*. Part of the reason this spring has felt so surreal is that that book came out in the midst of this—a book I sent off last year after my father said he could "never" have a relationship with me. So I'd thought fine, that's that, I can send this work out. It's very much about my alienation from him. I fear that some would read it reaffirming the stupid stereotypes of distant fathers as an etiology for homosexuality (though I'd question the cause-effect relationship even of that etiology: is it that gay sons look for some compensation for a distant father, or that fathers distance themselves early on from sons who seem so alien to them, unconsciously or otherwise). It's also about the range of male-male relationships. Needless to say, I haven't talked about this book at all here, other than to a cousin and an aunt with whom I can talk honestly—a rare blessing here.

An old friend and employee of my father's who stopped by Saturday said to me outside how my father's life now isn't really living. But looked at me and said, "But his being here now is really more for you all than for him." I think that's true.

I wrote this over the weekend.

PRODIGAL, RECONSIDERED

I was not that creature, begging to be absolved,
the bent son on his knees in the road's dirt. I thought
that's what he wanted, what I ought to do. Instead,
they wanted this: a man on his knees, lifting
his father's feet, one at a time, to the pedals of the chair,
wrapping the blanket around his thin legs, tucking his robe
around his back, unlocking the wheels to roll him out
of the house to the carport for the sun and a smoke.
Instead he wanted this: a son to light his last cigarette,
and after, to lift him back into the bed.[6]

Two more poems:

June 4
LANDSCAPE, WITH LEVEES
"If this is the middle, how long does it last?'
 Luisa A. Igloria

Yesterday, they put up levees in the field
across the road, the new rice a green sheen,
the levees ready for what's to come.
When I drive to town, I leave the windows
down, drink in the smell of well water,
metallic, cold. I remember the taste.
We think we've been close, but can't know.
That weekend he was away from us, his eyes
glazed and moving around the room, his hands
picking at the blanket, his feet and legs
twitching, jerking beneath the sheets.
That morning he couldn't breathe.
That night Norman decided he was dying,
said 'It's time for me to tell you goodbye,'
leaned back in bed and waited. Nothing
happened, and he was mad, the next morning,
that he hadn't been taken. 'I'm still alive?'
Outside, since we've been here, the floods have
receded from the fields, the men and tractors
taken over—landplanes leveled the field
for the rows, a red Case IH and
a huge John Deere pulling the yellow planes,
the long silver blades across the field.
Disk and plow have done their turn, turned
stubble under, and weeds, and the trees
along the ditch filled out thick and green.
The river has stalled, so much water
coming from up north, and the ditch ran
backward for two days, but that's passed.
The nurse blames the moon for dad's moods,
says it was a solar eclipse the day he decided
to die, though all his vital signs were fine.
We open the curtains so he can see.
We hear the tractors in the field. He's retired,
but sometimes doesn't remember, says
he wishes he could get up on a tractor,
get out there, help them finish up.

THEOLOGY LESSON
A brown thrasher eats the little grasshoppers;
it stalks the lawn, its beak open. The mockingbird

has taken off, twig in its beak almost
as long as it is, stopped its song for this,

though now I hear it singing again. My dad
says an old boy goes out of this world

and a little girl comes in. He's looking
at the picture of my cousin's baby,

her pink blanket, on the dresser near
his railed bed. He's taken off his oxygen

for the moment, though he'll need it again.
Under the flower bed out back, a thick

layer of stuff left over from the kitchen
feeds the roots, and along the surface

a slow watering of Miracle-Gro, the zinnias
open. The cosmos try on little blooms.

On June 14, I published an op-ed piece (Bishop 2011b) that I wanted to share with
Ed. It was written on the occasion of the death of Jack Kevorkian. The newspaper
articles announcing his death said that he had died alone, and I thought about how
most of the patients (or victims?) enlisting Kevorkian's services were left alone
with his Mercitron or Thanatron machines. I thought about how so many of the
patients in intensive care units died alone also surrounded by technology.

June 14
Thanks for the op-ed, Jeff. I will read it later.
  My dad hit 3 months at home yesterday, but today he's really very, very tired. The
nurse has refused to predict—said she hates that doctors do, and also says Norman has
proven to be totally unpredictable—but said today it will be soon. He's really out of it,
weak, not responding (or only in the most minimal ways). The nurse told my aunt what
she wouldn't tell my mom (my aunt has been with 3 siblings who died of cancer and has
been very much a part of our caregiving)—that if it were anyone else, she would say 24
hours, but with Norman, she knows it could be days. He's a tough old man.
  Ed

In the op-ed piece, I also shared a story about a patient of mine, a young woman
named Becky:

As I read her chart that day, a woman walked out of Becky's room; it was her sister, escort-
ing a boy of about 5 years of age. She was teary eyed; the boy did not seem to know what to
make of it all. A few minutes later, I walked into the room and into the middle of a conversation between Becky and her mother.
  "It is time," Becky said, with tears streaming down her face. She struggled to take off the
facemask delivering oxygen.
  "No, Becky," her mother said, as she struggled to put the mask back on.
  "Momma," Becky said, with her East Texas accent, "I told you that after I saw him one
more time, I would be ready. We have said our good-byes. Now it is time."
  Her mother, not knowing what to do, shook her head in defiance. "No, dear! He still
needs you. Please leave the oxygen on, honey."
  Within a few seconds, everything became clear. I realized that Becky was talking about
her death, that the boy was her son, and that she had made her peace with him. I sat down
next to Becky's bed, asking a few medical questions. She redirected me to existential questions. She wanted to stop the medications and to be allowed to die. It became clear that

Becky had been planning her death after she had one last visit with her five-year-old son. I stepped out, spoke with the attending physician, spoke with Becky's mother, and then returned to Becky's bedside to tell her that we would work to make her comfortable and to allow her to die.

To this day, I remember the relief on Becky's face, like I had taken from her a heavy load that she had carried up a long hill. I wrote orders to discontinue antibiotics, and to begin her on a little Morphine to reduce any air hunger. I changed her from the uncomfortable face-mask delivery of oxygen to oxygen delivered by nasal cannula.

Becky died rather quickly, as these things go. Her mother sat at the head of the bed, cradling Becky's head in her lap, stroking her hair. Her sister sat at the foot of the bed, tenderly holding her foot, occasionally kissing it. Becky died peacefully surrounded by those who loved her most.

. . . I do not know the details of Jack Kevorkian's death. The reports said he died alone at William Beaumont Hospital from pneumonia and renal failure. I hope the reports are wrong. I hope he had more than the trappings of medical technology with him. I hope he was surrounded by those whom he loved most, and those who loved him most. I hope that as he reached out, he did not find a cold machine, but a warm and loving hand. (Bishop 2011b)

June 14
Jeff, the op-ed is beautiful. My dad slept so peacefully today when my mom got in bed with him—they both did.

I am beside his bed now. He occasionally reaches out for my mom's hand—she's sitting on the other side.
  Ed

Norman E. Madden, Sr., died Saturday, June 18, 2011, surrounded by those who loved him most, and those whom he loved most.

POSTSCRIPT: CONCLUDING UNSCIENTIFICALLY

The spiritual work of dying is hard; it is messier than working the Arkansas soil. This kind of work is best not engaged in by scientists but by artisans; a *scientia mortis* is inferior to an *ars moriendi*. Do we not learn how to die in our own communities with our own resources, in the fertile soil of home and hearth, spirit and soul? In the *scientia mortis*, are we not seeking solutions that fit into some tidy psychological and sociological model? The truth is that all work of living is spiritual work, as well. But it is that fertile soil of the living that makes an *ars moriendi* possible, for it is what has come before in our lives that makes dying well possible.

There will no doubt be those in the medical/health humanities, those in palliative care, and those in chaplaincy practice (and even some in hospice)—those helping professions insisting that they must help—who will make two claims against what I have described. There will be the apologists of the *scientia mortis* who will claim that I have misrepresented what they do, that they do not discipline the body and spirit of their patients. And yet, august bodies of experts still insist that we must be there to offer spiritual care, spiritual assessments, and spiritual interventions. The *scientia mortis* is alive and well and yet does not make contact with the earthiness of dying. But it is a science that seems to operate quite apart from the realities of the spirit.

The second group of critics will claim: "Come on, Dr. Bishop. Ed is a professor of literature and a poet. He is well-educated and thoughtful, capable of navigating the experience of his father's death without much assistance. Besides, Dr. Bishop, you have mostly described Ed's journey and not Norman's journey." My response is this: Whoever said that intellectual expertise was necessary to live spiritually and to die well? Have we not died for millennia without doctors and therapeutic chaplains? Ed, like all of us, is a human with all the frailties and blindnesses that each of us carries, no matter how well educated. Our elitist education—our so-called knowledge of death and the dying process—does not give us insight into the *ars moriendi.*

Besides it is very likely that Norman and Ed and the rest of the family were all along practicing an *ars moriendi,* born in the soil and soul of Arkansas, slipping through the cracks of all our assessments. Norman held on for Ed's mother and brother and for Ed, perhaps trying to say what needed to be said to them, to Ed, even if it was never verbalized. Or perhaps he did say it without speaking it. Perhaps in receiving Ed's kindnesses and loving care, Norman was, in his own way, being reconciled to his son. Perhaps this is how sons of Arkansas live and die well. Perhaps this is their *ars moriendi* grounded in *their ars vivendi.*

Ed was there, focusing on Norman; so were Ed's mother and brother, Norman's sister, and Norman's pastor, among many other friends and family in their community. Surrounded by tractors, plows, and rice fields to be flooded, soil and soul were in harmony, working out their living and their dying. No need for the generic chaplains with generic assessments bent on plying their disciplinary power at Norman's bedside. As Ed wrote, "We wondered why we had a chaplain—it was a pretty worthless visit, and we don't really want him back." Perhaps the art of dying well is just this: two prodigals meeting in a field in Arkansas, holding each other up, not sure who left whom, and who is returning to whom. But then perhaps that doesn't matter once they are at home in each other's arms.

May the soul of Norman rest in peace, and may light perpetual shine upon him.

NOTES

1 Jean-Jacques Rousseau is one of those figures whose overall diagnosis of early modern philosophy was very accurate but whose therapy was utterly wrongheaded. Yet this statement, like many of his observations, rings true.
2 For a critical analysis of humanism that begins to point out some of the difficulties of *humanism,* see Jeffrey Bishop (2008).
3 Consider Wittgenstein's point from *Philosophical Investigations* that there can be no private language. Of course, there are those who would claim to be spiritual because they are religious, and there are even those who would claim that they are religious, but not spiritual.
4 Oddly enough, pain is the one vital sign that medical practitioners attempt to stamp out.
5 For a more in-depth analysis of the importance of an assessment both to define its objects and to define the subject, the one doing the assessing, see Bishop (2009).
6 Revised versions of some of the poems that appear in the correspondence between Ed and me are published in *My Father's House* (Madden 2013) and in the *Journal of the South Carolina Medical Association* (Madden 2012).

Chapter 38

MEDITATIONS OF AN ANESTHESIOLOGIST

Poem and Commentary

AUDREY SHAFER

MEDITATIONS OF AN ANESTHESIOLOGIST

The woman selling cotton candy is massive
solid as her wisps of spun sugar are slight
each uplift of her arm saps her breath—
while my own anxiety climbs the ziggurat folds of her chin

In the operating room
syringes brightly labeled
her nose and mouth bathed in oxygen
she would still scare me
her escaping soul could freeze my heart

Every day a blinding light tips a wand, pierces a body
illuminates a knobbed liver or inflamed tissue
floating in a knee joint like fan coral:
we do not see the person because we glimpse inside

In our separate uniforms
we barely remember we journey together—
harder yet to remember the patient who journeys still
who waits, suspended in hope and dread

I lie awake at night
rehash memories real and imagined
listen to my husband's breath, thrum his rolling hand veins
walk my fingertips along his trim beard
and settle into my good fortune:
that what I know could be is not
no parasite cancer, no welling blood, no choking myocardium
no downward spiral of desaturation
no devil's bargain to get the tube in
not this night, no please, not tomorrow either
not ever I would say
not yet

I pass the cotton candy stand
mutter a chant into the swirl of her confection
don't code here don't code here
she smiles at my glazed stare

My shed scrubs lie crumpled in the hamper—
cirrus prayers rise and
tiny pink crystals alight
like fairy dust across her titan flesh.

COMMENTARY

Medicine doesn't let you forget about disease or decrepitude or death. For all its classifications and nomenclature, protocols and hierarchy, medicine is basically untidy. Blood gets out, bugs get in. Lungs clog with fluid, veins collapse from dehydration. Bad tissue grows, good tissue fails to grow.

We are embodied creatures. Yet concentrating on the body is a surefire way to make the non-body, even if under-acknowledged, keenly important. What's more, medicine examines the body at the extremes—the flagging body reminds us of mortality, and the luminous newborn body reminds us of miracles and a sort of immortality.

"Meditations of an Anesthesiologist" is an exploration of wishful thinking, blurred boundaries, prejudice, shared humanity, and the consequences—including otherness—of embodiment. It is an acknowledgment that the doctor, nurse, social worker, and teacher do not stop being those professionals when exiting the hospital doors. Likewise, we bring all kinds of experience, expectation, bias, and relations (parent, spouse, daughter, and so on) in through the doors when we enter. Hopefully, the poem is an expression of gratitude for both a life in medicine and for life itself.

The poem is also a search for meaning in that life. Meaning permeates hospitals and clinics. Where one person may find meaning in the fantastic arborialization of neuronal dendrites, another may find meaning in filling a patient's pitcher with ice water. Look at the bald head of a pediatric cancer patient and try not to ask, "Why?"

A code call: teams rush to a patient's room; hard physical and mental work is done. After the code, the crowd disperses. House staff respond to beeping pagers or look up lab results at computer terminals; nurses tend to other patients; pharmacists return to complete inpatient medication dispensing. A physician calls the family. The particulars of the code, even the name of the patient, lodge so deeply into memory banks that this event, dramatic and the stuff of television entertainment, becomes as irretrievable as what was eaten for lunch three Tuesdays ago.

The difference in importance of that particular code, surgical procedure, worsening symptom, or new diagnosis to a patient and family as compared to the impact on the healthcare worker is vast. In the dailiness, the pressures and codification of tending to the sick, we can lose meaning and routinize our work. Seeking to understand another is not only the business of the health humanities but also the business of every healthcare worker. The humanities provide the tools, the rigor, and the context for such understanding. But it is up to the healthcare worker to renew the connection to the individual patient.

"Spirit" derives from the Latin *spiritus*, or breath. Anesthesiologists listen, all day long and sometimes through the night, to the breathing of their patients. When we brought our firstborn home from the hospital, we set up his crib in the bedroom of our small apartment. Listening to the normal stops and starts of his newborn breathing, I could not sleep. We moved him into the living room. I slept in blissful exhaustion while he slumbered.

Spirituality doesn't mean secure centering and knowledge of the holy. Like parenting and breathing, spirituality is a process. If spirituality were a punctuation mark, it wouldn't be a period. Spirituality is a quest, and a meandering one at that. It resists residence in a single form or belief system. The hospital chapel can offer respite and sanctuary, but it is not necessarily where meaning or spirituality begins or ends.

At its most transcendent, spirituality renews the awe of existence. Awe nourishes not only the individual but also the connections between us and around us. At these moments of wonder, we feel gratitude—for something as simple as the twirl of air and sucrose into cotton candy or as craved as one unencumbered breath in an ill loved one. The sense that meaning exists, call it spirituality if you will, is often ineffable or ethereal. At other times, particularly as related to health, illness, and the physical and emotional demands of medical care, that same awareness becomes achingly acute. It is an awareness that penetrates straight to the bone and allows us to rediscover awe, hiding in plain sight.

Part XI
SCIENCE AND TECHNOLOGY

Chapter 39

ANDROMEDA'S FUTURES

A Story of Humanities, Technology, Science, and Art

CATHERINE BELLING

Our technology and our science saved us in the end, yes, but it was our arrogant misuse of both that got us into this trouble in the first place. . . . What happens next is anybody's guess.

The Andromeda Strain (television mini-series, 2008)

Our futures are always imaginary. We can never know them with certainty since their events are, by definition, as yet nonexistent. No matter how much data we have for calculating predictive statistical probabilities, we still create the future as fiction. For this reason, arts and humanities—the creation *and* the interpretation of cultural object-texts—are integral to the future-oriented endeavors of science and technology. If we are to construct and test hypotheses in the production of new knowledge—*scientia*—or if we are to apply that knowledge in the invention and implementation of new practices—*techne*—we must first envisage and articulate nonexistent conditions. This epistemology of the future complicates any rigid distinction between the natural sciences and the humanities (the human sciences).

The epigraph above is spoken by an imaginary scientist after he and his colleagues contain a fictitious disease outbreak caused by an extraterrestrial organism. Viewers of this story are expected to ask, "Could this happen? And what if it does?" The danger of a global pandemic over for now, a reporter asks the scientist to comment and gets an ambivalent message, echoing the cultural narratives we often tell about science and technology, at once acknowledging—and inviting us to wonder at—the powerful capacities of applied science and warning us about the consequences of failure to control that power. The scientist's words are meant to circumscribe his story and, as in so many fictional accounts of ambitious science since Prometheus, Faust, and Frankenstein, to define it as a cautionary tale.

But like its alien organisms, the plot of *Andromeda Strain* escapes containment. Despite the apparent closure of the story in a call for humility and regulation, the scientist relinquishes control over "what happens next." The future, he says, is speculative, "anybody's guess." Such speculation demands imagining. In representing science and its futures, science fiction thus acts as translator, commentator, and critic, and as those futures become present (or past—or impossible), science and its representations assimilate the languages and plots of fiction, both in professional scientific discourse and in public and media accounts of science and technology as well as their ethical implications.

If we trace some of the cultural reproductions of *The Andromeda Strain*, it becomes clear that in considerations of foresight, it may be fruitless, even foolhardy, to treat science and the arts as distinct discourses or cultures. Science, stereotypically, is based on excluding what is not objectively true. Art, stereotypically, deals in the fantastical and imaginary. In considerations of the future, the two are inextricable, and the work of the humanities is to understand how they work together.

ANDROMEDA'S STORY

Questions about the power of wisdom and imagination in contrast to the power of information . . . rise from events within the novel.
   New York Times review of *The Andromeda Strain* (Schott 1969)

The 2008 television miniseries *The Andromeda Strain* was adapted from a 1969 novel of the same name by Michael Crichton. Its story concerns a NASA space capsule that crash-lands outside a small Arizona town, bringing with it a dangerous unknown pathogen given the name *Andromeda*. In both versions of the story as well as an earlier feature film (Wise 1971), the central action is procedural, representing the scientific work of Wildfire, a secret federal team established in anticipation of just such an event, because the U.S. space program's Project Scoop has actively been seeking alien life forms with the clandestine intent of developing them as biological weapons. In their underground lab, the Wildfire scientists work to identify and contain Andromeda, but they and their technologies are fallible. The outbreak ends not because of their efforts but because Andromeda mutates rapidly into a form harmless to humans.

The Andromeda Strain was widely influential, one of the first science fiction novels to become a mainstream bestseller (Sutherland 2007, 70). In it, Crichton popularized a quasi-documentary narrative form that deliberately challenges readers' ability to distinguish between fiction and fact. Aiming for realism at the level of the text itself, this first "techno-thriller" mimics a top-secret government report, complete with maps, graphs, and a bibliography of (invented) references. The 1971 film reinforces this realism by beginning with a sober disclaimer: "This film concerns the four-day history of a major American scientific crisis. We received the generous help of many people attached to Project Scoop. . . . The documents presented here are soon to be made public. They do not in any way jeopardize the national security."

Crichton described his efforts to make the novel seem artless and hard in the style of "factual, non-fiction writing," intended to yield "a very cold, detached book that was also weirdly convincing."[1] In the foreword, he disingenuously apologizes for the tough reading to come: "This is a rather technical narrative, centering on complex issues of science. . . . I have avoided the temptation to simplify both the issues and the answers, and if the reader must occasionally struggle through an arid passage of technical detail, I apologize" (1969, 4). In its specialist vocabulary and stylistic aridity lies the text's tantalizing verisimilitude.

In its plot, the novel echoes a present turned weirdly futuristic. Published on May 12, 1969, the story resonated with avid public interest in space exploration. In the week of the Moon landings in July, it sold a substantial eight thousand copies.[2] Critic John Sutherland argues that this success was "boosted by the chauvinist publicity for the Apollo moon landings," calling the novel a "celebration of American (specifically NASA's) science" (2007, 70). But, in fact, Crichton conveys more anxiety than enthusiasm. His explicit focus on the scientists' methods and on the errors and accidents that complicate the plot suggests that the novel fed off, and into, the very real fears accompanying such achievements: fears about science's power and knowledge, its fallibility and its lack of prescience.

One week after *The Andromeda Strain* was published, a *New York Times* editorial worried that plans to quarantine astronauts returning from the Moon were inadequate: "If there are lunar bacteria . . . different from anything known on earth then the plant and animal life here—including human beings—have not been prepared in any way . . . to resist the depredations of such extraterrestrial pathogens. The result could be disaster" ("Danger from the Moon" 1969). We can tell, now, that the Apollo mission brought no plague back from the Moon, but in May 1969 we could tell—narrate—only conditionally: *if* pathogens infect the astronauts in July, there *could be* a disaster. At the moment of publication, *before* the Moon landing, both Crichton's fictional account and the hypothetical disaster scenarios informing NASA's quarantine policy were unfalsifiable. Both were fiction.

However, this is not to say that either the novel or the preparatory scenarios are anti-science, a claim often used reflexively against cautionary tales. In both cases, imagining the future makes it possible to ask questions and develop strategies that would otherwise be unthinkable. In making up and interpreting stories, we—scientists and inventors and policy makers, as well as novelists and film makers—either constitute or prevent "what happens next." The bioethical role of fiction (and not only science fiction) lies, then, in its capacity to extrapolate from present circumstances and actions to the future outcomes they *may* cause. Fiction constitutes an imaginative consequentialism that exceeds the reductive and nonspecific calculations of statistical probability and risk assessment.

The Andromeda Strain, which became culturally endemic after its publication, illustrates how imaginative storytelling is itself integrated into the discourses of biotechnology, its public perception, and its regulation. Yet despite such deep conceptual interdependence, a rigid dualism between science and humanities continues to govern thinking at all levels of Western culture. Before tracing the proliferation of Andromeda, we must examine more closely the barriers set up to prevent its spread.

CULTURES AND FUTURES

> If the scientists have the future in their bones, then the traditional [literary] culture
> responds by wishing the future did not exist.
>   C. P. SNOW, *The Two Cultures* ([1959] 1993, 11)

The division of human thought and endeavor into two ostensibly antagonistic "cultures" congeals in C. P. Snow's 1959 description of physical scientists and literary intellectuals as polar opposites, between them "a gulf of mutual incomprehension" (4). Snow's overt purpose is to encourage education in the sciences, but the former lab scientist turned novelist seems more interested in asserting the power of science (and scientists) over what he considers an ignorant intellectual majority "on the point of turning anti-scientific" (11). In defining this dualism, Snow installs and entrenches a durable antagonism. Barbara Herrnstein Smith observes that Snow's account is not a description but an ideology, figuring difference "dichotomously, hierarchically, and invidiously" (2005, 20–21). The result is that the work of science and humanities, "more or less divergent but conceivably complementary and equally estimable," are cast dualistically as "superior and inferior, proper and improper, admirable and contemptible" (21). The dualism helps institutionalize tensions that continue to affect public culture in general and education in particular. In relation to health care, the humanities are still defined (and largely marginalized) by their difference from science and technology. In medical education, humanities work may be presented, positively, as a respite from the reductiveness of the scientific method and the inhumanness of mechanistic technology—but as respite, nonetheless, rather than an intellectual and practical value in its own right.

A particular focus of Snow's dichotomy is the orientation of each "culture" toward the future. For Snow, science's future is one of unquestionable progress, where literary culture seems neurotically fearful: "The non-scientists have a rooted impression that the scientists are shallowly optimistic" while "scientists believe that the literary intellectuals are totally lacking in foresight" ([1959] 1993, 5). He describes literary intellectuals as "natural Luddites," congenitally averse to and threatened by scientific and technological progress. By implication, their view of the future is conservative, the cautionary anticipation of regret.

But Snow is writing on the verge of a massive shift in public culture's attitude to expertise and power, and the publication of *The Andromeda Strain*, ten years after his manifesto, coincides with a far-from-conservative rise in resistance against a technoscience culture now seen as oppressive and paternalistic. Paul Goodman, reporting on 1969 campus anti-science demonstrations, mourns the "unblemished and justified reputation" of science and technology, long seen as "a wonderful adventure, pouring out practical benefits, and liberating the spirit from the errors of superstition and traditional faith" (1969). Goodman is amazed to find that science is seen now as "essentially inhuman, abstract, regimenting, hand-in-glove with Power, and even diabolical." Yet in the context of these interrogations, popular attention to science shifts from what Snow considers Luddite superstition to critique by progressive social scientists and humanities scholars who are deeply engaged in science and its epistemologies and practices, not as a threat but as an absorbing object of study in its own right. The first science studies university program is founded at Edinburgh in 1971.[3] Science, scientists, and their technologies are now subjected to the scrutiny of the social sciences and the humanities. Snow's cultures were—dare one say?—contaminated.

An especially problematic aspect of the "two cultures" ideology is its poorly defined account of the non-science side of the binary, which Snow simply calls "traditional culture." This has meant that the creative arts and the interpretive scholarly humanities (including history and the values-oriented social sciences) are clumped together as not- (and, by extension, anti-) science. It is because of this category error that the humanities in health care continue to be seen as object rather than subject of intellectual (in the broad sense, scientific) investigation.

Almost a century earlier, T. H. Huxley presented a more complex perspective on the relationships among science, art, and the work of the humanities. He established an allegory intended to caricature Matthew Arnold's arguments that science is a threat to liberal education: "I think there are many persons who look upon this new birth of our times [i.e., science] as a sort of monster rising out of the sea of modern thought with the purpose of devouring the Andromeda of art" ([1883] 1999, 628). This is Andromeda of Greek mythology. Her father is an Ethiopian king who sacrifices her to a sea monster. Her rescuer is the hero Perseus. Rather than a duel between art and science, Huxley's allegory constitutes a three-way meeting: "Perseus, equipped with the shoes of swiftness of the ready writer, with the cape of invisibility of the editorial article, and it may be said with the Medusa-head of vituperation, shows himself ready to try conclusions with the scientific dragon" (628). This hero is the critical public intellectual—ideally, the humanities scholar—expected to challenge hegemonic science with quick critical commentary and, where fitting, scolding invective. Problematic though Huxley's assumptions are, the figure of Perseus, mediating the dualism of art and science, is missing both from Snow's two cultures and from the subsequent models that take his binary as a given. For the humanities, art and science are both cultural texts, both objects for analysis, explanation, and critique.

This Perseus interprets and evaluates—and, frequently, defends—the human products that include both art and science in all their forms. Such work can be done in the form of fictional as well as overtly analytical genres. Crichton's work, in its imaginative but deliberate engagement with the implications of real science, carries out what Lorraine Daston has described as the work of science studies: estrangement by transparency. "By steadfastly and warily refusing to privilege the scientists' own accounts of how they did what they did," says Daston, science studies can "crack open the 'black boxes' of science and technology that had been opaque to public scrutiny—and hence to public surveillance" (2009, 805).

Where one reviewer could claim that *The Andromeda Strain* was a "chauvinist" celebration of science (Sutherland 2007, 70), another could use the novel as evidence that science fiction has turned against science, that where such writing "used to minister to our need for prophecy, now it ministers to our need for fear" (Comfort 1969). In framing his novel as an after-the-fact report on a completed event, Crichton situates narrator and reader together in the future, evaluating the outbreak in retrospect, and as a touchstone for some other still imaginary time: "In the near future, we can expect more crises on the pattern of Andromeda. Thus I believe it is useful for the public to be made aware of the way in which scientific crises arise, and are dealt with" (1969, 3). One may read this as deceitful, or paranoid, or one may read it as an effective tool, like any thickly imagined hypothetical future scenario used to prepare for otherwise-unforeseen disasters (or to take advantage of opportunities).

In telling what might happen next, the idea and the story of the Andromeda Strain were to prove more contagious than the fictitious life form to which the term strictly refers. In the next few decades, Andromeda would be used as a warning by virtue of its plausibility, and, by virtue of its fictionality, to reassure.

ANDROMEDA'S AFTERLIVES

The precore A1896 stop mutation was reported to be an Andromeda strain that markedly increased HBV virulence and contributed to the development of fulminant hepatitis.
GEORGE K. K. LAU ET AL. (2002, 2325)

In this passage from the hematology journal *Blood*, the fictitious biology of Andromeda is wholly integrated into scientific discourse. Discussing an exacerbation of liver disease affecting patients with hepatitis B after autologous bone marrow transplants (cells removed from their bodies and later returned), the authors use "Andromeda strain" not just generally to describe the virulence of mutated cells but specifically, conveying the process by which infected cells taken out of a patient mutate, making them more harmful when returned. This is directly analogous to the process in Crichton's novel by which Andromeda, thought to have terrestrial origins, is transported into the upper atmosphere by space travel and evolves into the virulent form later transplanted back to Earth on the satellite.

As this example shows, science can be omnivorously intertextual in its search for the meanings it needs. This is why the discourses of science should be read, attentively, not only for transparently referential meanings but also for the freight of connotation and allusion that embeds science, as much as any film or poem, within its cultural context.

While literary tropes function within scientific discourse at a variety of levels, most explicit references can be found in the meta-discourses that connect science and technology to their sociocultural implications. *The Andromeda Strain* is especially illuminating in relation to two concerns about our future: the emergence of new diseases and the generation of new life forms through DNA manipulation.

In the 1970s and 1980s, Andromeda's story was invoked both descriptively, as a plot structure against which to compare actual outbreaks of novel infectious disease, and normatively, as a cautionary tale about risky biotech activities. For example, a 1972 *New York Times* article warning that antibiotic use in meat production would encourage drug-resistant microbes was headlined: "Are We Breeding an 'Andromeda Strain'?" (Ubell 1972). Moreover, ten years after the novel came out, an *Annals of Internal Medicine* editorial on public health's response to newly discovered infectious diseases had this title: "Ebola Virus and Hemorrhagic Fever:

Andromeda Strain or Localized Pathogen?" (Johnson 1979, 117). The author, Karl Johnson of the Centers for Disease Control, does not explain the allusion; he takes its meaning for granted and uses it to make his final point: "Until effective vaccines are developed . . . , careful management of patients and surveillance of their close contacts . . . offer the only rational way to deal with agents sometimes viewed as Andromeda's children" (119). And this allusion is not idiosyncratic. A *New England Journal of Medicine* editorial headlined "Containing Andromeda" acknowledged that reports of the first Western outbreak of Lassa fever "may well remind readers of Michael Crichton's superb and suspenseful novel, *The Andromeda Strain*" (Eickhoff 1977, 836). Eickhoff compares the migration of Lassa from the developing world with the arrival of infection from outer space.

Andromeda could also be used to reassure, held up as an extreme against which to measure present threats. For instance, a *New York Times* report on a 1984 outbreak of Legionnaires' Disease in Brooklyn quoted from a pamphlet that the hospital issued to reassure its staff that the infection was not airborne: " 'It is not the Andromeda Strain or anything,' the pamphlet said" ("Two with Legionnaire's Disease Die at the Downstate Medical Center" 1984, 45). Another new transmissible disease also claimed comparisons with Andromeda. A 1983 *New York Times* editorial measured AIDS against Crichton's worst-case scenario in order to reassure readers—"AIDS is no Andromeda strain: the epidemic will doubtless peak at some time of its own accord" ("The Scourge of a New Disease" 1983, 20)—while another journalist tried to reassure by emphasizing *similarities* between AIDS and Andromeda—"The virus that causes AIDS is mutating much faster than previously thought. What may amount to a modern-day 'Andromeda strain' may eventually transform itself into something harmless to human beings" (Hailstone 1987). However, one feature in the *New York Times Magazine* was less sanguine: "AIDS: A New Disease's Deadly Odyssey" quoted an infectious-disease specialist at the National Institutes of Health who commented: "When people discuss this syndrome at scientific meetings, it sounds like something out of 'The Andromeda Strain' " (Henig 1983, 28).

As well as the obvious association between *The Andromeda Strain* and known but novel infectious diseases, Crichton's novel has been used as a warning against the uncertain potential of new biotechnologies, especially work on recombinant DNA (rDNA). The author of a 1974 *BioScience* editorial titled "Andromeda Strain?" creates a neat lexical connection between alien Andromeda and the terrestrial generation of genetically engineered organisms: "Alien genes from other species of bacteria and even viral DNA can now be grafted into a bacterium where it was not previously present. Because genes for resistance to antibiotics or for oncogenesis could be introduced into ubiquitous bacteria, appalling dangers to the human race are inherent in this discovery" (Moment 1974, 487).

Public anxieties about science have been reliably mobilized by invoking the novel's unsettling combination of threatening new biological forms and scientific fallibility. In 1976, a Cambridge (MA) City Council vote forced a temporary moratorium on rDNA research at Harvard and MIT, supported by the reported rhetoric of mayor Alfred Vellucci as "saying that with recombinant DNA 'those people in white coats' could build a Frankenstein or turn loose upon the populace a deadly organism like the fictional Andromeda strain" (Culliton 1976, 300).

Ten years later, these arguments continued to turn on the question of Andromeda's plausibility. Those in support of external regulation of research treated the novel as a credible monitory fable, while those supporting continued research relied on rigid genre distinctions between fact and fiction. A group of Harvard scientists wrote to the *New York Times*, objecting to recent coverage of anxiety about the use of rDNA in developing a new pig vaccine. Published under the headline, "The 'Andromeda Strain' Is Still Science Fiction," their letter accused the paper of "reviving fears that have long been settled" (Davis et al. 1986, 26). And yet, even as they object that the public is being frightened by "pseudorisks," the scientists themselves use the biology of Andromeda to buttress their argument: engineered organisms, they say, will, like Andromeda, be unable to survive in the external biosphere: "Since there is virtually no chance that artificially altered microbes will be competitive with the natural forms, which have been adapting for billions of years, *the 'Andromeda strain' remains science fiction*" (26, emphasis in original).

Even as they cling to the fictionality of Crichton's invention, they can find no scientific counternarrative about the future that is more verifiable. The accessible shorthand of the popular narrative is used and repudiated at the same time. The scientists claim that the newspaper is making "the remarkable suggestion that the deletion of a gene for virulence might create unforeseen hazards." But such a suggestion is remarkable only if one is absolutely certain that all possible hazards have already been foreseen and that what must be imagined before it can be known should never be a cause for concern. Andromeda, as artful invention, as hypothesis, and as analytical and critical commentary on both, breaks apart Snow's two neat categories.

"WHAT HAPPENS NEXT IS ANYBODY'S GUESS": FICTION, SCIENCE, AND SPECULATION

A characteristic of all crises is their predictability, *in retrospect.*
MICHAEL CRICHTON, *The Andromeda Strain* (1969, 19, emphasis added)

One reference to *The Andromeda Strain* in a medical journal best exposes the embeddedness of powerful fictions in the culture of factuality. In the novel, Crichton discusses the Andromeda outbreak as the world's first biological crisis, quoting the work of Alfred Pockran, author of *Culture, Crisis, and Change*, on the commonalities among crises and the role of foresight in anticipating them. In 1971, the author of an article in the *British Medical Journal*, predicting a crisis in British health care, used the same Pockran quotation that Crichton does (Special Correspondent 1971, 225).

Pockran, however, is entirely fictitious, his work and words invented by Crichton for the novel. They are found nowhere else, simply extracted from the novel by the *BMJ* writer who apparently did not see the need to check his sources further. Perhaps this is just a case of carelessness; perhaps it is a scandal. Perhaps the truth articulated by Crichton, in the guise of his narrator who makes use of the authority of a published but imaginary expert, quite beautifully reminds us that while crisis—or any aspect of the future—may be predictable, it is only so *in retrospect*. In *prospect*, our futures are inescapably as imaginary as the wise Mr. Pockran.

The 2008 television version of *The Andromeda Strain* has an added twist. In it, we learn that Andromeda came not from another space but another time: the object containing the pathogen is a coded message sent back in time by humans in a future blighted by a global Andromeda pandemic. They know that Andromeda's only natural enemy is *Bacillus infernus*, an archaeon being wiped out by deep-sea vent mining in the story's present. Our future selves, in other words, suffer as a result of our present technological activities. They can see, in retrospect, the harm we are doing now. Andromeda—the organism itself—is thus a message sent to us from the future. This captures a paradox implicit in all speculative and cautionary fiction: such texts invite us to read them as *messages from our future selves*. But Andromeda, as biological code and intentional message, is very hard to read. The thriller plot of this version of *The Andromeda Strain* turns on the scientists' failure to recognize that Andromeda is not an alien threat but a message. The future—our real future, which is always imaginary—works just this way. It demands methods of telling and reading that science alone cannot provide.

Embedded in Crichton's novel is a little parable about science and the problem of knowing the future and, hence, at an epistemological level, about the role of fiction making in the practices of science. When the contaminated satellite falls near a small Arizona town, the locals take it to the town doctor. He incautiously opens the thing with a chisel, releasing the pathogen and killing himself and almost everyone in the town. When Wildfire operatives Burton and Stone retrieve the capsule, they find evidence of the doctor's reckless curiosity. Stone exclaims, "The bastard opened it. . . . Stupid son of a bitch," and Burton replies with the essential question: "*How was he to know?*"

How *are* we to know, in advance, the consequences of our best intentions and most wondrous discoveries and inventions? Burton means that the doctor should be forgiven because he *could* not have known what harm he would cause. Crichton's novel, though, is arguably an attempt to take the question more literally: by what means might one know the future effects of attempting to satisfy our marvelous and inventive curiosity? How *does* one tell what happens next?

Crichton's science fiction novel and its future avatars (now, like all futures, eventually already past) can tell us something valuable about the essential—and inescapable—role of fictions in the development of wise—which is not necessarily conservative or Luddite or paranoid—foresight.

The role of the humanities is to ask meta-questions, to go beyond the rhetoric of referentiality and to decode the more complex meanings of our texts. We anxiously analyze all our objects—texts and narratives and practices that include the arts and sciences and technologies—as these all function together, interwoven in the complex matrix that constitutes our biocultural habitat. Only in this way can we hope to tell what might happen next.

NOTES

1 See "Andromeda Strain note" on Crichton's website (Crichton 1997–2000). Crichton attributes the idea for this form to his editor, Robert Gottlieb (1997).
2 "Fiction Review: Andromeda Strain by Michael Crichton" (1969).
3 Science, technology and society, or science and technology studies, refers to a multidisciplinary scholarly endeavor that takes as its object the epistemologies and practices of science and technology as they function inextricably from their social, cultural, representational, and historical contexts.

Chapter 40

KNOWING AND SEEING
Reconstructing Frankenstein

PAUL ROOT WOLPE

F EW works, even those designated as "classics," pervade the modern collective
Western mind as thoroughly as Mary Shelley's *Frankenstein*. Like most classics,
it has spawned a vast literature that analyzes the novel from almost every literary perspective and ideological approach. But even more than most other classic
works, *Frankenstein* has permeated popular culture, generating countless numbers
of films, books, references, spin-offs, visual images, and other cultural products.
Frankenstein's monster—usually rendered as Boris Karloff portrayed him—is
an instantly recognizable figure, iconic in the same sense as the silhouette of Che
Guevara or the Campbell's soup can.[1]

However, the image of Frankenstein's monster has become more than a pop
culture symbol. It has become a signifier of a set of ideological stances toward science and technology and represents a set of cultural conversations around scientific and medical hubris, unfettered technological advances, transgression of the
proper limits of human intervention, and experimentation without full knowledge
or appreciation of implications and consequences. Even the very name "Frankenstein" has been abridged into a prefix that designates those same set of concerns in
specific areas of life where technology has made inroads—frankenfoods, franken-
cells, and frankenfish (Thelwall and Price 2006).

So pervasive is the cultural penetration of the trope of Frankenstein that most
assume that the set of associated cautions and perspectives evoked by the image
of the monster are in Shelley's original work. Relatively few people actually read
the original novel, so most base their impressions on cinematic treatments (fifty
motion pictures have been made based on the story of *Frankenstein*) or cultural
osmosis. Yet very few adaptations of Shelley's *Frankenstein* are true to the original,
and few focus the dramatic tension of the story where Shelley does. Each retelling of *Frankenstein* carries with it the assumptions and constructions of its time
and place, reflecting its own concerns rather than Shelley's. Thus, the narrative
becomes the template on which modern threats can be projected, the base melody
from which each artist creates his or her own improvisation.

Shelley's *Frankenstein* is a work of dynamic tensions and contradictions. It
is about the creation of life, yet it is set in the Far North, which is devoid of life.
It is about the rejection of the nonhuman, yet it is the nonhuman who often

demonstrates, and remonstrates against, our most human traits. Victor Franken-stein himself lives between boundaries; his work in animating life is a violation of the boundary between religion and science, between the living and the dead. And it is about death precipitated by an unnatural birth. Moreover, *Frankenstein* is a transitional book, representing a historical moment when medieval alchemy was transforming into a modern chemistry of combination and construction. Its power lies in its ability to illuminate through its narrative the essential challenges and dangers of the scientific enterprise, seen purely, if somewhat naively, given how early it was written in the Scientific Age. *Frankenstein* remains so important because the same tensions and contradictions have become, if anything, more immediate and trenchant as the power to alter our nature has actually emerged.

It is natural that a novel written in 1818 has altered its meaning and impact over the ensuing 185 years, and that its message has been adapted to modern needs. And while it is true that most serious treatments of *Frankenstein* don't completely distort Shelley's message, they do selectively magnify her themes. Still, the startling thing about a careful reading of the original *Frankenstein* is how fully relevant and important are the themes that Shelley *is* trying to convey—themes that are often lost or minimized in modern adaptations of the story. It is worth taking an in-depth look at the rich messages of *Frankenstein* because of its remarkable insight into the challenges of twenty-first-century biotechnology.

THE STRUCTURE OF *FRANKENSTEIN*

The overall structure of the text is a series of letters written to his sister by Robert Walton, the captain of a ship trying to make its way through the North Pole to find a quicker passage to the New World. Trapped in ice, Walton's men spot Victor Frankenstein, who is cold and enfeebled from traveling a great distance by dogsled. Taken aboard, Victor tells his long and tragic tale to Walton, who then recounts it to his sister. Thus, *Frankenstein* contains a narrative within a narrative within a narrative (Benford 2010). The novel is structured around the letters of Captain Walton, the naïf of the story, who tries to understand the strange account being told to him by Victor Frankenstein (and seems to be using his letters to make sense of it all). But within Frankenstein's narrative is another narrative, that of the creature, told to Victor when they finally encounter one other. The tripartite nature of the story, as the lives of the three intertwine, allows each character to reflect the meaning of the other through the lens of his own account.

This rich and complex narrative has produced many interpretive schemas that situate the three characters differently. For example, one interpretation that has been suggested is that Frankenstein (born of wealth and station) represents the elite, the captain the bourgeois middle-class, and the creature the proletariat, with ensuing analyses of how their interactions evoke class relationships (Montag 2000). Similar analyses have used critical theories such as feminist, psychoanalytic, and disability studies approaches to interpret the relationship of these characters and suggest their metaphorical meanings. Such analyses often reveal as much about the scholars making them as about the book itself.

The three characters also tell their tales from their relative positions in the scientific enterprise: Frankenstein represents the scientist and, therefore, the scientific community; the creature is the scientific product; and Walton is the unsuspecting public, the ultimate consumer of science. The scientist not only creates the scientific product but also presents and interprets its meaning for the public. Frankenstein's account of the creation, purpose, and motivations of the monster is assumed by Walton to be unbiased and true. But Shelley does not leave us there; while the scientist may initially mediate the product, it (like all products) eventually stands on its own, creates its own relationship with the user. Thus, at the end of the novel, with Frankenstein lying dead in his cabin, Walton at last encounters the creature himself and finds the creature's narrative more complex, troubling, and ambiguous than Frankenstein's account.

Here we will examine *Frankenstein* through two prominent themes that emerge from the tale and that offer deep bioethical insights: the nature of scientific knowledge and appearance versus essence. Both offer narratives of caution that can be examined through the lenses of different critical theories but that remain beyond any particular theory. What ultimately strikes the reader is how contemporary Shelley's concerns are and how prescient.

THE PURSUIT OF KNOWLEDGE AND THE NATURE OF SCIENTIFIC WORK

Shelley's work is partially a meditation on the nature of the human pursuit of knowledge, especially by scientists, as well as its intoxications. Most important, it tells us that knowledge for knowledge's sake alone, untempered by moral virtue, is corrupt. If there is one overarching message to *Frankenstein*, this is it—not that human beings should not pursue knowledge, even forbidden knowledge, but that it must be done with humility and higher purpose.

At the beginning of the story, Victor Frankenstein is presented as a deeply committed scientist. "None but those who have experienced them can conceive of the enticements of science," he claims (50).[2] His scientific temperament is contrasted with that of Elizabeth, his childhood companion and erstwhile sibling. Nearly a century and a half before C. P. Snow, Shelley understands and contrasts two cultures, placing Frankenstein squarely in one of them. Victor Frankenstein reminisces:

Elizabeth was of a calmer and more concentrated disposition; but, with all my ardour, I was capable of a more intense application and was more deeply smitten with the thirst for knowledge. She busied herself with following the aerial creations of the poets; and in the majestic and wondrous scenes which surrounded our Swiss home—the sublime shapes of the mountains, the changes of the seasons, tempest and calm, the silence of winter, and the life and turbulence of our Alpine summers—she found ample scope for admiration and delight. While my companion contemplated with a serious and satisfied spirit the magnificent appearances of things, I delighted in investigating their causes. The world was to me a secret which I desired to divine. Curiosity, earnest research to learn the hidden laws of nature, gladness akin to rapture, as they were unfolded to me, are among the earliest sensations I can remember. (31)

Frankenstein is the true scientist, attracted neither to wealth nor beauty but to knowledge—though also to the glory attendant to great discovery. However, he realizes that such glory does not come to the timid. Determined to understand the basic nature of the "principle of life," a topic others shy away from, Frankenstein justifies his curiosity about this difficult and dangerous terrain by musing: "With how many things are we upon the brink of becoming acquainted, if cowardice or carelessness did not restrain our inquiries" (51).

We can hear the clear echoes of the modern critique of science here but also, more important—though less recognized—of *scientists*. Shelley's novel is not so much about the nature of science as it is about the character of scientists. Today, it seems, scholars and ethicists are far more apt to talk about the ethical challenges of science as a pursuit than about scientists as actors, yet to the public, their moral character is of equal concern. A report on a survey of the public's attitude toward the emergence of synthetic biology, for example, shows that the motivations of the scientists themselves was of key ethical concern in the public's attitudes toward synthetic biology (Biotechnology and Biological Sciences Research Council 2010). As new technologies emerge, safeguards are not sufficient; scientists stand as the gatekeepers, and the public wants to see that they are grappling with the moral questions that the power and danger of new technologies evoke.

Yet Frankenstein's considerations over whether to create the creature are purely practical; it never occurs to him to question whether the pursuit of the project is moral or even prudent. He takes no precautions; planning for any potential consequences of his creation never occurs to him, nor does he anticipate any responsibilities he might have to the resultant being. In fact, Frankenstein acknowledges that he is wholly caught up in his passions and is not thinking clearly. He understands that he is violating his own beliefs, that true science should be conducted in a peaceful dispassionate manner:

I pursued my undertaking with unremitting ardour. . . . A human being in perfection ought always to preserve a calm and peaceful mind and never to allow passion or a transitory desire to disturb his tranquility. I do not think that the pursuit of knowledge is an exception to this rule. If the study to which you apply yourself has a tendency to weaken your affections and to destroy your taste for those simple pleasures in which no alloy can possibly mix, then that study is certainly unlawful, that is to say, not befitting the human mind. (56)

He is besotted by the discovery of the nature of reanimating life. In a crucial passage, Shelley recognizes how the intoxication of discovery can cloud the process that leads to it, can subsume years of toil under the dazzle of the revelation:

The astonishment which I had at first experienced on this discovery soon gave place to delight and rapture. After so much time spent in painful labour, to arrive at once at the summit of my desires was the most gratifying consummation of my toils. But this discovery was so great and overwhelming that all the steps by which I had been progressively led to it were obliterated, and I beheld only the result. (52)

Victor re-imagines himself, endowed as he now is with the power to re-animate life. He sees himself as the potential father of a new species, armed with the ability to cure disease by repairing dying tissue. He will become the healer of the sick and bring the dead to life—a deistic analogy not lost on Frankenstein himself. As he imagines creating a perfect being, re-animating life into beauty and wholeness, the unexpected hideousness of the monster will not only dash his aesthetic fantasies but also his divine aspirations:

> No one can conceive the variety of feelings which bore me onwards, like a hurricane, in the first enthusiasm of success. Life and death appeared to me ideal bounds, which I should first break through, and pour a torrent of light into our dark world. A new species would bless me as its creator and source; many happy and excellent natures would owe their being to me. No father could claim the gratitude of his child so completely as I should deserve theirs. Pursuing these reflections, I thought that if I could bestow animation upon lifeless matter, I might in process of time (although I now found it impossible) renew life where death had apparently devoted the body to corruption. (54)

How much greater, then, and more understandable is his disappointment when the being he creates is not Adam, poised in the Garden with a fig leaf, but Satan, the hideous spawn of the corrupting influence Frankenstein convinces himself he can repair. The creature does refer to himself as the "Adam of your labors," but he also understands the irony: "I ought to be thy Adam, but I am rather the fallen angel" (114). Moreover, Frankenstein himself commonly addresses his creation as "daemon." It is precisely Frankenstein's self-delusion as savior and creator, his own misguided sense of divinity, that forces him to see his failed creation not as an imperfect result of science or a failed experiment on the way to perfecting his scientific method but as evil personified: God does not make mistakes; God does not have to try again.

The trope of scientist as "playing God" is old and established. But what is really meant when people wonder if scientists are "playing God" is not only the idea that they are manipulating forces of great power but that they are doing it thoughtlessly, without due reflection and humility. Frankenstein is seduced by the idea that "a new species would bless me as its creator and source," seduced by the power he now controls. And his motivations, he tells himself, are noble: he wants to cure, heal, to "pour light" into a dark world. But, of course, his self-justifications hide a darker motive, a narcissistic desire for control and power. Ultimately, that narcissism and grandiosity are counterbalanced by cowardice. One can see again and again that Victor has an opportunity to do the right thing, to put the lives of others before his own, but his concerns about reputation and status compel him to make the wrong choices (Lunsford 2010). Victor first hides his work and performs it in secret; he then denies the existence of the creature, hides its crimes, and seeks to destroy it in private; and finally, he refuses to divulge the secrets of animating life to Captain Walton. Victor's entire life is avoiding, hiding, denying responsibilities and colluding in silences.

However, by the end of that life, Frankenstein finally understands in his heart what he had averred, but did not practice, at the start: knowledge is dangerous, and its pursuit is a kind of folly if it is not tempered by humility and a sense of limits. When he begins the story of the monster's creation, he warns Walton that he will not reveal any secrets of the manner in which matter can be animated:

> I see by your eagerness and the wonder and hope which your eyes express, my friend, that you expect to be informed of the secret with which I am acquainted; that cannot be; listen patiently until the end of my story, and you will easily perceive why I am reserved upon that subject. I will not lead you on, unguarded and ardent as I then was, to your destruction and infallible misery. Learn from me, if not by my precepts, at least by my example, how dangerous is the acquirement of knowledge and how much happier that man is who believes his native town to be the world, than he who aspires to become greater than his nature will allow. (53)

Shelley wants to show us that Frankenstein's lesson was not in vain. As he lay dying, he addresses Walton assuming that—like Frankenstein himself—preserving life is less important to the captain than reputation and accomplishment (Lunsford 2010). He informs Walton that he is sure they will continue to look for the passage to the West: "You were hereafter to be hailed as the benefactors of your species, your names adored as belonging to brave men who encountered death for honour and the benefit of mankind" (266). Frankenstein echoes what Walton himself has said when they first met before Victor begins his story—that he is ready to sacrifice his life and that of his crew for his aspirations: "How gladly I would sacrifice my fortune, my existence, my every hope, to the furtherance of my enterprise. One man's life or death were but a small price to pay for the acquirement of the knowledge which I sought, for the dominion I should acquire and transmit over the elemental foes of our race" (19–20). Frankenstein is distraught at hearing how Walton is willing to subordinate human life to aspiration; he exclaims: "Unhappy man! Do you share my madness? Have you drunk also of the intoxicating draught? Hear me; let me reveal my tale, and you will dash the cup from your lips!" (20).

Despite his skepticism at the end, Frankenstein is right. Walton has been sobered by the tale, and he does plan to turn back. Frankenstein's folly has become a lesson, scientific hubris a model of all hubris. Walton is also in danger of pursuing knowledge at the expense of humility and humanity, and Frankenstein's lesson is learned.

UGLINESS AND HUMANITY

One of the key motifs of *Frankenstein* is the visual hideousness of the creature. For Frankenstein, it is the trait that makes the creature's existence unpalatable; for others, the creature's physical appearance provokes fear. That his deformities disqualify him for natural human regard is taken for granted in *Frankenstein*; disgust seems to be the natural and unquestioned response. In fact, given that the entire story is based on Frankenstein's decision, at the moment of creation, to repudiate and abandon the creature, it is remarkable how little he actually says about it and how little he feels the need to explain his reaction:

> How can I describe my emotions at this catastrophe, or how delineate the wretch whom with such infinite pains and care I had endeavoured to form? His limbs were in proportion, and I had selected his features as beautiful. Beautiful! Great God! His yellow skin scarcely covered the work of muscles and arteries beneath; his hair was of a lustrous black, and flowing; his teeth of a pearly whiteness; but these luxuriances only formed a more horrid

contrast with his watery eyes, that seemed almost of the same colour as the dun-white sockets in which they were set, his shrivelled complexion and straight black lips. The different accidents of life are not so changeable as the feelings of human nature. I had worked hard for nearly two years, for the sole purpose of infusing life into an inanimate body. For this I had deprived myself of rest and health. I had desired it with an ardour that far exceeded moderation; but now that I had finished, the beauty of the dream vanished, and breathless horror and disgust filled my heart. (58–59)

And later that night, he exclaims:

Oh! No mortal could support the horror of that countenance. A mummy again endued with animation could not be so hideous as that wretch. I had gazed on him while unfinished; he was ugly then, but when those muscles and joints were rendered capable of motion, it became a thing such as even Dante could not have conceived. (60)

It is clear that the objection is fundamentally aesthetic rather than religious or supernatural. Early in the novel, Frankenstein expresses that he is neither superstitious nor squeamish about the natural world:

In my education my father had taken the greatest precautions that my mind should be impressed with no supernatural horrors. I do not ever remember to have trembled at a tale of superstition or to have feared the apparition of a spirit. Darkness had no effect upon my fancy, and a churchyard was to me merely the receptacle of bodies deprived of life, which, from being the seat of beauty and strength, had become food for the worm. (51)

The use of physical difference to equal monstrosity in *Frankenstein* has led feminists, disability theorists, and others to examine the nature of deformity in the novel and its assumptions that deformity and monstrosity are uncomplicated equivalents (Joshua 2011). The use of the disfigured and the disabled as a literary device to set the normal against the deviant is well known; David Mitchell and Sharon Snyder call its use a *narrative prosthesis* and describe it as twofold: disability "lends a distinctive idiosyncrasy to any character that differentiates the character from the anonymous background of the 'norm'" and serves as a "metaphorical signifier of social and individual collapse" (2010, 274). *Frankenstein* serves as an almost canonical text in the classic use of disability and deformity as a signifier.

However, Shelley asks the reader to consider whether the "creature" is rightly designated as a human being or as a simulacrum of a human being. She makes the creature sufficiently brutal to have us question its base nature, but the narrative plays that physical brutality against Frankenstein's abandonment and neglect, tempering any judgment of the creature by soliciting the reader's sympathies. The novel sets up a constant dichotomy—Frankenstein versus the creature—and makes it clear, at times, that our sympathies should lie with the latter. It does this, not by stressing their differences, but their similarity. David Marshall (1988) writes that the creature "is in fact a being like his creator—and it this likeness that makes him so monstrous" (209).

Frankenstein asks the timeless question of what exactly it is that makes us human. It is it our form, our behavior, our inner life, our relationships? There is speculation as to whether Shelley ever read or heard the Jewish legend of the Golem—the creature of clay animated by Rabbi Judah of Prague and destroyed when it got out of hand. It was unlikely she was unfamiliar with discussions in the Talmud in which rabbis not only imagine all sorts of clay creatures and human figures animated into life, as well as hybrid creatures that were half-animal, half-human, but also discuss their nature and the degree to which they should be considered to have the rights and responsibilities of human beings. The question implicit throughout *Frankenstein*—What is the nature of our humanity, and does the creature fulfill it?—fits into a long philosophical and religious tradition.

It is a very current one as well, particularly in a number of areas of the ethics of biotechnology and neuroscience. We have grafted human neurons into rat brains and other animals, we have discussed engineering nonhuman genes into human beings, and we have created transgenic creatures that hint at the eventual possibility of transgenic humans. Transhumanists and their opponents have discussed the feasibility, and the ethicality, of creating a "humanzee," a genetic hybrid of a chimpanzee and a human being. Neuroscientists have begun to create neuronal networks in petri dishes, and artificial intelligence researchers are creating ever more sophisticated robotic intelligence. The questions of Shelley are even more valid in our day than in hers. In 1818, they were theoretical questions, while today they are practical ones. What is it that makes a creature human or less than human? Is it origins or traits that are of key importance? Or is it—as Frankenstein himself seems to think—the appearance of humanness that is most important?

This question of the creature's visual appearance resonates in a contemporary discussion in the fields of animation and robotics, called the "uncanny valley" phenomenon: when the appearance of robots or animation gets too close to precisely replicating human beings—looks almost exactly like a human, but something is off—the response of observers is revulsion. We enjoy human robots and animation that look somewhat human, and we like the look of creatures that are perfectly human. However, when replicants are just a little off, close to humans but not-quite-human, we don't like it. (The "valley" reference is to the dip in the graph that measure people's positivity in reaction to replicants as they get closer and closer to human likeness.) Shelley notes this in the monster's reflection that "God, in pity, made man beautiful and alluring, after his own image; but my form is a filthy type of yours, more horrid even from the very resemblance" (155). It is precisely the monster's simulacrum of humanity that makes him so repugnant in others' eyes.

Shelley's exploration of the boundaries between the human and nonhuman is based, not on technical definitions of humanity, but rather on our judgments of behavior, sympathy, emotional response, and responsibility. As Jeanne Britton writes:

Terms used for both Frankenstein's creation and human beings establish a semantic fluidity that makes distinctions between literal and figurative language, as well as those between human and inhuman, increasingly difficult to make. The monster is frequently described as "the figure of a man," and human beings, repeatedly called "creatures" or described as "wretched," are said to resemble "monsters" and carry "fiends" within them. The novel's terminology characterizes the boundary between human and inhuman, as well as the concept of monstrosity, as imprecise and elastic. For the language-learning monster, this imprecision hints at the possibility of sympathy only to give false hope. (2009, 11)

The monster of Shelley's *Frankenstein* is far more complex than the Franken-stein of the cinema. He represents neither pure evil nor complete victim; he is wronged, yet he has murdered. He demands justice for himself and, eventually, on himself. He is a monster because the acts of the human Frankenstein have made him one; he has a nobility, even a kind of integrity, that his creator lacks. We are torn between condemnation and sympathy, between the "creature" and the "mon-ster." And we share Frankenstein's dilemma. Moreover, it is not only Frankenstein but the monster himself who wonders at his own humanity. Hiding out in a hovel, the creature begins to learn language and human relations by observing a family through a small hole. The creature muses on the nature of Man, his strengths and weaknesses, his triumphs and failings:

Was man, indeed, at once so powerful, so virtuous and magnificent, yet so vicious and base? He appeared at one time a mere scion of the evil principle and at another as all that can be conceived of noble and godlike. To be a great and virtuous man appeared the highest honour that can befall a sensitive being; to be base and vicious, as many on record have been, appeared the lowest degradation, a condition more abject than that of the blind mole or harmless worm. For a long time I could not conceive how one man could go forth to murder his fellow, or even why there were laws and governments; but when I heard details of vice and free bloodshed, my wonder ceased and I turned away with disgust and loathing. (140–141)

But as he learns, he turns that reflective eye on himself. Now that he knows what Man is, he wonders, is he, himself, one? Comparing the traits he can see, he begins to consider the question:

And what was I? Of my creation and creator I was absolutely ignorant, but I knew that I possessed no money, no friends, no kind of property. I was, besides, endued with a figure hideously deformed and loathsome; I was not even of the same nature as man. I was more agile than they and could subsist upon coarser diet; I bore the extremes of heat and cold with less injury to my frame; my stature far exceeded theirs. When I looked around I saw and heard of none like me. Was I, then, a monster, a blot upon the earth, from which all men fled and whom all men disowned? . . . As I read, however, I applied much personally to my own feelings and condition . . . My person was hideous and my stature gigantic. What did this mean? Who was I? What was I? Whence did I come? What was my destination? These questions continually recurred, but I was unable to solve them. (141, 152–153)

His reflections are reinforced by discovering Frankenstein's journal in a pocket of clothes he had taken from the laboratory. Telling Frankenstein of both his discov-ery and reading of the journal, he recounts:

Everything is related in [the journal] which bears reference to my accursed origin; the whole detail of that series of disgusting circumstances which produced it is set in view; the minutest description of my odious and loathsome person is given, in language which painted your own horrors and rendered mine indelible. I sickened as I read. "Hateful day when I received life!" I exclaimed in agony. "Accursed creator! Why did you form a mon-ster so hideous that even you turned from me in disgust? God, in pity, made man beautiful and alluring, after his own image; but my form is a filthy type of yours, more horrid even from the very resemblance. Satan had his companions, fellow devils, to admire and encour-age him, but I am solitary and abhorred." (155)

The novel compels us to ask the same questions the monster asks of himself. The nature of a monster is to confront us with problem of classification. It is easy to make the monster a symbol, to refuse to consider him a monster but, instead, a deformed human, a metaphor, or an icon. Yet the difficult moment is to engage the creature precisely *as* a monster (Bissonette 2010), to allow him to inhabit that boundary between the human and nonhuman, the natural and synthetic, the moral and amoral. To treat the monster as a metaphor or symbol is to do to the monster exactly what Frankenstein has done to it: to deny it the integrity of existence as a being-in-itself and to treat it as an object onto which we project our confusions about human boundaries. To treat the monster as what he is, rather than a symbol of something else, is to confront the complexity of both the act of creation and the status of the created. The novel offers a critique of visuality as a means to know and understand (Joshua 2011). It implicitly critiques scientific method not only through the production of a monster that is a standing rebuke to Frankenstein's preoccupation with a detached scientific stance but also through its implicit suggestion that it is not through observation but through interaction and verbal interchange that true knowledge arises.

CONCLUSIONS

Frankenstein reminds us of the ways in which science is embedded in our social relationships and how dangerous it is to lose sight of that. The ultimate betrayals of Frankenstein are in his relationships: to his family, his friend, and—most important, perhaps—to the creature. Shelley demands that we establish a relationship to our creations. In the age of biotechnology, all of our creations are "monsters" that haunt, or should haunt, their creators. Scientists are altering the very plasms of life, as Frankenstein did, and then abandoning their creations to the marketplace.

The power and longevity of the novel is due to the primordial nature of its social and ethical insights about science. Our understandings of the capacity of scientific knowledge to alter our perceptions, our boundaries, and our relationships may have been stronger when those changes were just beginning than now when they are ubiquitous. The ability of science to create a new kind of monster, not an accidental one but a designed one, seems more startling in a time without such monsters than one where transgenic animals and cloned sheep seem like everyday occurrences.

Victor Frankenstein's final transgression against the creature comes when the creature tells him that his only solace would be a mate. He convinces Frankenstein to create one, but then Victor destroys it, fearful that a stronger, malevolent race may eventually destroy humankind. Therein lies the fear that underlies all our scientific hand-wringing: we worry that we will destroy ourselves at the hands of our creations. *Frankenstein* offers us an unrivaled opportunity to confront that fear head on. The power of Shelley's tale is in the directness and complexity with which it forces us to confront that fear, and through the ambiguity of monstrosity, to better understand ourselves as creators.

NOTES

1   In this article, *Frankenstein* (the title italicized) refers to the novel (Shelley [1818] 1994); Frankenstein (plain type) to Victor Frankenstein, the character; and the "monster" or "creature" to his famous creation.

2   All page references refer to the e-book edition of *Frankenstein* (Shelley [1818] 1994).

Chapter 41

A BRIEF HISTORY OF LOVE
A Rationale for the History of Epidemics

ALLISON B. KAVEY

CONSIDER how a minor malady like the common cold can reduce a healthy, young person to sitting on the couch, sucking on Nyquil and watching *America's Next Top Model* because it is the only plot she can follow. The previous day, perhaps, she was capable of moving around without a blaring sinus headache, endlessly runny nose, repetitive sneezing, and the mental capacity of a slow-witted reptile. Within ninety-six hours, she will, most likely, return to her status quo. If she had been infected with tuberculosis instead of the rhinovirus, however, that status quo would increasingly include a failure to get enough oxygen, then constant exhaustion and weakness. She would be less capable of physical and, over time, intellectual exertion. Without appropriate treatment (something that was not available until the discovery of antibiotics and that is increasingly difficult to accomplish given the rise of drug-resistant TB), she would slowly suffocate to death.

Historically, doctors might have assessed the progress of her symptoms with pinpoint accuracy, mapping her decline in order to frame her: perhaps, she came from "weak stock" and thus, was more susceptible to "bad air," or she had been harmed by conditions in her workplace or home. Those assessments would determine, in combination with her socioeconomic status, how she would be treated by medical professionals and even other patients. Had she been infected with Hansen's disease (at any time between the medieval period and the mid-twentieth century), her soft tissue and nerves would visibly deteriorate in a sea of external lesions. No available treatments would stop the progression of these symptoms, whose visible marks would increasingly determine how she was treated. The marks of her illness would be seen as the physical manifestations of her sins, her rotting skin interpreted as evidence of her rotting soul. She would be pushed out of her family to the outskirts of town, forced to live by begging or in a home with other lepers, and her disease would become her identity. Over the course of her life span, her individuality would be eclipsed, at least in the eyes of those who encountered, treated, and perhaps even loved her, by her disease; she would become a leper. Had she contracted cholera, Ebola, pneumonic or bubonic plague, typhoid, or a hundred other fast-moving killers, the ninety-six hours it would have taken to recover from the rhinovirus that began this chapter would have witnessed her death. Historically, medicine would have had no useful response, but the cultures surrounding the deaths described above would make sense of them using the most accessible available lenses: religion, magic, and stereotypes about race, ethnicity, sex, and class. Diseases, especially those that have had the biggest impact on human history because they were so common, have been so readily incorporated into our ways of understanding the world that they provide great insight into how we have made sense of unknowns.

The history of medicine can convincingly be told through the history of epidemic disease. From the ancient world forward, epidemics have defined medical practice, produced innovations in medicine and public health, changed ideas about the meaning of disease and its modes of transmission, and challenged cultural convictions about the charged relationship between morality and infection. Some of the most compelling work within the history of medicine uses epidemics as a lens for better understanding the theories influencing medicine, practitioners' approaches, and the complicated cultural milieu in which doctors and patients struggle with diseases that frequently seem more intelligent than the people they infect. The study of epidemics allows us to appreciate the significant effects that diseases have had on medicine, as a theoretical system, an institution, and a practice. The plague, for example, along with other transmissible diseases from colds to pneumonia, prompted the creation of the theories of contagion. Ancient medical theorists proposed ideas about miasma (bad air), poisonous environments (including water and landscapes), inherently weak races, and voracious "germs" (seeds of disease) to explain disease transmission. Similar diseases promoted the first institutional medical responses, including quarantine of affected cities, the closing of harbors and trade routes, and the burning of infected bodies and clothing. Medical practice also changed as physicians, surgeons, and lay practitioners attempted to protect themselves from contracting the diseases they were treating. These innovations were unsurprisingly related to ideas of disease transmission and included attempts to purify the practitioner's air supply or protect him from breathing bad air. Practitioners also realized that they could carry disease with them from one set of patients to another, which resulted in efforts to avoid using the same set of instruments on affected patients and the separation of patients to avoid transmission. Finally, epidemics often reflected the cultural anxieties and preoccupations of their time and place. In the medieval period, for example, plague and leprosy were frequently treated as punishments by God for those who had sinned against him or the rules of the Church; in the 1980s, the same was said about AIDS by many right-wing evangelicals.

Why should potential health professionals and even undergraduates study the history of medicine, and what perspective can they gain through the lens offered by epidemics? No other lens offers insight into so many different aspects of the role medicine and disease have played in global history and the ways in which we have shaped culture around the fear of death from disease such as ideas about the body and the way it works; constructs of disease; medicine as an evolving discipline and set of practices; ideas about public health as a government responsibility; and cultural anxieties surrounding contagion and death. Epidemics demonstrate the centrality of bodies, both sick and well, to being human. From infancy to the last stages of old age, we are defined by the ways our bodies work and look.

EPIDEMICS AND MEDICAL INNOVATIONS: FROM SMALLPOX TO HIV

If medicine is defined as the set of theories and practices amassed to combat disease, then it inherently responds most effectively or at least with greater alacrity and conviction to already encountered diseases. Unfamiliar diseases test existing practice and demonstrate the gaps in theories about transmission, treatment, and the nature of disease itself. Frequently, epidemics produce significant innovations in medicine, though not always with great success. The Black Death prompted great strides forward in public health management, including the formal institution of quarantine, because it ravaged medieval Europe with such ferocity that containment seemed the best possible option (Slack 1988). Smallpox raged across Europe and North America during the seventeenth and eighteenth centuries to such an extent that "pockmarked" became one of the most common descriptors in London ads for missing persons. It was a frightening disease for many reasons, not the least of which was its tendency to infect pediatric populations and its relatively high mortality rate. It was also a strange disease according to contemporary ideas about epidemics, since it could only be contracted once. If a patient survived smallpox, she was very unlikely to get it again. This observation prompted the development of the practice of inoculation, in which an uninfected person's arm is scored and bandaged with material from an infected person in an attempt to promote a mild case of the illness and prevent future serious ones. The idea of giving someone smallpox raised serious questions, since sometimes inoculation caused a serious outbreak. A secondary observation—that people who had exposure to cows and the related disease of cowpox also seemed protected from smallpox—promoted the spread of inoculation; cowpox was a less serious disease, and the potentially harmful impact of inoculation was minimal to patients, in comparison to the risks of vaccination.

In the case of smallpox, another critical aspect of medicine, the social structure surrounding it, changed history. An English aristocrat, Lady Mary Wortley Montague, chose to inoculate her children rather than see them suffer and die from a disease that had killed so many. Because of her social class and her wealth, she made inoculation a common practice among her peers; within a few decades, the Sutton family created a cheaper and less dangerous version of inoculation that made the practice available to all classes, including the poor. Those subject to the Poor Law were experimental subjects for the new inoculation program, and the approach significantly decreased the rate of infection throughout urban areas in Europe (Thomas 1980). The smallpox vaccination also offered physicians in the New World the opportunity to move across social boundaries and build new networks (Gherini 2010). By the twentieth century, smallpox existed solely in laboratories, including those of the Centers for Disease Control (CDC) in Atlanta; this once devastating disease had been reduced to a potential mechanism of biomedical terrorism and a subject of infectious disease research.

Perhaps the greatest vaccination story in the history of medicine belongs to Jonas Salk, who in 1952 tested and perfected the vaccine that prevented polio. Salk benefited from funding provided by the March of Dimes organization with the support of polio victim Franklin Delano Roosevelt. The March of Dimes chose to fund the development of a vaccination because case numbers were still increasing in the early 1950s, and no clear understanding of polio transmission or patterns of immunity had emerged. In 1949, Salk was able to grow the polio virus in a cell culture, rather than the traditional host, a monkey. Within three years, he had produced the three different viruses causing polio, making a vaccine with the use of formalin; by killing the viruses, he decreased the risk to patients of contracting polio in the effort to prevent it. However, the first round of clinical trials across the United States and Canada resulted in 260 cases of polio and 10 deaths. The vaccination campaign did, however, dramatically reduce the rate of polio in the test groups, and in 1955, the United States deemed vaccination required for all schoolchildren. The next round of vaccinations was thoroughly tested to ensure that the virus used for the vaccine was, in fact, dead. Polio cases dropped dramatically in the wake of the vaccination program. In 1960, there were 2,525 cases of polio in the United States; in 1965, there were 61, and in 1990, there were 8, all of which were induced by the vaccine. The Salk vaccine has been a consistently successful preventative with 70–90 percent efficacy even in immune-impaired patient populations. In combination with the oral vaccine developed by Joseph Sabin, it has effectively eliminated naturally transmitted polio in North America and dramatically decreased it across the world (Oshinsky 2006).

Some epidemics, such as the influenza epidemic of 1916–1918, do not prompt significant medical innovation because they are simply beyond the grasp of all available medical and public health tools. The flu, felling people in otherwise good health and in young to middle age, was an aggressive epidemic of related diseases, including pneumonia and encephalitis lethargica, made famous by Oliver Sacks ([1976] 1990). The most lasting impact of this epidemic, beyond the fact that it killed more people than did combat in World War I, was the medical research it promoted. Samples of the 1918 flu circulated throughout the world's laboratories and contributed to significant improvements in our understanding of viral mutation (Eyler 2009). Despite all of our best efforts, however, the factors that made this particular flu virus so deadly or well suited to attacking an otherwise resilient population remain beyond current medical knowledge. We did, however, learn to manage better a public health disaster of such proportion (Holmes 2011; MacDougall 2007).

There is currently no effective vaccine against HIV/AIDS, though in 2009 an attempt that combined two failed vaccines had a heartening prevention rate of approximately one-third (Dolgin 2009), and recent studies have demonstrated promising avenues to pursue even more effective vaccines (Walker et al. 2011). Three decades after it emerged in the United States and Europe, HIV/AIDS continues to prey on our most human characteristics—carelessness and trust in the face of addiction, desire, and love. Thirty million people have died worldwide since "gay cancer" traveled across the Atlantic in the body of a French flight attendant and landed in San Francisco (Avert, n.d.). The original public health efforts to control the spread of HIV focused on educating the gay male population, especially in bathhouses and clubs, where drug use and anonymous sex were common. It was not clear, however, what exactly they were being educated about, since the CDC physicians could not originally determine whether sex or drugs were spreading the disease. Early efforts to stop the use of stimulants called *poppers* reflect that confusion, and it would take additional cases in other populations, especially intravenous drug users and Haitian immigrants, to demonstrate that HIV/AIDS traveled through the transmission of all body fluids. Thirty years later, decades in which we moved from a senator deeming the disease to be divine punishment for gay sex to endless campaigns to get people of every sexual inclination to use condoms, we still can't make it stop.

PUBLIC HEALTH RESPONSES TO EPIDEMICS: SEVERAL LIGHTS AND A LOT OF DARKNESS

The bubonic plague took advantage of newly mobile populations to spread to pandemic proportions. The economic boom of the high medieval period resulted in trade moving beyond the Mediterranean coast into northern and eastern Europe. As caravans traversed Europe, frequently bringing with them the rats they had imported from Arabia, Asia, and North Africa, they carried the plague along with the chance for prosperity and a reinvigorated global economy. The price Europe paid for this opportunity was very high; between 1348 and 1350, one-half to two-thirds of the European population died from one of three forms of plague. It would take another century for the continent to regain its lost socioeconomic ground. Burgeoning market towns and cities were decimated, and existing institutions, including the monarchies, municipal governments, and various incarnations of the Catholic Church, were strained beyond their surviving personnel and resources. The most lasting effect of the plague, however, was not the devastation it wrought, but the public health efforts it prompted. The practice of holding ships in harbor for twenty-four hours before allowing anyone to disembark, coupled with the practice of refusing to allow ships with diseased passengers to unload for two weeks after the last patient had either died or recovered reflected the realization that contagion traveled by ship, just like goods. The practice of quarantine also represented an evolving notion of disease transmission that depended on land travel linking urban areas, villages, and market fairs. Once a town or city had experienced its first cases of plague, its doors would be closed by municipal authority; people could neither leave nor enter for forty days until after the last victim had died or recovered (Aberth 2005).

In reality, these rules were often applied too late to stem the tide of people who could afford to flee the plague, especially when those who tried to leave frequently commanded significant power and wealth within their societies. Ironically, doctors and priests were among the first to flee infected cities, leaving a dedicated few to tend the dying. In this case, cultural practices collided with public health interests, but the efficacy of the practice, when properly applied, was an elegant response to evolving ideas about how diseases travel. A similar rule was applied to individual homes; any house in which a plague victim lived was identified by a white cross, and people could neither enter nor leave until the house had been cleared. Physicians and religious officials were the exception to this rule, though frequently the dying were left with only their families, or just the corpses of their deceased loved ones, to accompany their last days (Ziegler 1971).

The final important public health practice to emerge from the plague pandemic of 1348–1350 was an old one with a new twist; the bodies, clothes, and even household furnishings of the dead were burned, frequently with their bodies, on the outskirts of the city. When the bodies were not burned, they were buried, but even then, they were entombed outside city walls. This practice reflects the belief that disease was enshrined within the body it killed and could be transmitted by the corpse or the things it touched. The unlucky few who were paid to move the corpses and burn their belongings were most frequently from the poorest level of society. Their poverty forced them to take such a repulsive and dangerous job, often hastening their own deaths because they frequently took the clothes they were supposed to burn. Rather than destroying the plague-carrying fleas, they generously provided them with a new feast—their own flesh. This essentially human act, preserving and using the belongings of someone who has died, nearly guaranteed the deaths of the corpse bearers (Ziegler 1971). Here, as in so many other instances, the disease seemed primed to take advantage of its victims' weaknesses. The corpse bearers' appropriation habits also demonstrate the radical difficulty of regulating people, especially in the face of a deadly disease. While all of these public health responses were thoughtful reactions to a virulent pandemic, their inconsistent application and resultant failures are due as much to the tremendous challenge of controlling people, especially terrified people, as to their own inadequacy.

The state played an even more important role in addressing the public health crisis posed by the influenza pandemic of 1918. Appearing nearly simultaneously in the military training facility at Fort Riley, Kansas, and on the battlefields of France and North Africa, this new form of influenza began taking advantage of young men weakened by the straitened circumstances of a long and painful war. The flu rapidly moved beyond the confines of the military, extending its deadly reach into urban centers like Paris, London, New York, and Philadelphia. Between the fall of 1917 and the end of 1919, it claimed more lives than the war itself, over one million in total. Moreover, 675,000 American military personnel died of the flu, ten times the number that died in World War I. It affected every continent with especially high mortality rates in urban areas across the globe, striking New Delhi, London, New York, and Shanghai with equal force (Afkhami 2003; Humphries 2005; Patterson 1983; Rice and Palmer 1993; Tompkins 1992). The five centuries intervening between the Black Death and the flu epidemic of 1918 witnessed the creation of much stronger local, state, and federal governments as well as their powers to direct and control populations. This was especially true in the militarized environment of

World War I, a period in which people had become accustomed to accepting, for their own and the public good, limits on their freedom, including curfews, black-out hours, and the draft. Similar measures were employed to limit the spread of the flu, especially in cities. Philadelphia, for example, imposed rules about hospitalizing all infected people, governing the disposal of the dead, compelling all medical personnel to remain at work until the end of the epidemic, and defining the actions to be taken regarding the clothes and belongings of the dead. They also attempted a mass vaccination campaign, though given the unreliable nature of the vaccine, it cannot have contributed much (Eyler 2009).

The mayor and the public health director of St. Louis produced the most significant decline in flu cases in the United States epidemic by closing all public gatherings, including schools, theaters, and libraries (Wilson 2011). First, there were inevitable responses to a disease that was already on the ground. Moreover, the flu resembled, in its early stages, the less terrifying rhinovirus, so many infected people continued to go to work, travel on public conveyances, and socialize while infectious. Finally, in a time of war, more people were moving with greater frequency and over longer, less predictable distances. This meant that the flu could jump from one city to another in the body of an infected soldier who traveled for his leave or from one area of the front to another. Civilian movements also contributed to the spread of the flu. Given that so many men were at the front or had already died, women's incomes were a significantly larger part of household budgets than before the war. These women—married and single, young and middle-aged—worked in offices and shops, bringing the flu back to their homes and the children and elderly who waited there. They were reluctant to miss a day of work for minor symptoms, since their jobs could easily pass to another anxious young woman trying to support her family. Given these factors, the efforts to control the spread of the flu were always significantly behind the progression of the disease itself and demonstrated the inefficacy of human interventions in the face of such extraordinary viral efficiency.

Polio was the next epidemic to challenge the public health infrastructure. During the summers of the forties and fifties, polio claimed the lungs, legs, and lives of hundreds of thousands of children. It also prompted one of the most coherent public health campaigns of the American twentieth century, now even more impressive given there was no consensus about how the disease was transmitted. Reflecting social anxieties rather than medical truths, local and state governments across the United States assigned the cause to the poor, especially non-white, non-Protestant people. The campaign targeted flies, which were believed to spread polio by landing on diseased refuse and carrying it to the cribs of helpless infants. Posters, newspaper advertisements, and other announcements brought this message to suburban housewives, whose job was to protect their children from invading insects. Disinfection became the housewife's most important weapon, since aggressive cleaning with sufficiently antibacterial products would both discourage flies from landing in the house and remove any traces left behind. The class aspect of this public health message could not be overlooked, since the practice of weekly trash removal thrived in wealthy suburbs but was nonexistent in most urban areas and poor neighborhoods. As a result, poor areas experienced significant fly problems every spring and summer, while the suburbs remained relatively insect-free. The poor were depicted as a direct threat to the health of upper- and middle-class children, a theory that reflects many of the same anxieties aired in the debates over how best to control tuberculosis. In this case, however, the threat was quite literally in suburban kitchens and nurseries, where maids and nannies from poor neighborhoods threatened the health of wealthy children with the disease they might have carried from their trash-strewn streets and perpetuated with unsanitary practices. Coupled with the racial and economic divides already separating urban and suburban areas and the prejudice surrounding "old-fashioned" (read: poor, black) approaches to child care, this public health campaign wreaked cultural havoc while doing nothing at all to regulate the spread of polio. Even some of the public health officials of the time, including those enmeshed in these prejudices, found it hard to ignore the significantly higher mortality rates from polio in wealthy suburbs than in poor urban areas (Tomes 1998).

Not every public health effort is as racially and culturally motivated as the campaigns against flies. Such efforts have met with mixed receptions, however, because of the limits they place on personal freedoms. The Federal Emergency Management Association (FEMA) has enormous power to limit movement within the United States to protect public health in case of an epidemic. The powers of FEMA are defined in the Robert T. Stafford Disaster and Emergency Assistance Act (Public Law 93-288). Among other powers, it maintains the right to define a hazard or disaster, control lighting and communications during and after a hazard, enforce passive defense regulations, purchase and maintain properties and equipment required to respond to disasters and hazards, review and coordinate all state disaster response efforts, and use the resources of any related federal agency. Since March 2003, FEMA (www.fema.gov) has been part of the Department for Homeland Security and commands the same powers as that agency. Those powers, if abused, could reduce fundamental constitutional rights, including the freedoms of association and speech, to unrecognizably low levels and pave the way for the rise of a fascist state.

The Centers for Disease Control (www.cdc.gov), founded in 1946 and successfully contributing to American public health in the areas of epidemiology, education, and laboratory research, also has the potential to derail the Constitution. It maintains experimental reserves of infectious diseases that pose a viable threat to national security if they are ever mistakenly released or used as agents of bioterrorism. It also has the power to impose orders of isolation to end the free movement of affected populations and prevent the spread of an infectious disease. In 2007, the CDC issued its first orders of isolation since 1963 in response to the H1N1 flu outbreak.

Finally, the research institute at the now closed Walter Reed Army Medical Hospital maintained samples of many contagious diseases for its own experiments to combat bioterrorism. Among other specimens finding a new home at the Bethesda Naval Hospital are lung tissue samples from the first American military victims of the 1918 influenza virus. The threats posed by studying these diseases are not inherently less than the potential for finding a cure or means of prevention, but they are real. No institution has infallible security, so the chance that a pathogen is stolen and weaponized is always present. Just as frightening, and equally real, is the risk of a scientist being mistakenly infected by a pathogen and quite literally walking out the door with it, ready to infect a host of new subjects on the way home before he feels a single symptom.

The means by which diseases pass from one affected individual to another also demonstrate their potential uses as weapons. A disease like pneumonic plague, for example, has nearly perfect transmissibility and a mortality rate near 90 percent. In nature, pneumonic plague is so efficient that it destroys itself, decimating its population until it runs out of victims. Imagine its efficacy, then, as a weapon of mass destruction. Unleashed upon an isolated population, pneumonic plague would eliminate it. And if one person manages to leave the area after being infected but before dying, a period of one to three days, pneumonic plague would move beyond its intended targets to destroy civilization itself. Any highly infectious disease would do the same, as Ebola and cholera have demonstrated under natural conditions. Ebola is particularly dangerous because of its potentially long (up to twenty-one days) incubation period. Less infectious agents are no less dangerous if weaponized. The Hanta virus could decimate the world if released from its traditional hosts, field mice, and given free access to human populations. From hit television series like *The X Files* (1994–2002) and *24* to Justin Cronin's (2010) novel *The Passage*, popular culture delights in describing how remarkably stupid the decision to weaponize infectious disease would be. Cronin's plot borrows the governmental conspiracy theory proposed by the writers of *The X Files*, following the impressively bad results of a governmentally funded military attempt to infect death row inmates with a virus to create a race of supersoldiers. Unsurprisingly, the virus escapes and spreads across the United States, leaving only a few isolated communities of survivors to attempt to survive complete colonization by vampire human hybrids. The rollicking plotline notwithstanding, the novel clearly illustrates that the military can neither predict nor control human nature, not to say the movement of populations, enough to make the weaponization of epidemic diseases anything other than an elaborate and bloody form of mass suicide.

THE SOCIAL AND CULTURAL FRAMEWORK OF EPIDEMICS

Even the best-understood diseases, those that derive from known etiologies and display consistent and understood symptom progression, can baffle us. Knowing that a loved one will die is not made much easier by knowing how and why that death will occur. The specter of an unknown epidemic raging through a city and destroying families with impunity, leaving medical and public health authorities helpless in its wake is, however, somehow much worse. It brings out the best and worst of humanity, from those who volunteer to serve the ill though they know they are likely to join their numbers to scapegoating zealots who use the instance of an epidemic to spread their hatred and fear. It also spawned a new discipline, epidemiology, in which diseases themselves became the object of scrutiny. Epidemiology moves beyond bodies and symptoms to a macroscopic examination of the movement of disease through populations. It reveals the elegance of transmission and the challenges facing public health policy. Epidemics take advantage of the most human aspects of populations, thriving on human contact, proximity, and sex to destroy their hosts. The exceptionally moving opening scene of the 1993 film *And the Band Played On* (Spottiswoode 1993) demonstrates the ways that an efficient, deadly disease can reduce a successful village to desperation and ashes. The Ebola virus, a pathogen so small that only exceptionally powerful microscopes can see it, invites explanations that look to magic, Satan, or God as the source of the illness. Resorting to similar magical explanations also seems more comprehensible when the film demonstrates the failure of our favorite modern explanatory system, science, to do anything but map the path of HIV/AIDS in every urban center of the United States. Maps were the best science could offer; after the virus was isolated nearly simultaneously in French and American labs, the most effective tactic that emerged was epidemiology. Doctors were left with no effective treatment, no means of prevention, and a front row seat at patients' bedsides as they died from a variety of opportunistic infections. Thirty years later, Tony Kushner's (2003) epic play, *Angels in America*, makes more sense of that virus than all of our laboratory failures because it makes real the people who have lived and died with AIDS, rather than reducing it to a series of mortality statistics and the ongoing unsuccessful hunt for a vaccine.

Epidemics also reinvigorate old and spark new debates about the contested cultural meanings of disease and the role of disease as a signal of the relationship between God and people. The Black Death promoted a wide array of xenophobia and anti-Semitism, including multiple attacks on Jewish communities that were blamed for causing the plague by poisoning wells or bringing down God's wrath by killing Christian children to drink their blood. The plague also spawned some of the most radical public forms of religious expression of the medieval period, including scourging and self-flagellation in which large groups of people whipped themselves into a frenzy to appease God and end the epidemic. Plague parades in towns begging for God's forgiveness through mass displays of piety also demonstrate the importance of the divine in causing and alleviating disease (Cohn 2002; Raspe 2004).

Smallpox, because it spawned the first practical medical approach to preventing disease, also prompted significant religious debates about the role of medicine in mediating divine will. If disease was sent by God to test personal faith, as most eighteenth-century Protestants believed, then a practice that prevented disease might violate divine will and interfere with providence (Walsham 1999). Promoters of inoculation, including Protestant minister and physician Cotton Mather, argued that God gave people the tools to manage disease so that they might live well and faithfully and that refusing to use those tools was itself a violation of divine will. Despite the fact that vaccination with cowpox protected the vast majority of those treated with very few bad effects, some people still refused to inoculate themselves and their children because they believed it to be a direct violation of God's plan (Burton 2001; Miller 1956; Warner 1981).

While these responses seem logical in the medieval and early modern period, they are perhaps more surprising in twentieth-century America. When HIV/AIDS reached epidemic proportions among urban gay men, several members of the U.S. Congress as well as President Ronald Reagan interpreted this as evidence of God's rage against homosexuals. That narrative only began to lose power among religious conservatives, to the extent that it has, when "innocent victims" such as Ryan White made AIDS into a disease that anyone could get, rather than direct divine punishment for sexual transgression. When this book goes to press, many members of the religious right will still maintain that AIDS is divine punishment, and like those who marched in plague parades and scapegoated Jews during the Black Death, they maintain that a society permissive of sin is to blame for the disease.

Many of the cultural responses to epidemics have been paranoid and angry, perhaps because a poorly understood contagious disease ravaging a population tends to bring out the tensions underlying human communities. Tuberculosis, an epidemic that tore through Europe and North America in the mid-twentieth century, highlighted many of the social anxieties that complicated medical understandings of contagious diseases. The fact that tuberculosis crossed class boundaries produced a compelling and disturbing narrative about potential means of transmission. The symptoms of tuberculosis became intertwined with class narratives at both ends of the social spectrum, including neurasthenic aristocrats and the urban poor (Lomax 1977). Good health and strong lungs increasingly became a means of undermining elite claims to superiority, especially as tuberculosis was said to be an inherited, rather than a contagious, disease. The same claim was made in the late nineteenth century against the urban poor by no lesser medical minds than some of the leading physicians of the Johns Hopkins Medical School and the University of Pennsylvania Medical School ("Discussion on the Advisability of the Registration of Tuberculosis" 1894; Flick 1888). The debate over whether tuberculosis was inherited, contagious, or possibly both became an integral part of medical and public health debates and certainly made managing the disease significantly more difficult. Given its frustrating refusal to respond to any existing treatments, the social arguments about tuberculosis provided rich fodder for medical experts to exercise their prejudices, which included suggestions to limit the reproduction of affected individuals in an early argument for eugenics ("Discussion on the Advisability of the Registration of Tuberculosis 1894; Flick 1888; Frost 1937; Lerner 1994).

That said, some institutions have managed to produce positive responses to disease, including epidemics. The Catholic Church, for example, has devoted several orders of nursing sisters to the care of those afflicted by disease. Members of these orders have cared for patients of nearly every epidemic from the Black Death forward, and Mother Teresa's work with cholera, malaria, and leprosy victims in India has reinvigorated modern interest in the role of the Church in caring for the sick. Volunteers with the Red Cross (www.redcross.org) and Les Médecins sans Frontières (Doctors without Borders; www.msf.org) have provided consistent, direct support for patients for over a century. Within the United States, the Red Cross has also provided emergency medical care, public health assistance, and poverty relief since its founding. Its clean water programs, public health nurse training institutes, and first aid courses remain important parts of its mission. Evidence of its leading role within the American public health movement is the fact that its membership jumped from 17,000 to 310,000 in 1918. Les Médecins sans Frontières was created in 1971 by doctors and journalists; it now serves people in nearly sixty countries with members on the frontlines of wars, epidemics, and famines throughout the world.

CONCLUSION

The very present nature of epidemics reminds us of our frailty. Another virulent strain of influenza would decimate our population with the same efficiency of the 1918 version, but it would do so with the help of an even faster moving global population. We would respond with our best medical, public health, and scientific tools, yet history shows us that only the public health response would have any chance of making a meaningful impact on the epidemic itself. Science and medicine would produce innovations to prevent deaths from later, similar diseases. Students would see their worlds more clearly by studying what has killed us and how we have responded in the past. They might also feel something that is generally reserved for historians: a genuine connection to the people who lived before us.

Sitting with a dying loved one, especially with the sure knowledge that nothing can be done to save her, is among the most humanizing experiences I can imagine. It reduces us to our purest emotional form, the part of us that exists across historical contexts and outside of superficial divisions of time, space, and language. Love, fear, loss, all without hope of reprieve: these might be the most powerful unifying forces in the history of the world. Every one of us will sit at that bedside, some as health professionals and all of us as spouses, siblings, and children. Some of us already have. All of us will find something in the stories of plague, flu, polio, smallpox, and AIDS that remind us of who we are because of who and how we love.

ACKNOWLEDGMENTS

This article is dedicated to Noel, who during the summer of 2011 reminded me with her grace and extraordinary strength how to love in the face of death. With great appreciation to Andrea Woodner and Dr. Paul Mountan: we fought with her and we lost her. We will never be the same.

Chapter 42

CALCEDONIES

JEFF NISKER

To the woman I call Ruth and to Catherine Frazee

PLAYWRIGHT'S NOTE

Calcedonies should be considered a work of fiction although it is completely based on true occurrences in my interactions with two women I have had the privilege of knowing, though not well. The first woman, whom I call Ruth, made me promise to write about her in order to bring attention to a broken system that could easily be beautiful. So I wrote *Calcedonies* with the permission of this never broken, always beautiful woman. She told me to make sure I use her real name, but I have not, so as not to presume more insight into her lived experience than I have. I regret that she did not live long enough to read even the first draft of *Calcedonies*. She succumbed to one of the injustices depicted in this play. I wrote the memorial service scenes just before and immediately following her memorial service. However, it has taken me more than a decade to complete this script. I hope I have written the play she wanted me to write.

The other woman is Catherine Frazee, a disabilities scholar, activist, and writer. Catherine's presence in this play exists as the powerful keynote speaker in the penultimate scene and permeates my writing throughout. Her insight inspired, her kindness encouraged, and I have tried to weave her wisdom into every line. I hope I have written a play worthy of her presence.

All the injustices inflicted on the central character are true occurrences, representing only a tiny fraction of the lack of accommodation and the list of inequalities endured by disabled citizens in one of the world's wealthiest countries and its supposedly wonderful health and social support systems.

SCENE 1

To Stage Left is a small table on which sits a large mid-1990s Apple computer in classic translucent green. Large calcedony bookends bookend the computer on either side. Also on the table is a calcedony paperweight. Further to Stage Left is a narrow lectern facing away from audience. At Stage Right is a hospital bed, head cranked to 75 degrees, facing audience. The bed is covered in white sheets and a hospital-blue blanket.

Three intravenous (IV) bags are suspended from two "T-poles" inserted into the head of the bed. A hospital television set is suspended from a similar pole on the right side of the bed. A semicircle of simple straight-back chairs perimeters the stage, open to the audience. A large picture of the calcedony bookends is suspended stage back behind the chairs and can be colored by lights to cathedral-like hues in the memorial service scenes.

FRIEND sits in the first chair of the semicircle Stage Front and Right, head bowed, eyes open. FRIEND wears a black sport jacket over a black T-shirt and tan slacks. Lights for group home up On Stage. Spot on RUTH as she zooms onto stage in her power wheelchair. From the power chair's right armrest extends a chin-operated joystick. RUTH charges across Stage Front and pirouettes. RUTH gets out of chair and walks to desk (with assistance if required). RUTH wears a peasant dress popular in the late 1960s and early 1970s. RUTH has a large colorfully patched and fringed handbag of that time that she either carries on her shoulder or on her chair. A large agate pendant hangs from her neck on a black leather strap.

RUTH   Calcedonies are rocks.
   Crusty-surfaced rocks.
   That open to amethyst, agate, onyx, chrysoprase.
   And become jewelry, paperweights, bookends.
   For into each one's core,
   Millennia have poured alloyed amazement.
   Depending on their community,
   They endow their bearers with wisdom,
   Courage,
   Healing powers.
   Spiritual powers,
   Each calcedony is unique
   Wonderfully one of a kind.
   Friends used to give me calcedonies as gifts.
   Because I love them.
   Calcedonies and them.
   Like this paperweight

     [Lifts paperweight and places it back on desk.]

And this agate,

     [Lifts pendant from neck.]

My favorite calcedonies are my bookends.

     [Lifts one in each hand, does three arm curls, feigns fatigue, returns them.]

My bookends now bookend my computer,
'Cause my books ended.
Seventeen years without turning a page.
My computer waits patiently for me
To press its power button.

And I will one day.
Then these arcs on my bookends will become my rainbow.
And my computer will fly me over my rainbow
To a better-than-emerald place,
From which I will never return.

[*Walks with assistance if required to picture of bookends and uses laser pointer.*]

Don't my bookends look like a brain
On a TV doctor's MRI screen?
The "cerebral cortex."

[*Indicates bookends poster Stage Back with laser pointer, as in medical lecture.*]

The fluid-filled "ventricles."
Their brain resemblance reminds me
That I have a neurological condition.

[*Walking to power chair.*]

Not that I need bookends to remind me
That my brain no longer speaks to my muscles.
Any of my muscles.
Except those that open my eyes,
Move my eyeballs,
Breathe me,
And, most important, move my jaw.
My other muscles are useless.
So you're probably wondering how I can walk around like this?
Fine, I'll sit down if it's bothering you.

[RUTH *sits in power chair and positions her chin on joystick.*]

My brain still works.
Exceptionally well, actually.
As I'm sure you've already noticed.
Even my doctors think my brain works exceptionally well.
But as they see the rest of my body as so un-well,
It's easy for them to see my brain as exceptional.
I guess it's better to have a well brain than a well body.
I mean if you had to choose one or the other.
At least I think so.

[*Quickly moves chair to other side of stage.*]

I know you can't wait to hear more about my amazing brain muscles,
But first I must tell you about my amazing jaw muscles.
My jaw muscles allow me to speak,
Albeit very quietly,
And seldom heard.

They open my mouth so I can eat,
Although an attendant at the group home
Has to shovel the food in.
And most important,
My jaw muscles work this joystick on my chair,
The magic wand that propels me to the joy I have left.
Like dancing.

[RUTH *dances around stage in power chair in graceful arcs to "Unchained Melody," Righteous Brothers' version, then to Michael Jackson's "Billie Jean."* RUTH *"moonwalks" the chair backward to a wing, then races it across the stage front, then turns to face audience.*]

Not bad, eh?
Now where was I?
Each morning I patiently wait to be cleaned up,
Bum loaded into chair,
Chin placed on joystick,
Head strapped down.
But when the patient wait is finally over,
Which might be noon,
My joystick frees me.
At least to dash around the group home:
TV room, dining room, back to bedroom.

[*Stands and walks across stage to hospital bed.*]

When I'm in hospital,
And recovered enough from what got me here,
Sometimes someone has the time
To get me into my chair.
Then I really have fun.

[*Walks back to chair facing audience and sits in it with chin on joystick and hands on imaginary steering wheel.*]

I bomb down the halls at full throttle,
Pick up some serious speed,
Pick off a doctor or two.
I've made a blood sport of it.
When I spot a doctor down the hall,
I stop my chair.
Slowly move my jaw left or right,
Turning my chair's front wheels
To aim at the doctor's white coat,
As if it was a matador's red cape.
My left foot stamps the sand of the bullring.

[*Uses left hand for stomping motion.*]

Then push my jaw as forward as possible,
Charging at the matadoctor like a ferocious bull.
Doctors never notice me until I'm almost on them,
Because patients are invisible to doctors.
But when they see me bearing down upon them,
With no intention of swerving from my bloody course,
Surprise then terror grips their eyes,
And they plaster themselves against the nearest wall,
Or dodge into a patient's room.
I love scaring the shit out of doctors.
It's the most fun I ever have.
And I really do scare the shit out of some doctors.
My sense of smell still works you know.
And I always take a quick sniff as I speed by.
Of course I'm used to the smell of shit,
Steeping in it as I do
While patiently waiting for someone to clean me up.
Anyway, unlike matadors,
Matadoctors never beckon me to another charge.
In fact they usually flee next time they see me.
But just like matadors kill bulls,
The matadoctors will kill me in the end.
The crowd may even cheer.

> [*RUTH sits in chair, places her chin on joystick and freezes.*]

SCENE 2

> [*Lights fade to memorial service with spot on* FRIEND *again.* FRIEND *slowly lifts head.*]

FRIEND I sit amidst a "Circle of Friends,"
Eight women,
None who know me.
"It will be a simple service,"
I was told on the phone.
I said I had "another commitment,"
"A son's soccer practice,"
And apologized.
"You might say a few words."
I apologized again.
"Only if you're so moved."
Rainbows pour from the simple windows,
Melting their art on the silent circle.
All eyes are open,

Staring downward.
All hearts are open,
Embracing her life;
Except my heart,
Fixed in the formaldehyde of her death.

SCENE 3

[*Lights up for hospital room.* RUTH *stands and walks to Stage Front.*]

RUTH   Let me tell you more about my body.
   I could be burned at the stake like Joan of Arc,
   And feel no pain.
   At least until my chin caught fire.
   The no-pain thing amazes medical students.
   They come to practice neurological exams on me all the time I'm in,
   Which always includes the infamous pinprick test.
   You don't know what the pinprick test is?
   Little pricks . . . prick your skin . . . with little pins . . . to determine
   Which areas of skin are still connected to your brain.
   I refer to all medical students as "little pricks,"
   Having no insight into their true prick size.
   And of course there're more women in medical school
   Than when I first became a voodoo doll.
   If a medical student acts like an arrogant prick,
   I mess him up a bit.
   Like by shrieking in pain when they prick me,
   Or screaming "Fuck!"
   It's a hoot watching them flinch,
   Apologizing profusely.
   One little prick actually pricked himself.

   [*Sits on bed*]

So why am I in hospital getting pricked?
I get pressure sores
"Down there."
Because we who can't feel pressure
"Down there,"
Can't shift the weight off our butts
The way you who can feel your butts
Do all the time without realizing it.
They sometimes call these things bedsores,
Though the bed doesn't get sore.
And if a bedsore gets infected,
We get admitted to hospital

For IV antibiotics.
I made a nurse show me
What my infected bedsore looks like once.
She had to use two mirrors
To show me a dollar-size circle of black, red, and yellow crud.
Sort of an angry archery target.
One look was enough, thank you very much.

> [RUTH *sits back in chair and moves along Stage Front with occasional loops,*
> *flourishes, and other waltz-like moves, and she stops Stage Center.*]

Before I went from "able-bodied" to chin-bodied,
From free spirit to—
Well I'm still a free spirit,
But could easily be much freer
If I could just fucking get my joystick connected to my computer.
Sorry about that.
I was a sculptor:
Amazed each day by the beauty
Glazes baked on my clay,
And colored enamel bits melted on my carved copper.
I formed a special relationship with my copper kiln.
He was my partner in creating jewelry.
Yes my kiln is a "he."
His name is Fred.
And he was so much my partner in creation
That the sign on my studio read "Ruth and Fred."
When I was moved into my first chronic care "facility,"
I gave away my furniture, clothes, kitchen things,
Even my books,
But I couldn't give Fred away.
So I asked a friend to keep him for me in her garage.
He might still be there.
I know that Fred will never help me create again.
But I will create again.
Through poetry.

> [*In voice from* "The Six Million Dollar Man."]

"We have the technology,"

> [RUTH *walks over to her computer and smiles.*]

It's an Apple.

> [*Looks fondly at computer.*]

Apple developed disability-friendly software years ago.
So I cashed in my life savings to buy this beauty.

[*Caresses computer.*]

My chin will operate it through my joystick
The way your hand uses a mouse.
Only I won't need a mouse pad.
The software platform will be my rocket-launching pad,
And I will blast off from this world of exclusion,
And I will never "reenter."
It has voice-activated software,
Called "Dragon."
Dragon will allow me to communicate with people
And to write the poems
I have collected in my heart for so many years.
I will speak a line,
See the words appear on the screen,
Spend all day gently massaging the words
As they gently massage me.
But a bio-med-i-cal engineer is required
To calibrate my jaw with the computer program
That will interface my face with my computer's face.
I've been on the waiting list for over a year now.
And was told it could be another two-year wait.
Because there're only two bio-med-i-cal engineers in our "Region"
Who can connect the umbilical cords of people "like me."
And no more can be hired.
Because of the fucking funding cutbacks.
Sorry again.
So I wait.
I patiently wait.

SCENE 4

[*RUTH stands, exits Stage Right, and returns quickly with a hospital gurney.
There are two IV poles attached to the head of the gurney, and three plastic IV
bags hang from the poles with their IV tubing pinned to the stretcher under
the white sheet. RUTH pushes the stretcher to Stage Front Center and orients it
parallel to Stage Front. RUTH then lies on the stretcher and covers herself with the
white sheet. Once RUTH covers herself with the sheet, FRIEND walks to behind
the center of stretcher and faces the audience. Light comes down on them.*]

FRIEND The patient's face seems familiar to me,
As the Clinical Fellow rapidly presents
The patient's history and clinical findings.
[*Rapidly*] "A 3 cm infected bedsore ulcerating skin of vulva,
Just south and to left of vagina.
Came in unconscious through ER three nights ago.

Total body sepsis from spread of infection from bedsore.
Triple antibiotic therapy.
Still out of it.
Nothing more we can do for bedsore,
Or for her for that matter.
Quadriplegic."
[*Pause*] Quadriplegic.
I knew I've seen this woman before.
In fact I've seen her several times over the years,
Racing down our hospital's halls in her electric wheelchair.
I remember once she lost control of her chair
And almost plowed me over.
I remind the Clinical Fellow to always treat my patients like they're fully
     awake.
He quips, "We're not in the operating room,"
An attempt at a joke as I am well known (and derided)
For insisting my anesthetized patients are treated as if they are awake.
I have insisted this ever since I was a Clinical Fellow,
And a large woman had written on her abdomen prior to surgery
"No fat jokes please," in indelible ink.
The Clinical Fellow urges, "She really can't hear us,"
Then shouts at her,
[*Shouting*] "Do—you—know—where—you—are?"
Then claps his hands in front of her face.

   [*Claps loudly three times.*]
   [*Pause with* FRIEND *staring at* RUTH's *eyes.*]

I ask our patient's name.
He replies, "Ruth ____."
"Hello, Ruth,
I'm sorry that you're not feeling well."
[*Pause*] "Ruth, I need to examine the bedsore on your vulva."
The Clinical Fellow gives me his "Don't you trust me" look.
[*Pause*] "You may not be able to give me your permission,
But it is important that I examine your bedsore."
The nurse helps me position the white sheet below Ruth's knees.
We gently lift the emaciated calf muscles
Upward and outward to the "frog leg" position.
I part the white curtains.
To the infected ulceration.
I say to myself, "I hope the antibiotics can ameliorate this,
I don't think surgery is the answer."
I close the curtains.
I say to Ruth, what I'm sure she has heard so many times before,
"I'm sorry, but there's nothing more we can do."

Then I pull the chart from the Clinical Fellow's hands.
He is taken aback.
Because I've never done this before.
He urges, "They must be ready to start our case in the OR."
I flip back the pages to the very beginning.
[*Pause*] Ruth's date of birth and mine are identical:
Same year, same month, same day.
My eyes rivet the hundreds of haunting pages.

SCENE 5

[*RUTH gets out of gurney and lies on hospital bed (60 degrees up) facing audience. FRIEND pushes gurney into wing, returns to his chair and sits.*]

RUTH I have another bedsore,
And this one got infected.
Really infected.
And the infection spread through my body so quickly
That by the time the ambulance got me to Emerg—

[*FRIEND stands and hesitantly takes a few steps toward RUTH.*]

I'll have to tell you about that later
Because some strange doctor has just come into my room,

[*FRIEND keeps looking over shoulder back at the door as he walks even more hesitantly to RUTH.*]

I think he's in the wrong room.
That happens sometimes.
His first words to me are,
FRIEND [*Hesitantly walks to bed.*]
"I am no longer your physician,"
RUTH Like God talking to Moses in *The Ten Commandments*.
So I carefully choose my first words to him.
"Who the fuck are you?"
But as I'm still weak from infection
"Fuck" comes out quieter than usual
So he's not sure he hears me right.
Or can't believe he hears me right.

[*FRIEND looks like he wants to leave, but he takes a chair, places it close to head of bed, sits on chair, and brings his ear close to RUTH's lips.*]

RUTH [*Loud*] "Who-the-fuck-are-you?"

[*FRIEND jolts back.*]

FRIEND I'm sorry, I'm Doctor _____.

RUTH   Let's leave out his name to protect the guilty.

FRIEND   "May I speak with you for a few minutes?"

RUTH   "Well, Doc, you're really lucky
  I just happen to have some free time in my crowded social calendar
  Because my Pilates class was cancelled."

FRIEND   [*Sheepishly*] "I want to apologize to you."

RUTH   "You should, Doc,
  It's late and I need my beauty sleep
  If I'm ever going to hump a pole again."

  [FRIEND *looks stunned, hesitates, then plods onward.*]

FRIEND   "I'm apologizing for watching the colors of your TV set
  Reflect on your face while you were sleeping last night."

RUTH   "Doc, if you were that interested in what was on TV,
  You could've turned the TV around to watch it."

  [FRIEND *looks stunned.*]

  No sense of humor,
  No doctors have a sense of humor.
  But get this, after watching my face for a bit,
  He, and these are his exact words,

FRIEND   "Felt like a voyeur."

RUTH   So he decided to leave.
  But before he left he shut off the TV,
  And separated its neckset arms from my ears.

FRIEND   "To let you sleep more peacefully."

RUTH   But when he stepped out of my room,

FRIEND   "I froze in a shower of stupidity."

RUTH   Because he realized that if I woke up

FRIEND   "You wouldn't be able to turn the TV back on."

RUTH   Nor press the button to call a nurse to turn it back on.

FRIEND   "You'd just stare at the dark screen
  Because of my ____"

RUTH AND FRIEND   "Misplaced assistance."

RUTH   I like "stupidity" better.

FRIEND   "So I returned and moved the TV back to where I thought it was,
  Turned it back on to the same channel I hope,
  And placed the audio pieces back in your ears."

RUTH   Very strange doctor.

FRIEND   "I also want to apologize
  For examining you last week when you were unconscious.
  [*Pause*] Without your permission."

RUTH   Whoa.
  "Really, Doc.
  And exactly what part of me

Did you examine without my permission?"

FRIEND "I examined the bedsore on your vulva."

RUTH [*Pause*] "O . . . K . . ."

I really thought doctors couldn't say anything to throw me off anymore.

So of course I make him explain in great detail what a "VULVA" is,

Insisting on all the anatomical and functional details.

[*To* FRIEND] "And what exactly did you do to my "VULVA," Doc?

Let me summarize:

He looked at my crotch,

And, yes, he touched my crotch.

I clearly must've been out of it

Because that's the sort of thing a gal remembers,

Even if she can't feel her "VULVA."

FRIEND "I'm glad you don't remember me.

I don't want any vestige of a doctor-patient relationship to exist."

RUTH "Vestige?"

FRIEND "Because I want to ask your permission to visit you as a friend.

You're free to say 'no,'

Or, if you say yes now,

You can change your mind at any time."

RUTH He's asking my permission in such a formal way,

That I'm surprised he doesn't shove a consent form in my face,

And put a pen in my hand to sign it.

Not that he wouldn't have, if I could have.

He says he's written a note on my chart

Dissolving our physician-patient relationship,

And asked a colleague to see me in follow-up.

"So why do you want to be my friend, Doc?

If you stay my doctor

You can bill the system for visiting me.

Even bill double for a Sunday night like tonight.

Even if you don't look at my VULVA anymore.

Although I must have one hell of a VULVA."

[FRIEND *tries to speak but freezes with stunned look again.*]

RUTH "Now why exactly did you want to be my friend instead of my doctor?"

FRIEND "We have identical dates of birth."

RUTH "What?"

FRIEND "We were born same year, same month, same day."

RUTH Born same day.

This is getting

[*Sings "Twilight Zone" tune.*]

"Don't tell me that in addition to looking at my VULVA

You actually looked at my chart.

Only nurses and medical students ever look at a patient's chart."
[*To audience*] Being exactly the same age has connected him with me in
    some way.
Probably in a there-but-for-the-grace-of-God-go-I way.

> [*FRIEND turns and begins to walk out but stops.*]

FRIEND   "Ruth, the arms of the TV's audioset in your ears last night
    Made it look like you were wearing a stethoscope,
    Listening to the TV's heartbeat."

> [*FRIEND turns again to leave.*]

RUTH   [*In "Rocky" voice*] "Yo, Doc
    If you're not too busy,
    Drop in after work tomorrow."
    [*To audience*] Better than boredom.
FRIEND   "I'd love to, but tomorrow is Monday."
RUTH   "Monday, no kidding Doc?
    Quads do know the days of the week."

> [*FRIEND looks stunned again.*]

FRIEND   "On Monday nights, I do an elective for our medical students."
RUTH   "An 'elective'?"
FRIEND   "It means that the students are not required to attend."
RUTH   "Then why would they?"
FRIEND   "I guess they come because they like what we discuss."
RUTH   "And what about those who don't come?"
FRIEND   "Most of the guys stay and watch Monday Night Football. Sorry, I really
    have to go."

> [*FRIEND quickly leaves.*]

SCENE 6

> [*Spot on* RUTH *as she gets into chair and wheels to beside back-facing lectern and
> faces audience. Second spot on* FRIEND *as he enters and hurries toward lectern
> but encounters* RUTH *on the way.*]

RUTH   He hurries into the hospital's lecture theater
    Seconds before he's scheduled to begin.
    He sees me right away.
    He has no choice,
    As my chair is right in front of the front doors.
    I have no choice,
    As wheelchairs can only enter at the front,
    And then there are steps.
    I can tell he wants to start his class,

But he just keeps staring at me,
Probably wondering how I got a doctor to write the order
For me to leave the ward.
(No order of course was ever written.)
And how I knew where the lecture theater was.
(I've been displayed here several times over the years.)
He forces his stare away from me
To smile at the hundred or so medical students behind me,
Who are also trying not to stare at me.
But stare anyway,
Looking for clues to what I have:
Half-filled piss bag beside my chair's left wheel,
No movement of limbs,
Head supported front and back.
Obviously something neuromuscular.
Car accident quads aren't interesting enough
To be displayed in large lecture hall.
His feet come even closer to mine,
So he's sure I can see him.
He thanks me for coming and tells me,
FRIEND   "You're looking very well tonight."
RUTH   Give me a break.
    Then he quickly asks my permission
    To introduce me to the students.
FRIEND   "Not as a patient here but as your friend."
RUTH   He wants my permission again.
    "Why not introduce me as someone born the identical day as you?"

    [*FRIEND starts to speak but stops.*]

"Hey Doc, what do you think of my slippers?"
He looks down at my furry bear paw slippers,
Complete with black felt claws.
He's just about to tell me how much he likes my slippers
When I interrupt again with, "I've had these for years."

    [*FRIEND opens mouth and freezes again.*]

He's trying to determine whether I'm making a joke
(Because slippers don't wear out when you don't walk on them),
Or am I innocently applauding the staff for not losing them
(Me, innocent),
Or am I trying to throw him off
His carefully thought-out introduction to tonight's "exploration."
Finally he forces his jaw to work
And fumblingly welcomes the students and introduces the topic.
He then smiles and takes a deep breath:

FRIEND "We have a guest with us tonight,
My friend, Ruth."

SCENE 7

[*RUTH gets onto the bed and covers herself.*]

RUTH Now that I've made my way back to my room,
Been lifted back into bed,
Piss bag changed,
Teeth brushed,
TV channel turned to the one I've calculated
To have the fewest bad shows till I fall asleep,
Let me tell you what the medical students got tonight.
Seven student "volunteers" came to the front
And took turns reading stanzas of two poems by Rilke.
I knew the one about the panther
Pacing the perimeter of its cage,
Paralyzed by the bars.
Then the students watched part of a film
About a man in Victorian England,
Who had these huge lumps on his body,
And had to hide or be taunted.

SCENE 8

FRIEND When I walked into the meeting room,
I was again asked to "Share a few words."
I repeated I could not.
"Only if you want to."
"I apologized again."
"Only when you're ready to."
I knew I never would be ready to,
Reeking of remorse about her life,
Guilt about her death.

[*Looks across at semicircle of chairs.*]

The woman who met me at the door lifts her eyes,
And tells a warm anecdote about "our Friend."
She finishes too soon for me.
The ensuing silence consumes me.
I feel all eyes upon me
Finally another woman lifts her eyes,
And speaks about "our Friend's" great sense of humor.
All smile, [*Pause*] Except me.

SCENE 9

[RUTH *in peasant dress sits in her chair and wheels to beside back-facing lectern and faces audience.*]

RUTH This time he runs in
  With a whole three minutes to spare.
  Of course, I sit in the same place.
  Of course, he gives me the same stunned look,
FRIEND "I'm sorry you're back in hospital."
RUTH "I'm not back in hospital.
  A van that moves us disableds
  Out of our storage facilities and back in again
  Got me here."
FRIEND "I'm glad you're not ill again."
RUTH Then he quickly welcomes the students before I can throw him off,
  And finishes with
FRIEND "Our friend Ruth has joined us again."
RUTH This Monday Night's not as powerful.
  Just one very long one-woman Victorian play
  About mental illness.
  The strange doc-who-wants-to-be-my-friend
  Told the students he adapted it from a short story
  With "permission of the estate of the author."
  I did like the way the play showed
  How women can be confined by the times in which they live,
  And by the medical profession.
  I also liked the medical student actor.
  She didn't miss one line
  Of those thousands and thousands of lines.
  I'll bet she'll remember every line of every medical textbook she reads.
  She also seemed very sensitive.
  I want her to be my doctor on both counts.
  When the "exploration" is over,
  A bunch of students surround me,
  Asking how I'm feeling,
  How I liked the play,
  What I thought of their buddy's memorization skill.
  Out of the corner of my eye I see my strange doctor,
  Grinning like a Cheshire cat.
  After all the students are gone,
  He walks over, still smiling,
  And asks if he can "accompany me" to the van.
  I rapidly lead onward.
  He stupidly walks behind my chair
  As if he's pushing it.

When we come to the closed doors
Separating the lecture halls from the rest of the hospital,
He dashes round my chair,
And bows as he opens the doors for me.
So *gal-lont.*

  [*Speeds wheelchair across Front Side of Stage.*]

I speed down the hall to the elevators.
He catches up puffing, blushing, apologizing.
Eventually it dawns on him to press the down button.
He smiles.
The elevator comes quickly as "Visiting hours are now over."
I pirouette my chair and quickly back in.
He presses G
Then proceeds to tell about his claustrophobia
Since a teenager because of a recurring dream.
Just as the elevator doors open to the ground floor.

  [*Speeds wheelchair to Center Stage*]

I make a beeline for the front doors
Even though I know the automatic doors don't work after nine.
He catches up and smiles.
I tell him, "I would like to wait outside,
It's a beautiful evening after all."
He proudly presses the door's "ALARM WILL SOUND" lever-bar,
Telling me, "It's okay, the alarm won't sound,
I always use this door at night to quickly get to my car."

  [*Speeds wheelchair to opposite side of stage.*]

I dash out, turn left, and stop before the sign
Prohibiting smoking near the doors.
My strange-doctor friend catches up
And asks my "permission" to wait with me.
I tell him, "The van's usually late,
May not be here for an hour."
FRIEND "I would still like to wait with you if that's okay,
  'It's a beautiful evening after all.'"
RUTH "Okay, Doc, then make yourself useful,
  Fetch me a cig from the sack behind my chair."
FRIEND "You smoke?"
RUTH "Of course not, smoking would be bad for my health."
  He tries not to glance at the no smoking sign.
  I don't tell him that I always smoke in front of this sign,
  Just to see if any security guard has the rocks
  To make me move further from the door.

They never do.
Afraid of me for some reason.
Maybe they think they'll catch what I got.
"My cigs please."

[FRIEND *hesitantly walks to back of chair and very gingerly places his hand in sack.*]

He's carefully feeling around in my sack,
Probably embarrassed to have his hand in a woman's purse,
Afraid of what he might touch.

[FRIEND *finally pulls out the pack of Marlboros and holds it in front of* RUTH's *face.*]

FRIEND I found them.
RUTH "Now take a cig out of the pack."

[FRIEND *slowly draws cigarette out of pack*]

He's drawing it out of the pack
As if it's a nuclear rod.
"Now into my mouth please,"
"Come on, I promise not to tell anyone that you're hastening my death."
He's a blushing iceberg,
But I'm getting really pissed off.
You'd be pissed off too if a cig was taunting you
Mere inches from your mouth.
"Just put the fucking thing in my mouth!"
FRIEND Fine.

[*Shoves cigarette deep into* RUTH's *mouth.*]

RUTH [*choking*] "Take it out."
FRIEND "Sorry, sorry, sorry, sorry _____."
RUTH "Just put it back in!
    But just a little way this time."

[FRIEND *very gently places the cigarette at the edge of* RUTH's *lips.* RUTH *tightly clamps on to cigarette, rotating her lips to move it further into her mouth.*]

FRIEND "In okay?"
RUTH "Would I be working my mouth like a camel if it's IN OKAY?"
FRIEND "Sorry."

[*Gently pushes cigarette in further.*]

RUTH He stands there like a dolt
    Staring at my cig,
    I sit here like a patient woman,
    Staring at his stupid face.

"You don't expect me just to suck on it
Like a fucking candy cigarette?"

FRIEND   "I'm sorry. Do you have any matches in your purse?"

RUTH   [*Glaring at* FRIEND] He cautiously excavates my purse again
While I'm dying here.

> [*FRIEND embarrassed with hand in purse. Then raises matches high in victory, proud of himself, and then holds them in front of* RUTH's *face.*]

FRIEND   "Do you want me to light your cigarette for you?"

RUTH   I'm ready to kill him but instead say,

> [*Billy Crystal's Fernando Lamas:*]

"That would be M-A-H-V-E-L-O-U-S,
That is if you think you can light it without burning my face."
But the joke's on me.
He fumbles with the matches like he's never lit one before.
He scratches and scratches,
Finally a flame,
But it goes out before it reaches my cig.
Because his hands are shaking like he has a neurological problem himself.
I'm glad he's never going to operate on me.
I wish I could steady his hands in mine like in the movies.
[*Next match gets to cigarette and* RUTH *frantically puffs.*]
The fucking flame went out.

FRIEND   Okay, okay.

> [*Scratches match after match and puts flame to cigarette.*]

RUTH   [*Puffs and puffs, then*] Ahh . . . Ahh . . . Ahh.

FRIEND   "You look like a movie gangster,
With the cigarette in the corner of your mouth like that."

> [RUTH *cradles cigarette in corner of mouth. Ignores him.*]

FRIEND   [*In movie gangster voice*] "Tell me everything."

RUTH   I think he's trying to make a gangster movie joke,
I go with it though.
"I've committed no crimes I know of."
Then instead of telling him "everything" about me,
I tell him "everything" about his healthcare system,
And what he can do with it.
I love how he flinches in pain
Each time I skewer his profession,
Which he apparently loves,
And definitely has endless excuses for.
Like,

FRIEND   "We've less than half the doctors per citizen of any developed country,"

RUTH Like,
FRIEND "We do the best we can under hospital funding cutbacks,"
RUTH Like,
FRIEND "Don't blame the physicians
Blame the politicians,
And the citizens who voted them in
For personal income tax cuts."
RUTH All the while he tries not to stare at the bobbing ash of my cig.
Or at the ash falling on my shawl
I know he wants to brush the ash off
But he's afraid to touch me.

    [*FRIEND timidly brushes air above shawl.*]

Now he's worrying the cig's getting too short
And my lips will burn.
FRIEND "Can I take it out?"
RUTH "Sure, if it's making you nervous,
But you're wasting good tobacco.

    [*FRIEND gently removes the butt and looks for a place to dump it.*]

Light me another thank-you-very-much."

    [*FRIEND searches purse again, then remembers Marlboros are on the ground
where he dropped them.*]

I usually have just one cig in the evening.
But it's such a riot watching this doctor struggle
That I keep asking him to light me cig after cig.
He tries not to look relieved when the van arrives.
I try not to look disappointed,
But I was hoping the driver forgot about me.
That happens you know.
Tonight's driver,
A burly guy about our age,
Walks round to our side of the van.
He smiles as he swings open the barn doors,
And presses the button that lowers the elevator platform.
I gun my chair forward onto the platform,
"Thanks for the drags, Doc."
And am hauled up and into the van.
As there's no room to turn my chair,
I stare out the window on the opposite side
At a vacant bus shelter and a yellowish street light.
I hear the ratcheting down of my chair to the van's floor,
Then the metallic thud of the closed doors.
The driver walks past the window.

His weight enters the van.
The motor rumbles on,
The bus shelter and street light move left and are gone.
Suddenly I see my strange-doctor friend running beside the window,
Frantically waving goodbye with both hands,
And mouthing like an orangutan,
"T-H-A-N-K Y-O-U F-O-R C-O-M-I-N-G"
He's going to get hit by a car.
He keeps this up for a while,
But finally disappears left.
Probably collapsed on the street.

SCENE 10

[RUTH wheels to Center Stage Front.]

RUTH   I'm back in hospital for some plumbing problems.
Nothing serious.
I saw my strange-doctor-supposed-friend today
While I was bombing down the halls on his floor.
Too bad he saw me coming,
And jumped out of the way,
Or I would have flattened him good.
With all his "I want to be friends" bullshit,
He never visited me at the group home.
Not once in six months.
And it's so close to the hospital.
Anyway after he peeled himself off the wall,
He asked my room number so he could visit me later,
And dashed off.

SCENE 11

[FRIEND walks to Center Stage Front, stands beside RUTH and talks to
the audience]

FRIEND   I saw Ruth while I was waiting for an elevator.
She was hurrying over to say hello,
But lost control of her wheelchair,
And almost crashed into me.
I told her how glad I was to see her,
But she misunderstood and said,
"You're glad I'm back in this ____
[Pause] Place."
She used an adjective before "place"
Because she doesn't like hospitals.

I was late for a meeting so couldn't talk to her,
But I'll try to see her after work.

SCENE 12

[*RUTH gets into bed*]

RUTH   All patients learn to be patient.
 That's why we're called "patients."
 We have no choice but to be patient patients,
 Except for some rich patients,
 Who are "connected."
 And patient patients are invisible while they wait:
 Invisible to doctors obviously,
 But also to nurses and receptionists.
 Family members also learn to be patient.
 And they don't get a dime for waiting room time,
 Or transportation time,
 Or help at home time.
 But I am "no longer patient."
 I need my joystick connected to my computer.
 Now.
 I've waited almost three years,
 And can't fucking wait any longer.
 There are things I want to learn,
 Places I want to see,
 Words I need to write.
 And no doctor thought I'd live this long.

SCENE 13

[*RUTH is sitting up in hospital bed. FRIEND rushes over and mimes caring and concern gestures while RUTH speaks.*]

RUTH   [*To audience*] He rushes into my room after six.
 Starts with his usual greeting, caring, concern for my health.
 But, like all doctors, he's already got one foot out the door.
 Doesn't even have time to draw the curtain around my bed.
 After less than a minute of the bullshit he looks at his feet,
 As he always does just before he starts apologizing for having to leave,
 Then, as usual, he asks me,
FRIEND   "Is there anything you need?"
RUTH   I always just stare.
 He always just leaves.
 But this time his feet don't move.
FRIEND   "Since you're back in hospital and looking so well"

RUTH [*To audience*] Something's coming.
    Probably wants some students to see me or something.
FRIEND "Would you give me permission to bring my children in to meet you?"
RUTH [*To audience*] Well, well, well.
    And he hasn't surprised me for a while.
FRIEND "It would only be for a few minutes.
    But I'd like you to say a few words to them.
    But only if you want to.
    And only if you're feeling well enough to.
    Please feel free to say no."
RUTH Does this nutbar think I could possibly say,
    No, I'd rather not meet your kids?
    "Permission" to bring in your kids,
    Give me a break.
    So of course I say
    [*To* FRIEND] "I'm dying to meet your kids."
FRIEND "Thank you, I'll bring them to your room in an hour or so."

        [*Turns and starts leaving.*]

RUTH "Wait a second,
    Let's meet in my favorite part of the hospital."
FRIEND [*Hesitantly*] "Favorite part?"
RUTH "You know where,"
FRIEND [*Hesitates again*] "I do?"
RUTH "Outside the front doors."
FRIEND "Well, I don't—ah—"
RUTH " 'It's a beautiful evening after all.' "
FRIEND "I'm not sure it's a—"
RUTH "I promise not to smoke in front of your kids."
FRIEND "Thank you."

        [*Turns and starts to leave.*]

RUTH "But only if you tell me about your recurring dream."
FRIEND "Recurring dream?"
RUTH "The one that makes you claustrophobic in elevators."
FRIEND "I can't."
RUTH "Then I might just ask you in front of your kids
    If you would join me in another cigarette.
    Marlboros are your favorites aren't they, Macho Man?"
FRIEND "I'd rather not talk about my dream."
RUTH "You'd rather not talk about anything having to do with you.
    But I really want to know about your dream.
    Maybe I can help you get over your claustrophobia."
FRIEND "You'll think I'm ridiculous."
RUTH "Not to worry.

I already find you ridiculous."
Now put your ass in that chair,
Pretend it's a couch,
And tell me your dream.

[FRIEND *sits tentatively and looks down.*]

FRIEND "There's a tumultuous lake."
RUTH "Very original."

[FRIEND *gets up.*]

RUTH "I'm sorry.
[*Yawns*] I promise not to interrupt again."
FRIEND [*Sits*] "We're standing on a pier,
We, being the neighbors on my childhood block.
A fourteen-year-old me
Stands between my mother and Mrs. Warner,
The beautiful woman who lives next door.
Mrs. Warner is holding the hand of her five-year-old son Jamie.
Suddenly a hard wave smashes into the pier
And sweeps Jamie into the roiling water.
He looks at me just before he's sucked down.
My mother grasps my arm and turns me toward her.
Her eyes beseech, "Don't."
I love my mother
But I'm the strongest swimmer on the street.
I dive in, but can't find Jamie.
I duck dive again and again.
I see a cave under the pier.
I swim in a ways and find Jamie.
He's very frightened.
I mouth, "Everything will be okay,"
Grasp his hand and turn to swim him out.
But there are two tunnels.
I choose one and swim Jamie down it,
But it gets narrower and narrower.
I have trouble turning us around.
I swim back as hard as I can.
I feel Jamie's body go limp.
I drag him with all that I have,
Running out of breath.
[*Gasping*] Fighting panic with every stroke,
[*Gasping*] And wake up gasping for air,
[*Gasping*] Drenched in water."
RUTH "You mean sweat."
FRIEND [*Pauses, still gasping.*]

RUTH "Okay, we're making progress here.
　　Besides elevators what else gives your claustrophobia?"
FRIEND "Being buried in the sand by my kids.
　　Being buried in the sand is the worst."
RUTH "For me, too."

　　[FRIEND *stares at* RUTH *then quickly leaves.*]

SCENE 14

RUTH [*Gets out of bed and goes to front of stage.*]
　　I wonder what he's told his kids about me.
　　Maybe she's like that guy in the *Star Trek* episode,
　　Where all that remains of him
　　Is his head mounted on a brainwave-operated wheelchair
　　After a radiation explosion.
　　I've seen that episode many times.
　　Seen all the *Star Trek*s many times
　　Like every other series in syndication.
　　You know, I think that episode is called "The Menagerie."
　　Well the nurses do call this place "a zoo" when things get crazy busy,
　　Which is most of the time.
　　So bring on the kids,
　　Let them see the most ferocious animal in this fucking zoo.

SCENE 15

FRIEND I pick up my sons,
　　Take them to "Wendy's Pick-up Window,"
　　Where they order grilled chicken with broccoli-cheddar baked potatoes,
　　As trained to,
　　And head back to the hospital.
　　There is silence in the car except for chewing jaws.
　　My mind is immersed in the novel *To Kill a Mockingbird,*
　　The part where Atticus Finch sends his twelve-year-old son Jem
　　To read to a seemingly unconscious woman.
　　Jem would rather be doing anything else during his summer holidays
　　Than reading all afternoon to a woman who can't even hear him.
　　A nurse comes in now and then and sends Jem out for a few minutes.
　　Over the weeks Jem notices that the nurse came in less frequently,
　　Then not at all,
　　And that the woman gradually acknowledges him more and more.
　　When the woman dies, Atticus explains to his son
　　That the woman had insisted on backing off the medicine
　　That took away her pain but made her sleepy

Because she wanted to fully experience life again before she died.
Atticus was teaching his son courage.

SCENE 16

[*RUTH sits in hospital bed. FRIEND sits beside her.*]

RUTH He's come alone to see me three nights in a row.
Three nights in a row is a new world's record,
And I guess his way of thanking me for permission to bring his kids in. They
    were very quiet.
I was very quiet.
That is until we started talking about movies.
I asked what their favorite movies are.
One said, "*The Great Escape*."
Another, "*The Bridge On the River Kwai*."
The third said, "*Ghostbusters*."
Tonight when my strange doctor friend asks before he leaves,

[*FRIEND stands and turns to leave*]

FRIEND "Is there anything you need?"
RUTH Instead of just staring,
I whisper, "Hey you born-the-identical-day-as-me,"
FRIEND "Yes."
RUTH "I need my chair's joystick hooked up to my computer."
FRIEND [*Laughing*] "I'm sorry but my experience with computers is confined
    To helping my kids find 'Carmen Sandiego.'"

[*FRIEND leaves but comes back in a few seconds and pulls up chair.*]

RUTH He draws the drapes around my bed.
FRIEND "I'm sorry. Tell me about—"

[*Blackout.*]

SCENE 17

[*Spot on FRIEND standing beside lectern.*]

FRIEND [*Urgency in voice*] I call our Regional Biomedical Engineering
    Department.
I leave a message on the answering machine
Requesting one of the engineers return my call as soon as possible.
I prefix my name with "Doctor" to ensure a response.
I hate playing the "Doctor" card.
But I've done it before.
An engineer almost immediately returns my call.

[*Speaks very rapidly*] I quickly plead Ruth's story,
Insisting that I'm not asking him to see Ruth ahead of someone else,
Rather to see her after hours,
And would be happy to pay him at an overtime rate,
And would consider it a personal favor.
[*Sheepishly*] He jumps in before I embarrass myself further with,
"Don't you think that every parent with financial means,
Whose child has cerebral palsy or a neuromuscular condition,
Offers to pay me to see their child after hours?
They all want their child in computerized education,
Rather than falling farther and farther behind kids their age.
Some parents without the money promise to 'beg, borrow, or steal' to pay me.
I stopped returning phone calls two years ago.
The only reason I'm returning yours
Is because you're a physician."

SCENE 18

> [*Lighting for bedroom at group home.* RUTH *flattens bed, removes hospital blanket and IV pole, and lies on her stomach facing audience.*]

RUTH Last week I developed another butt bedsore.
The nurse for the group home has me on my stomach all day
To expose my ass to the air.
Royal pain.
But I'll do anything to prevent it from getting infected
Two years ago infection spread from a butt bedsore
Through my entire body.
By the time they got me to the ER
The doctors thought I was unconscious.
But I was just too weak from infection to open my eyes,
Or speak.
And of course I couldn't feel them pinching me,
So I couldn't respond to "painful stimuli."
But I could sure hear them all right.
Hear them debate my fate:
"Death with dignity" now,
Or a "persistent vegetative state" in their "expensive care unit,"
Possibly denying the ICU bed to someone
Who could recover with a higher "quality of life."
"Quality-of-life" assessment can trap people "like me"
In lethal traps.

> [RUTH *stands and walks to stage front.*]

I really thought they were going to let me "die with dignity"

Right then and there;
Curtained off from help,
Where no one could hear my heart screaming
I want to live,
I want to live no matter what.

[*Sits in memorial service chair* FRIEND *usually sits in.*]

Because the ER can be a very dangerous place for someone "like me."
I considered having someone write me an "advance directive,"
Like I saw on *Chicago Hope.*
Except indicating the opposite:
I do want everything to be done to keep me alive,
No matter what.
Even "heroic measures."
But I heard there were problems with advance directives,
And began worrying that written words could be used against me
To permit my "death with dignity,"
Then I heard about "Life Story Decision Making."
You write down the names of people who know your life story
And who you trust to make decisions for you.
You need several names to ensure a few people can be contacted
And corroborate each other's' point of view.
Three women have already written their names and phone numbers
On the special card in my wallet.
And I'm also going to ask my strange-doctor friend.
[*Pause*] I know,
He doesn't know me very well.
And I don't think we've talked more than a dozen times.
But he was very upset when I told him about
The "death with dignity" debate in Emerg.
And he definitely knows I want to live no matter what.
And I believe his MD degree
Is my best defense against "death with dignity."
Doctors will listen to him when he tells them
She wants "to live no matter what."
He's a member of their club,
And doctors will have more trouble browbeating him
Than the women on my list,
One of whom has already written his name and phone numbers under hers.
I'll ask his permission next time I see him.

SCENE 19

FRIEND   I wonder what it would cost to take Ruth to the States.
   To get her hooked up to her computer there.

I know you can buy prompt health care in the States;
Why not biomedical engineer services?
I know if my children had to wait I would find the money.
But Ruth is not my child.
She is my friend.
Anyway, I don't have time to take Ruth to the States.
No, that's a cop out.
I could hire one of the caregivers at Ruth's home to take her.
I'm sure they'd like to make some extra money on a day off.
They're only paid minimum wage.

SCENE 20

[*Group home lighting.* RUTH *sits in her chair.*]

RUTH The antibiotics resolved the bedsore after a few weeks,
And I've been great for months,
And I have something very important to tell you.
I am in love.
I am completely and so deeply in love.
I have found the soulmate I sought for so many years.
I know, soap opera clichés,
But I've hoped to feel them for so long.

[*Walks to her desk.*]

I am so in love.
So Fuck'n A in Love
He listens to me so eagerly,
Longing to learn me.
He speaks to me so gently,
Calling me his calcedony,
Because he says I'm beautiful to the core,
Though a little crusty on the surface.
[*Pause*] Okay, I showed him my bookends.

[*Indicates. Walks to stage front.*]

I love the way he strokes the hair that sticks to my forehead,
Or moves my drinking straw to my lips when it goes amiss.
And the way he lovingly traces my jaw line to my chin.
With such soft, tender strokes.
Each caress of his fingers
Smoothes away years of loneliness.
I have never felt so alive.
His name is Alex but I call him Fred.
Fred had a stroke.

The left side of his body doesn't move.
He uses a chair,
But not a power chair like mine.
And even if he had a power chair,
He obviously wouldn't be able to go as fast as me.
But then few can.
Fred writes me poem after poem.
And he reads them so lovingly,
Although his speech is slurry.
I will write Fred poem after poem
As soon as I'm connected to my computer.
I will pour out the love collected in my heart,
The love bursting my heart
Every minute I am awake.
And I am so exquisitely awake.
Wait just one a sec,
An attendant's coming into my room.
[*Whispers*] I'll tell you more about Fred later.
She says,
[*Cheery voice*] "Ruth, good news
An engineer's coming to see you on Tuesday
To assess you for your computer."
She smiles and leaves.
The word "assess" terrifies me.
What if my jaw muscles aren't working well enough anymore?

SCENE 21

[*Lighting for memorial service.*]

FRIEND Another Friend lifts her eyes
And tells a story about helping "our Friend" smoke.
All smile, except me.
All eyes stare at me.
Encouraging me.
Waiting for me.
Waiting for me.

SCENE 22

[*Lighting for bedroom at group home. RUTH sits in her chair.*]

RUTH The biomedical engineer gently places my chin
Into a cold metal cup he calls a transducer.
It's connected by thin black and red wires to a little black box
That looks like a Geiger counter.

You know the things they use in old movies to test for radiation,
Little glass windshield over trembling red needle and all.
I don't hear any Geiger counter static, though.
And I sure don't want to give this guy any static.
Heaven is in his hands.
I'm on my best behavior.
I ask him if he thinks I'm hot.
Whoops.
He smiles and reminds me to only move my jaw when he asks.
He spends over an hour with me.
It's hard for me to be good that long.
As he gathers his stuff to leave I say,
[*In "Rocky" voice*] "Yo, Mr. Biomedical Engineer,
When do we hook up?"
He smiles, but apologetically.
"I'm sorry, you'll have to be patient."

SCENE 23

[*RUTH stands and walks to Stage Front and Center.*]

RUTH I've got another butt bedsore.
The nurse has me lying on my stomach again all day.
Ass-naked to the world.
The worst part is I won't let Fred into my room.
Not because I'm modest,
But I'm sure the bedsore looks awful,
And I'm worried it's starting to smell.

[*Blackout.*]

SCENE 24

[*FRIEND stands holding briefcase and walks to desk. Night time light or desk lamp on.*]

FRIEND I've just flown home from yet another conference.
Being away from my kids is hard,
And flying is claustrophobic.
But this time it was worth it.
A keynote speaker spoke softly into the microphone
The most powerful words I have ever heard.
She began by declaring,
RUTH "I am the healthiest person I know."
FRIEND Which surprised the more than five hundred attendees,
Because she is quadriplegic.

She uses a state-of-the-art power wheelchair,
The seat of which periodically raises, lowers, and tilts,
To rotate pressure off the weight-bearing points on her skin.
She credits her wonderful health
To financial means and education,
Two of the World Health Organization's social determinants of health
And most important love:
The love of her partner in everything she does.
The love of her parents in insisting and financing the type of education
Where pages could be turned and doors opened,
Physically and metaphorically.
Her voice is now heard all over the world.
She writes by speaking into her computer,
Her words transcribed into text through software
I think she called "Dragon."
At the end of this amazing talk,
She read a list of names and causes of death
Of persons killed by government cutbacks to social programs:
A woman starved to death
Because funding for someone to check in on her was cut off.
A man was burned to death
Because he was placed into a bath tub of scalding water
By a new and less costly attendant.
Many names and atrocities followed.
With each name, my heart heard a bell chime,
And saw a flame appear.
By the time she finished the stage seemed carpeted with candles
Of compassion [Chime],
Of equality [Chime],
Of purpose [Chime],
Of solidarity [Chime].
I have to tell Ruth about this amazing woman.
I haven't seen Ruth for a while.

   [Walks across stage to desk looking tired.]

No red light on my answering machine.
But there is a note from my fourteen-year-old son:
"The hospital called, going to bed."
I'm not on-call.

   [Picks up phone.]

I page the Clinical Fellow.
She's not looking for me.
Must be some confusion now rectified.

   [Puts down receiver, takes off jacket, phone rings, picks up.]

"Hello."

RUTH "Ruth's in trouble,
   Please come to the hospital right away."

   [*Dial tone.*]

FRIEND [*Walks to stage front speaking rapidly.*]
   I quickly drive to the hospital,
   Assuming the woman who called is on Ruth's list of people,
   Trusted to insist that all be done for her,
   "No matter what."
   I park illegally at the ER doors and dash in.
   Ruth's not here.
   At least she's been admitted.
   I ask the receptionist where,
   But her computer is taking too long.
   I run up the stairs to Intensive Care.
   The nurse at the desk is expecting me.
   She looks frightened,
   Says nothing,
   But the index finger of her right hand
   Is pointing to a draped-off area at the unit's far end,
   Where incandescent curtains project ominous shadows.
   I turn to dash,
   But she grips my right wrist,
RUTH "Why don't you stay here with me until they're finished?"
FRIEND I extricate my wrist and run.
   I clench the curtain's edge and take a deep breath.
   These drapes will not be Ruth's shrouds.
   I fling open the curtains.
   [*Pause*] To horror.
   Oh Ruth.
   Bacteria have blackened her skin,
   And swollen her body to a huge black balloon,
   Knotted at her neck, elbows, and wrists
   By a sadistic birthday party clown.
   Ruth's closed eyes bulge like black tennis balls.
   Her chin is gone.
   I see a black Michelin Man.
   The periphery of my underwater vision
   Sees a woman sitting to the left of Ruth's bed,
   Tears streaming down her face;
   And the ICU doc standing on Ruth's right,
   Acknowledging me as he draws drugs into syringes.
   Hollowness expands within me,
   Vacuuming me downward.

I fight it.
I can stop this.
Ruth wants "to live no matter what."
I stare at Ruth,
Working hard to see,
Working hard to breathe,
Drowning in what I see.
I turn to the doctor.
"You're not going to disconnect her?"
He puts his hand on my shoulder.
He was once one of my students,
A Monday Night regular.
I tell him, "Ruth wants to live no matter what."
He gently whispers, "There's nothing left."
"How can you be so sure?"
He squeezes my right arm and says,
"Look."
I put my body between Ruth's and his as I'm supposed to do.
But instead of insisting that she remain on the ventilator,
I place my lips where Ruth's ear should be and plead,
"Ruth, give me some sign.
Twitch an eyelid,
Something.
Please Ruth.
Please."

[*Freezes under spot.*]

SCENE 25

[*Memorial service lights.* FRIEND *sits in same memorial service chair. He looks up and unfolds sheet of paper from his pocket.*]

FRIEND   "It's not Ruth's life that I can share,
For I knew little of Ruth's life.
And I can't share Ruth's death,
Too painful for me to recount.
But I can share Ruth's beauty,
That beamed in the sound bites I permitted her."
Ruth gave me so much,
Asked so little,
Received much less
From me,
And from a health and social system
With limited capacity for compassion
And accommodation.

Her last words to me were,
"I am in love,
'Why don't you come on up and see me sometime,
And I'll tell you all about him."
Ruth was beautiful to her core,
Is beautiful to her core
Like the bookends that stood beside the computer
She was never permitted to use;
The bookends that now stand beside my computer.

[*Light on* RUTH *in peasant dress in memorial service chair on other side.*]

RUTH He tells them her bookends are calcedonies:
Rough-surfaced rocks,
That can open to amethyst,
Agate,
Onyx,
Chrysoprase.

[*Stands and walks to front of stage.*]

He tells them that each calcedony is unique.
That calcedonies have spiritual powers
Healing powers,
He tells them he will share her beauty.
He tells them he will always introduce her as "my friend,"
"My friend who wanted to be a poet,
But is a poem.
My friend . . ."

FINIS

ACKNOWLEDGMENTS

I would like to thank Catherine Frazee for her inspiration, wisdom, and encouragement; Lisa Balkan for her dramaturgical suggestions; and Sheila Boyd, Susan Cox, Les Friedman, Roxanne Mykitiuk, Jennifer Ryder, and Katharine Timmins for their suggestions and assistance in script preparation. Portions of *Calcedonies* were previously published as a narrative essay in the *Canadian Medical Association Journal* (Nisker 2001, 74–75) and *From the Other Side of the Fence: Stories from Health Care Professionals* (Nisker 2008, 172–176). An earlier version of the first few scenes was published in *Reflective Practice: International and Multidisciplinary Perspectives* (Nisker 2010, 417–432). *Calcedonies* will be published in a collection of Jeff Nisker's plays, *From Calcedonies to Orchids: Plays Promoting Humanity in Health Policy*, available from Iguana Books (www.iguanabooks.com).

Part XII

HEALTH PROFESSIONS
EDUCATION

Chapter 43

TEACHING AUTISM THROUGH NATURALIZED NARRATIVE ETHICS

Closing the Divide between Bioethics and Medical Humanities

JULIE M. AULTMAN

We cannot understand a life, and what it might mean, without referring to the individual's narrative and also to the social and cultural context in which it is lived.

CARL ELLIOTT (1999, 133)

T HE often unspoken, but ever-present social divide between medical ethicists and medical/health humanities scholars is created in part from the ways illness, disability, and death are conceptually, descriptively, and normatively examined. Medical ethicists use theories, principles, and approaches to ethical decision making to recognize, resolve, and reflect on ethical problems. The humanities scholar, in constrast, is not solely concerned with problem solving, per se, but seeks to understand the human condition—those who suffer, those who are disempowered by disease, those who want their children to be "normal." They also seek to understand the webs of relationships in which individuals are embedded, along with the meanings of those relationships. This is not to say that medical ethicists do not engage in similar activities, particularly those who identify themselves as theologians, philosophers, historians, and others whose training, knowledge, and scholarly activities are grounded in the humanities.

Still, medical ethics education and training are often distinguished from medical humanities curricula, and this distinction can be both beneficial and limiting to healthcare professionals. In closing the gap between medical ethics and humanities, the move toward a naturalized narrative ethics in health professions education can develop students' and professionals' critical thinking, self-reflection, communication, moral imagination, and sensitivity toward others, along with other skills, values, and attitudes that enhance and guide person-centered care in historical, social, political, and cultural contexts. At the same time, this approach to ethics can help students recognize the need for narrative inquiry, moral imagination, and self-reflection without dependency on traditional moral theories and principles. This approach reveals the importance of understanding ethics through the performance of storytelling by particular people in particular times, places, cultures, social structures, and professional settings.

This chapter is an examination of a naturalized narrative ethics (Chambers 2008) as a useful pedagogical tool for an ethics-driven curricular activity I initially developed in 2007 with the support of the Rich Center for Autism in Youngstown, Ohio. Fully implemented into an interprofessional curriculum at Northeast Ohio Medical University in 2009, "Narratives of Autism," is an opportunity for six to eight parents of children with autism to tell their stories to over two hundred first-year medical and pharmacy students. This activity follows a lecture on the clinical diagnosis of autism (as presented in the *Diagnostic and Statistical Manual of Mental Disorders* [*DSM-IV-TR* 2000]) and a brief description of ethical, clinical, and scientific issues surrounding its treatment and management. Parents tell their stories for over an hour, then student questions and comments follow, including their own stories of caring for their siblings or other family members with developmental disorders. Finally, students have the opportunity to interact with many of the children with autism who attend the session.

Students' experiential recognition of specific ethical issues in the context of families' struggles to understand and live with autism is successfully achieved through this academic activity in ways that traditional bioethics lectures and readings are unable to achieve. Narratives, especially those that lack restitution such as chaos narratives (Frank 1995), challenge students to understand moral inquiry as something more than the application of ethical principles and theories to dilemmas and cases. However, there are limitations to this and similar curricular activities that aim to close the divide between rule-based bioethics and medical/health humanities curricula with an emphasis on narrative. Thus, while I argue that naturalized narrative ethics is a significant step in closing the divide among bioethics and medical/health humanities, I conclude by briefly describing the limitations of this approach, using "Narratives of Autism" as a way to improve moral education and training for health professions students.

CHLOE'S CHAOS NARRATIVE

Chaos feeds on the sense that no one is in control. People living these stories regularly accuse medicine of seeking to maintain its pretense of control—its restitution narrative—at the expense of denying the suffering of what it cannot treat.
    ARTHUR FRANK (1995, 100)

Of the various illness narratives Arthur Frank describes in *The Wounded Storyteller* (1995), the chaos narrative is often told by individuals with autism and their caregivers, especially the mothers of young children with autism. Frank describes this narrative as the anti-narrative of time without sequence or discernable causality. These narratives are hard to hear because of their lack of coherence and ability to provoke anxiety among readers/listeners. From the reader/listener's perspective, the storyteller is not telling a "proper" story and is not perceived "to be living a 'proper' life, since in life as in story, one event is expected to lead another. Chaos negates that expectation" (1995, 97). The wounded storyteller is the teller of the chaos narrative, but as Frank explains, "Those who are truly *living* the chaos cannot express it in words. To turn the chaos into a verbal story is to have some reflective grasp of it.... The person living the chaos story has no distance from her life and no reflective grasp on it. Lived chaos makes reflection, and consequently storytelling, impossible" (98).

The stories told by the parents of children with autism reveal they have some "reflective grasp" on their lives and acquire both physical and emotional distance simply by removing themselves from familiar environments or participating in emotionally challenging activities such as storytelling. Other parents ignore the chaos and acquire emotional distance simply by denying that their child has autism or is "different." Regardless of the types of narratives, parents feel an overwhelming sense of purpose when telling their stories to future caregivers—students who will assume caregiver roles whether as physicians, pharmacists, parents, or others. The storytellers aim to guide future healthcare professionals to be cognizant of challenges in caring for persons with developmental disabilities or disorders, to be sensitive to the values of parents that may conflict with "experts" of autism, and to feel empathy, rather than frustration, pity, or disgust when confronted with parents and others who believe and act in ways that are counter to scientific and medical advice. These storytellers want to be heard and feel a sense of relief when students are willing to listen, question, and self-reflect on their own values, feelings, and attitudes.

Many of the stories told in "Narratives of Autism," however, are characteristic of the chaos narrative, which has an interesting pedagogical effect on the student-listeners. Students quickly recognize that life will not become "normal" for the teller of the chaos narrative, even becoming frustrated that the stories lack restitution. One of these life stories, Chloe's story, is particularly difficult for students to hear.

"Chloe" is in her late thirties. She moved from the West to be closer to her parents after having lost her house, a nursing career, her vintage Volkswagen beetle, and a marriage of ten years. She held onto the most important thing in her life—her nine-year-old son, "Michael," who was diagnosed with autism at age 3. His functionality and development were deemed "low to moderate" according to clinical standards. Chloe believes her son loves her, despite the lack of eye contact and affectionate embraces she desires. She knows Michael feels and exhibits frustration when placed in uncomfortable environments, for example, changes from his patterned walks through the grocery store. She used to feel embarrassed when he threw his small body on the floor of the store, kicking and screaming until shoppers questioned why she could not control her child "like most parents." These days, Chloe explains that Michael has autism to shoppers who criticize her parenting skills; she offers to educate them, instead of leaving the store without purchasing a single item, embarrassed, discouraged, and feeling alone. She used to blame the vaccines. And before that she blamed herself, assuming even her ex-husband's blame was rightly placed. Now Chloe feels even more despair because she has nothing to blame and no hope for her son to get better and to just be "normal":

Something caused my son to be this way. The doctors say it is not the vaccines. If it is not the vaccines, then what are the causes? I am not even sure if the doctors are right about his diagnosis of autism. They do not seem to know much about it, even after I describe what Michael eats, how he plays, why I cannot hug him. They don't listen to me. They just tell me to enroll him in speech therapy and all these other "therapies" I cannot afford. Nothing I do helps, anyway. He screams. He is bruised, and people, including my own family, think I have hurt him. I took care of myself and Michael as soon as I found out I was pregnant, but people still blame me. Maybe not the vaccines, but maybe his diet or toxins from the environment did something to him. I have ripped out my carpeting, removed the wallpaper, use only natural household cleaning products, and I feed him a gluten-free diet—just like some other parents I know—you know, those who are like me. I have very little government assistance and no health insurance. My old insurance company dropped me after my son was diagnosed with a disorder *they* did not see as real.

Chloe and other parents and their children with similar stories drive for over an hour to share their stories for the two-hour, discussion-based class. They are eager to share what it is like to be a parent of a child with autism and the social, economic, and moral struggles they face every day in the presence of future healthcare professionals. Since her first classroom appearance, Chloe's story changes with every new technology, influential news story, theory hypothesized and debunked, and personal experience. Her story lacks coherent sequence with the exception of those events that led her to move from the West Coast to the Great Lakes. As she tells her story, Chloe expresses her moral judgments, such as "vaccinating is wrong," actively altering her judgments based on new or unconsidered information about autism (e.g., the Wakefield studies; see Wakefield et al. 1998) or on what guiding values she may be following at the time (e.g., freedom not to vaccinate her children). Some of Chloe's ideas and judgments have even changed based on the immediacy of student questions and feedback during the class session as she thinks in real time about particular events or her life story. Students witness a living narrative about a mother raising a child with autism, but they also see the unfolding of a moral life that is not guided by absolute values. It is a narrative that exposes her humility in seeking, not the "right" answers, but the answers she can comfortably live with, and it is this ethics lesson that can teach future healthcare professionals that moral deliberation is dynamic, reflexive, and able to change when there is no actual or perceived resolution in sight.

Some would argue that Chloe is not a sufferer *of* autism or a sufferer of any medically diagnosable illness for that matter, and hence her story is one that may not fall under the definition of "illness narrative." However, her story is one of chaos told *through* a wounded body (Frank 1995, 2). Chloe is not wounded by an identifiable disease but by the emotional, social, and moral distress she experiences as a caregiver responding to her son's illness. The medical profession easily ignores these wounded bodies without a classifiable diagnosis, treatment, or prognosis, but such bodies are in need of recognition and care.

Chloe's life, as she narrates it, does not get better. There is no happy ending. Her story makes some students uncomfortable as they struggle to find resolution, not just for her or the other parents, but for themselves as well as they think, "How will I, a future healthcare professional, be able to 'fix' these families?" Some students also become angry with Chloe's story because they cannot understand why a former healthcare professional (a nurse practitioner) would blame vaccines for having caused her son's autism, alter a child's environment and diet, or use alternative medical therapies unsupported by scientific evidence, such as chelation and cranial sacral therapies. These students argue that Chloe is not a "good" parent because she allows "quack practitioners" to practice risky and harmful procedures on Michael. They see her, as well as many of the parents who share their stories, as desperate, uneducated, and prey to Internet propaganda, self-help books, and false beliefs. Many of the students question why these parents are able to listen to the narratives of uninformed public figures, instead of the advice of healthcare professionals and scientists who *know* more. Nonetheless, participation in the storytelling as listeners becomes a transformative experience for many other students. These students are able to recognize and confront their own biases and feelings of anger, frustration, and resentment and, in turn, feel a sense of belonging, purpose and duty. These are the students who are able to see the value of caregivers' life stories, not for purposes of diagnosing and treating the disease, but for understanding the social, political, moral, and cultural aspects of how autism affects and is affected by the storytellers. Students recognize they become part of the story as they confirm, alter, or abandon preexisting beliefs and attitudes about the nature of autism as it is told and understood by caregivers.

Chloe's story is complicated, chaotic, and, at times, incoherent. It is a story that many ethicists would not even consider to evaluate or use as a teaching tool about the dynamics of ethical thought. It does not fit in a neat package or "case study" that can be presented, discussed, and resolved in a fifty-minute class session by applying the principle-based, common morality theory of Tom Beauchamp and James Childress (1979) or a set of prima facie duties like those of W. D. Ross ([1930] 2002). This is not to say that principlism or moral intuitionism, like many other ethical theories and frameworks, cannot be useful for understanding ethical judgments and guiding resolution among value conflicts. However, if we are really to understand the moral complexities of Chloe's story and what we as educators, students, and members of a social community can learn from her story, we need to delve deeply into why and how her story and the telling of that story affects and is affected by us.

I use the chaos narrative as a way to show how bioethics often misses the mark in describing the moral complexities of a person's story and how such narratives may be independent from those moral principles that are commonly *applied* without understanding how they are interpreted or known by the storyteller, the reader/listener, or other. The chaos narrative is an important pedagogical example of real-life moral deliberation that does not require problem resolution. Sometimes ethical decisions need to be made, and moral problems resolved, as in many end-of-life situations in the clinical setting. And, while students should learn about those traditional ethical principles and moral theories that can guide decision making and case resolution, these ethical tools fall short when it comes to understanding not only the wounded storyteller but oneself in relation to the other. The medical/health humanities, including moral philosophy, have the power to shape bioethics into a discipline that does not measure success by "right" or "wrong" decision making or case resolution through compromise, consensus, and coherence among competing values and interests. And such shaping can occur through narrative ethics.

Initially, students expect to listen to the illness narratives of sufferers of autism to understand what it must be like to be autistic and to think critically about many of the ethical controversies surrounding the classification, diagnosis, and treatment of autism. This is because narratives in ethics have been used in these ways, and admittedly, I myself have used them in a very basic way to get students to think about the other. And, as medical educators, we have a tendency purposefully to expose our students to the stories of our ill patients so they may learn about the illness, and how "it" physically, emotionally, socially, and morally wounds the body. On occasion, our students are able to see beyond the disease entity. They are able to understand, even show concern for, the ill-embodied patient. As bioethicists, we have a tendency to direct students to attend to narratives and then identify the moral issues and dilemmas, apply principles in a top-down approach, arrive at a decision—which becomes evaluated as "right" or "wrong," "good" or "bad"—and then reflect on that decision. But in doing this step-by-step approach, we lose sight of the moral character of the narrative itself.

Frank explains that the need to honor chaos narratives is both moral and clinical. He writes: "To deny a chaos story is to deny the person telling this story, and people who are being denied cannot be cared for. People whose reality is denied can remain recipients of treatments and services, but they cannot be participants in empathic relations of care" (1995, 109). The moral lesson of "Narratives of Autism" is to guide students not only to recognize the person telling the story but to recognize themselves as listeners entering the "space of the story *for* the other" (Frank 1995, 18). Students learn about the ethics of autism as they inadvertently and mutually construct the narrative with the storyteller when they ask questions, tell their own stories, and make comments based on their initial social and moral judgments.

CAREGIVER NARRATIVES IN MEDICAL ETHICS

Narrative teaches that being human is the perpetual finding out of what is good and virtuous, whether the process of that moral inquiry is called the examined life or reflexive monitoring.
    ARTHUR FRANK (1995, 157)

Unfortunately, we often do not expose our students to caregiver narratives and the wounds they endure as their own stories become embedded, sometimes without discernment, in the narratives of their ill loved ones. We are especially forgetful of these important caregiver narratives in medical ethics. In most cases, medical ethics (specifically clinical ethics) tends to focus on the patient or, more broadly, the physician-patient relationship. Arthur Frank reiterates this point in response to Rita Charon's narrative contributions to ethics. While Charon's description of narrative can ultimately guide participants in "ethical deliberations to appreciate the coherence, the resonance, and the singular meaning of particular human events" (quoted in Frank 1995, 155), the focus is on the therapeutic relationship and the ill patient.

This approach to narrative ethics can be useful for guiding moral discussions and for adding more depth to the medical history; it is, however, a myopic ethical framework. The listener of the story is able to recognize the narrative coherence of a patient's life, but the focus is on the identity of the illness in relation to the patient rather than the ill embodied *person*. The difference between these frameworks partially rests on the meaning of coherence. Under Charon's description of narrative ethics, the emphasis is on how the listener understands the coherence of the *patient's* story. A deeper understanding of coherence reveals that it is about embodiment and how the *person's* story affects and is affected by relationships, medical advice, scientific theories, moral and cultural values, social expectations, and unfounded beliefs. Frank shows that stories "open up moral dimensions of the lives of ill persons when they are *not* being patients" and have the ability to "guide people, whether ill or healthy, lay or professional, in the moral commitments that illness calls them to" (quoted in Frank 1995, 156–157). Chloe's story expresses a moral commitment that her son's illness calls her to.

Unfortunately, stories have been typically understood in medical ethics as rich examples for teaching principle-based ethics and as moral guides to living a good life, but Anne Hudson Jones shows that narrative approaches to medical ethics can actually reconceptualize the practice of medical ethics by replacing principlism with a "paradigmatically different practice" of literary, critical analysis (1999, 255). Students are required to read (or listen) in the fullest sense to narratives, mastering literary analysis skills that can prepare them for listening to and interpreting patients' stories, identifying the gaps in their stories and possible ways to fill those gaps, and acknowledging the additional voices that ought to be heard to understand fully the patient's plight. Questions posed to learn about a literary text, Jones writes, can also be used in the examination of ethical texts and practices; for example, "Who is the narrator? Is the narrator reliable?" and so forth.

Jones describes how narrative contributes to medical ethics through mimetic content—for what narratives say—and through analysis of their diegetic form or "for the understanding of how stories are told and why it matters" (1999, 253). In addition, "narratives of witness" force us to reexamine and reflect upon medical practices and ethical precepts. To elaborate, Jones shows us that autobiographical accounts by patients or their family members and friends may "comment from the patient's point of view on ethical issues such as autonomy and respect for persons, truth-telling and informed consent, beneficence (and, sometimes, maleficence or negligence), incompetence, and error" (254). In the "Narratives of Autism" session, parents provide personal accounts of living and caring for a child with autism from a moral and social perspective, commenting on how this developmental disorder has negatively affected the way in which they are respected. For example, one mother spoke of how the mothers of "normal" children in her neighborhood would ignore, pity, or even blame her for having a "disruptive, cognitively delayed" child. A father, who to this day is in denial that his son has autism, described his own ethical dilemma in playing video games as a way to connect with his son.

These games were violent and often mistaken for reality by his son, who is a "high-functioning" adolescent with autism. Admittedly, the father recognized that if he did not play these games, he would have very limited interactions with his only child, inevitably leading to an unwanted acceptance that his son was not like other kids. He is still struggling with his own decisions and does not feel this issue has been resolved.

Students have the opportunity to ask questions, describe their own perspectives and opinions about autism, its causes, diagnosis, and treatment, but they are also challenged to think about the moment they, as future healthcare professionals, tell a mother for the first time her child has autism. They are challenged to assume the role as co-author in the mother's narrative and imagine what it would be like to construct a joint narrative of medical care: what treatment choices would be available, what social and economic resources would be needed, what existing beliefs and perspectives would need to be discussed. Underlying this relational ethic, as proposed by Howard Brody (1994) is the challenge to construct jointly an illness narrative without bias, anger, and frustration even when advice is not followed, when irrational beliefs overpower medical evidence, and when problems cannot be fixed. The class persuades students to imagine what it would be like to be healthcare professionals caring for the families seated before them, what it would be like to be a parent trying to care and cope, and what it would be like to be a child whose identity is tied to a disability that is not completely understood.

Students' moral judgments become better informed as they begin to understand the parents' perspectives of caring for their children with autism; their interactions with healthcare professionals, insurance companies, and others; and their role as storytellers. The power of stories, as Tom Tomlinson describes, "may awaken moral sensibilities, so that we more keenly feel the wrongfulness of circumstances we had become hardened or blind to" (1997, 132). Students often learn more about themselves through this curricular activity than they do when simply studying about the nature of autism as it is diagnosed, treated, and understood by parents, healthcare professionals, and others.

However, I did not realize the extent to which this activity really affected both the storytellers and the listening students until this last year, when I recognized how the stories and storyteller-listener interactions changed from previous years. As new information, such as the controversial and unethical Wakefield studies, emerged, students became more critical of parents' lack of acceptance of scientific evidence—for example, that vaccines do not cause autism. Yet, criticism aside, the storytellers anticipated that their medically oriented audience would question their beliefs and attitudes surrounding this new information, and some told their stories with this in mind. However, as Chloe retold her story for the third, consecutive year, I recognized the significance of her story at that moment, in front of this particular group of students, and with the recently acquired knowledge of those social, moral, political issues surrounding the Wakefield study. Chloe desperately wanted to find something or someone to blame for her son's autism, and so this was her story for that moment in time and place. Her story became shaped through students' questions, and what occurred was a mutual understanding of the other.

Students' negative attitudes and criticisms changed to respectful inquiry into the life of the storyteller. Chloe felt more at ease, less defensive, and was open to new perspectives and insight from her audience, while also expressing the power struggles she faced among those in "superior" positions in life, including those privileged student-listeners who initially criticized her beliefs and values.

NATURALIZED NARRATIVE ETHICS

Hilde Lindemann, Marian Verkerk, and Margaret Urban Walker, editors of *Naturalized Bioethics: Toward Responsible Knowing and Practice* (2008), advocate for naturalism in ethics, which Walker describes as "committed to understanding moral judgment and moral agency in terms of natural facts about ourselves and our world" (2008, 1). While their book is a compilation of chapters, each distinct with their own interpretation of naturalized bioethics, the overall purpose is to move us toward an ethic that is "empirically nourished but also acutely aware that ethical theory is the practice of particular people in particular times, places, cultures, and professional environments" (5). They ask bioethicists to move toward a "self-reflexive, socially inquisitive, politically critical, and inclusive ethics" as they abandon traditional moral theories and the principles that emerge from them (e.g., utilitarianism). It is a type of naturalism that allows for social and social scientific analysis in bioethics through which we are able to better understand the values of particular people and cultures, including those voices that are underrepresented or unrepresented. It "is also wary of idealizations that bypass social realities and of purely 'reflective' approaches to ethics that are apt to reflect only some, and usually the socially most privileged, points of view regarding the right, the good, and moral ideals such as autonomy, respect, beneficence, and justice" (5).

In support of a naturalized ethics, Jennifer Torres and Raymond DeVries (2009) propose "pay[ing] attention to everyday ethics and . . . look[ing] beyond narrow definitions of ethical problems and the solutions offered by bioethicists" when critically looking at ethical issues such as those surrounding birth (2009, 21). In their critique of principle-based ethics, with an emphasis on autonomy and patient empowerment, they describe how principles and a case-based model of bioethics can have adverse effects on patient care and our understanding of the various political, economic, social, and cultural aspects of ethical issues and problems. They further suggest that ethics "can be marshaled to protect the interests of a profession" (21), such as the case of autonomy as the driving principle to support the use of surgery to deliver healthy babies from healthy women (also see DeVries et al. 2008).

When looking specifically at the role of narrative with respect to a naturalized bioethics, Tod Chambers shows that stories do not exist to be "found" but "are continually engaged in rhetorical work" (2008, 128) and believes that Arthur Frank comes closest to analyzing a naturalized narrative medical ethics. Chambers asks us to focus not just on the story but also on the activity of storytelling, which "serves and is shaped by the particular settings in which it occurs, the ends for which it is done, and the authority or expectations of the one who tells the story or elicits it" (Walker 2008, 15). He explains that a naturalized narrative ethics uses stories as rhetorical tools in which one must—ask in addition to asking, What is the point of the story?—What is the point of *telling* the story?

Chambers describes folklorist Richard Bauman's approach to storytelling "that attends not merely to the narrative told but also to the event of narration" (Chambers 2008, 138). Citing Erving Goffman (Goffman et al. 1997, 153), Bauman shows that when individuals attend to any current situation, they encounter the question, "What is it that's going on *here*?" Bauman adds a second question, "What is it that's going on *there*?" (Bauman 1986, 6, cited in Chambers 2008, 138; emphasis added). It is the relationship between the narrative event and the narrated event that reveals the rhetoric of storytelling and pushes us to ask questions, not just about the story itself, but how, where, to whom it is being told, who the story teller is, and what she is trying to do with her story. In addressing these questions, Chambers writes:

> We can begin to thwart any attempt at the construction of a single narrative and instead keep the stories embedded in the ongoing social life of the people involved in the medical decision. Doing this forces us not only to notice how stories are naturally evoked in medical ethics decisions but also to attend to the power struggles with that decision making. Only by moving from a concern with stories to an integration of storytelling can we naturalize narrative medical ethics. (2008, 140)

In educating future healthcare professional students about ethical issues and problems, it is important to present them with complex narratives that are not easily reasoned or constructed into resolvable case studies. The narratives of autism, as told by mothers and fathers, are very much entangled with the social dynamics of a particular place and time (Chambers 2008, 139). The expectation for medical educators is to guide students to recognize these dynamics, as well as how they themselves become entangled within these stories as listeners and as participants who help shape the stories. The parents of children with autism want their voices to be heard among future healthcare professionals. They desire future physicians, pharmacists, bioethicists, medical researchers and others to understand the difficulties of getting health insurance, of taking a child with behavioral problems to a grocery store, of allowing strangers to perform holistic medicine, and having others criticize such efforts. These parents are not looking to these future healthcare professionals for answers to their moral and social problems. They simply want to tell their stories and connect with persons as persons.

One limitation to this approach and its application to "Narratives of Autism," is that one can fall into the trap of a relativistic-like understanding of values. Student listeners may identify that particular people in particular times, places, cultures, and professional environments as having different sets of moral values and that ethical theory will vary among individuals and groups without commonality and universality. However, to combat this type of thinking, it is important that medical educators who have an interest in ethics and the humanities guide students to locate stories in "the ongoing social life of the people involved in the medical ethics decisions," as Chambers explains (2008, 140), as well as to understand who the storyteller is, why she is telling the story, and to recognize oneself as the person to whom the story is being told. In my first attempt to implement "Narratives of Autism" I failed in preparing my students for these important questions and treated the parents' stories as narrative cases to be analyzed. It was Chloe's chaos narrative that guided my own thinking about stories and how they should not always be deconstructed for purposes of moral inquiry. Ethical issues are present, and it is up to the student to recognize these issues in both the narrative and narrated events. For me, "Narratives of Autism" is still a work in progress, as challenges of classroom space, scheduling, and finances seem to dominate its structure. Ideally, this activity should have breakout sections so students can talk about their experiences as listeners and participants, discuss the complex issues surrounding autism, and express their feelings, attitudes, and beliefs surrounding their future roles as healthcare professionals in responding to and caring for families living with autism.[1] However, the three-hour session, including a brief overview of the clinical and scientific views of autism, provides a rich, narrative approach to ethical and social inquiry that begins to close the divide between rule-based bioethics and medical humanities.

NOTES

1   These break-out sessions were implemented in 2011 and led by faculty with diverse expertise (pharmacists, physicians, literary scholars, administrators, ethicists, etc.).

Chapter 44

COURTING DISCOMFORT IN AN UNDERGRADUATE HEALTH HUMANITIES CLASSROOM

MICHAEL BLACKIE AND ERIN GENTRY LAMB

My goal isn't to shed the perspective that comes from my particular experience, but to give voice to it. I want to be engaged in the tribal fury that rages when opposing perspectives are let loose.

HARRIET MCBRYDE JOHNSON (2003, 79)

WITHIN health professions education, the inclusion of humanities within the curriculum is usually justified by the promise of better, more thoughtful, more compassionate healthcare practitioners. For example, a touchstone essay by several key figures in literature and medicine makes this case explicitly: "The introduction of literature and of literary studies to medicine will allow physicians to more accurately render the lives of their patients and to recognize the human dimensions of all of the experiences that occur within their gaze" (Charon et al. 1995, 604). The more recent approach of narrative medicine likewise focuses on the healthcare practitioner, combining close reading with reflective writing to "examine and illuminate four of medicine's central narrative situations: physician and patient, physician and self, physician and colleagues, and physicians and society" (Charon 2001a, 1897). Even medical humanities educators who critically revisit these rationales—such as Delese Wear and Julie Aultman, who call for a "radical hermeneutics" to address the "thorny, perplexing, and often unaddressed issues in medical education"—still narrowly aim to cultivate students who are "likely to provide skilled, compassionate, and optimal care to all their patients" (2007, 358–359).

As undergraduate health humanities educators, we recognize that many of our students do not desire careers in the health professions; consequently, the nuances of the physician-patient relationship typically hold little fascination for them. All of our students can, however, expect to interact with healthcare settings throughout their lives. This fact determines how we structure our classes: our goal is to prepare students to be critical, discerning participants in the future delivery of health care, whether they are receiving this care, providing it, shaping policy around it, or engaging with it in some other capacity. Thus, in our classrooms, medicine is the text but not the context; that is, we use medically relevant texts to improve students' abilities to ask critical questions about the world around them and about their own habituated ways of seeing it with the aim of becoming better prepared to negotiate the uncertain terrain of health care more generally. Through such questioning, we encourage our students to identify the myriad ways medicine functions as an ideological system that serves some better than others, how the biomedical model of health is one model among many, and particularly how their own participation and vested interests in this system contribute to its outcomes, both desirable and undesirable. Such inquiry rarely leads to simplified clarity or clear cut decision making; rather, it produces uncomfortable ambiguity that we see as an essential challenge for our students.

To illustrate our goals in the classroom and how we accomplish them, we focus on a moment of our own pedagogical failure. We revisit this moment—generated by a problematic student presentation on reproductive technology—through Megan Boler's (1999) "pedagogy of discomfort." Boler's work helps us identify missed opportunities to engage productively with the discomfort this presentation generated, thereby enabling our students to recognize the stakes they hold in the healthcare system and—through recognizing their interrelationships with others—the possible consequences of their actions within that system. We move from this unique situation to offer strategies for how to produce similar discomfort within other health humanities classrooms. We propose that courting discomfort in health humanities classrooms helps form students into discerning participants in the healthcare system able to engage critically with situations that challenge their deeply held beliefs and defy simple solution.

We teach at Hiram College, a small liberal arts college in northeast Ohio, within the biomedical humanities major, one of the few but increasing number of formalized undergraduate health humanities curricula. Hiram College is committed to team-taught, interdisciplinary classes. The moment under examination took place midway through a team-taught, discussion-driven course on narrative bioethics. We had two prospective students visit our classroom midway through the class session on the same day as a group presentation on the bioethical implications of pre-implantation genetic diagnosis (PGD), a technology used to screen embryos created via in vitro fertilization (IVF) for genetic conditions or abnormalities before selected embryos are implanted in a woman's uterus. The group offered an acceptable explanation of the science behind PGD but an incomplete overview of the technology's current and imagined uses, focusing primarily on uses typically represented as ethical extremes, such as screening for a condition like Tay-Sachs that will almost certainly be fatal for a child or selecting for sex in the interest of "gender balancing" a family. The group decided to (in their words) "stir things up" for discussion by presenting a dramatized dialogue of two people arguing about whether life begins at conception or at birth, ignoring the legally defined (albeit debatable) points in between. We, as instructors, found troubling the absence of nuanced thinking evidenced in the presentation and began imagining strategies for how we might improve the discussion once the presentation concluded.

The prospective students joined the class halfway through the hour-long presentation, just before the introduction of a case study involving "savior siblings," a term that refers to the use of PGD to select an embryo tissue-matched to a sick older child in need of a transplant. In keeping with their oversimplified approach, the presenters opened the floor to discussion with questions like: "Is it wrong to bring a child into the world for a purpose?" Or, "Would a savior sibling be wanted or loved less than another child?" While some of their peers (not to mention their professors) attempted to complicate these questions, many in the audience took them at face value, speculating on how deprived the life of such an instrumentally conceived child might be.

Following the presentation, one of the visiting students—let's call her Claire— appeared visibly upset to the point of tears. While Michael initiated the post-presentation discussion, Erin took Claire to the hallway. Claire disclosed that she was offended by some of the questions and comments presented by our students; she was, she indicated, a savior sibling, one of the first in Ohio, and was dismayed that anyone would question whether her parents love her any less than her brother.[1] "There are so few of us, and hardly any of us who are old enough to speak out," she said. After reassurances from Erin about the validity of her reaction, Claire agreed to rejoin the discussion—aware that she was welcome to speak out but would not need to if she preferred.

The discussion already under way was exploring the more contentious uses of PGD, including screening for nonfatal, nonguaranteed, or late-onset diseases (such as a predisposition to breast cancer or early-onset Alzheimer's); for disabilities or disorders (such as deafness or achondroplasia dwarfism); or for—in an imaginable future—factors like sexual orientation or personality traits. As Erin and Michael posed questions about the motivations behind and potential consequences of such screening, Claire joined the discussion asserting that autism is generally seen as a negative condition for which people might wish to screen, but people with autism are now speaking out about how they are simply different, not impaired. Our students paused respectfully for this comment although they did not accept its invitation to think through the ways difference and disability are socially defined. Instead, our students continued to speak in generalities about undesirable conditions for which one might screen and implied that people afflicted with such conditions were clearly Other from themselves. Even those who felt that PGD was unethical because it creates unused embryos did not question that, given the choice, one would not choose an embryo predisposed to be deaf or autistic. At this point, Claire once again joined the discussion, this time to read from a hastily written statement—in a semi-hostile manner—revealing that she is a savior sibling whose parents love her very much and that she also has Asperger syndrome.

Her disclosure stunned the class into silence. It took longer to reach some students' faces than others, but we could see, looking around the room, the dawning recognition that the hypothetical person whose fate the class had been cavalierly debating was in the room with them. We thanked Claire for her contribution and then attempted to guide the discussion toward considering how the voices of variously defined minorities might challenge our larger cultural assumptions about what is or is not a desirable difference. This attempt failed; in fact, most of our students retreated into silence. One of the presenters interjected with an awkward apology on behalf of the group. Several of our students nodded as he spoke; others looked critically at the presenters, seeking to distance themselves from their poor judgment shown throughout the presentation. All our further attempts to complicate the discussion met with stonewalling mantras of "every life is sacred" and "we can't judge others' difference." After a few more ineffectual attempts at improving the conversation, we reached 12:00 and ended class. Claire rushed out before we had a chance to talk to her.[2] This coincidental encounter left us dumbfounded and uneasy about how we handled it.

In reflecting on this incident and imagining how we could have responded more effectively, Boler's "pedagogy of discomfort" helps us identify several ways we might have productively pursued the discomfort generated during the presentation and by Claire's disclosure. As a classroom strategy, a pedagogy of discomfort "invites educators and students to engage in critical inquiry regarding values and cherished beliefs, and to examine constructed self-images in relation to how one has learned to perceive others," with a central goal being "to recognize how emotions define how and what one chooses to see, and conversely, not to see" (Boler 1999, 176–177). Put in the context of our narrative bioethics course, the "gut feelings" on which our students frequently draw when formulating their ethical responses do not provide solid ground for moral inquiry but, rather, mark a starting point for exploring and evaluating how one's gut feelings are habituated responses shaped by previous experiences and cultural forces (including, we must acknowledge, education). It is only through such ongoing inquiry that students can become aware of how these responses play a significant role in determining "what one chooses to see, and . . . not to see." The possibility of seeing in multiple ways simultaneously—and of seeing oneself in relation to others, for Boler insists this must be a "collective" process—requires that participants in this "culture of inquiry" become willing to "inhabit a more ambiguous and flexible sense of self" (1999, 176). In terms of our goals as undergraduate health humanities educators, a student at peace with his or her "morally ambiguous self" and adept at the critical inquiry necessary to get there is a student more likely to regard medicine and the biomedical model of health care not as "givens" from which to work outward but as texts whose founding assumptions are open to criticism and questioning (182).

Returning to the presentation with Boler in mind, we identify one early moment of our failure to court discomfort as our response to the presenters' "stirring things up" approach. Their framing of the debate with stark polarities—does life begin at conception or at birth?—was already a way of avoiding a sincere examination of the ambiguity engendered by the topic. By presenting an either/or option, the presentation elided the messy middle ground between these extremes where ethical stances, cut off from dogmatic retreats, become more difficult to defend, more morally ambiguous. Arguing that PGD is unethical because life begins at conception and the process of PGD creates unused embryos is perhaps the easiest position on PGD to defend; it is one we find many students readily adopt. We want to be clear that we see nothing objectionable with a student taking this stance; rather, we find problematic the presenters' framing of the question because it enabled, perhaps even encouraged, their peers to assume such a stance *without any critical investigation* of how they came to hold it.

Boler tells us that the value of discomfort lies in "questioning cherished beliefs and assumptions" (1999, 176). To question in this manner means recognizing how we protect such beliefs and assumptions by calling them "private." Thus, in reflecting on the presentation, we should have insisted that the presenters look beyond the polarities they had erected to acknowledge the morally ambiguous terrain between them. We should have facilitated inquiry into *why* they believe life begins at a given point and from *where* their beliefs have arisen. Such inquiry would likely have exposed parental, religious, political, and educational influences, the examination of which many undergraduates, not to mention educators, would rather not pursue precisely because to do so requires being open to the discomforting possibility of seeing familiar things made disturbingly unfamiliar. And yet it is through this form of exploration that we, as a class, could have begun to appreciate the degree to which specific cultural influences have shaped our "private" beliefs and determined—in the public sphere as well as in our classroom—the form discussions of reproductive technology take. Recognizing the historical and cultural contingency of one's attitudes and of public debate facilitates seeing medicine itself as an ideological system responsive to the ever-shifting forces of culture. In turn, the recognition of medicine as a contingent, ideological system is a key step in empowering students to be critical and questioning participants in the health-care system.

The most important moment of our failure to court discomfort came after Claire's disclosure when we let our students take refuge in the simple binary of guilt or innocence. Students either joined in the expression of contrition or blamed the presenters' insensitivity to affirm their own innocence. These simplified positions permitted students to retreat from discomfort—"I'm sorry I offended you/that you were offended"—and maintain their separation from the Other responsible (in their minds) for generating that discomfort. Rather than accept our students' easy admission of guilt, we should have challenged them to revisit the conversation that prompted Claire's disclosure in order to question the beliefs and assumptions motivating it. Such exploration would have required students to recognize that while they were insisting post-disclosure that "we can't judge others' difference," their earlier comments were clearly implying that, given the option, they would not have selected to bring a child like Claire into existence. Exposing such contradictions makes it clear that "guilt" and "innocence" are inadequate positions to take up in response to such a complex situation.

Instead, we should help our students recognize the importance of inhabiting "a morally ambiguous self" because it allows them to appreciate how their beliefs and assumptions determine how they respond to others and to take responsibility for the consequences of their actions. In their earlier discussions, students were evaluating the ethicality of PGD from the framework that seemed most obvious and relevant to them: that of the individual. Seen this way, preventing illness, disability, or other conditions construed as socially disadvantaged seems like a logical response to the difficulties people with these health differences face and *should* be done in the best interests of the child. And yet this view is premised on the problematic yet widespread assumption, based squarely on a biomedical model of "health," that one can know with certainty that such a child will experience a "lower quality of life" (Asch 1998). Additionally, frequently hidden behind the "best interests of the child" are the vested interests of potential parents who cannot imagine caring for a "disadvantaged" child and of society wherein such individuals may require more resources. Here disability studies becomes quite useful as it provides a clear model for how changing the frame of evaluation—changing, in Boler's terms, *what we choose to see*—makes an ethical difference.

Disability rights activists view disability as a social rather than medical problem, suggesting the difficulties faced by persons with disabilities are due to societal barriers ranging from unaccommodating architecture to "social beliefs, attitudes, policies, and practices" (Cox-White and Boxall 2009, 558). With regards to PGD, this reframing from the level of the individual to the level of society requires consideration that, given the oppression and stigmatization persons with disabilities have faced, forms of prenatal screening like PGD "may be regarded as yet another form of social abuse" (Kaplan 1994, 60). This societal-level frame raises very practical concerns about reduced funding of programs for persons with disabilities, an increase in negative attitudes toward disability, and a shift in societal understanding of the "causes" of disability such that parents might be blamed for *not* selecting *against* disabilities for their children (Kaplan 1994, 57–58). By pushing students to consider these larger ramifications of an "individual" choice, they are forced to confront the moral ambiguity of wishing to "not judge difference" while simultaneously desiring to ensure their own children are "healthy" and to recognize that their "private" choices are complicit in defining differences like disability as undesirable. Claire's presence in the classroom offered a catalyst for shifting the frame beyond the individual in order to see the larger, collective stakes of their choices.

Recognizing one's stakes in an ethically charged situation and especially acknowledging the implications of one's actions is uncomfortable work. Boler insists that this labor is not just for students: "A pedagogy of discomfort is a mutual transaction. The educator's own beliefs and assumptions are by no means immune to the process of questioning and 'shattering.' Similarly, it is important that the educator explore what it means to 'share' the students' vulnerability and suffering" (Boler 1999, 188). We interpret Boler as calling for educators to model this difficult process of self-investigation for their students; at a minimum, it is an insistence that we must be aware of how our beliefs and assumptions shape our own views on the subjects we teach, the ways that we teach them, and how we respond to our students. By publicly engaging with our own pedagogical failure, this essay is one way in which we are responding to Boler's call. We also have to recognize that even while "we" have been writing in a collective voice about our shared failure, the two of us were motivated to action (or inaction) by different factors.

For example, at the time of the class, Erin was thirty-three weeks pregnant and had learned that same morning that good friends had given birth to twins— conceived via PGD to avoid the spinal muscular atrophy that had killed their son before his first birthday—at a terrifyingly early twenty-five weeks gestation. The twins' lives were uncertain, and if they survived, their chances of severe disability were extremely high. When the student presenters asked when life begins, all she could see were the snapshots of two preemies weighing just over one pound apiece. When the discussion moved to children with disabilities, she inwardly questioned if it might not be better for the twins to die than for her friends to face more endless rounds of hospitals and specialists, even while she recognized the problematic assumptions she was making about the twins' and her friends' quality of life. At one point during the presentation, students put Erin on the spot by asking if she would have aborted her child if she learned it had Down syndrome, a question that recalled uncomfortable conversations with her husband and evoked her own moral ambiguity. Rather than own up to and model how to engage this ambiguity at a moment when she was already feeling emotionally vulnerable, she deflected the question and instead modeled the same sort of retreat from discomfort the students would take after Claire's disclosure. Had she been willing to put her own visibly pregnant body on display and charge students with the task of determining the fate of *this child*—or to share the story and snapshots of the twins alongside statistics of preemie outcomes and require students to talk about *these children's* lives and issues of distributive justice—she could have evoked some of the same discomfort produced by Claire's presence.

For Michael, an openly gay man, the ability to screen for diseases or particular traits conjures up nightmarish scenarios in which parents eliminate embryos destined to be gay or lesbian. Such a possibility came to him almost immediately after the initial reports first appeared in the early 1990s that homosexuality may be genetically determined. Should this be the case, few parents would be likely to choose to bring a gay or lesbian child into the world either because of their own deeply held homophobic assumptions or because, they reason, such a child would surely have a tougher time growing up than would a heterosexual child. This latter justification is particularly troubling for Michael because, on one level, it amounts to nothing more than heterosexist reasoning masquerading as beneficence and, on another, it perpetuates the very conditions that often make the lives of gay and lesbian children difficult. Although Michael briefly introduced these possibilities for discussion, he received only a few nods from students. Rather than challenge them with his personal stake in these questions and insist they not back away from the topic, he let it drop entirely and, like Erin, avoided producing any more discomfort.

In that moment, Claire's disclosure rattled us, just as it did our students. Here was a young woman visiting our class because she was considering attending Hiram College, and in minutes, she was able to silence all of us in the room. Her contributions to the class discussion had, however, even greater significance than simply reminding us that there is always more at stake in discussing health care than mere ideas, concepts, and rules. The great opportunities Claire's disclosure generated show us that we need to work actively to create similar forms of discomfort within our classrooms if we want to help students become truly discerning participants in the delivery of health care. Encouragingly, we do not need a Claire to create this kind of discomfort. In addition to the modeling we might have offered, we had rich texts on the table for that day's discussion—Jeff Nisker's (2005) play *Orchids* and Harriet McBryde Johnson's (2003) article "Unspeakable Conversations"—which we could have used to generate discomfort and illustrate moral ambiguity.

Orchids, by physician and playwright Jeff Nisker (2005), explores the consequences of assisted reproductive technologies through the personal lives of two female patients, Rose and Heather, and the professional lives of two physicians, Doctors Blume and Staiman. The play invokes discomfort through the increasingly tense discussion between the two women in the doctors' waiting room. Rose is seeking PGD to ensure that her child does not have Tourette's syndrome, like her twin brother, whose condition allegedly caused tremendous suffering for Rose and her parents, while Heather, who has Tourette's syndrome, requires IVF to get pregnant because of damaged fallopian tubes. Rose and Heather's conversation offers rich opportunities for discussing the social consequences of one's personal reproductive choices.

Rose refuses to take responsibility for the wider implications of her decision not to have a child with Tourette's. Soon after Rose discovers Heather has Tourette's, she apologizes for being "insensitive" while characterizing her brother's condition as a "disease" that "really made life hell" for her family (Nisker 2005, 22), but Rose refuses to concede that her choice challenges Heather's "right to exist" (43). She insists on seeing her choice as entirely individual: "Can't you see I would be less of a mother if my child's life was less than it could be?" (43). Exploring the legitimacy of Heather's challenge to the logic of Rose's decision offers a useful means of asking students to enter the discussion with more at stake than deliberating over the fate of either character's unborn child. To make the discomfort of such stakes personally relevant, we might ask students to choose some quality about themselves that could be perceived as negative and imagine what it would mean if others in the room wanted to ensure people like themselves never existed. While such an exercise risks trivializing the reasons prospective parents seek PGD,[3] challenging students to overcome the distance between themselves and Others by inhabiting uncomfortable or foreign subject positions can offer insight into the interests and assumptions motivating all subject positions, including their own.

Heather's character affords students opportunities to acknowledge the challenges that arise when inhabiting a morally ambiguous self. When Rose protests to Heather that she can't let her child be "less than it could be," she then asks, "Can't you see that, Heather?" To which Heather offers the concluding line of dialogue: "No. I can't allow myself to go there" (Nisker 2005, 44). Here we have another form of refusal, this one motivated largely by fear. Heather is unable or unwilling to accept the legitimacy of views antithetical to her own; she thus provides us with a useful transition to Harriet McBryde Johnson's first-person account of viewing the world through the beliefs and assumptions of someone who doubts the value of her life.

In "Unspeakable Conversations," Johnson (2003), a disability rights lawyer with a congenital degenerative neuromuscular disease, recounts her experiences publicly disagreeing with the Utilitarian philosopher Peter Singer over her life's value. She went to Princeton as Singer's guest to dialogue on the subject of terminating the lives of severely disabled infants. In her moving narrative, she models what it means to understand the Other, in this case, a man who, in her own words, "thinks it would have been better, all things considered, to have given my parents the option of killing the baby I once was, and to let other parents kill similar babies as they come along and thereby avoid the suffering that comes with lives like mine" (2003, 50).

Unlike the fictional Heather who cannot "go there," Johnson willingly enters Singer's "conceptual world," where she has to admit some of his ideas make sense (2003, 52). Nowhere are the stakes of such a move more apparent than in a conversation Johnson recounts having with her sister after returning home from Princeton. Her sister likens Singer to a Nazi—"He's advocating genocide"—and Johnson uncomfortably finds herself defending the "terrible purity of Singer's vision" (79). Her willingness to inhabit his point of view—and the moral ambiguity required to do so—leads her to the most valuable outcome of her visit: a clearer sense of what she brings to her own life and her community by being a discerning participant in both. In response to Singer's cold logic, she looks "to the corruption that comes from interconnectedness" and invokes "the muck and mess and undeniable realities of disabled lives well lived" (79). Through her willingness to inhabit another's point of view, Johnson models for students the insights that follow making peace with moral ambiguity.

We have tried to show how the "morally ambiguous self" that Johnson illustratively inhabits can be achieved through a pedagogy of discomfort. Asking students to identify and evaluate their habituated ways of seeing the world—by exploring the foundations of their beliefs, values, and assumptions—trains them to ask discerning questions about biomedicine: Whom does this system best serve or not serve? What assumptions about health and the value of life drive current medical practices? What power, authority, and vested interests do I have in this system, and how does my participation within it influence how the system serves others? Additionally, becoming comfortable with moral ambiguity is a key part of becoming discerning participants in the delivery of health care. Health care does not present a world of polarized extremes for one to choose between; rather, navigating health care requires negotiation of a constantly shifting middle ground. Students who are able to "see" the healthcare system from many perspectives are more prepared for these negotiations. In debates about healthcare reform, their positions will be founded on consideration of larger stakes than just their own limited interests. They will more readily recognize there is no one correct solution to the problem of deciding what course of treatment to pursue for inoperable cancer, what to do with a parent who has Alzheimer's, or what a "healthy" child is and to what lengths they would go to have one.

The goal of preparing undergraduates to be critical and discerning participants in the healthcare system is commensurate with the goal of shaping better healthcare practitioners expressed at the professional level of health humanities education. Undergraduates who become discerning healthcare participants are more likely to be the kind of professional school students who welcome humanities coursework in health professions education; that is, they will readily accept that an investigation of human values will help them become better practitioners. For those students who go on to medical school, the time spent in a classroom where the centrality of the physician is always in question exposes them to ways of seeing the practice of medicine as less rigidly hierarchical. Healthcare practitioners who can comfortably inhabit a morally ambiguous self are more ready to interact with patients whose beliefs do not match their own and more prepared to navigate thorny healthcare problems that defy simple solutions.

Ultimately, however, we promote a pedagogy of discomfort as an approach to serve all of our students, including those with no interest in delivering health care. Traditional undergraduates are in a period of the life course designated as "emerging adulthood," a time in which their worldviews are most formatively shaped (Arnett 2004).[4] What better moment, then, to encourage students to "see" the healthcare system in which they are a participant with more complexity? As undergraduate health humanities educators, we, too, are in a uniquely nimble position to raise critical questions of the healthcare system from many of our peers located in professional schools. As our space in the curriculum and our jobs are not dependent on the support of these professional institutions, we are freer to criticize, challenge, and imagine ways of changing these professions.[5] Little has been written exploring the role of health humanities education and educators at the preprofessional, undergraduate level; we hope to see more of this in the future. For now, following Johnson's lead, we will continue to court discomfort in our classrooms and seek to engage our students "in the tribal fury that rages when opposing perspectives are let loose."

NOTES

1 While Claire verbally identified herself as a "savior sibling," it is far more likely that she was either conceived naturally in the hopes she would be a donor match for her sibling or that she was more generally identifying herself as having been conceived through the process of PGD. While children have been successfully born via PGD free of the screened-against diseases since the early 1990s (Handyside et al. 1992), the first recognized "savior sibling," Adam Nash, was born in 2000 (Belkin 2001). As a high school senior in 2010, Claire was probably born in 1992 or 1993.

2 Given Claire's hasty departure, we were left uncertain about her experience. Anecdotal evidence from the admissions department suggests Claire felt positively about the experience.

3 While students' potential concerns about acne or obesity are not equivalent to fatal or degenerative diseases, disability, or sexual identity, such an exercise may provide a bridge to truly thoughtful consideration of the implications of screening for such concerns. Nisker authorizes the value of such an exercise in his use of Tourette's syndrome within *Orchids*, as it is not a condition that can currently be screened for: "By focusing on Tourette Syndrome, Nisker explored the problems of genetically selecting against disability without having to speak to a real experience but rather a metaphorical and imagined one" (Johnston 2010, 283).

4 Events experienced during this period, as stated by Jennifer Tanner and Jeffrey Arnett, "are integrated into individuals' identities and memories more so than those events occurring during younger and older life stages" (2009, 40).

5 This observation is indebted to Diane Price Herndl's analysis of the different approaches toward disability used by medical humanists and used by those in disability studies (2005, 595).

Chapter 45

THE MEDICAL HUMANITIES IN MEDICAL EDUCATION

Toward a Medical Aesthetics of Resistance

ALAN BLEAKLEY

DIAGNOSING MEDICINE'S ILLS

In April 2011, the internationally celebrated Chinese artist Ai Weiwei was detained by Beijing police, ostensibly for tax evasion but more likely for persistent political dissidence through his art. *The Times* newspaper in London published responses from public figures as a collective open letter of protest to the Chinese government. Sir Nicholas Serota, director of the Tate Gallery, observed in his response

that the health of a society is indicated, in part, by the freedom of its artists and writers to express their views without fear of suppression. Diversity of view generates creativity and occurs through meeting of opposing ideas, a respect for differing viewpoints and the expression of distinctive visions. A society that tolerates difference will remain creative as its values are challenged. A society that cannot accommodate points of view will stagnate and become an empty husk. (Serota 2011)

The first part of what Serota suggests—that an indicator of the "health of a society" is its level of democracy—is familiar to proponents of "open" societies (Popper 2002). The second part, however, is more radical—that it is particularly the work of artists that protects a liberal democracy. Indeed, as Gilles Deleuze suggests, using Friedrich Nietzsche's cultural analysis, artists are physicians in another realm—as "diagnosticians" and "symptomatologists" of the body of culture (Smith 2005).

Medicine has traditionally been a closed society, a self-regulating profession, only recently forced to account publicly for its practices and mistakes (Ludmerer 1999). And while medicine is undergoing an invigorating (post)modernization, there are conservative legacies, such as autocratic relationships with other professions and patients, where hierarchies persist, although they are often disguised as meritocracies (Bleakley et al. 2011). Such autocracy is evident even within medicine's own specialties, with surgery as the most authority-conscious (Fisher and Peterson 1993). And there is a strong, evidence-based argument that such lingering autocracies generate work structures that place patients' safety and health at risk: an estimated "70–80% of healthcare errors are caused by human factors associated with poor team communication and understanding" (Xyrichis and Ream

2008, 232). Physicians themselves reinforce such autocracies, characteristically viewing "teamwork as a form in which nurses (are) subordinate" (236). It has been estimated that effective teamwork can halve the risk of medical error (Kohn et al. 1999) where both cross-team and within-team communication are important (Engeström 2008). Moreover, better coordinated teamwork in hospitals correlates with reduced patient mortality as well as an improvement in practitioner morale (Borrill et al. 2000; West and Borrill 2002).

Medical errors in hospitals worldwide place an estimated one in ten patients at risk (National Patient Safety Agency 2010). The seminal 1999 Institute of Medicine (IOM) report on patient safety concluded that medical errors caused as many as 98,000 deaths annually in the United States (Kohn et al. 1999). While this estimate was initially questioned on the basis of methodological rigor (Sox and Woloshin 2000), subsequent studies and reports suggest that the IOM study underestimated the level of error (Aspden et al. 2004; Department of Health 2000; National Audit Office 2005; National Patient Safety Agency 2010; Zhan and Miller 2003). For example, the "Health Grades Quality Study" (2004) of 37 million patient records in the United States doubled the top end of the IOM estimate, suggesting that as many as 195,000 Medicare patients died owing to potentially preventable, hospital-based medical errors in each of the years 2000, 2001, and 2002, constituting a national epidemic. Thus, the transition from high-risk to high-reliability service requires culture change, one involving a transformation of values and institutional structures (Vincent 2010).

What has this got to do with the medical/health humanities? Serota's implicit assertion that art is a democratising force is elegantly articulated in Martha Nussbaum's *Not for Profit: Why Democracy Needs the Humanities* (2010). She argues for the humanities (including the arts) as the chief cultural force for promoting democracy, in which they diagnose social ills, such as questionable authority that supports unproductive habits; suggest cures, such as tolerance of difference; and offer creative debate about quality of life. Nussbaum's argument can be readily transposed to medical education.

Where medicine remains structurally undemocratic, dysfunctional hierarchies and autocracies will persist in clinical teamwork, and paternalism will prevail in consultations, placing patients at risk by compromising communication essential for effective systems-based health care that includes accurate diagnoses and referrals. The instrumental response to patient safety and optimal care issues in medical education has been to place greater emphasis upon teaching medical students communication skills in the hope that a new generation of doctors will emerge who can communicate well with colleagues and patients. However, the patient safety agenda has yet to have an impact on undergraduate medical education, and thirty years of communication skills training have failed to produce significant impact. For example, a meta-review by Debra Roter and Judith Hall shows that physician-patient communication is still relatively poor, suggesting that structural issues are not being addressed (2006).

Good communication with patients and colleagues goes beyond instrumental skills training to engage with values-driven ways of being. In order to inform their practice, health professionals must reflexively account for culture-specific values. In medical education, it is common to teach communication skills integrated with clinical skills such as the physical examination. This sounds good in principle, but in practice, clinical skills are increasingly taught in the bubble of the simulation center, so communication skills are also learned by simulation and as protocols, bracketing out context-based, values-laden, and feelings-laden responses (Bligh and Bleakley 2006). This pedagogy is counterproductive, serving to frustrate transfer to real clinical contexts. Medical students, for example, are rarely taught about complexities in professional communication, such as the dynamics of erotic transference and countertransference. And although they are systematically taught how to take a patient's history, which is often integrated with "communication skills," there remain an estimated 15–20 percent of misdiagnoses by physicians leading to medical error. Such misdiagnoses are usually grounded in poor history taking that fails to draw from the patient's narrative (Sanders 2010).

Also taught through communication skills training is empathy. Although empathy is a contested term (Macnaughton 2009; Marshall and Bleakley 2009), understanding of and connection to a patient's perspective is fundamental to good doctoring, and communication can act as a health intervention in its own right (Roter and Hall 2006). Empathy, however, has been shown to be on the decline generally amongst young people in the United States (Zaki 2011), and in medicine, "empathy decline" (Hojat et al. 2009) and "moral erosion" (Liebowitz 2011) are noted as common, as idealistic students meet the realities of clinical work and the pervasive cynicism within medical culture. While the evidence for empathy decline in medical student education has been challenged on reexamination of validity of studies (Colliver et al. 2010), we must ask why empathy does not increase and also face the other end of the career spectrum—where physicians suffer from relatively high rates of anxiety, depression, burnout, substance abuse, and suicide (Council on Science and Public Health 2010). Communication skills training in medical education may be necessary, but such training is not sufficient to offer a democratizing force. Something else is needed.

Reading literature has long been associated with gaining empathy—and claims are persistently made for the value of this association within medical education (Charon 2011b); however, it is only relatively recently that we have empirical evidence for the connection (Mar et al. 2006). The volume of stories that preschoolers read predicts their ability to understand others' emotions, and adults who read less fiction report themselves to be less empathic. For instance, in the United States, "the number of adults who read literature for pleasure sank below 50 percent for the first time ever in the past 10 years, with the decrease occurring most sharply among college-age adults" (Zaki 2011, 12). Importantly, where reading narrative fiction correlates positively with improved social abilities, this is not the case for nonfiction reading.

If we transpose Nussbaum's argument for the humanities and the arts as a democratizing force in wider culture to medical culture in particular, the medical/ health humanities may play a bigger role in medical education than we imagine. They might provide the contextual media through which the lessons of the science of communication are best learned. Where good medical practice depends upon both technical (clinical knowledge and skills) and nontechnical (cognition, communication, and teamwork) elements, the non-technical realm will not be fully realised until and unless medicine is changed structurally—shifting from autocracy to democracy. As an elective course or fringe compensation for science, the medical/health humanities will not be powerful enough to effect such a structural change. This chapter offers a rationale for how such change might be achieved through a core and integrated provision of the medical/health humanities, and we begin with the evidence of the senses.

MAKING SENSE OF DIAGNOSIS

Consider this description of a clinical practitioner at work:

> Around midnight he started getting a bit more pale . . . and his lung sounds were ok . . . by about 2am he was looking quite a bit worse and very wet. . . . So I got blood gas and the pH was 7.2. . . . I finished giving the bicarb about a half hour previously and I looked at the baby and he looked much worse than he had before. . . . His mouth was just open slightly. He was gasping to try to breathe. He just looked awful, looked absolutely terrible. . . . So I gave the Lasix (a diuretic), but at that point the baby was looking so bad that I didn't even wait for the Lasix to take effect before I went ahead and did another blood gas. (Benner et al. 1996, 126–127)

The decisions made to treat this sick baby were based on a close noticing of qualities, primarily visual—"getting a bit more pale," "looking quite a bit worse." Ways of "looking" are central to diagnostic acumen and may best be taught with clinicians working together with those whose primary work is also "looking," such as visual artists and art historians. Where physicians teaching students in clinical settings affords relevance, the addition of artists affords meaningfulness. Thus, ingredients for a successful core medical/health humanities provision are education of sensibilities and sensitivities set in live clinical contexts—with physicians, artists, humanities scholars, patients, and students working democratically to improve patient care.

The practitioner looking at the sick baby above is a nurse, and the example of such sensitive close noticing is purposefully chosen to raise three issues:

1 to question casual and exclusive use of the common descriptor "the medical humanities,"
2 to ground the artistry of clinical practice in the senses, in aesthetic work, and
3 to address the issue of democratizing clinical practice.

The first issue can be dealt with briefly. Although this chapter concentrates on medicine, the continued use of the term *medical humanities* is exclusive and undemocratic in an era of collaborative, patient-centered, interprofessional teamwork. The generic term *health* (or *healthcare*) *humanities* is explicitly inclusive, especially when *humanities* includes the arts.

The second issue—grounding practice artistry in the senses—also involves making a case for the shared praxis of the health humanities, to democratize the previously exclusive domain of the "medical gaze." The medical/health humanities can be summarized as the humanity (*sensitivity*) and artistry (*sensibility*) of medicine and health care. How this is taught depends, again, upon a structured collaboration among clinicians, artists, humanities scholars, students, patients, and the public. Sensitivity encompasses *ethical care*, where sensibility is *aesthetic labor*, such as the expressive close noticing of the nurse in the example above. *Medical aesthetics* complements the established field of *medical ethics*. Moreover, we must unhook ourselves from the legacy of aesthetics as "high art" confined to "pleasure." The root of "aesthetics" is the ancient Greek *aisthesis*, which means perception by means of the senses, or "sense impression." Thus aesthetics is to do with *quality* of life as experienced through the senses, including not just the pleasurable but also the perplexing, disgusting, sublime, perverse, and abject. For Nietzsche, ill health paradoxically provides the conditions of sensitivity needed to become an acute diagnostician of culture, problematizing the notion of "health" humanities (1998). Education of the senses in terms of "lay" connoisseurship (close noticing) or "professional" connoisseurship (pattern recognition and close diagnosis in expertise) is an educated bodily event. The arts and humanities create ambiguity, destabilizing and challenging habit and abuse of authority, so that creative ways of living can emerge. This, again, is a basis of democracy.

But there is a prerequisite for both citizenship and professionals working in democratic team settings—persons must be sensitized and aestheticized to notice closely, not dulled or anaesthetized. Without the evidence of the senses, debate cannot ensue about the logic of practice, and tolerance of uncertainty and ambiguity is central to performing that debate. Intolerance of ambiguity is the central character trait of the authoritarian personality type resistant to democracy (Adorno et al. 1950). Thus, an *aesthetics of resistance* is needed to counter such authoritarianism (Weiss 2005).

Let us return to the nurse above, making qualitative judgements based on sense impressions. In 1859, Florence Nightingale wrote that close noticing is "the *sine qua non* of being a nurse," where "attending to . . . one's own senses . . . should tell the nurse how the patient is" (Quain 1883, 1038). This is the aesthetic labor of health care—elegant, inspiring, beautiful, imaginative, animated, dignified, graceful, sensitive, distinctive, and passionate. Who would wish for an anaesthetic healthcare service—dull, uninspired, ugly, unimaginative, flat, ungracious, clumsy, insensitive, tiresome, and numbing? In the context of art history, Rudolf Arnheim describes a sophisticated kind of looking as "intelligent vision" but reminds us that this "cannot be confined to the art studio" (1969, 206). He suggests that such intelligent vision can succeed in other disciplines "only if the visual sense is not blunted." We must, in Arnheim's phrase, "think with the senses" and think acutely, as art historian James Elkins suggests: "Most sciences have specific visual competencies and these present 'ways of seeing' waiting to be explored" (2003, preface, 7).

Michael Polanyi and Harry Prosch argue that education of the senses is essential for good science: "No science can predict observed facts except by relying with confidence upon an art: the art of establishing by the trained delicacy of eye, ear, and touch a correspondence between the explicit predictions of science and the actual experience of our senses to which these predictions shall apply" (1975, 31). Charles Bardes and colleagues also note that "clinical diagnosis involves the observation, description, and interpretation of visual information"; such skills "are also the special province of the visual arts" (2001, 1157). Moreover, observational skills in medicine can be significantly improved through tutored examination of images in art galleries and transferred back to the clinic (Bardes et al. 2001; Naghshineh et al. 2008; Reilly et al. 2005), similar to arts-based observation for diagnosis in family practice settings (Kirklin et al. 2007). While such studies are exciting and offer the kind of evidence needed to convince skeptics of the value of the humanities, we need a theoretical rationale to understand their effects.

Bleakley and colleagues describe a research project on "ways of seeing" that attempts to anatomize and theorize sense perception within the domain of medical expertise (Bleakley et al. 2003a, 2003b). The method involves analysis of videotaped conversations between artists and physicians about profession-specific ways of looking and seeing, where artists visited clinics and physicians visited studios. One element emerging from this research was how expertise may either reach a comfortable plateau that becomes habitual or may continue to develop as a generative connoisseurship. Experienced physicians said that comparing their work with that of experienced artists had challenged their comfort zones and rekindled their passion in the artistry of visual diagnosis. In Japanese, a distinction is made between *ordinary seeing* and *active seeing*; in English, this is equivalent to the distinction between mere *looking* and active *seeing*. *Active seeing* in Japanese is used, for example, to describe a doctor looking at a patient. The same word (*miru*) also means "to have sexual relations" and a "stolen look." This deeper kind of seeing is then eroticized as *passionate*, or life giving.

DEMOCRATIZING THE MEDICAL GAZE

Much of medical work is sense-based diagnosis and ongoing diagnostic treatment informed by *illness scripts*, science-informational cognitive maps shaping and informing clinical reasoning. In novices, this work is analytic; in experts, it is largely synthetic, as pattern recognition (Norman et al. 2007). The acquisition of such expertise, characterized as the *medical gaze*, constitutes socialization into medical culture and the identity construction of the "doctor" (Bleakley et al. 2011). Physicians first call on the power of science to see "into" the body beyond symptom to cause and then separate objectified "disease" from experienced "illness," patient from person.

The medical gaze, or "perception," the key performance element described in Michel Foucault's account of the birth of the clinic (modern diagnostic medicine in the teaching hospital), rests on an idiosyncratic, socialized connection between "seeing" and "saying" (1989). The act of looking deep into bodies through literal dissection is linked with an exclusive diagnostic vocabulary that affords an imperialism of the gaze. What the doctor says is "true" (knowledge is power), which is reinforced by it being said in the doctor's exclusive professional domain of the clinic (authority), which in turn reinforces identities (that of the doctor and that of the patient). The "gaze" is not confined to literal sense-based diagnosis but offers a metaphor for professional solidarity, making sense of medicine as a cultural discourse.

Central then to the project of the democratization of medicine is dispersal of the medical gaze (Bleakley and Bligh 2009). Where public respect for medicine has gradually eroded through high-profile examples of error and misjudgment as well as growing concern about medicine's arrogance and lack of accountability (Ludmerer 1999), the medical gaze is resisted, dispersed, and reallocated. Greater public and patient involvement in medicine shows not only a participative democracy at work but also a monitory democracy (Keane 2009), in which public response affords surveillance and quality control. This public aesthetics/ethics of resistance has forced medicine to diagnose its own limits through adopting internal accountability practices such as appraisal and revalidation. Moreover, as the penetrative medical gaze has been gendered male, the shift toward a majority of women studying medicine further resists and democratizes this gaze (Bleakley et al. 2011). The medical gaze is also democratized with the general public's ability now to self-diagnose and self-medicate (expert patients, Internet-led information, medical soap operas with associated helplines, pregnancy testing kits, etc.) and by the establishment of interprofessional clinical teamwork in which a range of healthcare practitioners take on some of the traditional work of doctors.

MAKING SENSE OF DEMOCRACY IN MEDICINE

To summarize the argument so far: medicine infects wider health care with its historical, structural legacy of autocracy and autonomy that is realized in hierarchies and results in a range of iatrogenic symptoms. An absence of democratic structures provides the conditions that place patients at risk for an unacceptably high rate of medical error, where such error is largely due to underperformance in communication with colleagues and patients. While such "hypocompetence" (Platt and McMath 1979) is partly remediable through, for example, improving clinical teamwork, this treats symptom and not cause. The structural cause of such relatively poor communication is the legacy of medical imperialism realized in hierarchies. A meritocracy based on a level of technical knowledge and skill is translated into an autocracy that, paradoxically, encroaches on shared, nontechnical work such as communication and decision making with colleagues in team settings. This symptom is repeated in relationships with patients where paternalism is still the norm, despite the "patient-centered" movement (Bleakley forthcoming).

Progress toward forms of democracy is both tacitly and explicitly resisted in medical discourse, where militaristic metaphors are common (the "war on disease"), and clinical practice, where management is often configured as the bureaucratic "enemy" as a strategy to gain alliances with grassroots practitioner colleagues (Bleakley 2006). A state of exception allows the ruler (operating surgeon, attending physician) to exert autonomous decisions and bypass the established democratic processes of assembly (open debate) and representation (election; see Agamben 1998; Keane 2009), embodied in good team practices such as briefing and debriefing (Bleakley et al. 2004).

A century of medical education has worked within, rather than diagnosed and healed, the fault line that runs through medical culture. Abraham Flexner's (1910) root-and-branch professionalization of medical education at the beginning of the twentieth century involved closing down medical schools that did not reach a certain standard. However, one of the perhaps unintended but far-reaching consequences of this was to shutter the only schools offering places to women and minority groups, already underresourced and inevitably at risk (Hodges 2005). At the Flexner centenary, medical education is undergoing a transformation (Cooke et al. 2010), yet doctors nevertheless continue to repeat the habits of their teachers in exerting paternalistic control and modelling humiliation (through "pimping"), resulting in a culture-wide neurotic denial of vulnerability. Junior doctors often see asking for help as a sign of lack (Brennan et al. 2010; Illing et al. 2008) that possibly translates into iatrogenic symptoms: for example, the reported 10 percent spike of fatal medication errors in teaching hospitals that occurs in July in the United States, when interns begin their first jobs (Phillips and Barker 2010), and the reported 6 percent spike in death rates for emergency cases, as well as 8 percent spike in mortality rates for patients with general medical conditions, that occur in August in the United Kingdom when Foundation Doctors (junior doctors) begin their first jobs (Rose 2009).

WHY A DEMOCRATIC MEDICINE NEEDS THE HUMANITIES

The medical/health humanities as core, integrated provision in medical education can provide what pediatrician and psychoanalyst Donald Winnicott describes as a "potential space" of "play," necessary for learning social or collaborative expertise and grounded in tolerance of difference and ambiguity (1971). In the case of medical students' development from novices to relative experts at graduation, this "potential space" is now often described instrumentally, as "protoprofessionalism" (Hilton and Slotnick 2005). A carefully designed medical/health humanities curriculum can provide the platform for development of sensibilities (diagnostic acumen) and sensitivities (ethical personal and interpersonal behavior) to shape an elegant clinical practice (Bleakley et al. 2006). Central to this, again, is aesthetic labor—the design of a surgery and medicine curriculum as an aesthetic text (Bleakley 2009; Pinar et al. 1995) in order to provide the conditions of possibility for the emergence of expressive practices of close noticing within democratic structures. This includes the democratizing of the medical gaze that is at the heart of interprofessionalism and patient involvement. Where this is informed by the arts and humanities, it affords an aesthetic of resistance necessary to challenge medical education's habitual instrumentalism and lack of imagination. Perhaps the medical/health humanities as a whole can be seen as a permanent revolution within healthcare by offering a fluid aesthetic resistance movement.

In posing the question, "What is it about human life that makes it so hard to sustain democratic institutions based on equal respect . . . and so easy to lapse into hierarchies of various types?" Nussbaum makes a compelling case for "why democracy needs the humanities" (2010, 28). Drawing on Winnicott's developmental psychology, she notes that where play and the use of transitional objects (such as cuddly toys and imaginary friends) are essential for children to acquire social capability, including the capacity to understand others, so the arts and humanities offer a sophisticated and challenging adult field of play, extending social collaboration into democratic structures. This development is based around the dynamic of two permeating feeling states—shame and disgust—expressed as the need to control in tension with the need for social collaboration.

The young child's initial narcissism and helplessness can be effectively extended to make slaves of the adults who care for him or her. This is the first developmental ground for the emergence of an autocratic character, and Nussbaum notes that "the narcissistic child's original desire to turn their parents into slaves finds fulfilment—by the creation of a social hierarchy. This dynamic is a constant threat to democratic equality" (2010, 33). A healthy developmental process involves gradual achievement of a personal mastery, freeing the child from a need to make slaves of others; as the child also recognizes limits to autonomy, he or she must actively pursue help, laying the foundation for sociability. As a consequence of limits and lack of mastery, the child feels both shame and disgust—the latter, specifically where this is related to the lack of control of bodily functions. Curiosity and wonder are laced with anxiety. It is psychoanalytic orthodoxy that the greater the unresolved tension around the dynamic between disgust and shame, the more the adult will be drawn to control as a way of keeping feelings of disgust and shame at bay. Unresolved tensions concerning self-loathing will be projected as prejudice—a form of control where the Other becomes the "abject," an object of disgust (Kristeva 1982).

In healthy development, the adult not only shows acceptance of his or her own limits and subsequent lack of desire to control but also cultivates a desire to understand the Other. Mutual respect and interdependency arise from this transition as a basis to democratic habits—tolerance of difference and sensitivity to another's vulnerability. When imaginative play is denied in childhood, the adult shows residual effects, such as difficulties in forming loving, intimate, and empathic relations. Further, the transition from child's play to adult forms of creativity through the arts and humanities is frustrated, so that the value of these cultural forms is denied (Bleakley 2004). In adult life, residual effects of childhood use of imaginative play go beyond the complex, consensual intimacy of sexual relationships to the ethics of professional relationships and to wider active citizenship through engagement with cultural forms such as the arts, humanities, and popular culture. Affording high levels of ambiguity, these cultural forms promote democratic debate.

Where childhood play develops into adult "potential spaces" necessary for social experimentation, so creative imagination engages critical thinking. Citizens participating in democracy are capable of dissent and resistance to forms of authority and peer pressure. The arts and humanities, perhaps more so than communication skills-based "assertiveness training," can foster the moral courage needed to speak out when one is lower on the hierarchy and spots a potential error by a senior colleague through a more developed and imaginative "situation awareness" (Bleakley 2006).

Moreover, democracy brings a necessary vulnerability when it asks, "How shall we proceed without the parental figure, the mother or the father?" Autocracies, as controlling parental figures with unresolved issues, resist seeing the function of the arts as offering a fluid medium for reflexive critique and improvisation. Theodor Adorno's work suggests that authoritarians use the arts and the humanities to resolve ambiguity when the function of art is primarily to create ambiguity (1997). When Hitler annexed Czechoslovakia in the late 1930s, the first art form that he banned was jazz. In public, bands were forced to play militaristic marching music, square to the beat, squashing improvisation. Jazz was also seen as the degenerate musical providence of blacks, Jews, and Gypsies (Skvorecky 1994).

While this psychoanalytic reading is one story among many of the vicissitudes of human life, it has compelling parallels in medicine. If we put medicine on the couch, we see many of the symptoms discussed above. Medical culture has been in denial of its necessary flaws, what Ivan Illich called the "limits to medicine" (1997). Medicine's nemesis is unacceptably high levels of iatrogenic effects, so the democratizing of medicine through the arts and humanities can thus be seen as both an educational and therapeutic intervention.

But surely medicine's primary calling—to relieve and cure symptoms—shows that its altruism far outweighs its hubris? Medical students and physicians surely sacrifice themselves in the service of others, on oath? The more critical view is that medicine has been concerned with treating symptoms, not persons. Medicine's persistent desire to transcend its limits is a technical goal, not necessarily a humane one. Otherwise, we would not still be debating what it is to have a proper collaboration between the medical profession and the patients it serves, centered on principles of collaboration, democratic participation, equality, equity, and good communication.

While Nussbaum talks of the "creation of a decent world culture" (2010, 142), Jacques Derrida perceptively describes democracy as a work in progress, a "democracy-to-come" (1997). In a groundbreaking series of books, Michael Hardt and Antonio Negri provide a blueprint for how new kinds of democratic structures can emerge in a globalized world, moving from old forms of colonialism and imperialism to learning how to tolerate a multitude of cultural forms and voices in the adoption of a global "common wealth" (2001, 2006, 2009). Is it too much to ask to have not only a decent, functional global medical culture but also one that pursues quality and equality through a collaborative use of common "wealth" or expertise and feelings in common, such as recognition and care for vulnerability? Surely we are up to the task of democratizing our health care. But to do this, let us extend our interests from instrumental communication skills interventions and weak forms of "professionalism" to develop the medical/health humanities as a form of aesthetic resistance through a poetics of relations.

Chapter 46

IN DEFENSE OF CHEAPER
STETHOSCOPES

JAY BARUCH

I was working alongside an emergency medicine colleague when she surprised me with this confession: she'd been using my stethoscope when I wasn't on duty. Her stethoscope had vanished months before, and she expressed no immediate plans to replace it. Our white coats shared the coat rack in a tiny room that smelled of whatever refrigerated mystery was both growing and decomposing inside long-abandoned Tupperware. She liked my lower-end Littman, with its rubber missing from around the bell. "The earpieces fit my ears just so," she said, and then sighed. "And your stethoscope has the spirit of an older physician." This shift, she'd borrowed the magnificent acoustic instrument belonging to another physician in our group. "But it's a younger doc's stethoscope." A sly grin hid her dismay. "It's not the same."

Older physician? When did that happen? And what exactly did she mean by older? I hope it implied a wise physician, perhaps someone savvy enough not to waste money on an expensive stethoscope. My colleague's stethoscope was high-end, though she was an older physician, too, and should have known better.

A dizzying assortment of objects have disappeared from the ED. Coffee. Donuts. White coats. Cell phones. Purses. Even cardiac monitors and computer screens. Over the years I've lost my hair, a permanent state, along with my idealism, which graces me with frequent and quite pleasant visits. Stethoscopes, I've observed, respect the same gravitational forces as sunglasses and pens. Expensive models float away into the furthest gone; the functional versions return like boomerangs.

Apart from the physics of neglect and appropriation, the noise that fills EDs neutralizes the acoustic advantages of premium stethoscopes. Not necessarily loud, but distracting and numbing, like the mall at holiday season, except there are caroling monitors overdubbed with conversations, yells, moans, and ringing phones. Hearing isn't the only problem, but not hearing, sorting through the mash of sounds and voices, simultaneously tuning out and tuning in and hoping your ears are making the right choices.

When René Laennec, the renowned French physician and inventor of the stethoscope, rolled a sheath of papers to conduct the chest sounds of a young woman on rounds in 1816, he ushered in a vibrant era of modern medicine. Derived from the Greek *stethos* for chest and *skopos* for observer, the stethoscope, more than any other instrument, has symbolized my chosen career. The stethoscope I received on entering medical school embodied for me all the knowledge and skills I was responsible to master, the gravity and immensity of my future life's work. More than the white coat, which always felt like a straitjacket, constraining and starched from the persona I was expected to force-fit into.

The stethoscope offers opportunities for personal expression, too. Pediatricians hang furry creatures from the tubing like it's a tree limb in paradise. Young physicians have delicious colors such as raspberry, peach, and orange. A few physicians who served with the Indian Health Service dress their tubing in intricate, Native American handiwork, like tight sweaters on handbag dogs. The internists and cardiologists bear the stethoscope on their person like Indiana Jones's whip, a tool for rooting out the wiliest heart murmur, disarming the most combative surgeon, and escaping from a pit of poisonous snakes. The orthopedists, meanwhile, stride like proud nudists, not knowing when the last time they wore a stethoscope, or where it was hidden should they ever need it.

For those of us who use a stethoscope as part of our daily work, it becomes a body part. That my colleague found comfort placing my earpieces inside her ears made me uneasy. Certain objects and experiences are valued more intimately than others, and don't share well. Baseball mitt? Sure. Underwear. Forget it. A five iron? Go ahead. A putter? Over my dead body. Particular transgressions defy rational explanations. I willingly accept the smells, secretions, and sights of sick and unfortunate bodies as a necessary part of my daily work, and yet I get the creeps squeezing my feet into rented bowling shoes.

So much of what's valuable and special about medical education involves sharing experiences, both personal and clinical, that we find disturbing and uncomfortable: mistakes in judgment or behavior; opportunities lost through doubt or fear or fatigue; even successes that shocked us with good fortune. So vast and complex is medicine and our role in it that we must, by necessity, learn from the experiences of others. Medical school and residency for me involved every third or every fourth night call, but many of my teachers boasted of working every other night at the hospital. Inevitably they'd ask, "Do you know the worst part of being on call every other night?" The answer was always: "You miss half the interesting cases."

My stethoscope had acquired talismanic properties, time-earned luck, along with a memory of the thousands of patients we'd listened to together, their mischievous language and the deceiving dialects issued by these bodies. During critical moments when uncertainty or panic pushed into my head, my trusted stethoscope helped focus my attention. Slow down and close your eyes, it advised me. We've been here before. Listen to what the body is telling you, and what it's not.

With time, the stethoscope becomes your child, and a loving, responsible parent doesn't share his child with anyone else. But my colleague had my blessing to continue plundering the pocket of my white coat. She's a wonderful parent. She and her partner have all boys, and one has autism. She has the patience, the resolve, the tested love that makes me strive to be a better person. Wouldn't my stethoscope benefit from working with someone who was more understanding and fully evolved as a caregiver, who engaged the most difficult of patients without judgment or an edge in her voice?

In turn, when my stethoscope sat around my neck, my colleague's light touch relaxed my shoulders. Facing the belligerent intoxicated, or a young woman who insisted she wasn't pregnant even after giving birth in the bathroom, I channeled my colleague's calm, her nuclear-powered empathy. I lowered my voice as she would, slumped deferentially until I looked like a slow drip. The stethoscope didn't make me a better doctor; it allowed me to tap into that place where a better doctor could be found.

Regardless of how old, or wise, or kind a doctor you are, there is always room to do it better the next time. To that end, you must understand your own heart before you can listen to others; more importantly, you need to listen *with* your heart. So relinquish all ego, which serves as vacuum packaging, preserving certainty and protecting against ambiguity and doubt. This seal, I surmise, might explain why the most egotistical physicians, even the really old ones, appear so fresh, their skin flush, their decisions crisp. But it's effective for only so long. Remember, the Tupperware festering in the refrigerator once contained a delicious and nutritious meal.

Becoming an older physician means achieving the inevitable consolation that you'll be humbled again and again. The body doesn't read the textbooks, and it's safe to assume patients haven't read the script either.

When I was younger, I copied this quote from Ralph Waldo Emerson upon a three-by-five notecard and taped it above my desk (sadly, it's true. I did.): "Shall I tell the secret of the true scholar? It is this: Every man I meet is my master in some point, and in that I learn of him."

Teachable moments and pricks of insight often strike without warning, usually outside the carefully constructed knowledge delivery systems of lecture halls or ward rounds.

Nurses and ward clerks, social workers and translators, security guards and custodians have all served as my "masters" throughout my career. They have offered winking approvals, as well as casting a hot spotlight on behaviors, attitudes, and actions that *weren't* me.

Patients have also imparted sharp and unexpected lessons: this is how you die with grace; this is how you survive on the streets; this is how you *don't* talk to patients, even when the ED is crazy and there's a cardiac arrest pulling through the door; this is how you earn my trust. Teaching such knowledge and insight in its many forms can be difficult. Each situation feels new and particular, expected and surprising.

When first entering medical school, I never imagined the most influential teacher in my medical career would come in the form of the late Walter James Miller, an New York University professor, author, poet, critic, radio personality. He was not a physician. His mentorship, and later friendship, began during my year away from medical school and flourished as I wrote a terrible novel. He knew that to write well, you must first write poorly. But you must write. He rarely took a sharp knife to my prose. Years later, I accused him of being too kind to my early work. He said I wasn't ready for that type and depth of criticism. Instead, I needed encouragement, the license to stay true to what he knew was so important to me. Only now, twenty years later, do I recognize mentoring so deftly wrought that I didn't know it was going on. The right knowledge at the right time. He set the conditions that permitted me to discover what I needed to learn. I've "borrowed" more from his mentoring style than that of any other physician/educator.

I'm now an older physician and still a work-in-progress, thirsty for ways to become a better version of myself.

What does this have to do with my beat-up stethoscope?

For all its grandeur, its many functions as instrument, adornment, and friend, the stethoscope is limited to unidirectional conduction of the body's objective sounds. It captures narrative fragments, tiny statements. What really matters is how we process these sounds—intellectually and emotionally—and then translate them into meaningful action. That's why a less expensive stethoscope achieves a perfect balance for me. It's light and flexible, and the acoustics allow space for suggestion, permits me to hear judiciously what I need to hear and to filter out that which I don't. Listening through and around the earpieces—an idea that winks at Laennec's original definition of the stethoscope as a *chest observer*—is the only way to reconcile the multiple streams of sounds into a coherent story.

My year writing fiction in medical school was marked by intense anxiety and fear that I wasn't becoming the doctor I expected myself to be. Little did I realize that what I was learning about finding voice, committing to craft, obeying passions, pushing boundaries, embracing mistakes, welcoming uncertainty, and accepting rejection was developing the essential pieces that would give shape to this older physician.

To become an excellent doctor, one must take care of patients, an endless train of them. Along the way, as doctors-in-training master clinical skills and cultivate emotional attunement, it's imperative that they also find their voice. Otherwise, there is danger of becoming a high-end stethoscope. The writer/critic Anatole Broyard said it best: "There is a paradox here at the heart of medicine, because a doctor, like a writer, must have a voice of his own, something that conveys the timbre, the rhythm, the diction, and the music of his humanity that compensates us for all the speechless machines" (1992, 53).

Medical school can make students feel like suffocating victims in a knowledge avalanche. But the practice of medicine is more nuanced and oblique, with room for personality to take fully authentic breaths. I'm still working on finding my voice in medicine. After all these years, patients continue to surprise me, and as a consequence, I continue to surprise myself. I've become more comfortable with that, as I was with sharing a stethoscope with a colleague I respect so much. She eventually moved on to a job that better fit her clinical and teaching skills, and I did as well. My treasured stethoscope, fulfilling its fate, vanished. I'd like to imagine a younger physician using it, channeling the experience of two older physicians while acquiring and accumulating his or her own, but I'm doubtful. It was only a fair conductor of pure sounds. But if you knew what to listen for, there was no better guide.

ACKNOWLEDGMENTS

Special thanks to Betsy Biggs, whose work and ideas have deepened my understanding of sound.

REFERENCES

Aaron, Deborah J., Akira Sekikawa, Francois Sauer, John Patrick, Rimei Nishimura, Benjamin Acosta, and Ronald LaPorte. 1998. "The Reincarnation of Biomedical Journals as Hypertext Comic Books." *Nature Medicine,* vol. 4. www.nature.com/nm/web_specials/comics/index.html.

Aarons, Victoria. 2007. " 'There's No Remaking Reality': Philip Roth's *Everyman* and the Ironies of Body and Spirit." *Xavier Review* 21 (1): 116–127.

Aberth, John. 2005. *The Black Death: The Great Mortality of 1348–1350: A Brief History with Documents.* New York: Palgrave Macmillan.

Abraham, Abraham S. 2000. *Nishmat Avraham,* vol. 2: *Yoreh De'ah: Medical Halachah for Doctors, Nurses, Health-Care Personnel, and Patients.* Artscholl Halachah Series. 1st ed. Translated by Abraham S. Abraham. Brooklyn, NY: Mesorah Publications. www.torah.org/advanced/shulchan-aruch/classes/chapter30.html.

Accordino, Robert E., Danielle Engler, Iona H. Ginsburg, and John Koo. 2008. "Morgellons Disease." *Dermatologic Therapy* 21 (3): 8–12.

Adorno, Theodor W. 1973. *Negative Dialectics.* Translated by E. B. Ashton. New York: Seabury Press. (Originally published in 1966 by Suhrkamp Verlag, Frankfurt, under the title *Negative Dialektik.*)

———. 1997. *Aesthetic Theory.* Minneapolis: University of Minnesota Press.

Adorno, Theodor W., Else F. Frenkel-Brunswik, Daniel J. Levinson, and R. Nevitt Sanford. 1950. *The Authoritarian Personality.* New York: Harper & Row.

Afkhami, Afir. 2003. "Compromised Constitutions: The Iranian Experience with the 1918 Influenza Pandemic." *Bulletin of the History of Medicine* 77 (2): 367–392.

Agamben, Giorgio. 1998. *Homo Sacer: Sovereign Power and Bare Life.* Palo Alto, CA: Stanford University Press.

Albrecht, Gary L., Katherine D. Seelman, and Michael Bury. 2001. *Handbook of Disability Studies.* Thousand Oaks, CA: Sage.

Alcoff, Linda Martin. 1991–1992. "The Problem of Speaking for Others." *Cultural Critique* 20: 5–32.

Ali, A. Yusef. 2001. *An English Interpretation of the Holy Quran.* New York: Lushena Books.

Altavilla, Gina M. LeVasseur. 2010. "Queer Narrative Prosthesis: Disability and Sexuality in *Richard III* and *House M.D.*" Master's thesis, California State University San Marcos.

Alvarez, Walter C. 1961. *Minds That Came Back.* New York: J. B. Lippincott. www.archive.org/stream/mindthatcameback007026mbp/mindthatcameback007026mbp_djvu.txt.

American College of Obstetricians and Gynecologists. 2004, October 15. *Multiple Gestation: Complicated Twin, Triplet, and High-Order Multifetal Pregnancy.* ACOG Practice Bulletin no. 56. Washington, DC: American College of Obstetricians and Gynecologists.

American Public Health Association. 2008. "At the Intersection of Public Health and Transportation: Promoting Health Transportation Policy." www.apha.org/NR/rdonlyres/43F10382-FB68-4112-8C75-49DCB10F8ECF/0/TransportationBrief.pdf.

Anderson, Charles M. 1989. *Richard Selzer and the Rhetoric of Surgery.* Carbondale: Southern Illinois University Press.

Anderson, Laurie M., Susan C. Scrimshaw, Mindy T. Fullilove, Jonathan E. Fielding, Jacques

Normand, and the Task Force on Preventive Services. 2003. "The Effectiveness of Early Childhood Development Programs: A Systematic Review." *American Journal of Preventive Medicine* 24 (3): 32–46.

Andrews, Lori B. 1999. *The Clone Age: Adventures in the New World of Reproductive Technology.* New York: Henry Holt & Co.

The Andromeda Strain. 2008. Television miniseries. Directed by Mikael Salomon. Los Angeles: Scott Free Productions.

Angela. n.d. *Inflamed: Living with Rheumatoid Arthritis.* Blog. http://inflamed.wordpress.com. Accessed July 10, 2013.

Angell, Marcia. 2005. *The Truth about Drug Companies: How They Deceive Us and What to Do about It.* New York: Random House.

———. 2011a, June 23. "The Epidemic of Mental Illness: Why?" *New York Review of Books.* www.nybooks.com/articles/archives/2011/jun/23/epidemic-mental-illness-why.

———. 2011b, July 14. "The Illusions of Psychiatry." *New York Review of Books.* www.nybooks.com/articles/archives/2011/jul/14/illusions-of-psychiatry/?pagination=false.

Antze, Paul, and Michael Lambek. 1996. *Tense Past: Cultural Essays in Trauma and Memory.* New York: Routledge.

Appel, Jacob M. 2009, July 15. "Motherhood: Is It Ever Too Late?" *Huffington Post.* www.huffingtonpost.com/jacob-m-appel/motherhood-is-it-ever-too_b_233916.html.

Applbaum, Kalman. 2006. "Educating for Global Mental Health: The Adoption of SSRIs in Japan." In *Global Pharmaceuticals: Ethics, Markets, Practices,* edited by Adriana Petryna, Andrew Lakoff, and Arthur Kleinman, 85–111. Durham, NC: Duke University Press.

———. 2009. "Getting to Yes: Corporate Power and the Creation of a Psychopharmaceutical Blockbuster." *Culture, Medicine, and Psychiatry* 33 (2): 185–215.

Apted, Michael, dir. 1994. *Blink.* Los Angeles: New Line Cinema.

Ariès, Philippe. (1981) 2008. *The Hour of Our Death: The Classic History of Western Attitudes toward Death over the Last One Thousand Years.* Translated by Helen Weaver. New York: Vintage Books.

Arnett, Jeffrey Jensen. 2004. *Emerging Adulthood: The Winding Road from the Late Teens through the Twenties.* Oxford: Oxford University Press.

Arnheim, Rudolf. 1969. *Visual Thinking.* Berkeley: University of California Press.

Arnoff, Stephen. 2006, June. "Live by No Man's Code: The Religious Forms of Philip Roth's *Everyman.*" *Zeek: A Jewish Journal of Thought and Culture.* www.zeek.net/606roth.

Arnold P. Gold Foundation. 2010. "Planning for a White Coat Ceremony." www.humanism-in-medicine.org/index.php/programs_grants/gold_foundation_programs/white_coat_ceremony/planning_for_a_wcc.

Arthurs, Deborah. 2011. "Girl Gets Boob Job Voucher for Her SEVENTH Birthday from Surgery-Addicted Mother Dubbed 'the Human Barbie.'" *Daily Mail.* www.dailymail.co.uk/femail/article-2000871/Sarah-Burge-Human-Barbie-gives-daughter-boob-job-voucher-7th-birthday.html#ixzz1ep86NeKh.

Asch, Adrienne. 1995. "Can Aborting 'Imperfect' Children Be Immoral?" In *Ethical Issues in Modern Medicine,* edited by John D. Arras and Bonnie Steinbock, 523–533. Mountain View, CA: Mayfield Publishing Co.

———. 1998. "Distracted by Disability." *Cambridge Quarterly of Healthcare Ethics* 7: 77–87.

Ashby, Hal, dir. 1978. *Coming Home.* Beverly Hills, CA: United Artists.

Aspden, Philip, Janet M. Corrigan, Julie Wolcott, and Shari M. Erickson, eds. 2004. *Patient Safety: Achieving a New Standard for Care.* Institute of Medicine. Washington, DC: National Academies Press.

Astrow, Alan B., Ann Wexler, Kenneth Texeira, M. Kai He, and Dennis P. Sulmasy. 2007. "Is Failure to Meet the Spiritual Needs Associated with Cancer Patients' Perceptions of Quality of Care and Their Satisfaction with Care?" *Journal of Clinical Oncology* 25 (36): 5753–5757.

Atkinson, Jim. 2006. "Under My Skin." *Texas Monthly* 34 (10): 48–49.

Auden, W. H. (1938) 1991. "Musée des Beaux Arts." In *On Doctoring: Stories, Poems, Essays,* 1st ed., edited by Richard Reynolds and John Stone, 128–129. New York: Simon & Schuster.

Avert. n.d. "Worldwide HIV and AIDS Statistics:Global HIV and AIDS estimates, 2011." www.avert.org/worldstats.htm. Accessed July 15, 2011.

Avrahami, Einat. 2007. *The Invading Body: Reading Illness Autobiographies.* Charlottesville: University of Virginia Press.

AXIS Dance Company. 2009. "The Beauty . . ." [excerpt from "The Beauty That Was Mine, through the Middle, without Stopping"]. YouTube video. http://youtu.be/eX8fGbUWdIo.

Babbie, Earl. 2004. *The Practice of Social Research,* 10th ed. Belmont, CA: Wadsworth/Thomson.

"Babies Aborted for Not Being Perfect." 2006, May 30. *Daily Mail.* www.dailymail.co.uk/news/article-388114/Babies-aborted-perfect.html.

Backer, Leigh Ann. 2007. "The Medical Home: An Idea Whose Time Has Come . . . Again." *Family Practice Management* 14 (8): 38–41.

Bäckman, Lars, Sari Jones, Anna-Karin Berger, E. J Laukka, Erika Jonsson, and Brent Small. 2004. "Multiple Cognitive Deficits during the Transition to Alzheimer's Disease." *Journal of Internal Medicine* 256:195–204.

Bacon, Lloyd, dir. 1930. *Moby Dick.* Burbank, CA: Warner Bros.

Baggs, Amanda. 2007. *In My Language.* YouTube video. http://youtu.be/JnylM1hI2jc.

Baker Brown, Isaac. 1854. *On some Diseases of women admitting of surgical Treatment: Illustrated by coloured Plates and wood Engravings.* London: Churchill. (Subsequently published as *Surgical Diseases of Women.*)

———. 1866. *On the Curability of Certain Forms of Insanity, Epilepsy, Catalepsy, and Hysteria in Females.* London: Cox & Wyman.

Balboni, Tracy A., Mary Elizabeth Paulk, Michael J. Balboni, Andrea C. Phelps, Elizabeth T. Loggers, Alexi A. Wright, Susan D. Block, Eldrin F. Lewis, John R. Peteet, and Holly Gwen Prigerson. 2010. "Provision of Spiritual Care to Patients with Advanced Cancer: Associations with Medical Care and Quality of Life near Death." *Journal of Clinical Oncology* 28 (3): 445–452.

Balboni, Tracy A., Lauren C. Vanderwerker, Susan D. Block, M. Elizabeth Paulk, Christopher S. Lathan, John R. Peteet, and Holly Gwen Prigerson. 2007. "Religiousness and Spiritual Support among Advanced Cancer Patients and Associations with End-of-Life Treatment Preferences and Quality of Life." *Journal of Clinical Oncology* 25 (5): 555–560.

Balint, Enid. 1969. "The Possibilities of Patient-Centered Medicine." *Journal of the Royal College of General Practitioners* 17 (82): 269–276.

Banks, Russell. 2002. "Bodies in the Basement: An Ars Poetica with Attitude." In *Unholy Ghost: Writers on Depression,* edited by Nell Casey, 29–38. New York: Harper Perennial.

Barad, Karen. 2007. *Meeting the Universe Halfway: Quantum Physics and the Entanglement of Matter and Meaning.* Durham, NC: Duke University Press.

Bardes, Charles L., Debra Gillers, and Amy E. Herman. 2001. "Learning to Look: Developing Clinical Observational Skills at an Art Museum." *Medical Education* 35:1157–1161.

Barker, Pat. 1995. *The Regeneration Trilogy.* 3 vols. Harmondsworth: Plume.

Barker-Benfield, G. J. 1978. "Sexual Surgery in Late Nineteenth-Century America." In *Seizing Our Bodies: The Politics of Women's Health,* edited by Claudia Dreifus, 13–41. New York: Harper & Row. (Originally published in *International Journal of Health Services* 5 [1976]: 279–298.)

Barnard, David. 1985. "The Physician as Priest, Revisited." *Journal of Religion and Health* 24: 272–286.

Baron-Cohen, Simon, ed. 1993. *Understanding Other Minds: Perspectives from Autism.* Oxford: Oxford University Press.

———. 1997. *Mindblindness: An Essay on Autism and Theory of Mind.* Cambridge, MA: MIT Press.

Baron-Cohen, Simon. 2001. "Theory of Mind and Autism: A Review." Special issue of *International Review of Mental Retardation* 23:169–184.

———. 2004. *The Essential Difference*. London: Penguin.

Barton, Adriana. 2010, September 13. "Disagreements over Childrearing are Growing Cause of Divorce." *Globe and Mail* (Vancouver). www.theglobeandmail.com/life/family-and-relationships/disagreements-over-childrearing-are-growing-cause-of-divorce/article 1705528.

Bauby, Jean-Dominique. 1998. *The Diving Bell and the Butterfly: A Memoir of Life in Death*. New York: Vintage.

Baudrillard, Jean. 1993. *The Transparency of Evil: Essays on Extreme Phenomena*. Translated by James Benedict. London: Verso Books.

Bauman, H-Dirksen. 2004. "Audism: Exploring the Metaphysics of Oppression." *Journal of Deaf Studies and Deaf Education* 9 (2): 239–246.

———. 2008. "Introduction: Listening to Deaf Studies." In *Open Your Eyes: Deaf Studies Talking*, edited by H-Dirksen L. Bauman, 1–34. Minneapolis: University of Minnesota Press.

Bauman, Richard. 1986. *Story, Performance, and Event: Contextual Studies of Oral Narrative*. Cambridge Studies in Oral and Literate Culture. Cambridge: Cambridge University Press.

Bazzana, Kevin. 1997. *Glenn Gould, the Performer in the Work: A Study in Performance Practice*. Oxford: Clarendon Press.

———. 2004. *Wondrous Strange: The Life and Art of Glenn Gould*. Oxford: Oxford University Press.

Beach, Mary Catherine, Eboni G. Price, Tiffany Gary, Karen A. Robinson, Aysegul Gozu, Ana Palacio, Carole Smarth, Mollie W. Jenckes, Carolyn Feuerstein, and Eric Bass. 2005. "Cultural Competence: A Systematic Review of Health Care Provider Institutional Interventions." *Medical Care* 43:356–373.

Beagan, Brenda L. 2003. "Teaching Social and Cultural Awareness to Medical Students: 'It's All Very Nice to Talk about It in Theory, But Ultimately It Makes No Difference.'" *Academic Medicine* 78:605–614.

Beal, Anne C., Michelle M. Doty, Susan E. Hernandez, Katherine K. Shea, and Karen Davis. 2007. *Closing the Divide: How Medical Homes Promote Equity in Health Care. Results from the Commonwealth Fund 2006 Health Care Quality Survey*. New York: Commonwealth Fund. www.commonwealthfund.org/usr_doc/1035_Beal_closing_divide_medical_homes.pdf.

Beal, Anne, Susan Hernandez, and Michelle Doty. 2009. "Latino Access to the Patient-Centered Medical Home." *Journal of General Internal Medicine* 24 (suppl. 3): 514–520.

Beauchamp, Tom L., and James F. Childress. 1979. *Principles of Biomedical Ethics*, 1st ed. New York: Oxford University Press.

———. 1994. *Principles of Biomedical Ethics*, 4th ed. New York: Oxford University Press.

———. 2008. *Principles of Biomedical Ethics*, 6th ed. New York: Oxford University Press.

Beauvoir, Simone de. 1970. *La Vieillesse*. Paris: Gallimard.

Becker, Ernest. 1973. *The Denial of Death*. New York: Free Press.

Belcham, C. 2004. "Spirituality in Occupational Therapy: Theory in Practice?" *British Journal of Occupational Therapy* 67 (1): 39–46.

Belkin, Lisa. 2001, July 1. "The Made-to-Order Savior." *New York Times Magazine*.

Bell, Charles. 1824. *Essays on the Anatomy and Philosophy of Expression*. London: John Murray. (Originally published in 1806 as *Essays on the Anatomy of Expression in Painting* by Longman, Hurst, Rees, & Orme, London.)

Bell, Susan E., and Susan M. Reverby. 2005. "Vaginal Politics: Tensions and Possibilities in *The Vagina Monologues*." *Women's Studies International Forum* 28:430–444.

Belling, Catherine. 2006a. "Hypochondriac Hermeneutics: Medicine and the Anxiety of Interpretation." *Literature and Medicine* 25 (2): 376–401.

———. 2006b. "Medicine and the Silent Oracle: An Exercise in Uncertainty." *Journal for Learning through the Arts*, 2(1). http://escholarship.org/uc/item/4hq6k738.

———. 2010. "Narrating Oncogenesis: The Problem of Telling When Cancer Begins." *Narrative* 18 (2): 229–247.

Belmonte, Matthew K. 2008. "Human, but More So: What the Autistic Brain Tells Us about the Process of Narrative." In *Autism and Representation,* edited by Mark Osteen, 166–180. New York: Routledge.

Benedetti, Fabrizio. 2009. *Placebo Effects: Understanding the Mechanisms in Health and Disease.* New York: Oxford University Press.

Benesch-Granberg, Barbara, Kate Harding, Rachel Richardson, Fillyjonk, and Vesta44. n.d. *First, Do No Harm: Real Stories of Fat Prejudice in Health Care.* http://fathealth.wordpress.com.

Benford, Criscillia. 2010. "'Listen to My Tale': Multilevel Structure, Narrative Sense Making, and the Inassimilable in Mary Shelley's *Frankenstein.*" *Narrative* 18:324–346.

Benner, Patricia, Christine A. Tanner, and Catherine A. Chesla. 1996. *Expertise in Nursing Practice: Caring, Clinical Judgment, and Ethics.* New York: Springer.

Bennett, Amanda. 1992, October 14. "Lori Schiller Emerges from the Torments of Schizophrenia." *Wall Street Journal,* A1, A10.

Bennett, Joshua. 2009, November 2. "Tamara's Opus." *White House Poetry Jam.* YouTube video. youtube.com/watch?v=_U5BwD8zOeM.

Benson, Peter, and Bernard Spilka. 1973. "God Image: A Function of Self-Esteem and Locus Control." *Journal for Scientific Study of Religion* 12:297–310.

Bentham, Jeremy. 1823. *Introduction to the Principles of Morals and Legislation.* 2nd ed. London: E. Wilson.

Berkenkotter, Carol. 2008. *Patient Tales: Case Histories and the Uses of Narrative in Psychiatry.* Columbia: University of South Carolina Press.

Bergman, Ingmar. (1987) 1988. *The Magic Lantern: An Autobiography.* Translated by Joan Tate. New York: Viking.

Berlin. Richard. 2008. *Poets on Prozac: Mental Illness, Treatment and the Creative Process.* Baltimore: Johns Hopkins University Press.

Bernhardt, Curtis, dir. 1955. *Interrupted Melody.* Beverly Hills, CA: Metro-Goldwyn-Mayer.

Bewley, A. P., P. Lepping, R. W. Freundenmann, and R. Taylor. 2010. "Editorial: Delusional Parasitosis: Time to Call It Delusional Infestation." *British Journal of Dermatology* 163 (1): 899.

Biotechnology and Biological Sciences Research Council. 2010. *Synthetic Biology Dialogue.* www.bbsrc.ac.uk/syntheticbiologydialogue.

Bishop, Jeffrey P. 2008. "Rejecting Medical Humanism: Medical Humanities and the Metaphysics of Medicine." *Journal of Medical Humanities* 29 (1): 15–25.

———. 2009. "Biopsychosociospiritual Medicine and Other Political Schemes." *Christian Bioethics* 15 (3): 254–276.

———. 2011a. *The Anticipatory Corpse: Medicine, Power and the Care of the Dying.* South Bend, IN: University of Notre Dame Press.

———. 2011b, June 14. "Love Is Stronger than Death." *St. Louis Post-Dispatch.*

Bissonette, Melissa Bloom. 2010. "Teaching the Monster: Frankenstein and Critical Thinking." *College Literature* 37:106–120.

Black, John. 1997. "Female Genital Mutilation: A Contemporary Issue, and a Victorian Obsession." *Journal of the Royal Society of Medicine* 90:402–405.

Bleakley, Alan. 2004. "'Your Creativity or Mine?' A Typology of Creativities in Higher Education and the Value of a Pluralistic Approach." *Teaching in Higher Education* 9:463–475.

———. 2005. "Stories as Data, Data as Stories: Making Sense of Narrative Inquiry in Clinical Education." *Medical Education* 39 (5): 534–540.

———. 2006. "A Common Body of Care: The Ethics and Politics of Teamwork in the Operating Theatre Are Inseparable." *Journal of Medicine and Philosophy* 31:1–18.

———. 2009. "Curriculum as Conversation." *Advances in Health Sciences Education: Theory and Practice* 14:297–301.

Bleakley, Alan. (Forthcoming). *The Heart of the Matter: Patient-Centredness in Transition.* Dordrecht: Springer.

Bleakley, Alan, and John Bligh. 2009. "Who Can Resist Foucault?" *Journal of Medicine and Philosophy* 34:368–383.

Bleakley, Alan, John Bligh, and Julie Browne. 2011. *Medical Education for the Future: Identity, Power, and Location.* Dordecht: Springer.

Bleakley, Alan, Richard Farrow, David Gould, and Robert Marshall. 2003a. "Making Sense of Clinical Reasoning: Judgment and the Evidence of the Senses." *Medical Education* 37: 544–552.

———. 2003b. "Learning How to See: Doctors Making Judgments in the Visual Domain." *Journal of Workplace Learning* 15:301–306.

Bleakley, Alan, Adrian Hobbs, James Boyden,and Linda Walsh. 2004. "Safety in Operating Theatres: Improving Teamwork through Team Resource Management." *Journal of Workplace Learning* 16:83–91.

Bleakley, Alan, Robert Marshall, and Rainer Brömer. 2006. "Toward an Aesthetic Medicine: Developing a Core Medical Humanities Undergraduate Curriculum." *Journal of Medical Humanities* 27:197–214.

Bleckner, Jeff, dir. 1998. *Rear Window.* New York: American Broadcasting Company and Hallmark Entertainment.

Bley, Liza. 2008. "Defining Sex and Virginity." *Not Your Mother's Meatloaf,* issue no. 1. http://sexedcomicproject.blogspot.com. Accessed September 29, 2011.

———. 2008. "Take A Peak." *Not Your Mother's Meatloaf,* issue no. 1. http://sexedcomic project.blogspot.com. Accessed September 29, 2011.

Bligh, John, and Alan Bleakley. 2006. "Distributing Menus to Hungry Learners: Can Learning by Simulation Become Simulation of Learning?" *Medical Teacher* 8:606–613.

Block, Marcelline, and Angela Laflin, eds. 2010. *Gender Scripts in Medicine and Narrative.* Newcastle upon Tyne: Cambridge Scholars.

Block, Susan. 2011, March 8. "Helping Patients Make Peace with Death." HBR Blog Network, *Harvard Business Review.* http://blogs.hbr.org/innovations-in-health-care/2011/03/-the -stuff-i-do.html.

Blow, Frederic C., John E. Zeber, John F. McCarthy, Marcia Valenstein, Leah Gillon, and C. Raymond Bingham. 2004. "Ethnicity and Diagnostic Patterns in Veterans with Psychoses." *Social Psychiatry and Psychiatric Epidemiology* 39 (10): 841–851.

Bockoven, John S. 1956. "Moral Treatment in American Psychiatry." *Journal of Nervous and Mental Diseases* 124:167–194.

Boler, Megan. 1999. *Feeling Power: Emotions and Education.* New York: Routledge.

Bonham, Vence L. 2001. "Race, Ethnicity, and Pain Treatment: Striving to Understand the Causes and Solutions to the Disparities in Pain Treatment." *Journal of Law, Medicine, and Ethics* 29 (1): 52–68.

Boorse, Christopher. 1997. "Health as a Theoretical Concept." *Philosophy of Science* 44:542–573.

Borrill, Carol S., Jean Carletta, Angela J. Carter, Jeremy F. Dawson, Simon Garrod, Anne Rees, Ann Richards, David Shapiro, and Michael A. West. 2000. *The Effectiveness of Health Care Teams in the National Health Service.* Birmingham: Aston Business School, University of Aston.

Bosk, C. 1979. *Forgive and Remember: Managing Medical Failure.* Chicago: University of Chicago Press.

Boston Women's Health Book Collective. 1973. *Our Bodies, Our Selves.* New York: Touchstone.

Bourgois-Chacón, Emiliano. 2004. "My Body Is My Temple." *Bringing the Noise 3.* Audio CD.

Bouwsma, William J. 1973."Lawyers and Early Modern Culture." *American Historical Review* 78:303–327.

Bowling, Ann. 2005. *Measuring Health: A Review of Quality of Life Measurement Scales.* Maidenhead: Open University Press.

Braff, Zach, dir. 2004. *Garden State.* Los Angeles: Fox Searchlight Pictures.

Braithwaite, Dawn O. 1994. "Viewing Persons with Disabilities as a Culture." In *Intercultural Communication: A Reader,* edited by Larry A. Samovar and Richard E. Porter, 148–154. Belmont, CA: Wadsworth.

Branagh, Kenneth, dir. 1994. *Frankenstein.* Culver City, CA: TriStar Pictures.

Brashler, Anne. (1988) 1990. "He Read to Her." In *Vital Lines: Contemporary Fiction about Medicine,* edited by John Mukand, 84–87. New York: Ballantine.

Breitbart, William. 2001. "Spirituality and Meaning in Supportive Care: Spirituality- and Meaning-Centered Group Psychotherapy Interventions in Advanced Cancer." *Supportive Care in Cancer* 10 (4): 272–280.

Brennan, Nicola, Oonagh Corrigan, Jon Allard, Julian Archer, Rebecca Barnes, Alan Bleakley, Tracey Collett, and Sam Regan De Bere. 2010. "The Transition from Medical School to Junior Doctor: Today's Experiences of Tomorrow's Doctors." *Medical Education* 44: 449–458.

Brenner, M. Harvey. 1973. *Mental Illness and the Economy.* Cambridge, MA: Harvard University Press.

Brimlow, Deborah L., Jennifer S. Cook, and Richard Seaton. 2003. "Stigma & HIV/AIDS: A Review of the Literature." Rockville, MD: Health Resources and Services Administration, HIV/AIDS Bureau. http://test.stigmaactionnetwork.org/atomicDocuments/SANDocuments/20110330164904-HRSA_2003_Stigma%20and%20HIV-AIDS%20-%20A%20Review%20of%20the%20Literature.pdf. Accessed August 10, 2001.

Briski, Zana, and Ross Kauffman, dirs. 2004. *Born into Brothels.* Red Light Films. New York: HBO/Cinmax.

Britton, Jeanne. 2009. "Novelistic Sympathy in Mary Shelley's *Frankenstein.*" *Studies in Romanticism* 48:3–24.

Brody, Howard. 1981. "Hope." *Journal of the American Medical Association* 246:1411–1412.

———. 1987. *Stories of Sickness.* New Haven, CT: Yale University Press.

———. 1993. *The Healer's Power.* New Haven, CT: Yale University Press.

———. 1994. " 'My Story Is Broken; Can You Help Me Fix It?' Medical Ethics and the Joint Construction of Narrative." *Literature and Medicine* 13 (1): 79–92.

———. 2000. "The Placebo Response: Recent Research and Implications for Family Medicine." *Journal of Family Practice* 49:649–654.

———. 2003. *Stories of Sickness,* 2nd ed. New York: Oxford University Press.

———. 2009. *The Future of Bioethics.* New York: Oxford University Press.

Brody, Howard, and Daralyn Brody. 2000. *The Placebo Response: How You Can Release the Body's Inner Pharmacy for Better Health.* New York: HarperCollins.

Brody, Jane E. 2011, November 29. "It Could Be Old Age, or It Could Be Low B12." *New York Times,* D7.

Bromberg, Walter, and Frank Simon. 1968. "The 'Protest' Psychosis: A Special Type of Reactive Psychosis." *Archives of General Psychiatry* 19:155–160.

Books, Mel, dir. 1977. *High Anxiety.* Los Angeles: 20th Century Fox.

Brown, Judith B., Moira Stewart, Eric McCracken, Ian R. McWhinney, and Joseph Levenstein. 1986. "The Patient-Centred Clinical Method: 2. Definition and Application." *Family Practice* 3 (2): 75–79.

Browning, Barbara. 2010. "Rethinking Technique and the Body 'Proper.' " In "Dialogues: The State of the Body." *Dance Research Journal,* 42 no. 1 (Summer): 81–83.

Browning, Tod, dir. 1927. *The Unknown.* Beverly Hills, CA: Metro-Goldwyn-Mayer.

———, dir. 1928. *West of Zanzibar.* Beverly Hills, CA: Metro-Goldwyn-Mayer.

———, dir. 1931. *Dracula.* Universal City, CA: Universal Pictures.

———, dir. 1932. *Freaks.* Beverly Hills, CA: Metro-Goldwyn-Mayer.

———, dir. 1936. *The Devil-Doll.* Beverly Hills, CA: Metro-Goldwyn-Mayer.

Broyard, Anatole. 1990. "Good Books Abut Being Sick." *New York Times,* April 1. www.nytimes.com/1990/04/01/books/good-books-abut-being-sick.html?pagewanted=all.

Broyard, Anatole. 1992. *Intoxicated by My Illness: And Other Writings on Life and Death.* New York: Ballantine.

Brozan, Nadine. 1994, October 4. "Chronicle." *New York Times,* Style section. www.nytimes .com/1994/10/04/style/chronicle-427284.html?emc=eta1.

Bruegel, Pieter. ca. 1558. *Landscape with the Fall of Icarus.* Oil on canvas, mounted on wood, 73.5 × 112 cm. Brussels: Musées Royaux des Beaux-Arts de Belgique.

Bruner, Edward M. 1986. "Introduction." In *The Anthropology of Experience,* edited by Victor Witter Turner and Edward M. Bruner, 3–30. Urbana: University of Illinois Press.

Brunner, Eric, and Michael Marmot. 2006. "Social Organization, Stress, and Health." In *Social Determinants of Health,* 2nd ed., edited by Michael Marmot and Richard G. Wilkinson, 6–30. New York: Oxford University Press.

Buck v. Bell. 1927. 274 US 200. Supreme Court of the United States.

Budbill, David. 2008. "The Uses of Depression: The Way Around Is Through." In *Poets on Prozac: Mental Illness, Treatment and the Creative Process,* edited by Richard Berlin, 80–91. Baltimore: Johns Hopkins University Press.

Bureau of Democracy, Human Rights, and Labor. 2008, March 11. "China (includes Tibet, Hong Kong, and Macau)." U.S. Department of State. www.state.gov/g/drl/rls/ hrrpt/2007/100518.htm.

Burke, Kenneth. 1973. *The Philosophy of Literary Form: Studies in Symbolic Action.* Berkeley: University of California Press.

Burke, Ross David. 1995. *When the Music's Over: My Journey into Schizophrenia,* edited by Richard Gates and Robin Hammond. New York: Basic Books.

Burnham, Scott. 2001. "Beethoven, Ludwig van: Posthumous Influence and Reception." In *The New Grove Dictionary of Music and Musicians,* 2nd ed., edited by Stanley Sadie, 3:110–114. London: Macmillan.

Burris, Scott. 2002. "Disease Stigma in U.S. Public Health Law." *Journal of Law, Medicine and Ethics* 30:179–190.

Burris, Scott. 2011. "Law in a Social Determinants Strategy: A Public Health Law Research Perspective." *Public Health Reports* 126 (Suppl. 3): 22–27.

———. Forthcoming. "From Health Care Law to the Social Determinants of Health: A Public Health Law Research Perspective." *University of Pennsylvania Law Review.*

Burris, Scott C., Ichiro Kawachi, and Austin Sarat. 2002. "Integrating Law and Social Epidemiology." *Journal of Law, Medicine and Ethics* 30:510–521.

Burton, John D. 2001. "'The Awful Judgments of God upon the Land': Smallpox in Colonial Massachusetts." *New England Quarterly* 74 (3): 495–506.

Bury, Michael. 1991. "The Sociology of Chronic Illness: A Review of Research and Prospects." *Sociology of Health and Illness* 13 (4): 451–468.

Butler, Judith. 1993. *Bodies That Matter: On the Discursive Limits of Sex.* New York: Routledge.

———. 2006. *Gender Trouble: Feminism and the Subversion of Identity.* New York: Routledge.

Butler, Robert N. 1963. "The Life Review: An Interpretation of Reminiscence in the Aged." *Psychiatry* 26:65–76.

Byock, Ira. 1997. *Dying Well: The Prospect for Growth at the End of Life.* New York: Riverhead Books.

Cameron, James, dir. 2009. *Avatar.* Los Angeles: 20th Century Fox.

Campo, Rafael. 2005. "'The Medical Humanities,' for Lack of a Better Term." *Journal of the American Medical Association* 294 (9): 1009.

Carey, Benedict. 2011, June 23. "Expert on Mental Illness Reveals Her Own Fight." *New York Times,* A1, A17.

Carmichael, Stokely. 1968. "Black Power: A Critique of the System of International White Supremacy and International Capitalism." In *The Dialectics of Liberation,* edited by David Cooper, 150–174. New York: Penguin.

Carr, Tracy Jean. 2010. "Facing Existential Realities: Exploring Barriers and Challenges to Spiritual Nursing Care." *Qualitative Health Research* 20 (10): 1379–1392.

Carter, Bernie. 2004. "Pain Narratives and Narrative Practitioners: A Way of Working 'in-Relation' with Children Experiencing Pain." *Journal of Nursing Management* 12 (3): 210–216.

Cartwright, Samuel A. 1851. "Report on the Diseases and Physical Peculiarities of the Negro Race." *New Orleans Medical and Surgical Journal,* 691–751.

Carver, Raymond. 1989. *Where I'm Calling From.* New York: Random House.

Casey, Nell. 2002. *Unholy Ghost: Writers on Depression.* New York: Harper Perennial.

Cassell, Eric J. 1982. "The Nature of Suffering and the Goals of Medicine." *New England Journal of Medicine* 306 (11): 639–645.

———. 1991. *The Nature of Suffering and the Goals of Medicine.* New York: Oxford University Press.

———. 2004. *The Nature of Suffering and the Goals of Medicine.* New York: Oxford University Press.

Cassileth, Barrie R., Robert V. Zupkis, Kathering Sutton-Smith, and Vicki March. 1980. "Information and Participation Preferences among Cancer Patients." *Annals of Internal Medicine* 92:832–836.

Centers for Disease Control and Prevention. 2009a, November 4. "Preliminary Report on Progress of External Peer Review of CDC's Unexplained Dermopathy Project to the CCID Board of Scientific Counselors." Atlanta, GA: Centers for Disease Control and Prevention. www.cdc.gov/unexplaineddermopathy/. Accessed August 27, 2011.

———. 2009b, November 5. "Unexplained Dermopathy (also Called "Morgellons)." www.cdc.gov/unexplaineddermopathy/updates.html. Accessed August 27, 2011.

Chambers, Tod. 2008. "Toward a Naturalized Narrative Bioethics." In *Naturalized Bioethics: Toward Responsible Knowing and Practice,* edited by Hilde Lindemann, Marian Verkerk, and Margaret Urban Walker, 125–142. New York: Cambridge University Press.

———. 2009. "The Virtue of Incongruity in the Medical Humanities." *Journal of Medical Humanities* 30 (3): 151–154.

Chambliss, D. F. 1996. *Beyond Caring: Hospitals, Nurses, and the Social Organization of Ethics.* Chicago: University of Chicago Press.

Chaplin, Charles, dir. 1931. *City Lights.* Charles Chaplin Productions. Beverly Hills, CA: United Artists.

———. 1964. *My Autobiography.* New York: Simon & Schuster.

Chapman, C. R., K. L. Casey, R. Dubner, K. M. Foley, R. H. Gracely, and A. E. Reading. 1985. "Pain Measurement: An Overview," *Pain* 22:1–31.

Charmaz, Kathy. 2006. "Measuring Pursuits, Marking Self: Meaning Construction in Chronic Illness." *International Journal of Qualitative Studies on Health and Well-Being* 1: 27–37.

Charon, Rita. 1994. "Narrative Contributions to Medical Ethics: Recognition, Formulation, Interpretation, and Validation in the Practice of the Ethicist." In *A Matter of Principles: Ferment in U.S. Bioethics,* edited by Edwin R. DuBose, Ronald P. Hamel, and Laurence J. O'Connell, 260–283. Valley Forge, PA: Trinity International Press.

———. 2001a. "Narrative Medicine: A Model for Empathy, Reflection, Profession, and Trust. *Journal of the American Medical Association* 286:1897–1902.

———. 2001b. "Narrative Medicine: Form, Function, and Ethics." *Annals of Internal Medicine* 143 (1): 83–87.

———. 2004. "Narrative and Medicine." *New England Journal of Medicine* 350:862–864.

———. 2006. *Narrative Medicine: Honoring the Stories of Illness.* New York: Oxford University Press.

———. 2008. "Illness and the Limits of Expression." *Biography* 31 (4): 740–744.

———. 2011a, February 23. "The Clearings of Narrative Medicine." Presented at "New Teaching in Medical Education Conference." Toronto, ON: Associated Medical Services.

———. 2011b. "The Novelization of the Body, or, How Medicine and Stories Need One Another." *Narrative* 19:33–50.

Charon, Rita, Joanne Trautmann Banks, Julia E. Connelly, Anne Hunsaker Hawkins, Kathryn Montgomery Hunter, Anne Hudson Jones, Martha Montello and Suzanne Poirer.

1995. "Literature and Medicine: Contributions to Clinical Practice." *Annals of Internal Medicine* 122 (8): 599–606.

Chew, Kristina. 2008. "Fractioned Idiom: Metonymy and the Language of Autism." In *Autism and Representation,* edited by Mark Osteen, 133–144. New York: Routledge.

Chibnall, John T., and Christy A. Brooks. 2001. "Religion in the Clinic: The Role of Physician Beliefs." *Southern Medical Journal* 94 (4): 374–379.

Chochinov, Harvey Max, Thomas Hack, Thomas Hassard, Linda Kristjanson, Susan Mc-Clement and Mike Harlos. 2005. "Dignity Therapy: A Novel Psychotherapeutic Intervention for Patients near the End of Life." *Journal of Clinical Oncology* 23(24): 5520–5525.

Chowkwanyun, Merlin. 2011. "The Strange Disappearance of History from Racial Health Disparities Research." *DuBois Review: Social Science Research on Race* 8:253–270.

Chute, Hillary. 2010. *Graphic Women: Life Narrative and Contemporary Comics.* New York: Columbia University Press.

Cicero. 1909–1914. *De Senectute.* Translated by Charles W. Eliot. Harvard Classics. New York: P. F. Collier & Son. www.bartleby.com/9/2/1.html.

Clare, Eli. 2009. *Exile and Pride: Disability, Queerness and Liberation.* Cambridge, MA: South End Press.

Clark, Anna. 2008. *Desire: A History of European Sexuality.* New York: Routledge.

Clark, Hillary. 2008. *Narratives and Depression: Telling the Dark.* Albany: State University of New York Press.

Clark, Paul A., Maxwell Drain, and Mary P. Malone. 2003. "Addressing Patients' Emotional and Spiritual Needs." *Joint Commission Journal on Quality and Safety* 29 (12): 659–670.

Clouser, K. Danner. 1972. "Humanities and the Medical School." In *Proceedings of the First Session, Institute on Human Values in Medicine,* edited by L. L. Hunt, 50–59. Philadelphia: Society for Health and Human Values.

———. 1980, April. Keynote address for a conference entitled "The Allied Health Training Institute on the Role of the Humanities in Allied Health Education." Philadelphia: Thomas Jefferson University. http://weberstudies.weber.edu/archive/archive%20A%20%20Vol.%201-10.3/Vol.%203/3.1Clauser.htm.

Cohn, Samuel K. Jr. 2002. "The Black Death: End of a Paradigm." *American Historical Review* 107:703–738.

Cole, Thomas R. 1991. *The Journey of Life: A Cultural History of Aging in America.* New York: Cambridge University Press.

Collins, Wilkie. 1868. *The Moonstone.* London: Tinsley Brothers.

———. 1875. *The Law and the Lady.* London: Chatto & Windus.

Colliver, Jerry A., Melina J. Conlee, Steven J. Verhulst, J. Kevin Dorsey. 2010. "Reports of the Decline of Empathy during Medical Education Are Greatly Exaggerated: A Reexamination of the Research." *Academic Medicine* 85:588–593.

Comfort, Alex. 1969, June 15. "*The Andromeda Strain.*" *Book World.*

Commander X and Tim R. Swartz. 2007. *Morgellons: Level 5 Plague of the New World Order.* New Brunswick, NJ: Global Communications.

Commission on Social Determinants of Health. 2009. "Closing the Gap in a Generation: Health Equity through Action on the Social Determinants of Health." www.who.int/social_determinants/thecommission/finalreport/en/index.html.

Cooke, Molly, David M. Irby, and Bridget C. O'Brien. 2010. *Educating Physicians: A Call for Reform of Medical School and Residency.* San Francisco: Jossey-Bass.

Cooley, Donald. 1947, July. "Don't Tell Them We're All Going Crazy." *Better Homes and Gardens,* 122–125.

Cooper, Lisa A., and Neil R. Powe. 2004. "Disparities in Patient Experiences, Health Care Processes, and Outcomes: The Role of Patient-Provider Racial, Ethnic, and Language Concordance." New York: Commonwealth Fund. www.commonwealthfund.org/Publications/Fund-Reports/2004/Jul/Disparities-in-Patient-Experiences--Health-Care-Processes--and-Outcomes--The-Role-of-Patient-Provide.aspx.

Cooper, Lisa A., Debra L. Roter, Rachel L. Johnson, Daniel E. Ford, Donald M. Steinwachs, and Neil R. Powe. 2003. "Patient-Centered Communication, Ratings of Care, and Concordance of Patient and Physician Race." *Annals of Internal Medicine* 139:907–915.

Cooper-Patrick, Lisa, Joseph J. Gallo, Junius J. Gonzales, Hong Thi Vu, Neil R. Powe, Christine Nelson, and Daniel E. Ford. 1999. "Race, Gender and Partnership in the Patient-Physician Relationship." *Journal of American Medical Association* 282:583–589.

Coulehan, Jack. 1991. "Eleven Steps" In *The Knitted Glove.* Troy, ME: Nightshade Press.

———. 2003. "Metaphor and Medicine: Narrative in Clinical Practice." *Yale Journal of Biology and Medicine* 76 (2): 87–95.

Coulehan, Jack L., Frederic W. Platt, Barry Egener, Richard Frankel, Chen-Tan Lin, Beth Lown, William H. Salazar. 2001. " 'Let Me See If I Have This Right . . .': Words That Help Build Empathy." *Annals of Internal Medicine* 135 (3): 221–227.

Council on Science and Public Health. "Suicide in Physicians and Physicians-in-Training." Report 2 (A-10). 2010. www.ama-assn.org/resources/doc/csaph/a10csaph2ft.pdf.

Couser, Thomas G. 1997. *Recovering Bodies: Illness, Disability, and Life Writing.* Madison: University of Wisconsin Press.

Covert Affairs. 2010–. Television series. New York: USA Network.

Covey, Herbert. 1985. "Old Age Portrayed by the Ages-of-Life Models from the Middle Ages to the 6th Century." *Gerontologist* 29:692–698.

Cox-White, Becky, and Susanna Flavia Boxall. 2009. "Redefining Disability: Maleficent, Unjust, and Inconsistent."*Journal of Medicine and Philosophy* 33:558–576.

Craig, Kenneth D., and Christopher J. Patrick. 1985. "Facial Expression during Induced Pain." *Journal of Personality and Social Psychology* 48:1080–1091.

Crawford, Paul, Brian Brown, Victoria Tischler, and Charlotte Baker. 2010. "Health Humanities: The Future of Medical Humanities?" *Mental Health Review Journal* 15:4–10.

Crenshaw, Kimberle. 1991. "Mapping the Margins: Intersectionality, Identity Politics, and Violence against Women of Color." *Stanford Law Review* 43:1241–1299.

Crichton, Michael. 1969. *The Andromeda Strain.* New York: Knopf.

———. 1997–2000. "Andromeda Strain Note." *Michael Crichton: The Official Site.* Constant C Productions. www.michaelcrichton.net/books-andromedastrain.html. Accessed January 11, 2012.

Cromwell, John, dir. 1944. *Since You Went Away.* Beverly Hills, CA: United Artists.

———, dir. 1945. *The Enchanted Cottage.* New York: RKO Radio Pictures.

Cronin, Justin. 2010. *The Passage.* New York: Ballantine Books.

Crowther, Bosley. 1963, September 12. "The Screen." *New York Times,* 32.

Culler, Jonathan. 2005. "In Need of a Name? A Response to Geoffrey Harpham." *New Literary History* 36:37–42.

Curtiz, Michael, dir. 1933. *Mystery of the Wax Museum.* Burbank, CA: Warner Bros.

———, dir. 1946. *Night and Day.* Burbank, CA: Warner Bros.

Culliton, Barbara J. 1976. "Recombinant DNA: Cambridge City Council Votes Moratorium." *Science* 193 (4250): 300–301.

Dalai Lama and Paul Ekman. 2008. *Emotional Awareness: Overcoming the Obstacles to Psychological Balance and Compassion.* New York: New York Times Books.

Dally, Ann. 1991. *Women under the Knife: A History of Surgery.* New York: Routledge.

Damasio, Antonio R. 1994. *Descartes' Error: Emotion, Reason, and the Human Brain.* New York: Putnam.

"Danger from the Moon." 1969, May 18. *New York Times,* E-16.

Daniels, Cynthia R. 1997. "Between Fathers and Fetuses: The Social Construction of Male Reproduction and the Politics of Fetal Harm." *Signs* 22 (3): 579–616.

———. 1999. "Fathers, Mothers, and Fetal Harm: Rethinking Gender Difference and Reproductive Responsibility." In *Fetal Subjects, Feminist Positions,* edited by Lynn M. Morgan and Meredith W. Michaels, 83–98. Philadelphia: University of Pennsylvania Press.

Dannelly, Brian, dir. 2004. *Saved!* Beverly Hills, CA: United Artists.

Danquah, Meri Nana-Ama. 1999. *Willow Weep for Me: A Black Woman's Journey through Depression*. New York: One World/Ballantine.

Darabont, Frank, dir. 1999. *The Green Mile*. Burbank, CA: Warner Bros. Pictures.

Darby, Robert. 2007. "The Benefits of Psychological Surgery: John Scoffern's Satire on Isaac Baker Brown." *Medical History* 51:527–544.

Darwin, Charles. 1872. *The Expression of the Emotions in Man and Animals*. London: John Murray.

DasGupta, Sayantani. 2008. "Narrative Humility." *Lancet* 371:980–981.

DasGupta, Sayantani, and Rita Charon. 2004. "Personal Illness Narratives: Using Reflective Writing to Teach Empathy." *Academic Medicine* 79 (4): 351–356.

Daston, Lorraine. 2009. "Science Studies and the History of Science." *Critical Inquiry* 35: 798–813.

Daves, Delmer, dir. 1945. *Pride of the Marines*. Burbank, CA: Warner Bros.

David B. 2006. *Epileptic*. New York: Pantheon.

David, Larry. 2011, July 4. "Fore." *New Yorker*.

Davidson, Clifford. 2007. *"Everyman" and Its Dutch Original, "Elkerljic."* Kalamazoo, MI: Medieval Institute Publications.

Davidson, Larry. 2003. *Living outside Mental Illness: Qualitative Studies of Recovery in Schizophrenia*. New York: New York University Press.

Davidson, Larry, Maria J. O'Connell, Janis Tondora, Martha Lawless, and Arthur C. Evans. 2005. "Recovery in Serious Mental Illness: A New Wine or Just a New Bottle?" *Professional Psychology: Research and Practice* 36(5): 480–487.

Davidson, Larry, and Priscilla Ridgway. 2011. "The Community Support Movement and Its Demise (1977–1997)." In *Classics of Community Psychiatry: Fifty Years of Mental Health outside the Hospital*, edited by Michael Rowe, Martha Lawless, Kenneth S. Thompson, and Larry Davidson, 225–232. New York: Oxford University Press.

Davidson, Larry, and John S. Strauss. 1995. "Beyond the Bio-psychosocial Model: Integrating Disorder, Health and Recovery." *Psychiatry* 58:44–55.

Davidson, Larry, Janis Tondora, Martha Staeheli Lawless, Maria J. O'Connell, and Michael Rowe. 2009. *A Practical Guide to Recovery-Oriented Practice: Tools for Transforming Mental Health Care*. New York: Oxford University Press.

Davis, Andrew, dir. 1993. *The Fugitive*. Burbank, CA: Warner Bros.

Davis, Bernard D., Bernard N. Fields, Edward O. Wilson, and Harlyn O. Halvorson. 1986, May 31. "The 'Andromeda Strain' Is Still Science Fiction." *New York Times*, sec. 1, 26.

Davis, Dena S. 1997. "Genetic Dilemmas and the Child's Right to an Open Future." *Rutgers Law Journal* 28 (3): 549–552.

Davis, Kathy. 2007. *The Making of "Our Bodies, Ourselves": How Feminism Travels across Borders*. Durham, NC: Duke University Press.

Davis, Lennard. 2002. *Bending over Backwards: Disability, Dismodernism, and Other Difficult Positions*. New York: New York University Press.

———. 2010a. "Constructing Normalcy." In *The Disability Studies Reader*, 3rd ed., edited by Lennard Davis, 3–19. New York: Routledge.

———, ed. 2010b. *The Disability Studies Reader*, 3rd ed. New York: Routledge.

De Bont, Jan, dir. 1994. *Speed*. Los Angeles: 20th Century Fox.

Decety, Jean, Kalina Michalska, and Yuko Aktsuki. 2008. "Who Caused the Pain? An fMRI Investigation of Empathy and Intentionality in Children." *Neuropsychologia* 46:2607–2614.

Delahanty, J. 2001. "Differences in Rates of Depression in Schizophrenia by Race." *Schizophrenia Bulletin* 152 (1): 29–38.

Deleuze, Gilles. 1997. *Essays Critical and Clinical*. Minneapolis: University of Minnesota Press.

Dellasega, Cheryl, Paula Milone-Nuzzo, Katherine M. Curci, J. O. Ballard, and Darrell G. Kirch. 2007. "The Humanities Interface of Nursing and Medicine." *Journal of Professional Nursing* 23 (3): 174–179.

Delphin, Miriam, and Michael Rowe. 2008. "Continuing Education in Cultural Competence for Community Mental Health Practitioners." *Professional Psychology: Research and Practice* 39 (2): 182–191.

Dennett, Daniel C. 1995, August 25. "Review of Damasio, Descartes' Error." *Times Literary Supplement*, 3–4.

Department for Children and Families, Region IV. 2009. "Grandparents Raising Grandchildren: A Call to Action." Washington, DC: U.S. Department of Health and Human Services. http://www.wmich.edu/grandparenting/docs/Grandparentsbroch2-8.pdf. Accessed December 28, 2011.

Department of Health. 2000. *An Organization with a Memory: Report of an Expert Group on Learning from Adverse Events in the NHS.* London: Her Majesty's Stationery Office.

Derkatch, Colleen, and Judy Z. Segal. 2005. "Realms of Rhetoric in Health and Medicine." *University of Toronto Medical Journal* 82:138–142.

Derrida, Jacques. 1997. *Politics of Friendship.* London: Verso.

———. 1998. *Archive Fever: A Freudian Impression.* Chicago: University of Chicago Press.

Deutsch, Albert. 1948. *The Shame of the States.* New York: Arno Press.

Deutsch, Helen. 2002. "Exemplary Aberration: Samuel Johnson and the English Canon." In *Disability Studies: Enabling the Humanities,* edited by Sharon L. Snyder, Brenda Jo Brueggemann, and Rosemarie Garland-Thomson, 197–210. New York: Modern Language Association of America.

DeVita-Raeburn, Elizabeth. 2007. "Morgellons Mystery." *Psychology Today* 40 (2): 96–102.

DeVries, Raymond G., Lisa Kane Low, and Elizabeth Bogdan-Lovis. 2008. "Choosing Surgical Birth: Desire and the Nature of Bioethical Advice." In *Naturalized Bioethics: Toward Responsible Knowing and Practice,* edited by Hilde Lindemann, Marian Verkerk, and Margaret Urban Walker, 42–64. New York: Cambridge University Press.

DeVries, Raymond, and Janardan Subedi, eds. 1998. *Bioethics and Society: Constructing the Social Enterprise.* Upper Saddle River, NJ: Prentice-Hall.

Dewan, P., J. Miller, C. Musters, R. E. Taylor, and A. P. Bewley. 2011. "Delusional Infestation with Unusual Pathogens: A Report of Three Cases." *Clinical and Experimental Dermatology* 36:745–748.

DiCillo, Tom, dir. 1995. *Living in Oblivion.* JDI Productions. New York: Sony Pictures Classics.

Dickens, Charles. 1839. *The Life and Adventures of Nicholas Nickleby.* London: Chapman & Hall.

———. 1843. *A Christmas Carol.* London: Chapman & Hall.

Dickinson, Robert Latou. 1949. *A Topographical Hand Atlas of Human Sex Anatomy.* Baltimore: Williams & Wilkins.

Diehl, Matt. 2010, April 22. "It's a Joni Mitchell Concert, sans Joni," *Los Angeles Times.* http://jonimitchell.com/library/view.cfm?id=2235&from=search.

Digby, Anne. 1989. "Women's Biological Straitjacket." In *Sexuality and Subordination,* edited by Susan Mendus and Jane Rendall, 192–220. New York: Routledge.

"Discussion on the Advisability of the Registration of Tuberculosis." 1894. *Transactions of the College of Physicians of Philadelphia* 16:1–27.

Dmytryk, Edward, dir. 1946. *Till the End of Time.* New York: RKO Pictures.

Dolgin, Elie. 2009, September 24. "Vaccine Protects against AIDS Virus." *Nature.* www.nature.com/news/2009/090924/full/news.2009.947.html.

Doller, Jane. 1994. Foreword. In *The Quiet Room,* by Lori Schiller and Amanda Bennett, xi–xiii. New York: Warner Books.

Donehue, Vincent J., dir. 1960. *Sunrise at Campobello.* Burbank, CA: Warner Bros.

Donner, Richard, dir. 1980. *Inside Moves.* London: ITC Entertainment.

Don't Pull My Leg. 1908. Chicago: Essanay Film Manufacturing Co.

Dormen, Lesley. 2002. "Planet No." In *Unholy Ghost: Writers on Depression,* edited by Nell Casey, 229–242. New York: Harper Perennial.

Douglas, Mary. 1966. *Purity and Danger: An Analysis of the Concepts of Pollution and Taboo.* New York: Routledge & Kegan Paul.

Douglas, Mary. 1996. *Natural Symbols: Explorations in Cosmology: With a New Introduction.* London and New York: Routledge.

———. 2002. *Purity and Danger: An Analysis of Concepts of Pollution and Taboo.* New York: Routledge.

Doukas, David J., Laurence B. McCullough, and Stephen Wear. 2010. "Reforming Medical Education in Ethics and Humanities by Finding Common Ground with Abraham Flexner." *Academic Medicine* 85:318–323.

Doyle, Derek, Geoffrey Hanks, Nathan Cherny, and Keneth Calman. 2004. *Oxford Textbook of Palliative Medicine.* Oxford: Oxford University Press.

Drake, Robert E., Howard H. Goldman, Steven H. Leff, Antony F. Lehman, Lisa Dixon, Kim T. Mueser, and William C. Torrey. 2001. "Implementing Evidence-Based Practices in Routine Mental Health Settings." *Psychiatric Services* 52 (2): 179–182.

Dreger, Alice Domurat. 1998a. *Hermaphrodites and the Medical Invention of Sex.* Cambridge, MA: Harvard University Press.

———. 1998b. " 'Ambiguous Sex'—or Ambivalent Medicine? Ethical Issues in the Treatment of Intersexuality." *Hastings Center Report* 28 (4): 24–35.

Dreifus, Claudia, ed. 1978. *Seizing Our Bodies: The Politics of Women's Health.* New York: Vintage.

Dr. Quinn, Medicine Woman. 1993–1998. Television series. New York: CBS.

DSM-II (Diagnostic and Statistical Manual of Mental Disorders, 2nd ed.). 1968. Washington, DC: American Psychiatric Association Press.

DSM-IV-TR (Diagnostic and Statistical Manual of Mental Disorders, 4th ed., text revision). 2000. Washington, DC: American Psychiatric Association Press.

DSM-5 (Diagnostic and Statistical Manual of Mental Disorders, 5th ed.). 2013. Washington, DC: American Psychiatric Association Press.

Duchenne de Boulogne, G.-B. 1990. *The Mechanism of Human Facial Expression.* Translated by R. Andrew Cuthbertson. Studies in Emotion and Social Interaction. Cambridge: Cambridge University Press.

Duden, Barbara. 1993. *Disembodying Women: Perspectives on Pregnancy and the Unborn.* Translated by Lee Hoinacki. Cambridge, MA: Harvard University Press.

———. 1999. "The Fetus on the 'Farther Shore': Toward a History of the Unborn." In *Fetal Subjects, Feminist Positions,* edited by Lynn M. Morgan and Meredith W. Michaels, 13–25. Philadelphia: University of Pennsylvania Press.

Dugdale, David C., Ronald Epstein, and Steven Z. Pantilat. 1999. "Time and the Physician-Patient Relationship." *Journal of General Internal Medicine* 14 (suppl. 1): S34–S40.

Duke, Patty, and Gloria Hochman. 1992. *A Brilliant Madness: Living with Manic-Depressive Illness.* New York: Bantam Books.

Dumit, Joseph. 2006. "Illnesses You Have to Fight to Get: Facts as Forces in Uncertain, Emergent Illnesses." *Social Science and Medicine* 62:577–590.

Duncan, Barry L., Scott D. Miller, Bruce E. Wampold, and Mark A. Hubble, eds. 2009. *The Heart and Soul of Change: Delivering What Works in Therapy.* Washington, DC: American Psychological Association Press.

Dyer, Wayne W. 2006, April 19. "The Moment of Change." *Forbes.* www.forbes.com/2006/04/15/wayne-dyer-reinvention_cx_wd_06slate_0418dyer.html.

Eastwood, Clint, dir. 2004. *Million Dollar Baby.* Burbank, CA: Warner Bros.

Edson, Margaret. 1999. *W;t.* New York: Faber & Faber. (Also titled as *Wit.*)

Ehman, John W., Barbara B. Ott, Thomas H. Short, Ralph C. Ciampa, and John Hansen-Flaschen. 1999. "Do Patients Want Their Physicians to Inquire about Their Spiritual or Religious Beliefs If They Become Gravely Ill?" *Archives of Internal Medicine* 159:1803–1806.

Ehrenreich, Barbara, and Deidre English. 1989. *For Her Own Good: 150 Years of the Experts' Advice to Women.* New York: Anchor.

———. 1973. *Complaints and Disorders: The Sexual Politics of Sickness.* New York: Feminist Press.

Eickhoff, Theodore C. 1977. "Containing Andromeda." *New England Journal of Medicine* 297: 835–836.

Einstein, Gillian, and Margrit Shildrick. 2009. "The Postconventional Body: Retheorizing Women's Health." *Social Science and Medicine* 69:293–300.

Eisenberger, Naomi I., Matthew D. Lieberman, and Kipling D. Williams. 2003, October 10. "Does Rejection Hurt? An fMRI Study of Social Exclusion." *Science* 302 (5643): 290–292.

Ekman, Paul, ed. 1973. *Darwin and Facial Expression: A Century of Research in Review.* New York: Academic Press.

Ekman, Paul, and Wallace V. Friesen. 1969. "The Repertoire of Nonverbal Behavior: Categories, Origins, Usage, and Coding." *Semiotica* 1:49–98.

———. 1971. "Constants across Cultures in the Face and Emotion." *Journal of Personality and Social Psychology* 17:124–129.

Elikann, Larry, dir. 1994, January 16. *Out of Darkness.* Made-for-TV movie. New York: ABC.

Eliot, George. 1860. *The Mill on the Floss.* Edinburgh and London: William Blackwood & Sons.

Eliot, T. S. 1968. *Four Quartets.* Orlando, FL: Houghton Mifflin Harcourt.

Elkins, James. 2003. *Visual Studies: A Skeptical Introduction.* London: Routledge.

Elliot, Carl. 1999. *A Philosophical Disease: Bioethics, Culture, and Identity.* New York: Routledge.

Ellis, Mark R., Daniel C. Vinson, and Bernard Ewigman. 1999. "Addressing Spiritual Concerns of Patients: Family Physicians' Attitudes and Practices." *Journal of Family Practice* 48 (2): 105–109.

Ellison, C. W. 1983. "Spiritual Well-Being: Conceptualization and Measurement." *Journal of Psychology and Theology* 11:330–340.

Emanuel, Ezekiel J., and Linda L. Emanuel. 1992. "Four Models of the Physician-Patient Relationship." *Journal of the American Medical Association* 267: 2221–2226.

Engel, George L. 1977. "The Need for a New Medical Model: A Challenge for Biomedicine." *Science* 196 (4286): 129–136.

Engel, John D., Joseph Zarconi, Lura L. Pethtel, and Sally A. Missimi. 2008. *Narrative in Health Care: Healing Patients, Practitioners, Profession, and Community.* Oxford: Radcliffe Publishing.

Engelhardt, H. Tristram. 1991. *Bioethics and Secular Humanism: The Search for a Common Morality.* Philadelphia; London: SCM Press and Trinity Press International.

———. 1996. *The Foundations of Bioethics,* 2nd ed. New York: Oxford University Press.

———. 1998. "Generic Chaplaincy: Providing Spiritual Care in a Post-Christian Age." *Christian Bioethics* 4:231–238.

Engels, Friedrich. (1845) 2005. *On the Condition of the Working-Class in England in 1844.* Translated by Florence Kelley Wischnewetzky. Project Gutenberg e-book. www .gutenberg.org/ebooks/17306. (Originally published in 1845. Transcribed from the January 1943 George Allen & Unwin reprint of the March 1892 edition by David Price.)

Engeström, Yrjö. 2008. *From Teams to Knots.* Cambridge: Cambridge University Press.

Ensler, Eve. 2001. *The Vagina Monologues.* New York: Villard Books.

ER. 1994–2009. Television series. New York: NBC.

Eugenides, Jeffrey. 2001. *Middlesex: A Novel.* New York: Farrar, Straus, & Giroux.

Evans, Martyn. 2002. "Reflections on the Humanities in Medical Education." *Medical Education* 36(6): 508–513.

Evans, Timothy, Margaret Whitehead, Finn Diderichsen, Abbas Bhuiya and Meg Wirth. 2001. "Introduction." In *Challenging Inequities in Health: From Ethics to Action,* edited by Timothy Evans Margaret Whitehead, Finn Diderichsen, Abbas Bhuiya and Meg Wirth, 2–11. New York: Oxford University Press.

Evarts, A. B. 1914. "Dementia Praecox in the Colored Race." *Psychoanalytic Review* 1:388–403.

Ewbank, Douglas. 2004. "From Alzheimer's Disease to a Demography of Chronic Disease: The Development of Demographic Synthesis for Fitting Multistate Models." In *Aging Health and Public Policy: Demographic and Economic Perspectives,* edited by Linda J. Waite. (Reprinted in *Population and Development Review* 30:63–80.)

Eyal, Gil, Brendan Hart, Emine Onculer, Neta Oren, and Natasha Rossi. 2010. *The Autism Matrix: The Social Origins of the Autism Epidemic.* Cambridge: Polity Press.

Eyler, John M. 2009. "The Fog of Research: Influenza Vaccine Trials during the 1918–19 Epidemic." *Journal of the History of Medicine and Allied Sciences* 64 (4): 401–428.

Faden, Ruth R., and Tom L. Beauchamp. 1986. *A History and Theory of Informed Consent.* New York: Oxford University Press.

Fadiman, Anne. 1997. *The Spirit Catches You and You Fall Down: A Hmong Child, Her American Doctors, and the Collision of Two Cultures.* New York: Noonday Press.

Fahnestock, Jeanne. 1986. "Accommodating Science: The Rhetorical Life of Scientific Facts." *Written Communication* 3 (3): 275–296.

Fair, Brian. 2010. "Morgellons: Contested Illness, Diagnostic Compromise and Medicalisation." *Sociology of Health and Illness* 32 (4): 597–612.

Family Guy. 1999–. Television series. Los Angeles: 20th Television.

Farmer, Paul. 2005. *Pathologies of Power: Health, Human Rights and the New War on the Poor.* Berkeley: University of California Press.

Farrelly, Peter, and Robert Farrelly, dirs. 1994. *Dumb and Dumber.* Los Angeles: New Line Cinema.

———, dirs. 1998. *There's Something about Mary.* Los Angeles: 20th Century Fox.

———, dirs. 2000. *Me, Myself, and Irene.* Los Angeles: 20th Century Fox.

———, dirs. 2001. *Shallow Hal.* Los Angeles: 20th Century Fox.

———, dirs. 2003. *Stuck on You.* Los Angeles: 20th Century Fox.

Fausto-Sterling, Anne. 1992. *Myths of Gender: Biological Theories about Women and Men,* 2nd ed. New York: Basic Books.

"FBI Adds Negro Mental Patient to '10 Most Wanted' List." 1966, July 6. *Chicago Tribune,* A4.

Fellner, Michael J., and Muhammad Hassan Majeed. 2009. "Tales of Bugs, Delusions of Parasitosis, and What to Do." *Clinics in Dermatology* 27:135–138.

Ferguson, Warren, and Lucy M. Candib. 2002. "Culture, Language, and the Doctor-Patient Relationship." *Family Medicine* 34:353–361.

"Fiction Review: Andromeda Strain by Michael Crichton." 1969. Publisher's Weekly, August 4.

Fiedler, Leslie. 1986. "More Images of Eros and Old Age: The Damnation of Faust and the Fountain of Youth." In *Memory and Desire,* edited by Kathleen Woodward and Murray M. Schwartz, 40. Bloomington: Indiana University Press.

Field, D. 2000, March. "What Do We Mean by 'Psychosocial'?" Briefing no. 4. London: National Council for Hospice and Specialist Palliative Care Services.

Finger, Anne. 1990. *Past Due: A Story of Disability, Pregnancy, and Birth.* Berkeley: Seal Press.

Fisher, Bradley J., and Constance Peterson. 1993. "She Won't Be Dancing Much Anyway: A Study of Surgeons, Surgical Nurses, and Elderly Patients." *Qualitative Health Research* 3: 3165–3183.

Fisher, Elliott S., Daniel E. Wennberg, Thérèse A. Stukel, Daniel J. Gottlieb, F. L. Lucas, and Étoile L. Pinder. 2003a. "The Implications of Regional Variations in Medicare Spending: Part 1. The Content, Quality, and Accessibility of Care." *Annals of Internal Medicine* 138 (4): 273–287.

———. 2003b. "The Implications of Regional Variations in Medicare Spending: Part 2. Health Outcomes and Satisfaction with Care." *Annals of Internal Medicine* 138 (4): 288–298.

Fisher, Patricia. 2004. "The Importance of Variable Names." In *The Practice of Social Research,* edited by Earl Babbie. Belmont, CA: Wadsworth/Thomson.

Fleder, Gary, dir. 2003. *Runaway Jury.* Regency Enterprises. Los Angeles: 20th Century Fox.

Fleischman, Suzanne. 1999. "I am . . . , I have . . . , I suffer from . . .": A Linguist Reflects on the Language of Illness and Disease." *Journal of Medical Humanities* 20 (1): 3–32.

Flexner, Abraham. 1910. *Medical Education in the United States and Canada.* New York: Carnegie Foundation for the Advancement of Teaching.

Flick, Lawrence F. 1888, June. "The Contagiousness of Pthisis (Pulmonary Tubercolosis)." *Transactions of the Medical Society of the State of Pennsylvania* 20:164–186.

Flores, Glenn, Denise Gee, and Beth Kastner. 2000. "The Teaching of Cultural Issues in U.S. and Canadian Medical Schools." *Academic Medicine* 75:451–455.

Forman, Milos, dir. 1975. *One Flew Over the Cuckoo's Nest.* Berkeley, CA: Fantasy Films.

Foucault, Michel. (1966) 1994. *The Order of Things: An Archaeology of the Human Sciences.* New York: Vintage.

———. 1973. *The Birth of the Clinic: An Archaeology of Medical Perception.* Translated by Alan Sheridan. London: Routledge.

———. 1980. *A History of Sexuality*, vol. 1: *An Introduction.* Translated by Robert Hurley. New York: Vintage.

———. 1989. *The Birth of the Clinic: An Archaeology of Medical Perception.* London: Routledge.

———. 1994. *The Birth of the Clinic: An Archaeology of Medical Perception.* New York: Vintage.

———. 1995. *Discipline and Punish: The Birth of the Prison.* 2nd ed. New York: Vintage.

Fowler, J. 2004. "Mysterious Parasite Striking Bay Area Residents." San Francisco: KTVU-FOX. April 30.

Fowler, James W. 1995. *Stages of Faith: The Psychology of Human Development.* New York: HarperCollins.

Fox, Daniel. 1985. "Who We Are: The Political Origins of the Medical Humanities." *Theoretical Medicine* 6:327–342.

Fox, Renée C. 2005. "Cultural Competence and the Culture of Medicine." *New England Journal of Medicine* 353:1316–1319.

Francis, Leslie J., and Michael T. Stubbs. 1987. "Measuring Attitudes towards Christianity: From Childhood to Adult." *Personality and Individual Differences* 8:741–743.

Frank, Arthur W. (1991) 2002. *At the Will of the Body*, 2nd ed. Boston: Houghton Mifflin.

———. 1995. *The Wounded Storyteller.* Chicago: University of Chicago Press.

———. 1997. *The Wounded Storyteller: Body, Illness, and Ethics.* Chicago: University of Chicago Press.

———. 2000. "Illness and Autobiographical Work: Dialogue as Narrative Destabilization." *Qualitative Sociology* 23 (1): 135–136.

———. 2001. "Can We Research Suffering?" *Qualitative Health Research* 3:353–362.

———. 2004. *The Renewal of Generosity: Illness, Medicine, and How to Live.* Chicago: University of Chicago Press.

———. 2007. "Five Dramas of Illness." *Perspectives in Biology and Medicine* 50:379–394.

———. 2009. "Tricksters and Truth Tellers: Narrating Illness in an Age of Authenticity and Appropriation." *Literature and Medicine* 28:185–199.

———. 2010. *Letting Stories Breathe: A Sociology-Narratology.* Chicago: University of Chicago Press.

———. 2012. "Support, Advocacy, and the Selves of People with Cancer." In *Malignant: Medical Ethicists Confront Cancer,* edited by Rebecca Dresser, 166–178. New York: Oxford.

Frankl, Vicktor E. 1969. *The Will to Meaning: Foundations and Applications of Logotherapy.* New York: New American Library.

Freeman, John. 2006, May 5. "Philip Roth: Intimations of Mortality." *Independent.* www.independent.co.uk/arts-entertainment/books/features/philip-roth-intimations-of-mortality-476808.html.

Freeman, Richard, and Michael Rowe. 2011. Introduction. In *Classics of Community Psychiatry: Fifty Years of Mental Health outside the Hospital,* edited by Michael Rowe, Martha Lawless, Kenneth S. Thompson, and Larry Davidson, xix–xx. New York: Oxford University Press.

Freespirit, Judy. 2003. "On Ward G." In *The Strange History of Suzanne Lafleshe and Other Stories of Women and Fatness,* edited by Suzanne Koppelman, 153–160. New York: Feminist Press at CUNY.

Freire, Paolo. 2000. *Pedagogy of the Oppressed*. New York: Continuum.

Freud, Sigmund. 1955–1974. *Standard Edition of the Complete Psychological Works of Sigmund Freud*. 24 vols. Edited and translated by J. Strachey, A. Freud, A. Strachey, and A. Tyson. London: Hogarth.

Freud, Sigmund, and Sándor Ferenczi. 2000. *The Correspondence of Sigmund Freud and Sándor Ferenczi*, vol. 3: *1920–1933*, edited by Ernst Falzeder, Eva Brabant, with Patrizia Giampieri-Deutsch; translated by Peter Hoffer. Cambridge, MA: Harvard University Press.

Freudenreich, Oliver, Nicholas Kantos, Constantin Tranulis, and Corinne Cather. 2010. "Morgellons Disease, or Antipsychiotic-Responsive Delusional Parasitosis, in an HIV Patient: Beliefs in the Age of the Internet." *Psychosomatics* 51:453–457.

Frey, Rebecca J. 2003. "Dementia." *Gale Encyclopedia of Mental Disorders*. Detroit: Gale Group.

Fridlund, Alan J. 1994. *Human Facial Expression: An Evolutionary View*. San Diego: Academic Press.

Fries, Kenny, ed. 1997. *Staring Back: The Disability Experience from the Inside Out*. New York: Plume.

———. 2007. *The History of My Shoes and the Evolution of Darwin's Theory*. New York: Carroll & Graf.

Frith, Uta. 2003. *Autism: Explaining the Enigma*, 2nd ed. Oxford: Blackwell Publishing.

Frith, Uta, and Francesca Happé. 1999. "Theory of Mind and Self-Consciousness: What Is It Like to Be Autistic?" *Mind and Language* 14:1–22.

Frost, Robert. 1915. "The Death of the Hired Man." In *North of Boston*. New York: Henry Holt & Co. www.bartleby.com/118/.

Frost, Wade Hampton. 1937. "How Much Control of Tuberculosis?" *American Journal of Public Health* 27:759–766.

Fugazzotto, Martina. n.d. "Martina Fugazzotto's Comics." www.martinamartina.com/martina-fugazzottos-comics.html.

Fulford, Bill. 2004. "Facts/Values: Ten Principles of Values-Based Medicine." In *The Philosophy of Psychiatry: A Companion*, edited by Jennifer Radden, 205–237. Oxford: Oxford University Press.

Fulford, Bill, and Tony Colombo. 2004. "Six Models of Mental Disorder: A Study Combining Linguistic-Analytic and Empirical Methods." *Philosophy, Psychiatry, and Psychology* 11 (2): 129–144.

Fulford, Bill, Tim Thornton, and George Graham. 2006. *Oxford Textbook of Philosophy and Psychiatry*. Oxford: Oxford University Press.

Fuller, Sam, dir. 1963. *Shock Corridor*. Los Angeles: Allied Artists Pictures Corp.

Gabbard, Glen O., and Krin Gabbard. 1999. *Psychiatry and the Cinema*, 2nd ed. Washington, DC: American Psychiatric Press.

Galarneau, Charlene. 2010. " 'The H in HIV Stands for Human, Not Haitian': Cultural Imperialism in U.S. Blood Donor Policy." *Public Health Ethics* 3:210–219.

Galloway, Terry. 2010. *Mean Little Deaf Queer: A Memoir*. Boston: Beacon Press.

Gallup Daily News. 2011. "Religion." www.gallup.com/poll/1690/Religion.aspx. Accessed June 22, 2011.

García Márquez, Gabriel. (1985) 1988. *Love in the Time of Cholera*. New York: Knopf.

Garden, Rebecca. 2007. "The Problem of Empathy: Medicine and the Humanities." *New Literary History* 38 (3): 551–567.

———. 2008. "Expanding Clinical Empathy: An Activist Perspective." *Journal of General Internal Medicine* 24 (1): 122–125.

———. 2010. "Disability and Narrative: New Directions for Medicine and the Medical Humanities." *Medical Humanities* 36 (2): 70–74.

Garland-Thomson, Rosemarie. 1997. *Extraordinary Bodies: Figuring Physical Disability in American Culture and Literature*. New York: Columbia University Press.

———. 2001. "Seeing the Disabled: Visual Rhetorics of Disability in Popular Photography."

In *The New Disability History: American Perspectives,* edited by Paul K. Longmore and Lauri Umansky, 335–374. New York: New York University Press.

———. 2002. "The Politics of Staring: Visual Rhetorics of Disability in Popular Photography." In *Disability Studies: Enabling the Humanities,* edited by Sharon L. Snyder, Brenda Jo Brueggeman, and Rosemarie Garland-Thomson, 56–75. New York: Modern Language Association.

———. 2004. "The Cultural Logic of Euthanasia: 'Sad Fancyings' in Herman Melville's 'Bartelby.'" *American Literature* 76:777–806.

———. 2009. *Staring: How We Look.* New York: Oxford University Press.

Gawande, Atul. 2010, August 2. "Letting Go." *New Yorker.* www.newyorker.com/reporting/2010/08/02/100802fa_fact_gawande.

Gay, Lesbian, and Straight Educational Network (GLSEN). 2002. "Talking the Talk." http://www.glsen.org/cgi-bin/iowa/all/home/index.html.

Gayen, Swapna. 2005, March 15. "Nightmares on Celluloid." [Letter to the editor.] *Telegraph* (Calcutta, India). www.telegraphindia.com/1050315/asp/opinion/story_4491793.asp.

Geddes, Elizabeth R. C., and Rashid M. Rashid. 2008. "Delusional Tinea: A Novel Subtype of Delusional Parasitosis." *Dermatology Online Journal* 14 (2): 16.

Gee, Gilbert C., and Chandra L. Ford. 2011. "Structural Racism and Health Inequities: Old Ideas, New Directions." *DuBois Review: Social Science Research on Race* 8 (1): 115–132.

Geertz, Clifford. 1973a. "Ethos, World View, and the Analysis of Sacred Symbols." In *The Interpretation of Cultures,* 126–141. New York: Basic Books.

———. 1973b. "Religion as a Cultural System." In *The Interpretation of Cultures,* 87–125. New York: Basic Books.

———. 1983. "Blurred Genres: The Refiguration of Social Thought." In *Local Knowledge: Further Essays in Interpretive Anthropology,* 19–35. New York: Basic Books.

Geiger, H. Jack. 2001. "Racial Stereotyping and Medicine: The Need for Cultural Competence." *Canadian Medical Association Journal* 164:1699–1700.

Geller, Jeffrey L. 2000. "The Last Half-Century of Psychiatry Services as Reflected in Psychiatric Services." *Psychiatric Services* 51 (1): 41–67.

Gennep, Arnold van. 1960. *The Rites of Passage.* London: Routledge & Kegan Paul.

Gereben, Janos. 2002, July 7. "Quasthoff; a Hero's Journey Transforms the Festival Concert Hall." *Oakland Post.*

Gerhard, Jane. 2000. "'The Myth of the Vaginal Orgasm': The Female Orgasm in American Sexual Thought and Second Wave Feminism." *Feminist Studies* 26 (2): 449–476.

Gherini, Claire. 2010. "Rationalizing Disease: James Kilpatrick's Atlantic Struggles with Smallpox Inoculation." *Atlantic Studies* 7 (4): 421–446.

Gilb, Dagoberto. 2010, June. "please, thank you." *Harper's Magazine,* 65–70.

Gilbert, Sandra. 2006. *Death's Door.* New York: W. W. Norton.

Gill, Carol J. 2000. "Health Professionals, Disability, and Assisted Suicide: An Examination of Relevant Empirical Evidence and Reply to Batavia (2000)." *Psychology, Public Policy, and Law* 6 (2): 526–545.

Gilman, Sander L. 1982. *Seeing the Insane: A Cultural History of Psychiatric Illustration.* New York: Wiley Interscience.

———. 1983. "Why Is Schizophrenia 'Bizarre': An Historical Essay in the Vocabulary of Psychiatry." *Journal of the History of the Behavioral Sciences* 19:127–135.

———. 1988. *Disease and Representation: Images of Illness from Madness to AIDS.* Ithaca, NY: Cornell University Press.

Gleick, Elizabeth. 1997, June 30. "Triumph of the Spirit: German Singer Thomas Quasthoff Is Thrilling Audiences with His Voice—and His Courage." *Time.*

Glennie, Evelyn. 1990. *Good Vibrations: An Autobiography.* London: Arrow Books.

———. 1993. "Hearing Essay." www.evelyn.co.uk/Resources/Essays/Hearing%20Essay.pdf. Accessed July 13, 2013.

Gloeckner, Phoebe. 1998. *A Child's Life and Other Stories.* Berkeley, CA: Frog.

———. 2011. Keynote address. "Comics and Medicine: The Sequential Art of Illness" Conference. Chicago: Northwestern University, Feinberg School of Medicine, June 10. www.graphicmedicine.org/comics-and-medicine-conferences/2011-chicago-comics-and-medicine-conference.

Godwin, William. 1794. *Things as They Are; or, The Adventures of Caleb Williams.* London: R. Crosby.

Goffman, Erving. 1961. *Asylums: Essays on the Social Situation of Mental Patients and Other Inmates.* New York: Anchor Books.

———. 1963. *Stigma: Notes on the Management of Spoiled Identity.* Englewood Cliffs, NJ: Prentice-Hall.

Goffman, Erving, Charles C. Lemert, and Ann Branaman. 1997. *The Goffman Reader.* Cambridge, Mass: Blackwell.

Goldberg, Daniel S. 2009. "In Support of a Broad Model of Public Health: Disparities, Social Epidemiology, and Public Health Causation." *Public Health Ethics* 2:70–83.

———. 2011, May 20–21. "Global Health Care Is Not Global Health: Populations, Inequities, and Law as a Social Determinant of Health." Paper presented at Conference on Globalization and Health Care, Petrie-Flom Center for Health Law Policy, Biotechnology and Bioethics at Harvard Law School, Cambridge, MA.

———. 2012, October 31. American Society for Bioethics and Humanities Literature and Medicine Listserv. litmed@listserv.com.

Golden, Joshua S., and Edward H. Liston. 1972. "Medical Sex Education: The World of Illusion and the Practical Realities." *Journal of Medical Education* 47:761–771.

Gonick, Larry, and Christine DeVault. 1999. *The Cartoon Guide to Sex.* New York: Collins Business.

Gonzalez, Susan. 2001, March 2. "Director Spike Lee Slams 'Same Old' Black Stereotypes in Today's Films." *Yale Bulletin and Calendar.* www.yale.edu/opa/arc-ybc/v29.n21/story3.html.

Good, Bryon J. 1994. *Medicine, Rationality, and Experience: An Anthropological Perspective.* Cambridge: Cambridge University Press.

Good, Mary Jo DelVecchio, Byron J. Good, Cynthia Schaffer, and Stuart E. Lind. 1990. "American Oncology and the Discourse of Hope." *Culture, Medicine and Psychiatry* 14:59–79.

Goodman, Leo A. 1961. "Snowball Sampling." *Annals of Mathematical Statistics* 32 (1): 148–170.

Goodman, Paul. 1969. "Can Technology Be Humane?" *New York Review of Books* 13 (9). www.nybooks.com/articles/11145.

Graham, Hilary. 2004. "Social Determinants and Their Unequal Distribution: Clarifying Policy Understandings." *Milbank Quarterly* 82:101–124.

Gramaglia, Tony. 1996. "Okay, So I'm in This Bed." In *From a Burning House: The AIDS Project LA Writers Workshop,* edited by Irene Borger, 196–197. New York: Washington Square Press.

Grandin, Temple. 1995. *Thinking in Pictures, and Other Reports from My Life with Autism.* New York: Doubleday.

———. 1996. *Thinking in Pictures and Other Reports from My Life with Autism.* New York: Vintage.

Grandin, Temple, and Margaret M. Scariano. 1996. *Emergence: Labeled Autistic.* New York: Warner Books.

Gray, Denise. 1994, July. "The New Way to Predict Your Future Health." *Redbook Magazine.*

Grealy, Lucy. 1994. *Autobiography of a Face.* Boston: Houghton Mifflin.

———. 2003. *Autobiography of a Face.* New York: HarperPerennial.

Greenberg, Joanne [Hannah Green]. 1964. *I Never Promised You a Rose Garden.* New York: Signet.

Green, Justin. 1972. *Binky Brown Meets the Holy Virgin Mary.* Berkeley: Last Gasp.

Greenhalgh, Trisha, and Brian Hurwitz. 1998. *Narrative-Based Medicine.* London: BMJ Books.

Griffith, D. W., dir. 1921. *Orphans of the Storm*. Beverly Hills, CA: United Artists.

Grimes, Ronald L. 1990. *Ritual Criticism*. Columbia: University of South Carolina Press.

———. 2000. *Deeply into the Bone: Re-inventing Rites of Passage, Life Passages*. Berkeley: University of California Press.

Grinker, Roy. 2007. *Unstrange Minds: Remapping the World of Autism*. New York: Basic Books.

Grob, Gerald N. 1991. *From Asylum to Community: Mental Health Policy in Modern America*. Princeton, NJ: Princeton University Press.

———. 1994. *The Mad among Us: A History of the Care of America's Mentally Ill*. New York: Free Press.

Groce, Nora Ellen. 1985. *Everyone Here Spoke Sign Language: Hereditary Deafness on Martha's Vineyard*. Cambridge, MA: Harvard University Press.

Gronfein, William. 1985. "Psychotropic Drugs and the Origins of Deinstitutionalization." *Social Problems* 32 (5): 437–454.

Groopman, Jerome. 2004. *The Anatomy of Hope: How People Prevail in the Face of Illness*. New York: Random House.

Grumbach, Kevin, Thomas Bodenheimer, and Paul Grundy. 2009, August. *The Outcomes of Implementing Patient-Centered Medical Home Interventions: A Review of the Evidence on Quality, Access and Costs from Recent Prospective Evaluation Studies*. Washington, DC: Patient-Centered Primary Care Collaborative. www.pcdc.org/resources/patient -centered-medical-home/pcdc-pcmh/pcdc-pcmh-resources/toolkit-appendix/1_outcomes -of-implementing-pcmh.pdf. Accessed May 24, 2011.

Gullette, Margaret. 1997. *Declining to Decline: Cultural Combat and the Politics of Midlife*. Charlottesville: University Press of Virginia.

Hager Cohen, Leah. 1995. *Train Go Sorry: Inside a Deaf World*. New York: Vintage.

Hailstone, Barry. 1987, June 26. "Fast Virus Slows AIDS Fight." *Advertiser*.

Haines, Randa, dir. 1986. *Children of a Lesser God*. Hollywood, CA: Paramount Pictures.

———, dir. 1991. *The Doctor*. Touchstone Pictures. Burbank, CA: Buena Vista Pictures.

Hajdu, David. 2008. *The Ten-Cent Plague: The Great Comic-Book Scare and How It Changed America*. New York: Farrar, Straus & Giroux.

Hall, Donald. 1998. *Without*. New York: Houghton Mifflin.

Handyside, Alan H. 1995. "Genetic Testing and Screening: Pre-implantation Diagnosis." In *Encyclopedia of Bioethics*, edited by Warren T. Reich, 990–1005. New York: Simon & Schuster / Macmillan.

Handyside, Alan H., John G. Lesko, Juan J. Tarín, Robert M. L. Winston, and Mark R. Hughes. 1992. "Birth of a Normal Girl after in vitro Fertilization and Preimplantation Diagnostic Testing for Cystic Fibrosis." *New England Journal of Medicine* 327:905–909.

Haraway, Donna. 1990. *Simians, Cyborgs, and Women: The Reinvention of Nature*. New York: Routledge.

Harding, Courtenay M., George W. Brooks, Takamura Ashikaga, John S. Strauss, and Alan Brier. 1987. "The Vermont Longitudinal Study of Persons with Severe Mental Illness, II: Long-term Outcome of Subjects who Retrospectively Met DSM-III Criteria for Schizophrenia." *American Journal of Psychiatry* 144:727–735.

Harding, Nancy, and Colin Palfrey. 1997. *The Social Construction of Dementia: Confused Professionals?* London: J. Kingsley Publishers.

Hardt, Michael, and Antonio Negri. 2001. *Empire*. Cambridge, MA: Harvard University Press.

———. 2006. *Multitude: War and Democracy in the Age of Empire*. Harmondsworth: Penguin.

———. 2009. *Commonwealth*. Cambridge, MA: Harvard University Press.

Harlan, Chico. 2006, July 23. "Mom Fights for Answers on What's Wrong with Her Son." *Pittsburgh Post-Gazette*. www.post-gazette.com/stories/news/health/mom-fights -for-answers-on-whats-wrong-with-her-son-443228.

Harrington, Anne. 2008. *The Cure Within: A History of Mind-Body Medicine*. New York: W. W. Norton.

Hartouni, Valerie. 1999. "Epilogue: Reflections on Abortion Politics and the Practice Called

Person." In *Fetal Subjects, Feminist Positions,* edited by Lynn M. Morgan and Meredith W. Michaels, 296–303. Philadelphia: University of Pennsylvania Press.

Harvey, William T., Robert C. Bransfield, Dana E. Mercer, Andrew J. Wright, Rebecca M. Ricchi, and Mary M. Leitao. 2009. "Morgellons Disease: Illuminating an Undefined Illness, A Case Series." *Journal of Medical Case Reports* 3:8243. http://link.springer.com/article/10.4076%2F1752-1947-3-8243.

Hauerwas, Stanley, Carole Bailey Stonking, Keith Meador, and David Cloutier eds. 2003. *Growing Old in Christ.* Grand Rapids, MI: Eerdmans Publishing Co.

Hausman, Bernice L. 2011. *Viral Mothers: Breastfeeding in the Age of HIV/AIDS.* Ann Arbor: University of Michigan Press.

Havel, Václav. 1990. *Disturbing the Peace: A Conversation with Karel Hvížďala.* Translated by Paul Wilson. New York: Alfred A. Knopf.

Hawkins, Anne Hunsaker. 1999. *Reconstructing Illness: Studies in Pathography,* 2nd ed. West Lafayette, IN: Purdue University Press.

Hawkins, Anne Hunsaker, and Marilyn Chandler McEntyre. 2000. "Teaching Literature and Medicine: A Retrospective and a Rationale." In *Teaching Literature and Medicine,* edited by Anne Hunsaker Hawkins and Marilyn Chandler McEntyre, 1–25. New York: Modern Language Association.

Hawkins, Seth Collings. 2004. "Emergency Medicine Narratives: A Systematic Discussion of Definition and Utility." *Academic Emergency Medicine* 11 (7): 761–765.

Headlam, Dave. 2006. "Learning to Hear Autistically." In *Sounding Off: Theorizing Disability in Music,* edited by Neil Lerner and Joseph N. Straus, 109–120. New York: Routledge.

"Health Grades Quality Study: Patient Safety in American Hospitals." 2004, July. www.healthgrades.com/media/english/pdf/HG_Patient_Safety_Study_Final.pdf.

Healy, David. 2004. "Shaping the Intimate: Influence on the Experience of Everyday Nerves." *Social Studies of Science* 34 (2): 219–245.

———. 2006. "Manufacturing Consensus." *Culture, Medicine and Psychiatry.* 30:135–156.

Healy, Melissa. 2011, May 16. "An Infestation That Begins in the Mind." *Los Angeles Times.* http://articles.latimes.com/2011/may/16/health/la-he-morgellons-disease-20110517.

Hebert, Randy S., Mollie W. Jenckes, Daniel E. Ford, Debra R. O'Connor, and Lisa A. Cooper. 2001. "Patient Perspectives on Spirituality and the Patient-Physician Relationship." *Journal of General Internal Medicine* 16 (10): 685–692.

Hefferman, Virginia. 2002. "Delicious Placebo." In *Unholy Ghost: Writers on Depression,* edited by Nell Casey, 8–21. New York: Harper Perennial.

Helman, Cecil G. 1981. "Disease versus Illness in General Practice." *Journal of the Royal College of General Practitioners* 31 (230): 548–552.

Henig, Robin Marantz. 1983, February 6. "AIDS: A New Disease's Deadly Odyssey." *New York Times,* sec. 6, 28.

Henry, Julie, Peter G. Rendell, Amanda Scicluma, Michelle Jackson, and Louise H. Phillips. 2009. "Emotion Experience, Expression, and Regulation in Alzheimer's Disease." *Psychology and Aging* 24 (1): 252–257.

Herek, Gregory M., John P. Capitanio, and Keith F. Widaman. 2002. "HIV-Related Stigma and Knowledge in the United States: Prevalence and Trends, 1991–1999." *American Journal of Public Health* 92:371–377.

Hermelin, Beate, N. O'Connor, and S. Lee. 1987. "Musical Inventiveness of Five Idiots-Savants." *Psychological Medicine* 17:79–90.

Herrnstein Smith, Barbara. 2005. "Figuring and Reconfiguring the Humanities and the Sciences." *Profession* 10:18–27.

Hesse, Mary. 2000. "The Explanatory Function of Metaphor." In *Philosophies of Science: From Foundations to Contemporary Issues,* edited by Jennifer McErlean, 349–355. Belmont, CA: Wadsworth.

Hewitt, Bill. 1994, January 24. "Turning Back the Clock." *People.* www.people.com/people/archive/article/0,,20107350,00.html.

Heyland, Daren K., Deborah J. Cook, Graeme M. Rocker, Peter M. Dodek, Demetrios J. Kutsogiannis, Yoanna Skrobik, Xuran Jiang, Andrew G. Day, and S. Robin Cohen. 2010. "Defining Priorities for Improving End-of-Life Care in Canada." *Canadian Medical Association Journal* 182 (16): E747–E752.

Hill, Peter C., and Ralph W. Hood Jr. 1999. *Measures of Religiosity.* Birmingham, AL: Religious Education Press.

Hilton, Sean R., and Henry B. Slotnick. 2005. "Proto-professionalism: How Professionalisation Occurs across the Continuum of Medical Education." *Medical Education* 39:58–65.

Hoberman, John. 2012. *Black and Blue: The Origins and Consequences of Medical Racism.* Berkeley: University of California Press.

Hodges, Brian. 2005. "The Many and Conflicting Histories of Medical Education in Canada and the USA: An Introduction to the Paradigm Wars." *Medical Education* 39:613–621.

Hodgkiss, Andrew. 2000. *From Lesion to Metaphor: Chronic Pain in British, French and German Medical Writings, 1800–1914.* Atlanta, GA: Rodopi.

Hojat, Mohammadreza, Michael J. M. Vergare, Kaye Maxwell, George Brainard, Steven K. Herrine, Geral A. Isenberg, Jon Veloski, and Joseph S. Gonnella. 2009. "The Devil is in the Third Year: A Longitudinal Study of Erosion of Empathy in Medical School." *Academic Medicine* 84:1182–1191.

Holman Foundation. 2011, July. "Morgellons Disease Awareness and Support." www.thecehf .org. Accessed August 27, 2011.

———. 2012, July. "Morgellons Disease Awareness and Support." www.thecehf.org. Accessed March 13, 2012.

Holmes, Frederick. 2011. "The Last Irish Plague: The Great Flu Pandemic in Ireland, 1918–1919." *Journal of the History of Medicine and Allied Sciences* 66 (4): 589–591.

Holmes, Martha Stoddard. 2001. "Performing Affliction: Physical Disabilities in Victorian Melodrama." *Contemporary Theatre Review* 12 (3): 5–24.

———. 2004. *Fictions of Affliction: Physical Disability in Victorian Culture.* Ann Arbor: University of Michigan Press.

Holy Scriptures. 1955. Philadelphia: Jewish Publication Society of America.

Honisch, Stefan Sunandan. 2010, January. "Claiming the Speechless Space Surrounding Us: Tempo, Rhythm and Phrasing as Metaphors of Embodied Experience." Paper presented at the CUNY Symposium on Music and Disability.

hooks, bell. 1994. *Teaching to Transgress: Education as the Practice of Freedom.* New York: Routledge.

Hooper, Tom, dir. 2010. *The King's Speech.* London: Momentum Pictures.

Hopper, Kim. 2007. "Rethinking Social Recovery in Schizophrenia: What a Capabilities Approach Might Offer." *Social Science and Medicine* 65 (5): 868–879.

Hopper, Kim, Glynn Harrison, Aleksander Janca, and Norman Sartorius. 2007. *Recovery from Schizophrenia: An International Perspective.* New York: Oxford University Press.

Hornstein, Gail. 2000. *To Redeem One Person Is to Redeem the World: The Life of Frieda Fromm-Reichman.* New York: Free Press.

———. 2002, January 25. "Narratives of Madness, as Told from Within." *Chronicle of Higher Education.*

———. 2011. "Bibliography of First-Person Narratives of Madness in English," 5th ed. www .gailhornstein.com/_i_to_redeem_one_person_is_to_redeem_the_world__the_life _of_frieda_fromm_reichma_78431.htm.

House, M.D. 2004–2012. Television series. Los Angeles: Fox.

Huber, Samuel J. 2003. "The White Coat Ceremony: A Contemporary Medical Ritual." *Journal of Medical Ethics* 29:364–366.

Huizinga, Mary Margaret, Lisa A. Cooper, Sara N. Bleich, Jeanne M. Clark, and Mary Catherine Beach. 2009. "Physician Respect for Patients with Obesity." *Journal of General Internal Medicine* 24 (11): 1236–1239.

Humphries, Mark Osbourne. 2005. "The Horror at Home: The Canadian Military and the

'Great' Influenza Pandemic of 1918." *Journal of the Canadian Historical Association* 16: 235–260.

Hunter, Kathryn Montgomery. 1991a. "Toward the Cultural Interpretation of Medicine." *Literature and Medicine* 10:1–17.

———. 1991b. *Doctors' Stories: The Narrative Structure of Medical Knowledge.* Princeton, NJ: Princeton University Press.

Hunter, Kathryn Montgomery, Rita Charon, and John L. Coulehan. 1995. "The Study of Literature in Medical Education. *Academic Medicine* 70:787–794.

Hurt-Thaut, Corene. 2009. "Clinical Practice in Music Therapy." In *The Oxford Handbook of Music Psychology,* edited by Susan Hallam, Ian Cross, and Michael Thaut, 503–514. Oxford: Oxford University Press.

Huxley, Thomas H. (1883) 1999. "Science and Art." In *The World's Great Speeches,* 4th ed., edited by Lewis Copeland, Lawrence W. Lamm, and Stephen J. McKenna, 682–683. New York: Dover Publications.

Hyde, Michael J. 1993. "Medicine, Rhetoric, and Euthanasia: A Case Study in the Workings of a Postmodern Discourse." *Quarterly Journal of Speech* 79:201–224.

Hydén, Lars-Christer, and Jens Brockmeier. 2008. *Health, Illness, and Culture: Broken Narratives.* London: Routledge.

Hylwa, Sara A., Jessica E. Bury, Mark D. P. Davis, Mark Pittelkow, and J. Michael Bostwick. 2011. "Delusional Infestation, Including Delusions of Parasitosis." *JAMA Dermatology* [formerly *Archives of Dermatology*], May 16. http://archderm.jamanetwork.com/article.aspx?articleid=1105158.

Iezzoni, Lisa I., and Vicki A. Freedman. 2008. "Turning the Disability Tide: The Importance of Definitions." *Journal of the American Medical Association* 299 (3): 332–334.

"I'll Be Your Mirror." 2008. *Not Your Mother's Meatloaf,* issue no. 1. http://sexedcomicproject.blogspot.com. Accessed September 29, 2011.

Illich, Ivan. 1975. "The Medicalization of Life." *Journal of Medical Ethics* 1:73–77.

———. 1997. *Limits to Medicine: Medical Nemesi—the Expropriation of Health.* Harmondsworth: Penguin.

Illing, Jan, Gill Morrow, Charlotte Kergon, Bryan Burford, and John Spencer Warwick. 2008. *How Prepared Are Medical Graduates to Begin Practice? A Comparison of Three Diverse UK Medical Schools.* Final Report for the GMC Education Committee. London: General Medical Council.

"Insanity: Mental Illness among Negroes Exceeds Whites, Overcrowds Already-Jammed 'Snake Pits.'" 1949. *Ebony* (April), 19–23.

The Invalid's Adventure. 1907. San Francisco: Miles Bros.

Irwin, Lori G., Arjumand Siddiqi, and Clyde Hertzman. 2007. "Early Childhood Development: A *Powerful* Equalizer." Final Report for the World Health Organization's Commission on the Social Determinants of Health. http://whqlibdoc.who.int/hq/2007/a91213.pdf.

Ishiguro, Kazuo. 2005. *Never Let Me Go.* London: Faber & Faber.

Ivanova, Velichka. 2011. "The Ordinary Life of Ivan Ilych Levov: American Pastoral in Dialog with Tolstoy." In *Reading Philip Roth's American Pastoral,* edited by Ivanova Velichka, 241–254. Toulouse: Presses Universitaires du Mirail.

Jackson, Michael. 1989. *Paths toward a Clearing: Radical Empiricism and Ethnographic Inquiry.* Bloomington: Indiana University Press.

James, William. 2010. *The Heart of William James,* edited by Robert Richardson. Cambridge MA: Harvard University Press.

Jamison, Kay Redfield. 1995. *An Unquiet Mind: A Memoir of Moods and Madness.* New York: Alfred A. Knopf.

Jayasinghe, Saroj. 2011. "Conceptualizing Population Health: From Mechanistic Thinking to Complexity Science." *Emerging Themes in Epidemiology* 8. www.ete-online.com/content/8/1/2.

Jeeves and Wooster. 1990–1993. Television series. London: ITV.

Jeffries, Stuart. 2009, July 1. "Orlan's Art of Sex and Surgery." *Guardian.* www.guardian.co.uk/artanddesign/2009/jul/01/orlan-performance-artist-carnal-art.

Jimenez, Neal, and Michael Steinberg, dirs. 1992. *The Waterdance.* New York: Samuel Goldwyn Co.

Joan of Arcadia. 2003–2005. Television series. New York: CBS/Toronto: CTV.

John Paul II. 1995. "Evangelium Vitae: Encyclical Letter on the Value and Inviolability of Human Life." Vatican: Libreria Editrice Vaticana. www.vatican.va/edocs/ENG0141/_INDEX.HTM.

———. 2000, May 25. "Address to a New Ambassador of New Zealand to the Holy See." Vatican: Libreria Editrice Vaticana.

———. 2004, March 20. Address to the Participants in the International Congress on "Life-Sustaining Treatment and Vegetative State: Scientific Advances and Ethical Dilemma." www.vatican.va/holy_father/john_paul_ii/speeches/2004/march/documents/hf_jp-ii_spe_20040320_congress-fiamc_en.html.

Johnson, Harriet McBryde. 2003, February 16. "Unspeakable Conversations, or How I Spent One Day as a Token Cripple at Princeton University." *New York Times Magazine,* 50–55, 77–79.

Johnson, Karl M. 1979. "Ebola Virus and Hemorrhagic Fever: Andromeda Strain or Localized Pathogen?" *Annals of Internal Medicine* 91:117–119.

Johnson, Mark. 1987. *The Body in the Mind: The Bodily Basis of Meaning, Imagination, and Reason.* Chicago: University of Chicago Press.

Johnson, Rachel L., Debra Roter, Neil R. Powe, and Lisa A. Cooper. 2004. "Patient Race/Ethnicity and Quality of Patient-Physician Communication during Medical Visits." *American Journal of Public Health* 94:2084–2090.

Johnson, Rachel L., Somnath Saha, Jose J. Arbelaez, Mary Catherine Beach, and Lisa A. Cooper. 2004. "Racial and Ethnic Differences in Patient Perceptions of Bias and Cultural Competence in Health Care." *Journal of General Internal Medicine* 19:101–110.

Johnston, Kirsty. 2010. "Grafting *Orchids* and *Ugly:* Theatre, Disability and Arts-Based Health Research." *Journal of Medical Humanities* 31:279–294.

Jones, Anne Hudson. 1984. "Reflections, Projections, and the Future of Literature-and-Medicine." In *Literature and Medicine: A Claim for a Discipline,* edited by Delese Wear, Martin Kohn, and Susan Stocker, 29–40. Proceedings of the Northeastern Ohio Universities College of Medicine Literature and Medicine Conference, May 1984. Rootstown: Northeastern Ohio Universities College of Medicine.

———. 1990. "Literature and Medicine: Traditions and Innovations." In *The Body and the Text,* edited by Bruce Clarke and Wendell Aycok, 11–24. Lubbock, TX: Texas Tech University Press.

———. 1993. "Asylum—from the Patient's Point of View." *Texas Journal of Ideas, History and Culture* 15 (2): 16–19, 64.

———. 1995, Spring. "Voices from the Darkness: Narratives of Mental Illness." *Medical Humanities Review* 9 (1): 9–24.

———. 1998, September 26. "Mental Illness Made Public: Ending the Stigma?" *Lancet* 352: 1060.

———. 1999. "Narrative in Medical Ethics." *BMJ* 318 (7178): 253–256.

Jones, David S. 2004. *Rationalizing Epidemics: Meanings and Uses of American Indian Mortality since 1600.* Cambridge, MA: Harvard University Press.

Jones, Therese. 2007. "Ending in Wonder: Replacing Technology with Revelation in Margaret Edson's *W;t.*" *Perspectives in Biology and Medicine* 50 (3): 395–409.

Joshua, Essaka. 2011. " 'Blind Vacancy': Sighted Culture and Voyeuristic Historiography in Mary Shelley's *Frankenstein.*" *European Romantic Review* 22:49–69.

Juengst, Eric T. 1991. "The Human Genome Project and Bioethics." *Kennedy Institute of Ethics Journal* 1 (1): 71.

Kafka, Franz. (1915) 1972. *The Metamorphosis,* translated and edited by Stanley Corngold. New York: Bantam.

Kalter, Joanmarie. 1986, May 31. "The Disabled Get More TV Exposure, but There's Still Too Much Stereotyping." *TV Guide,* 42.

Kaminsky, Josephine, and Dominick Gadaleta. 2002. "A Study of Discrimination within the Medical Community as Viewed by Obese Patients." *Obesity Surgery* 12 (1): 14–18.

Kaplan, Deborah. 1994. "Prenatal Screening and Diagnosis: The Impact on Persons with Disabilities." In *Women and Prenatal Testing: Facing the Challenges of Genetic Technology,* edited by Karen Rothenberg and Elizabeth Thomson, 49–61. Columbus: Ohio State University Press.

Karp, David. 2006. *Is It Me or My Meds? Living with Antidepressants.* Cambridge, MA: Harvard University Press.

Kasdan, Lawrence, dir. 1983. *The Big Chill.* Culver City, CA: Columbia Pictures.

Kass, Leon. 1997. "The Wisdom of Repugnance." *New Republic* 216 (22): 17–26.

Katz, Stephen. 2005. *Cultural Aging: Life Course, Lifestyle, and Senior Worlds.* Ontario: Broadview Press.

Katzman, Robert. 1986. "Alzheimer's Disease." *New England Journal of Medicine* 314:964–973.

Kaysen, Susanna. 1994. *Girl, Interrupted.* New York: Vintage.

———. 2002. "Three Cheers for Melancholy." In *Unholy Ghost: Writers on Depression,* edited by Nell Casey, 38–44. New York: Harper Perennial.

Keane, Helen. 1996. "The Toxic Womb: Fetal Alcohol Syndrome, Alcoholism, and the Female Body." *Australian Feminist Studies* 11 (24): 263–276.

Keane, John. 2009. *The Life and Death of Democracy.* New York: Simon & Schuster.

Keats, John. (1818) 1958. Letter to J. H. Reynolds, 3 May 1818. In *The Letters of John Keats, 1814– 1821,* edited by Hyder Edward Rollins, 1:279. Cambridge, MA: Harvard University Press.

Kellett, C. E. 1935. "Sir Thomas Browne and the Disease Called Morgellons." *Annals of Medical History,* n.s., 7:467–479. Available at http://penelope.uchicago.edu/letter/kellett.html.

Keränen, Lisa. 2007. "'Cause Someday We All Die': Rhetoric, Agency, and the Case of the 'Patient' Preferences Worksheet." *Quarterly Journal of Speech* 93:179–211.

———. 2010a. *Scientific Characters: Rhetoric, Trust, and Character in Breast Cancer Research.* Tuscaloosa: University of Alabama Press.

———. 2010b. "Rhetoric of Medicine." *Encyclopedia of Science and Technology Communication,* edited by Susanna Hornig Priest, 2:639–642. Thousand Oaks, CA: Sage.

Kesey, Ken. 1962. *One Flew over the Cuckoo's Nest.* New York: Viking.

Kevles, Daniel J. 1995. "Eugenics: Historical Aspects." In *Encyclopedia of Bioethics,* edited by Warren T. Reich, 848–853. New York: Simon & Schuster/Macmillan.

Kinderman, William. 2009. *Beethoven,* 2nd ed. Oxford: Oxford University Press.

King, Pamela M. 1994. "Morality Plays." In *The Cambridge Companion to Medieval English Theatre,* edited by Richard Beadle, 240–264. Cambridge: Cambridge University Press.

Kirklin, Deborah, J. Duncan, Sandy McBride, Sam Hunt, and Mark Griffin. 2007. "A Cluster Design Controlled Trial of Arts-Based Observational Skills Training in Primary Care." *Medical Education* 41:395–401.

Kirmayer, Laurence. 2004. "The Cultural Diversity of Healing: Meaning, Metaphor, and Mechanism." *British Medical Bulletin* 69:33–48.

Kitt, Tom, and Brian Yorkey. 2010. *next to normal.* New York: Theatre Communications Group.

Kleinman, Arthur. 1978a. "Clinical Relevance of Anthropological and Cross-Cultural Research: Concepts and Strategies." *American Journal of Psychiatry* 135 (4): 427–431.

———. 1978b. "Concepts and a Model for the Comparison of Medical Systems as Cultural Systems." *Social Science and Medicine* 12 (2B): 85–95.

———. 1988. *The Illness Narratives: Suffering, Healing, and the Human Condition.* New York: Basic Books.

———. 1989. *The Illness Narratives.* New York: Basic Books.

———. 1998. *The Illness Narratives: Suffering, Healing and the Human Condition.* New York: Basic Books.

Kleinman, Arthur, Leon Eisenberg, and Bryon Good. 1978. "Culture, Illness, and Care: Clinical Lessons from Anthropologic and Cross-Cultural Research." *Annals of Internal Medicine* 88 (2): 251–258.

———. 2006. "Culture, Illness, and Care: Clinical Lessons from Anthropologic and Cross-Cultural Research." *Focus* 4 (1): 140–149. (Reprint of Kleinman et al. 1978.)

Kline, T. C. 2004. "Moral Cultivation through Ritual Participation: Xunzi's Philosophy of Ritual." In *Thinking through Rituals: Philosophical Perspectives,* edited by Kevin Schilbrack, 188–206. London, New York: Routledge.

Klugman, Craig. 2012, October 31. American Society for Bioethics and Humanities Literature and Medicine Listerv. listmed@listserv.com.

Knittel, Kay M. 1995. "Imitation, Individuality, and Illness: Behind Beethoven's Three Styles." *Beethoven Forum* 4:17–36.

Koblenzer, Caroline A. 2006. "Commentary: The Challenge of Morgellons Disease." *Journal of the American Academy of Dermatology* 55:920–922.

Koenig, Harold G., Lucille B. Bearon, and Richard Dayringer, 1989. "Physician Perspectives on the Role of Religion in the Physician–Older Patient Relationship." *Journal of Family Practice* 28 (4): 441–448.

Kohn, Linda T., Janet M. Corrigan, and Molla S. Donaldson, eds. 1999. *To Err Is Human: Building a Safer Health System.* Washington, DC: National Academies Press.

Kong, J., T. J. Kaptchuk, G. Polich, I. Kirsch, M. Vangel, C. Zyloney, B. Rosen, and R. Gollub. 2009. "Expectancy and Treatment Interactions: A Dissociation between Acupuncture Analgesia and Expectancy Evoked Placebo Analgesia." *NeuroImage* 45:940–949.

Krasnik, Martin. 2005, December 4. "It No Longer Feels a Great Injustice That I Have to Die." *Guardian.* www.guardian.co.uk/books/2005/dec/14/fiction.philiproth.

Krieger, Nancy. 2003. "Does Racism Harm Health? Did Child Abuse Exist before 1962? On Explicit Questions, Critical Science, and Current Controversies: An Ecosocial Perspective." *American Journal of Public Health* 93:194–199.

———. 2010. "Workers Are People Too: Societal Aspects of Occupational Health Disparities —an Ecosocial Perspective." *American Journal of Industrial Medicine* 53:104–115.

Krieger, Nancy, and Stephen Sidney. 1996. "Racial Discrimination and Blood Pressure: The CARDIA Study of Young Black and White Adults." *American Journal of Public Health* 86: 1370–1378.

Krieger, Nancy, and George Davey Smith. 2004. "'Bodies Count,' and Body Counts: Social Epidemiology and Embodying Inequality." *Epidemiologic Reviews* 26:92–103.

Kristeller, Jean L., Collette S. Zumbrun, and Robert F. Schilling. 1999. "'I Would If I Could': How Oncologists and Oncology Nurses Address Spiritual Distress in Cancer Patients." *Psycho-oncology* 8 (5): 451–458.

Kristeva, Julia. 1982. *Powers of Horror: An Essay on Abjection.* New York: Columbia University Press.

Kristof, Nicholas D. 2010, July 9. "Youtube Question on Africa Coverage." *New York Times* opinion column. Accessed Aug. 4, 2011. http://kristof.blogs.nytimes.com/2010/07/09/youtube-question-on-africa-coverage.

Kroplick, Lois. 2003, January–February 1. "The Stress of Being a Psychiatrist." *Synapse: The West Hudson Psychiatric Newsletter.* www.rfmh.org/nki/pubs/pubsearch_extended.cfm.

KTVU News. 2006, May 24. "Doctors Make Progress with Mysterious Disease." www.ktvu.com/news/9264350/detail.html.

Kübler-Ross, Elizabeth. (1969) 1997. *On Death and Dying.* New York: Simon & Schuster.

Kuczewski, Mark. 1996. "Reconceiving the Family: The Process of Consent in Medical Decision Making." *Hastings Center Report* 26 (2): 30–37.

Kukla, Rebecca. 2005. *Mass Hysteria: Medicine, Culture, and Mothers' Bodies.* Lanham, MD: Rowman & Littlefield.

Kumagai, Arno K. 2008. "A Conceptual Framework for the Use of Illness Narratives in Medical Education." *Academic Medicine* 83 (7): 653–658.

Kumagai, Arno K., and Monica L. Lypson. 2009. "Beyond Cultural Competence: Critical Consciousness, Social Justice, and Multicultural Education." *Academic Medicine* 84 (6): 782–787.

Kumagai, Arno K., Elizabeth A. Murphy, Paula T. Ross. 2009. "Diabetes Stories: Use of Patient Narratives of Diabetes to Teach Patient-Centered Care." *Advances in Health Sciences Education* 14 (3): 315–326.

Kunz, Miriam, Kenneth Prkachin, and Stefan Lautenbacher. 2009. "The Smile of Pain." *Pain* 145:273–275.

Kushner, Tony. 2003. *Angels in America: A Gay Fantasia on National Themes: Part One: Millennium Approaches. Part Two: Perestroika.* New York: Theatre Communications Group.

Kutchins, Herb, and Stuart A. Kirk. 1997. *Making Us Crazy: DSM: The Psychiatric Bible and the Creation of Mental Disorders.* New York: Free Press.

Kuuppelomaki, Merja. 2001. "Spiritual Support for Terminally Ill Patients: Nursing Staff Assessments." *Journal of Clinical Nursing* 10 (5): 660–670.

Kuusisto, Stephen. 1998. *Planet of the Blind.* New York: Dial Press.

Ladd, Paddy. 2003. *Understanding Deaf Culture: In Search of Deafhood.* Buffalo, NY: Multilingual Matters, 2003.

LaFraniere, Sharon. 2009, April 10. "Chinese Bias for Baby Boys Creates a Gap of 32 Million." *New York Times.* www.nytimes.com/2009/04/11/world/asia/11china.html.

Laing, R. D., and Aaron Esterson. (1964) 1990. *Sanity, Madness and the Family: Families of Schizophrenics.* New York and London: Penguin Books.

Lakoff, George. 1987. *Women, Fire, and Dangerous Things: What Categories Reveal about the Mind.* Chicago: University of Chicago Press.

Lakoff, George, and Mark Johnson. 1980. *Metaphors We Live By.* Chicago: University of Chicago Press.

Landsman, Gail. 2005. "Mothers and Models of Disability." *Journal of Medical Humanities* 26 (2–3): 121–139.

Lane, Harlan. 1999. *The Mask of Benevolence: Disabling the Deaf Community.* DawnSignPress.

Lang, Walter, dir. 1952. *With a Song in My Heart.* Los Angeles: 20th Century Fox.

Lantz, Paula M., Richard L. Lichtenstein, and Harold A. Pollack. 2007. "Health Policy Approaches to Population Health: The Limits of Medicalization." *Health Affairs* 26:1253–1257.

Laqueur, Thomas. 1990. *Making Sex: Body and Gender from the Greeks to Freud.* Cambridge, MA: Harvard University Press.

Lau, George K. K., Yu-hung Leung, Daniel Y. T. Fong, Wing-yan Au, Yok-lam Kwong, Albert Lie, Jii-lin Hou, Yu-mei Wen, Amin Nanj, and Raymond Liang. 2002. "High Hepatitis B Virus (HBV) DNA Viral Load as the Most Important Risk Factor for HBV Reactivation in Patients Positive for HBV Surface Antigen Undergoing Autologous Hematopoietic Cell Transplantation." *Blood* 99:2324–2330.

Lawless, Martha Staeheli, and Michael Rowe. 2011. "The Recovery Era (1998–Present)." In *Classics of Community Psychiatry: Fifty Years of Mental Health outside the Hospital,* edited by Michael Rowe, Martha Lawless, Kenneth S. Thompson, and Larry Davidson, 597–610. New York: Oxford University Press.

Leach, Joan, and Deborah Dysart-Gale, eds. 2011. *Rhetorical Questions of Health and Medicine.* Lanham, MD: Lexington Books.

Leader, Darian. 2008. *The New Black: Mourning, Melancholia, and Depression.* Minneapolis: Gray Wolf Press.

Lee, Ang, dir. 1995. *Sense and Sensibility.* Culver City, CA: Columbia Pictures.

The Legless Runner. 1907. Neuilly-sur-Seine: Société des Etablissements L. Gaumont.

Lerner, Barron H. 1994. "Constructing Medical Indications: The Sterilization of Women with Heart Disease or Tuberculosis, 1905–1935." *Journal of the History of Medicine and Allied Sciences* 49:362–379.

LeRoy, Mervyn, dir. 1944. *Thirty Seconds over Tokyo.* Beverly Hills, CA: Metro-Goldwyn-Mayer.

Levenstein, Joseph H., Eric McCracken, Ian R. McWhinney, Moira A. Stewart, and Judith B. Brown. 1986. "The Patient-Centred Clinical Method: 1. A Model for the Doctor-Patient Interaction in Family Medicine." *Family Practice* 3 (1): 24–30.

Levine, Judith. 2004. *Do You Remember Me? A Father, a Daughter, and a Search for Self.* New York: Free Press.

Levine-Clark, Marjorie. 2004. *Beyond the Reproductive Body: The Politics of Women's Health and Work in Early Victorian England.* Columbus: Ohio State University Press.

Levinson, Bruce Lubotsky, Kevin D. Hennessy, and John Petrila. 2010. *Mental Health Services: A Public Health Perspective.* New York: Oxford University Press.

Lewis, Bradley. 2006. *Moving beyond Prozac, DSM, and the New Psychiatry: The Birth of Postpsychiatry.* Ann Arbor: University of Michigan Press.

———. 2011. *Narrative Psychiatry: How Stories Can Shape Clinical Practice.* Baltimore: Johns Hopkins University Press.

———. 2012. *Depression: Integrating Science, Culture, and Humanities.* New York: Routledge.

Lewis, C. S. 1961. *A Grief Observed.* New York: Harper & Row.

Lidz, Charles W., Paul S. Appelbaum, and Alan Meisel. 1988. "Two Models of Implementing Informed Consent." *Archives of Internal Medicine* 148 (6): 1385. doi:10.1001/archinte.1988.00380060149027.

Liebowitz, Jason. 2011. "Moral Erosion: How Can Medical Professionals Safeguard against the Slippery Slope?" *Medical Humanities* 37:53–55.

Lind, J. E. 1914. "The Color Complex in the Negro." *Psychoanalytic Review* 1:404–414.

Lindemann, Hilde, Marian Verkerk, and Margaret Urban Walker, eds. 2008. *Naturalized Bioethics: Toward Responsible Knowing and Practice.* New York: Cambridge University Press.

Lindemann Nelson, Hilde. 2001. *Damaged Identities, Narrative Repair.* Ithaca, NY: Cornell University Press.

Link, Bruce G., and Jo C. Phelan. 1995. "Social Conditions as Fundamental Causes of Disease." *Journal of Health and Social Behavior* 35 (special issue): 80–95.

———. 2006. "Stigma and Its Public Health Implications." *Lancet* 367:528–529.

Linton, Simi. 1998. *Claiming Disability: Knowledge and Identity.* New York: New York University Press.

———. 2005. *My Body Politic: A Memoir.* Ann Arbor: University of Michigan Press.

Little, Margaret Olivia. 1999. "Cosmetic Surgery, Suspect Norms, and the Ethics of Complicity." In *Enhancing Human Traits: Ethical and Social Implications,* edited by Erik Parens, 162–176. Washington, DC: Georgetown University Press.

Litvak, Anatole, dir. 1948. *The Snake Pit.* Los Angeles: 20th Century Fox.

Lomax, Elizabeth. 1977. "Hereditary or Acquired Disease? Early Nineteenth Century Debates on the Cause of Infantile Scrofula and Tuberculosis." *Journal for the History of Medicine and Allied Sciences* 32 (4): 356–374.

Lombardi, Kate Stone. 1994, October 2. "Breaking the Deadly Hold of Schizophrenia." *New York Times.* www.nytimes.com/1994/10/02/nyregion/breaking-the-deadly-hold-of-schizophrenia.html.

Longmore, Paul. 1985. "Screening Stereotypes: Images of Disabled People in Television and Motion Pictures." *Social Policy* 16 (1): 31–37.

Lorber, Judith. 2000. *Gender and the Social Construction of Illness.* Lanham, MD: Rowman & Littlefield, 2000.

Lorde, Audre. 1980. *The Cancer Journals.* San Francisco: Spinsters, Ink/Aunt Lute.

Lubet, Alex. 2011. *Music, Disability, and Society.* Philadelphia: Temple University Press.

Ludmerer, Kenneth M. 1999. *Time to Heal: American Medical Education from the Turn of the Century to the Era of Managed Care.* Oxford: Oxford University Press.

Lunsford, Lars. 2010. "The Devaluing of Life in Shelley's *Frankenstein*." *Explicator* 68:174–176.

Luoma, Minna-Liisa, and Liisa Hakamies-Blomqvist. 2004. "The Meaning of Quality of Life in Patients Being Treated for Advanced Breast Cancer: A Qualitative Study." *Psycho-oncology* 13 (10): 729–739.

Lupton, Deborah. 2003. *Medicine as Culture: Illness, Disease, and the Body in Western Societies.* London: Sage.

Luria, A. R. 1979. "Romantic Science." In *The Making of Mind: A Personal Account of Soviet Psychology,* edited by Michael Cole and Sheila Cole, 174–189. Cambridge, MA: Harvard University Press. http://luria.ucsd.edu/intro.html.

Lustig, Andrew, Sherri Mackay, and John Strauss. 2009. "Letter to the Editor: Morgellons Disease as Internet Meme." *Psychosomatics* 50:90.

Lyne, John. 2001. Contours of Invention: How Rhetoric Matters to Biomedicine." *Journal of Medical Humanities* 22 (1): 1–13.

MacDougall, Heather. 2007. "Reinventing Public Health: A New Perspective on the Public Health of Canadians and Its International Impact." *Journal of Epidemiology and Public Health* 61 (11): 955–959.

Maciejewski, Paul K., Andrea C. Phelps, Elizabeth L. Kacel, Tracy A. Balboni, Michael Balboni, Alexi A. Wright, William Pirl, and Holly G. Prigerson. 2011. "Religious Coping and Behavioral Disengagement: Opposing Influences on Advance Care Planning and Receipt of Intensive Care Near Death." *Psychooncology* 21 (7) 714–723. http://onlinelibrary.wiley.com/doi/10.1002/pon.1967/full.

MacIntyre, Alasdair C. 1984. *After Virtue: A Study in Moral Theory,* 2nd ed. Notre Dame, IN: University of Notre Dame Press.

MacLean, Charles D., Beth Susi, Nancy Phifer, Linda Schultz, Deborah Bynum, Mark Franco, Andria Klioze, Michael Monroe, Joanne Garrett, and Sam Cykert. 2003. "Patient Preference for Physician Discussion and Practice of Spirituality." *Journal of General Internal Medicine* 18 (1): 38–43.

Macnaughton, Jane. 2009. "The Art of Medicine: The Dangerous Practice of Empathy." *Lancet* 373:1940–1941.

Madden, Ed. 2011. *Prodigal: Variations.* Maple Shade, NJ: Lethe Press.

———. 2012. "Thirteen Weeks." *Journal of the South Carolina Medical Association* 108 (February): 7.

———. 2013. *My Father's House.* Lewisburg, PA: Seven Kitchens Press.

Maher, Jane-Maree. 2001."The Promiscuous Placenta: Crossing Over." In *Contagion: Historical and Cultural Studies,* edited by Alison Bashford and Claire Hooker, 201–216. London: Routledge.

Mahowald, Mary B. 1997. *Genes, Women, Equality.* New York: Oxford University Press.

Mairs, Nancy. 1996. *Waist-High in the World: A Life among the Nondisabled.* Boston: Beacon Press.

Maloney, S. Timothy. 2006. "Glenn Gould, Autistic Savant." In *Sounding Off: Theorizing Disability in Music,* edited by Neil Lerner and Joseph Straus, 121–136. New York: Routledge.

Mann, Ronald D., ed. 1988. *The History of the Management of Pain: From Early Principles to Present Practice.* Park Ridge, NJ: Parthenon.

Mann, Thomas. 1912. *Death in Venice.* Berlin: S. Fischer Verlag.

Manning, Martha. 1994. *Undercurrents: A Therapist's Reckoning with Her Own Depression.* San Francisco: HarperSanFrancisco.

Mar, Raymond A., Kieth Oatley, Jacob Hirsch, Jennifer dela Paz, and Jordan B. Peterson. 2006. "Bookworms versus Nerds: Exposure to Fiction versus Non-fiction, Divergent Associations with Social Ability, and the Simulation of Fictional Social Worlds." *Journal of Research in Personality* 40:694–712.

Marcus Welby, M.D. 1969–1976. Television series. New York: NBC Universal Television Distribution.

Marmot, Michael. 2003. "Understanding Social Inequalities in Health." *Perspectives in Biology and Medicine* 46:S9–S23.

———. n.d. "The Whitehall Study." *Job Stress Network.* www.workhealth.org/projects/pwhitew.html.

Marsden, Alicia, and James Adams. 1949, March. "Are You Likely to Be a Happily Married Woman?" *Ladies' Home Journal*, 31.

Marshall, David. 1988. *Surprising Effects of Sympathy: Marivaux, Diderot, Rousseau, and Mary Shelley.* Chicago: University of Chicago Press.

Marshall, Robert, and Alan Bleakley. 2009. "The Death of Hector: Pity in Homer, Empathy in Medical Education." *Medical Humanities* 35:7–12.

Martin, Emily. 1991. "The Egg and the Sperm: How Science Has Constructed a Romance Based on Stereotypical Male-Female Roles." *Signs* 16:485–501.

———. 2006. "The Pharmaceutical Person." *BioSocieties* 1:273–287.

Martin, Francesca, and Elizabeth H. Flanagan. 2011. "The Pre-community Psychiatry Period (1850–1953)." In *Classics of Community Psychiatry: Fifty Years of Mental Health outside the Hospital,* edited by Michael Rowe, Martha Lawless, Kenneth S. Thompson, and Larry Davidson, 1–8. New York: Oxford University Press.

Martin, James C., Robert F. Avant, Marjorie A. Bowman, John R. Bucholtz, John C. Dickinson, Kenneth L. Evans, Larry A. Green, et al. 2004. "The Future of Family Medicine: A Collaborative Project of the Family Medicine Community." *Annals of Family Medicine* 2 (suppl. 1): S3–S32.

Massumi, Brian. 1995. "The Autonomy of Affect." *Cultural Critique* 31 (1995): 83–109.

———. 2002. "The Autonomy of Affect." In *Parables for the Virtual: Movement, Affect, Sensation,* 22–45. Durham, NC: Duke University Press.

Matheson, Alastair. 2008. "Corporate Science and the Husbandry of Scientific and Medical Knowledge by the Pharmaceutical Industry." *BioSocieties* 3:355–382.

Mattingly, Cheryl. 1998. *Healing Dramas and Clinical Plots: The Narrative Structure of Experience.* Cambridge: Cambridge University Press.

Mattingly, Cheryl, and Linda C. Garro. 2000. *Narrative and the Cultural Construction of Illness and Healing.* Berkeley: University of California Press.

May, William F. 1991. *The Patient's Ordeal.* Bloomington: Indiana University Press.

———. 2000. *The Physician's Covenant: Images of the Healer in Medical Ethics,* 2nd ed. Lexington, KY: Westminster John Knox Press.

McCarthy, Thomas, dir. 2003. *The Station Agent.* SenArts Films. New York: Miramax Films.

McCloud, Scott. 1994. *Understanding Comics: The Invisible Art.* New York: HarperPerennial.

———. 2000. *Reinventing Comics: How Imagination and Technology Are Revolutionizing an Art Form.* New York: Perennial.

McFerran, Katrina, Ju-Young Lee, Megan Steele, and Andrea Bialocerkowski. 2009. "A Descriptive Review of the Literature (1990–2006) Addressing Music Therapy with People Who Have Disabilities." *Musica Humana* 1:45–80.

McGrath, Charles. 2006, April 26. "Roth, Haunted by Illness, Feels Fine." *New York Times.* www.nytimes.com/2006/04/25/books/25roth.html.

McGuire, Dennis. 2005. "If People with Down Syndrome Ruled the World." *National Association for Down Syndrome.* www.nads.org/pages_new/news/ruletheworld.html.

McHugh, Heather. (1988) 1991. "What Hell Is." In *On Doctoring: Stories, Poems, Essays,* 1st ed., edited by Richard Reynolds and John Stone, 347–348. New York: Simon & Schuster.

McKenny, Gerald P. 1997. *To Relieve the Human Condition: Bioethic and the Technological Utopianism of Modern Medicine.* Albany: State of New York Press.

McLellan, Joseph. 1981, March 19. "Perlman to the Defense." *Washington Post.*

McMillen, Christian W. 2008. "'The Red Man and the White Plague': Rethinking Race, Tuberculosis, and American Indians, ca. 1890–1950." *Bulletin of the History of Medicine* 82: 608–645.

McRuer, Robert, and Anna Mollow, eds. 2012. *Sex and Disability.* Durham, NC: Duke University Press.

McSherry, Wilfred, and Steve Jamieson. 2011. "An Online Survey of Nurses' Perceptions of Spirituality and Spiritual Care." *Journal of Clinical Nursing* 20 (11–12): 1757–1767.

McWhinney, Ian R. 1989. "The Need for a Transformed Clinical Method." In *Communicating with Medical Patients,* edited by Moira Stewart and Debra Roter, 25–42. London: Sage.

"The Measurement of Pain." 1940. *Lancet* (August 10): 167.

Mechanic, David, and David A. Rochefort. 1992. "A Policy of Inclusion for the Mentally Ill." *Health Affairs* 11 (1): 128–150.

Mehlman, Maxwell J., and Jeffrey R. Botkin. 1998. *Access to the Genome: The Challenge to Equality.* Washington, DC: Georgetown University Press.

Meisel, Alan, and Mark Kuczewski. 1996. "Legal and Ethical Myths about Informed Consent." *Archives of Internal Medicine* 56 (December): 2521–2526.

Mental Disorders: Diagnostic and Statistical Manual. 1952. Washington: American Psychiatric Association Press.

Metzl, Jonathan M. 2010. *The Protest Psychosis: How Schizophrenia Became a Black Disease.* Boston: Beacon.

Meyers, Jeffrey. 1985. "Solzhenitsyn: *Cancer Ward.*" In *Disease and the Novel, 1880–1960.* New York: St. Martin's Press.

Michaels, Meredith W. 1999. "Fetal Galaxies: Some Questions about What We See." In *Fetal Subjects, Feminist Positions,* edited by Lynn M. Morgan and Meredith W. Michaels, 113–132. Philadelphia: University of Pennsylvania Press.

Michell, Roger, dir. 1999. *Notting Hill.* Universal City, CA: Universal Pictures.

Milgram, Stanley. 1963. "Behavioral Study of Obedience." *Journal of Abnormal and Social Psychology* 67 (1963): 371–378.

Millay, Edna St. Vincent. 1921. "Spring." In *Second April.* New York: Mitchell Kennerley. http://digital.library.upenn.edu/women/millay/april/second-april.html.

Miller, Arthur. 1998. *The Death of a Salesman.* New York: Penguin.

Miller, Genevieve. 1956. "Smallpox Inoculation in England and America: A Reappraisal." *William and Mary Quarterly* 13 (2): 476–496.

Miller, Leon K. 1989. *Musical Savants: Exceptional Skill in the Mentally Retarded.* Mahwah, NJ: Lawrence Erlbaum Publishers.

Miller, Rebecca, Allison N. Ponce, and Kenneth S. Thompson. 2011. "Deinstitutionalization and the Community Mental Health Center Movement (1954–1976)." In *Classics of Community Psychiatry: Fifty Years of Mental Health outside the Hospital,* 9–20. New York: Oxford University Press.

Mills, Bruce. 2008. "Autism and the Imagination." In *Autism and Representation,* edited by Mark Osteen, 117–132. New York: Routledge.

Mitchell, David T., and Sharon L. Snyder. 2003. *Narrative Prosthesis: Disability and the Dependencies of Discourse.* Ann Arbor: University of Michigan Press.

———. 2010. "Narrative Prosthesis." In *The Disability Studies Reader,* 3rd ed., edited by Lennard J. Davis, 275–287. New York: Routledge.

Mitchell, W. J. T. 1994. *Picture Theory.* Chicago: University of Chicago Press.

Moadel, Alyson, Carole Morgan, Anne Fatone, Jennifer Grennan, Jeanne Carter, Gia Laruffa, Anne Skummy, and Janice Dutcher. 1999. "Seeking Meaning and Hope: Self-Reported Spiritual and Existential Needs among an Ethnically-Diverse Cancer Patient Population." *Psychology* 8 (5): 378–385.

Molina, Natalia. 2006. *Fit to Be Citizens? Public Health and Race in Los Angeles, 1879–1939.* Berkeley: University of California Press.

Mollow, Anna. 2012. "Is Sex Disability? Queer Theory and the Disability Drive." In *Sex and Disability,* edited by Robert McRuer and Anna Mollow, 285–312. Durham, NC: Duke University Press.

Molloy, Seaneen. n.d. *Being Mentally Interesting.* Blog. http://thesecretlifeofamanicdepressive
.wordpress.com.

Molyneux, Jacob. 2008. "AKA 'Morgellons.'" *American Journal of Nursing* 108 (5): 25–26.

Moment, G. B. 1974. "Andromeda Strain?" *Bioscience* 24 (9): 487.

Montag, Warren. 2000. "The 'Workshop of Filthy Creation': A Marxist Retelling of *Frankenstein.*" In *Frankenstein,* edited by Johanna M. Smith, 384–394. Boston: Bedford.

Montaigne, Michel de. (1588) 2003. *The Complete Works.* Translated by Donald Frame. New
York: Alfred A. Knopf.

Morgan, Lynn. 1997. "Imagining the Unborn in the Ecuadoran Andes." *Feminist Studies* 23
(2): 323–350.

Morgellons Research Foundation. 2011. www.morgellons.org. Accessed August 27, 2011.

Morris, David B. 1993. *The Culture of Pain.* Berkeley: University of California Press.

———. 1998. *Illness and Culture in the Postmodern Age.* Berkeley: University of California
Press.

Morrison, David S., Melinda Petticrew, and Hilary Thomson. 2003. "What Are the Most
Effective Ways of Improving Population Health through Transport Interventions? Evidence from Systematic Reviews." *Journal of Epidemiology and Community Health* 5:
327–333.

Morrissey, Joseph P., and Howard H. Goldman. 1986. "Care and Treatment of the Mentally
Ill in the United States: Historical Developments and Reform." *Annals of the American
Academy of Political and Social Science* 484:12–27.

Morton, D. B. and P. H. M. Griffiths. 1985, April 20. "Guidelines on the Recognition of Pain,
Distress and Discomfort in Experimental Animals and an Hypothesis for Assessment."
Veterinary Record 166 (16): 431–436.

Moscucci, Ornella. 1993. *The Science of Woman: Gynaecology and Gender in England, 1800–
1929.* New York: Cambridge University Press.

———. 1996. "Clitoridectomy, Circumcision, and the Politics of Sexual Pleasure in Mid-
Victorian Britain." In *Sexualities in Victorian Britain,* edited by Andrew H. Miller and
James Eli Adams, 60–78. Bloomington: Indiana University Press.

Moss, Stephen. 2000, October 20. "'I'm Lucky. Everyone Can See My Disability': Thomas
Quasthoff Was Born a 'Thalidomide Baby' but He Has a Voice Sublime Enough to Overcome Any Prejudice." *Guardian.*

Mossman, Mark. 2001, May. "Acts of Becoming: Autobiography, Frankenstein, and the
Postmodern Body." *Postmodern Culture* 11(3). www.pmc.iath.virginia.edu/issue.501/11
.3mossman.html.

Mottron, Laurent, Isabelle Peretz, Sylvie Belleville, and N. Rouleau. 1999. "Absolute Pitch in
Autism: A Case-Study." *Neurocase* 5:485–501.

Mueller, Lisel. (1986) 1994. "Monet Refuses the Operation." In *Articulations: The Body and
Illness in Poetry,* edited by Jon Mukand. Iowa City: University of Iowa Press.

Mukherjee, S., S. Shukla, J. Woodle, A. M. Rosen, and S. Olarte. 1983. "Misdiagnosis of
Schizophrenia in Bipolar Patients: A Multiethnic Comparison." *American Journal of Psychiatry* 140:1571–1574.

Mullan, Fitzhugh, Ellen Ficklen, and Kyna Rubin, eds. 2006. *Narrative Matters: The Power of
the Personal Essay in Health Policy.* Baltimore: Johns Hopkins University Press.

Munch, Edvard. 1893. *The Scream.* Casein/waxed crayon and tempera on paper (cardboard),
91 × 73.5 cm. (35 7/8 × 29 inches). Nasjonalgalleriet (National Gallery), Oslo.

Munro, Alice. 2001. "The Bear Came over the Mountain." In *Hateship, Friendship, Courtship,
Loveship, Marriage: Stories,* 275–323. New York: Alfred A. Knopf.

———. 2007. *Away from Her.* Toronto: Penguin Canada, 2007.

Murase, Jenny E., Jashin J. Wu, and John Koo. 2006. "Notes and Comments: Morgellons
Disease: A Rapport-Enhancing Term for Delusions of Parasitosis." *Journal of the American
Academy of Dermatology* 55:913–914.

Murphy-Shigematsu, Stephen. 2009. "Teaching Cross-Cultural Competence through Narrative." *Family Medicine* 41 (9): 622–624.

Murray, Stuart. 2008. *Representing Autism: Culture, Narrative, Fascination.* Liverpool: Liverpool University Press.

Myers, David G. 2008. "Religion and Human Flourishing." In *The Science of Subjective Well-Being,* edited by Michael Eid and Randy J. Larsen, 323–344. New York: Guilford Press.

Nadeson, Majia Holmer. 2005. *Constructing Autism: Unraveling the "Truth" and Understanding the Social.* New York: Routledge, 2005.

"Nadya Suleman." 2011. *Wikepedia, the Free Encyclopedia.* http://en.wikipedia.org/wiki/Nadya_Suleman. Accessed December 28, 2011.

Naghshineh, Sheila, Janet P. Hafler, Alexis R. Miller, Maria A. Blanco, Stuart R. Lipsitz, Rachel P. Dubroff, Khosbin Shahram, and Joel T. Katz. 2008. "Formal Art Observation Training Improves Medical Students' Visual Diagnostic Skills." *Journal of General Internal Medicine* 23:991–997.

National Alliance of Multi-ethnic Behavioral Health Associations. 2008. *Blueprint for the National Network to Eliminate Disparities in Behavioral Health.* Washington, DC: National Alliance of Multi-ethnic Behavioral Health Associations.

National Association of State Mental Health Program Directors. 2006. *Morbidity and Mortality in People with Serious Mental Illness.* Alexandria, VA: National Association of State Mental Health Program Directors.

National Audit Office. 2005. *A Safer Place for Patients: Learning to Improve Patient Safety.* London: Her Majesty's Stationery Office.

National Consensus Project for Quality Palliative Care. 2009. *Clinical Practice Guidelines for Quality Palliative Care,* 2nd ed. Pittsburgh: National Consensus Project for Quality Palliative Care.

National Patient Safety Agency. 2010. *Medical Error. What to Do If Things Go Wrong: A Guide for Junior Doctors.* London: National Patient Safety Agency.

Nauert, Charles G. 2006. *Humanism and the Culture of Renaissance Europe,* 2nd ed. New York: Cambridge University Press.

Nead, Lynda. 1988. *Myths of Sexuality: Representations of Women in Victorian Britain.* Cambridge, MA: Basil Blackwell.

NHS Executive. 1998. *The New NHS Modern and Dependable: A National Framework for Assessing Performance.* Consultation document. London: Department of Health. Accessed January 12, 2012. http://webarchive.nationalarchives.gov.uk/20130107105354/http://www.dh.gov.uk/prod_consum_dh/groups/dh_digitalassets/@dh/@en/documents/digital asset/dh_4014486.pdf.

Niccol, Andrew, dir. 1997. *Gattaca.* Culver City, CA: Columbia Pictures.

Nichols, Mike, dir. 2001. *Wit.* New York: HBO.

Nietzsche, Friedrich. 1998. *Twilight of the Idols; or, How to Philosophize with a Hammer.* Oxford: Oxford University Press.

Nisker, Jeffrey A. 2001. "Calcedonies." *Canadian Medical Association Journal* 164 (1):74–75.

———. 2005, August 26. *Orchids.* Production Draft.

———. 2008. "Calcedonies." In *From the Other Side of the Fence: Stories from Health Care Professionals,* edited by Jeffrey A. Nisker, 172–176. Halifax: Pottersfield Press.

———. 2010. "*Calcedonies:* Critical Reflections on Writing Plays to Engage Citizens in Health and Social Policy Development." *Reflective Practice: International and Multidisciplinary Perspectives* 11 (4): 417–432.

Norden, Martin F. 1994. *The Cinema of Isolation: A History of Physical Disability in the Movies.* New Brunswick, NJ: Rutgers University Press.

Norman, Geoffrey R., Meredith E. Young, and Lee R. Brooks. 2007. "Non-analytical Models of Clinical Reasoning: The Role of Experience." *Medical Education* 41:1140–1145.

Not Your Mother's Meatloaf. 2011a. Issue nos. 1–5. http://sexedcomicproject.blogspot.com. Accessed September 23, 2011.

Not Your Mother's Meatloaf. 2011b, May 20. "NYMM at Comics and Medicine Conference." http://sexedcomicproject.blogspot.com/2011/05/nymm-at-comics-medicine-conference .html. Accessed July 14, 2013.

Noyes, Arthur P. 1927. *A Textbook of Psychiatry.* New York: Macmillan.

Nuland, Sherwin. 1988. *The Doctors: The Biography of Medicine.* New York: Vintage.

Nurse Jackie. 2009–. Television series. New York: Showtime.

Nussbaum, Martha C. 1995. *Poetic Justice: The Literary Imagination and Public Life.* Boston: Beacon Press.

———. 2010. *Not for Profit: Why Democracy Needs the Humanities.* Princeton, NJ: Princeton University Press.

Ockelford, Adam. 2007. *In the Key of Genius: The Extraordinary Life of Derek Paravicini.* London: Hutchinson.

O'Farrell, Mary Ann. 2001. "Self-Consciousness and the Psoriatic Personality: Considering Updike and Potter." *Literature and Medicine* 20 (2): 133–150.

Oldham, John, Daniel Carlat, Richard Friedman, Andrew Nierenberg, with response by Marcia Angell. 2011, August 18. " 'The Illusions of Psychiatry': An Exchange." *New York Review of Books.* www.nybooks.com/articles/archives/2011/aug/18/illusions-psychiatry -exchange.

Oshinsky, David M. 2006. *Polio: An American Story.* New York: Oxford University Press.

Osler, William. 1950. *Sir William Osler: Aphorisms from His Bedside Teachings and Writings,* edited by William Bennett Bean. New York: Henry Schuman.

Oyebode, Femi. 2003. "Autobiographical Narrative and Psychiatry." *Advances in Psychiatric Treatment* 9 (4): 265–270.

Padden, Carol, and Tom Humphries. 1988. *Deaf in America: Voices from a Culture.* Cambridge, MA: Harvard University Press.

———. 2006. *Inside Deaf Culture.* Cambridge, MA: Harvard University Press.

Palfrey, Judith S., Lisa A Sofis, Emily J. Davidson, Jihong Liu, Linda Freedman, and Michael L. Ganz. 2004. "The Pediatric Alliance for Coordinated Care: Evaluation of a Medical Home Model." *Pediatrics* 113:1507–1516.

Paloutzian, R. F., and C. W. Ellison. 1982. "Loneliness, Spiritual Well-Being, and Quality of Life." In *Loneliness: A Sourcebook of Current Theory, Research, and Therapy,* edited by La Peplau and D. Perman, 224–237. New York: Wiley Interscience.

Parens, Eric, and Adrienne Asch, eds. 2000. *Prenatal Testing and Disability Rights.* Washington, DC: Georgetown University Press.

Pargament, Kenneth I. 1997. *The Psychology of Religion and Coping.* New York: Guilford Press.

Pargament, Kenneth I., Harold G. Koenig, and Lisa M. Perez. 2000. "The Many Methods of Religious Coping: Development and Initial Validation of the RCOPE." *Journal of Clinical Psychology* 56 (4): 519–543.

Parker-Pope, Tara. 2011, October 23. "Studying Successful People with Mental Illness." *New York Times.* http://well.blogs.nytimes.com/2011/10/23/studying-successful-people-with -mental-illness.

Passer, Ivan, dir. 1981. *Cutter's Way.* Beverly Hills, CA: United Artists.

Patterson, K. David. 1983. "The Influenza Epidemic of 1918–19 in the Gold Coast." *Journal of African History* 24 (4): 485–502.

"Paul Farmer: 'Accompaniment' as Policy." 2011, May 25. *Harvard Magazine.* http://harvard magazine.com/2011/05/paul-farmer-accompaniment-as-policy.

Peabody, Francis W. 1927. "The Care of the Patient." *Journal of the American Medical Association* 88:877–882.

Peace, William. n.d. *Bad Cripple.* Blog. http://badcripple.blogspot.com.

Pearson, Michele L., Joseph V. Selby, Kenneth A. Katz, Virginia Cantrell, Christopher R. Braden, Monica E. Parise, Christopher D. Paddock, Michael R. Lewin-Smith, Victor F. Kalasinsky, Felicia C. Goldstein, Allen W. Hightower, Arthur Papier, Brian Lewis, Sarita

Motipara, and Mark L. Eberhard, for the Unexplained Dermopathy Study Team. 2012. "Clinical, Epidemiologic, Histopathologic and Molecular Features of an Unexplained Dermopathy." *PLoS ONE* 7 (1): e29908, 1–12. doi:10.1371/journal.pone. 0029908.

Pediatric Urology Clinics of Weill Cornell Medical College. 2011. "Genitoplasty." www.cornellurology.com/clinical-conditions/pediatric-urology/genitoplasty-surgery/. Accessed August 22, 2011.

Peerce, Larry, dir. 1975. *The Other Side of the Mountain.* Universal City, CA: Universal Pictures.

———, dir. 1978. *The Other Side of the Mountain, Part 2.* Universal City, CA: Universal Pictures.

Pekar, Harvey, Joyce Brabner, and Frank Stack. 1994. *Our Cancer Year.* New York: Four Walls Eight Windows.

Pellegrino, Edmund. 2001. "The Caring Ethic: The Relation of Physician to Patient." In *Physician and Philosopher: The Philosophical Foundation of Medicine.* Charlottesville, VA: Carden Jennings Publishing.

———. 1972. "Welcoming Remarks." In *Proceedings of the First Session, Institute on Human Values in Medicine,* edited by L. L. Hunt, 3–9. Philadelphia: Society for Health and Human Values.

Penn, Arthur, dir. 1962. *The Miracle Worker.* Beverly Hills, CA: United Artists.

Pernick, Martin S. 1985. *A Calculus of Suffering: Pain, Professionalism, and Anesthesia in Nineteenth-Century America.* New York: Columbia University Press.

———. 1995. *The Black Stork: Eugenics and the Death of "Defective" Babies in American Medicine and Motion Pictures since 1915.* Oxford: Oxford University Press.

Pescarmon, Denee. 2003. "The Performances/Surgeries." www.english.ucsb.edu/faculty/ecook/courses/eng114em/surgeries.htm.

Petchesky, Rosalind. 1987. "Fetal Images: The Power of Visual Culture in the Politics of Reproduction." *Feminist Studies* 13 (2): 263–292.

Peterkin, Allan. 2008. "Medical Humanities for What Ails Us." *Canadian Medical Association Journal* 178 (5): 648.

Peterkin, Allan, and Cathy Risdon. 2003. *Caring for Lesbian and Gay People: A Clinical Guide.* Toronto: University of Toronto Press.

Phelan, Jo C., Bruce G. Link, and Parisa Tehranifar. 2010. "Social Conditions as Fundamental Causes of Health Inequities: Theory, Evidence, and Policy Implications." *Journal of Health and Social Behavior* 51:S28–S40.

Phelps, Andrea C., Paul K. Maciejewski, Matthew Nilsson, TracyA. Balboni, Alexi A. Wright, M.Elizabeth Paulk, Elizabeth Trice, Deborah Schrag, John R. Peteet, and Susan D. Block. 2009. "Religious Coping and Use of Intensive Life-Prolonging Care near Death in Patients with Advanced Cancer." *Journal of American Medical Association* 301 (11): 1140.

Phillips, David P., and Gwendolyn E. C. Barker. 2010. "A July Spike in Fatal Medication Errors: A Possible Effect of Few Medical Residents." *Journal of General Internal Medicine* 25:774–779.

Piercy, Marge. 1976. *Woman on the Edge of Time.* New York: Fawcett Crest.

Pil, Tricia. 2011. *Babel: Voices from Medical Trauma.* YouTube video. http://youtu.be/LWTesIihoQY. (See also the text version at *Pulse Magazine,* www.pulsemagazine.org/Archive_index.cfm?content_id=119 .)

Pimp My Ride. 2004–2007. Television series. New York: MTV.

Pinar, William F., William M. Reynolds, Patrick Slattery, and Peter M. Taubman. 1995. *Understanding Curriculum: An Introduction to Historical and Contemporary Curriculum Discourses.* New York: Peter Lang.

Pitzer, Andrea. 2009, June 23. "U.S. Eugenics Legacy: Ruling on Buck Sterilization Still Stands." *USA Today.* http://usatoday30.usatoday.com/news/health/2009-06-23-eugenics-carrie-buck_N.htm?csp=usat.me.

Plath, Sylvia. 1978. *The Bell Jar.* New York: Faber & Faber.

Plato. 1968. *The Republic.* Edited by Allan Bloom. New York: Perseus Books.

———. 1989. *The Collected Dialogues*. Edited by Edith Hamilton and Huntington Cairns. Princeton, NJ: Princeton University Press.

———. 2003. *The Republic*. Translated by Desmond Lee. London: Penguin.

Platt, Frederic W., and Jonathan C. McMath. 1979. "Clinical Hypocompetence: The Interview." *Annals of Internal Medicine* 91:898–902.

Poirier, Suzanne, and Daniel J. Brauner. 1990. "The Voices of the Medical Record." *Theoretical Medicine* 11 (1): 29–39.

Polanyi, Michael, and Harry Prosch. 1975. *Meaning*. Chicago: University of Chicago Press.

Pollack, Andrew. 2010, March 20. "Consumers Slow to Embrace the Age of Genomics." *New York Times*. www.nytimes.com/2010/03/20/business/20consumergene.html?page wanted=all.

Polley, Sarah, dir. 2006. *Away from Her*. Santa Monica, CA: Lionsgate.

Pollock, George. 1989. *The Mourning-Liberation Process*. Madison, CT: International Universities Press.

Poore, Carol. 2009. *Disability in Twentieth-Century German Culture*. Ann Arbor: University of Michigan Press.

Poovey, Mary. 1986. "Scenes of an Indelicate Character: The Medical 'Treatment' of Victorian Women." *Representations* 14:137–168.

Popper, Karl. 1985. "Knowledge: Objective Versus Subjective." In *Popper Selections*, edited by D. Miller, 58–77. Princeton, NJ: Princeton University Press.

———. 2002. *The Open Society and Its Enemies*, 7th ed. London: Routledge.

Portelli, Alessandro. 2001. "Research as an Experiment in Equality." In *The Death of Luigi Trastulli and Other Stories: Form and Meaning in Oral History*, 29–44. Albany: SUNY Press.

Porter, Katherine Anne. (1930) 1958. "The Jilting of Granny Weatherall." In *Flowering Judas and Other Stories*. New York: Random House.

Porter, Liza. 2008. "Down the Tracks: Bruce Springsteen Sang to Me." In *Poets on Prozac: Mental Illness, Treatment and the Creative Process*, edited by Richard Berlin, 147–161. Baltimore: Johns Hopkins University Press.

Porter, Roy. 1997. *The Greatest Benefit to Mankind: A Medical History of Humanity*. London: HarperCollins.

———. 2002. *Madness: A Brief History*. Oxford: Oxford University Press.

Porter, Roy, and William Bynum, eds. 1993. *Companion Encyclopedia of the History of Medicine*, vols. 1 and 2. New York: Routledge.

Porter, Roy, and Lesley A. Hall. 1995. *The Facts of Life: The Creation of Sexual Knowledge in Britain, 1650–1950*. New Haven, CT: Yale University Press.

Porter, Roy, and Dorothy Porter. 1988. *In Sickness and in Health: The British Experience, 1650–1850*. London: Fourth Estate.

Powers, Madison, and Ruth Faden. 2006. *Social Justice: The Moral Foundations of Public Health and Health Policy*. New York: Oxford University Press.

Preminger, Otto, dir. 1970. *Tell Me That You Love Me, Junie Moon*. Otto Preminger Films. Hollywood, CA: Paramount Pictures.

President's New Freedom Commission on Mental Health. 2003. *Achieving the Promise: Transforming Mental Health Care in America*. Final Report. Rockville, MD: Department of Health and Human Services.

Price, Janet, and Margrit Shildrick. 1999. *Feminist Theory and the Body: A Reader*. New York: Routledge.

Price, Reynolds. 2003. *A Whole New Life*. New York: Alfred A. Knopf.

Price Herndl, Diane. 1993. *Invalid Women: Figuring Feminine Illness in American Fiction and Culture, 1840–1940*. Chapel Hill: University of North Carolina Press.

———. 2005. "Disease versus Disability: The Medical Humanities and Disability Studies." *PMLA* 120 (2): 593–598.

Prkachin, Kenneth M. 2005. "Facial Expressions of Pain: A Comparison across Modalities." In *What the Face Reveals: Basic and Applied Studies of Spontaneous Expression Using the*

Facial Action Coding System (FACS), edited by Paul Ekman and Erika L. Rosenberg, 181–197, and afterword, 198–202. New York: Oxford University Press.

"Psychiatrists Are Told of 'Literary Artists' Who Evidence Schizophrenia: Grandiloquence Is Sign." 1935, May 15. *New York Times,* 23.

Puchalski, Christina, Betty Ferrell, Rose Virani, Shirley Otis-Green, Pamela Baird, Janet Bull, Harvey Chochinov, George Handzo, Holly Nelson-Becker, and Maryjo Prince-Paul. 2009. "Improving the Quality of Spiritual Care as a Dimension of Palliative Care: The Report of the Consensus Conference." *Journal of Palliative Medicine* 12 (10): 885–904.

Puhl, Rebecca, and Kelly D. Brownell. 1991. "Bias, Discrimination, and Obesity." *Obesity Research* 9 (12): 788–805.

Puhl, Rebecca, Christopher Wharton, and Chelsea Heuer. 2009. "Weight Bias among Dietetics Students: Implications for Treatment Practices." *Journal of the American Dietetic Association* 109 (3): 438–444.

Purdy, Laura M. 1996. "Loving Future People." In *Reproducing Persons: Issues in Feminist Bioethics,* edited by Laura M. Purdy, 50–74. Ithaca, NY: Cornell University Press.

Quain, Richard. 1883. *Quain's Dictionary of Medicine,* 5th ed. New York: Appleton.

Quasthoff, Thomas. 2008. *The Voice: A Memoir.* Translated by Kirsten Stoldt Wittenborn. New York: Pantheon.

Quayson, Ato. 2007. *Aesthetic Nervousness: Disability and the Crisis of Representation.* New York: Columbia University Press.

Quincy, M.E. 1976–1983. Television series. New York: NBC.

Quindlen, Anna. 1994. *One True Thing.* New York: Random House.

Racine Eric, Ofek Bar-Ilan, and Judy Illes. 2005. "Science and Society: fMRI in the Public Eye." *Nature Reviews Neuroscience* 6:159–164.

Radstone, Susannah, and Bill Schwarz, eds. 2010. *Memory: Histories, Theories, Debates.* New York: Fordham University Press.

Ramsey, Paul. 1970. *The Patient as Person: Explorations in Medical Ethics.* New Haven, CT: Yale University Press.

Raphael, Dennis G. 2011. "Poverty in Childhood and Adverse Health Outcomes in Adulthood." *Maturitas* 69:22–26.

Raspe, Lucia. 2004. "The Black Death in Jewish Sources." *Jewish Quarterly Review* 94: 471–489. www.jstor.org/discover/10.2307/1455650?uid=3739672&uid=2129&uid=2&uid=70&uid=4&uid=3739256&sid=21102533469997.

Redford, Robert, dir. 2000. *The Legend of Bagger Vance.* Universal City, CA: DreamWorks Pictures.

Rees, Geoffrey. 2010. "The Ethical Imperative of Medical Humanities." *Journal of Medical Humanities* 31:267–277.

Regier, D. A., W. E. Narrow, and D. S. Rae. 1993. "The De Facto US Mental and Addictive Disorders Service System: Epidemiologic Catchment Area Prospective 1-Year Prevalence Rates of Disorders and Services." *Archives of General Psychiatry* 50 (2): 85–94.

Reich, Wilhelm. 1983. *Children of the Future: On the Prevention of Sexual Pathology.* New York: Farrar, Straus & Giroux.

Reilly, Jo Marie, Jeffrey Ring, and Linda Duke. 2005. "Visual Thinking Strategies: A New Role for Art in Medical Education." *Family Medicine* 37:250–252.

Remer, Gary. 1996. *Humanism and the Rhetoric of Toleration.* University Park: Pennsylvania State University Press, 1996.

Révész, Geza. 1925. *The Psychology of a Musical Prodigy.* New York: Harcourt Brace.

Rey, Roselyne. 1993. *History of Pain.* Translated by Louise Elliott Wallace and J. A. Cadden and S. W. Cadden. Paris: La Découverte.

Rice, Geoffrey W., and Edwina Palmer. 1993. "Pandemic Influenza in Japan, 1918–1919: Mortality Patterns and Official Responses." *Journal of Japanese Studies* 19:389–420.

Richardson, Robert. 2006. *William James: In the Maelstrom of American Modernism.* Boston: Houghton Mifflin.

Ricoeur, Paul. 1984. *Time and Narrative,* vol. 1. Chicago: University of Chicago Press.

———. 1991. "Life in Quest of Narrative." In *On Paul Ricouer: Narrative and Interpretation,* edited by David Wood, 20–187. London: Routledge.

———. 1992. *Oneself as Another.* Chicago: University of Chicago Press.

Ridge, Damien. 2009. *Recovery from Depression Using the Narrative Approach: A Guide for Doctors, Complementary Therapists, and Mental Health Professionals.* London: Jessica Kingsley Publishers.

Ridge, Damien, and Sue Zeibland. 2006. "'The Old Me Could Never Have Done That': How People Give Meaning to Recovery following Depression." *Qualitative Healthcare Research* 16 (8): 1038–1053.

Riding, Richard, and Indra Cheema. 1991. "Cognitive Styles—an Overview and Integration." *Educational Psychology* 11 (3): 193–215.

Riedelsheimer, Thomas, dir. 2004. *Touch the Sound: A Sound Journey with Evelyn Glennie.* New York: New Video Group.

Rieselbach, Richard E., Byron J. Crouse, and John G. Frohna. 2010. "Teaching Primary Care in Community Health Centers: Addressing the Workforce Crisis for the Underserved." *Annals of Internal Medicine* 152:118–122.

Risse, Gunter, and John Harley Warner. 1992. "Reconstructing Clinical Activities: Patient Records in Medical History." *Social History of Medicine* 5:183–205.

Ritvo, Lucille B. 1990. *Darwin's Influence on Freud: A Tale of Two Sciences.* New Haven, CT: Yale University Press.

Roberts, Melinda A. 2006, Winter. "Supernumerary Pregnancy, Collective Harm, and Two Forms of the Nonidentity Problem." *Journal of Law, Medicine, and Ethics* 34 (4): 776–792.

Robertson, John A. 1994. *Children of Choice: Freedom and the New Reproductive Technologies.* Princeton, NJ: Princeton University Press.

Robinson, Bruce, dir. 1992. *Jennifer 8.* Hollywood, CA: Paramount Pictures.

Robles, David T. 2008. "Morgellons Disease and the 'Tweezer Sign.'" *Clinical and Experimental Dermatology* 33 (6): 793–794.

Robles, David T., Jonathan M. Olson, Heidi Combs, Sharon Romm, and Phil Kirby. 2011. "Morgellons Disease and Delusions of Parasitosis." *American Journal of Clinical Dermatology* 12 (1): 1–6.

Robson, Mark, dir. 1951. *Bright Victory.* Universal City, CA: Universal Pictures.

Rodgers, Bernard, and Derek Parker Royal. 2007. "Grave Commentary: A Roundtable Discussion on *Everyman.*" *Philip Roth Studies* 3 (1): 3–25.

Roney, Lisa. 1999. *Sweet Invisible Body: Reflections on Life with Diabetes.* New York: Henry Holt.

Roof, Wade Clark, and Richard B. Perkins. 1975. "On Conceptualizing Salience in Religious Committment." *Journal of the Scientific Study of Religion* 14:111–128.

Rose, David. 2009, September 23. "Higher Hospital Death Rate Coincides with Junior Doctors' First Week." *Times.* www.thetimes.co.uk/tto/health/article1965186.ece.

Rose, Nicholas. 2003, November/December. "Neurochemical Selves." *Society,* 46–59.

Rosenbaum, Edward. 1988. *A Taste of My Own Medicine: When the Doctor Is the Patient.* New York: Random House.

Rosenthal, Thomas C. 2008. "The Medical Home: Growing Evidence to Support a New Approach to Primary Care." *Journal of the American Board of Family Medicine* 21 (5): 427–440.

Ross, Catherine L., and Nancy Green Leigh. 2000. "Planning, Urban Revitalization, and the Inner City: An Exploration of Structural Racism." *Journal of Planning Literature* 14: 367–380.

Ross, Linda. 2006. "Spiritual Care in Nursing: An Overview of the Research to Date." *Journal of Clinical Nursing* 15 (7): 852–862.

Ross, W. D. (1930) 2002. *The Right and the Good.* Edited, with an Introduction, by Philip Stratton-Lake. New York: Oxford University Press.

Roter, Debra L., and Judith A. Hall. 2006. *Doctors Talking with Patients/Patients Talking with Doctors: Improving Communication in Medical Visits,* 2nd ed. London: Praeger.

Roth, Philip. 1972. *The Breast.* New York, Holt, Rinehart & Winston.

———. 1977. *The Professor of Desire.* New York: Farrar, Straus & Giroux.

———. 1979. *The Ghost Writer.* New York: Farrar, Straus & Giroux.

———. 1991. *Patrimony.* New York: Random House.

———. 1995. *Sabbath's Theater.* Boston: Houghton Mifflin.

———. 1997. *American Pastoral.* Boston: Houghton Mifflin.

———. 1998. *I Married a Communist.* Boston: Houghton Mifflin.

———. 2000. *The Human Stain.* Boston: Houghton Mifflin.

———. 2001. *The Dying Animal.* Boston: Houghton Mifflin.

———. 2006. *Everyman.* Boston: Houghton Mifflin.

———. 2007. *Exit Ghost.* Boston: Houghton Mifflin.

———. 2009. *The Humbling.* Boston: Houghton Mifflin Harcourt.

Rousseau, Jean-Jacques. (1762) 1979. *Emile, or On Education.* Translated by Allan Bloom. New York: Basic Books.

Rowe, Michael. 1999. *Crossing the Border: Encounters between Homeless People and Outreach Workers.* Berkeley: University of California Press.

———. 2002. "*Metamorphosis*: Defending the Human." *Literature and Medicine* 21 (2): 264–280.

Rowe, Michael, Patty Benedict, David Sells, Thomas Dinzeo, Charles Garvin, Lesley Schwab, Madelon Baranoski, Vincent Girard, and Chyrell Bellamy. 2009. "Citizenship, Community, and Recovery: A Group- and Peer-Based Intervention for Persons with Co-occurring Disorders and Criminal Justice Histories." *Journal for Groups in Addiction and Recovery* 4 (4): 224–244.

Rowe, Michael, Bret Kloos, Matthew Chinman, Larry Davidson, and Anne Boyle Cross. 2001. "Homelessness, Mental Illness, and Citizenship." *Social Policy and Administration* 35 (1): 14–31.

Rowe, Michael, Martha Lawless, Kenneth S. Thompson, and Larry Davidson. 2011. *Classics of Community Psychiatry: Fifty Years of Mental Health outside the Hospital.* New York: Oxford University Press.

Rowe, Michael, and Kenneth S. Thompson. 2011. Conclusion: "Community Psychiatry and the Future." In *Classics of Community Psychiatry: Fifty Years of Mental Health outside the Hospital,* edited by Michael Rowe, Martha Lawless, Kenneth S. Thompson, and Larry Davidson, 597–610. New York: Oxford University Press.

Rowold, Katharina, ed. 1996. *Gender and Science: Late Nineteenth-Century Debates on the Female Mind and Body.* Bristol: Thoemmes Press.

Rümke, H. C. (1941) 1990. "The Nuclear Symptom of Schizophrenia and the Praecox Feeling." Translated by Jan Neeleman. *History of Psychiatry* 1:331–341.

Rushdie, Salman. 1991. *Haroun and the Sea of Stories.* New York: Penguin.

Russell, James A. 1994. "Is there Universal Recognition of Emotion from Facial Expression? A Review of the Cross-Cultural Studies." *Psychological Bulletin* 115:102–141.

Russett, Cynthia Eagle. 1989. *Sexual Science: The Victorian Construction of Womanhood.* Cambridge, MA: Harvard University Press.

Russo, Mary. 1994. *The Female Grotesque: Risk, Excess, and Modernity.* New York: Routledge.

Rutenberg, Jim, and Jackie Chalmes. 2009, August 13. "False 'Death Panel' Rumor Has Some Familiar Roots." *New York Times.* www.nytimes.com/2009/08/14/health/policy/14panel.html.

Sack, Kevin. 2008, June 10. "Doctors Miss Cultural Needs." *New York Times,* D1.

Sacks, Oliver. (1976) 1990. *Awakenings.* New York: Vintage Books.

———. 1985. "Witty Ticcy Ray." In *The Man Who Mistook His Wife for a Hat and Other Clinical Tales.* New York: Perennial Library.

———. 1986. "Clinical Tales." *Literature and Medicine* 5:16–23.

———. 1995. *An Anthropologist on Mars: Seven Paradoxical Tales.* New York: Alfred A. Knopf.

———. 2007. *Musicophilia: Tales of Music and the Brain.* New York: Alfred A. Knopf.

"SAG, AFTRA, and AEA Announce the I AM PWD Campaign." 2008, October 6. Press release. www.iampwd.org/sag-aftra-and-aea-announce-i-am-pwd-campaign.

Saks, Elyn R. 2007. *The Center Cannot Hold: My Journey through Madness.* New York: Hyperion.

Sanders, Linda. 2010. *Diagnosis: Dispatches from the Frontlines of Medical Mysteries.* London: Icon Books.

Sandoz, Andrea, Matteo LoPiccolo, Daniel Kusnir, and Francisco A. Tausk. 2008. "A Clinical Paradigm of Delusions of Parasitosis." *Journal of the American Academy of Dermatology* 59:698–704.

Satcher, David. 1999. *Mental Health: A Report of the Surgeon General.* Rockville, MD: Department of Health and Human Services, Substance Abuse and Mental Health Services Administration, Center for Mental Health Services, National Institutes of Health, National Institute of Mental Health.

Savage, Jon. n.d. *Lenois.* Vlog. http://lenois.com.

Savarese, Ralph James. 2007. *Reasonable People: A Memoir of Autism and Adoption: On the Meaning of Family and the Politics of Neurological Difference.* New York: Other Press.

Savely, Virginia. 2010. "Guest Editorial: Delusions May Not Always Be Delusions." *Archives of Psychiatric Nursing* 24 (1): 215.

Savely, Virginia R., Mary M. Leitao, and Raphael B. Stricker. 2006. "The Mystery of Morgellons Disease: Infection or Delusion?" *American Journal of Clinical Dermatology* 7 (1): 1–5.

Saxton, Marsha. 1997a. *Access to Medical Care: Adults with Physical Disabilities.* World Institute on Disability. www.wid.org/publications/access-to-medical-care-adults-with -physical-disabilities.

———. 1997b. *Access to Medical Care: People with Developmental Disabilities.* World Institute on Disability. www.wid.org/publications/access-to-medical-care-people-with -developmental-disabilities.

Scarry, Elaine. 1985. *The Body in Pain: The Making and Unmaking of the World.* New York: Oxford University Press.

Schechner, Richard. 1985. *Between Theater and Anthropology.* Philadelphia: University of Pennsylvania Press.

Schemmer, Cynthia. 2008. "Holes." *Not Your Mother's Meatloaf,* issue no. 1. http://sexed comicproject.blogspot.com. Accessed September 23, 2011.

Scheper-Hughes, Nancy. 1991. "Virgin Territory: The Male Discovery of the Clitoris." *Medical Anthropology Quarterly* 5 (1): 25–28.

Schiebinger, Londa. 1989. *The Mind Has No Sex? Women in the Origins of Modern Science.* Cambridge, MA: Harvard University Press.

Schiller, Lori, and Amanda Bennett. 1994. *The Quiet Room: A Journey out of the Torment of Madness.* New York: Warner Books.

Schott, Webster. 1969, June 8. "The Andromeda Strain." *New York Times,* BR4.

Schulte, Brigid. 2008, January 20. "Figments of the Imagination?" *Washington Post.* www .washingtonpost.com/wp-dyn/content/article/2008/01/16/AR2008011603134.html.

Schwartz, Marlene, Heather O'Neal Chambliss, Kelly D. Brownell, Steven N. Blair, and Charles Billington. 2003. "Weight Bias among Health Professionals Specializing in Obesity." *Obesity Research* 11 (9): 1033–1039.

Schweik, Susan. 2009. *The Ugly Laws: Disability in Public.* New York: New York University Press.

Schweinhardt, P., and M. C. Bushnell. 2010. "Pain Imaging in Health and Disease—How Far Have We Come?" *Journal of Clinical Investigations* 120:3788–3797.

Schweitzer, Albert. (1931) 1933. *Out of My Life and Thought: An Autobiography.* Woking: George Allen & Unwin.

Scott, J. Blake. 2003. *Risky Rhetoric: AIDS and the Cultural Practices of HIV Testing*. Carbondale: Southern Illinois University Press.

Scott, Ridley, dir. 2001. *Hannibal*. Beverly Hills, CA: Metro-Goldwyn-Mayer; Universal City, CA: Universal Pictures.

"The Scourge of a New Disease." 1983, May 15. *New York Times*, sec. 4, 20.

Scully, Jackie Leach. 2008. *Disability Bioethics: Moral Bodies, Moral Difference*. Lanham, MD: Rowman & Littlefield.

Sedgwick, Eve Kosofsky. 1992. *Between Men: English Literature and Male Homosocial Desire*. New York: Columbia University Press.

Seeleman, Conny, Jeanine Suurmond, and Karien Stronks. 2009. "Cultural Competence: A Conceptual Framework for Teaching and Learning." *Medical Education* 43 (3): 229–237.

Segal, Judy Z. 2007. *Health and the Rhetoric of Medicine*. Carbondale: Southern Illinois University Press.

———. 2009a. "Internet Health and the 21st-Century Patient: A Rhetorical View." *Written Communication* 26:351–369.

———. 2009b. "Rhetoric of Health and Medicine." In *The Sage Handbook of Rhetorical Studies*, edited by Andrea Lunsford et al., 227–246. Thousand Oaks, CA: Sage.

Segal, S. P., J. R. Bola, and M. A. Watson. 1996. "Race, Quality of Care, and Antipsychotic Prescribing Practices in Psychiatric Emergency Services." *Psychiatric Services* 47:282–286.

Selzer, Richard. 1987a. "Four Appointments with the Discus Thrower." In *Confessions of a Knife*. East Lansing: Michigan State University Press.

Selzer, Richard. 1987b. "Tube Feeding." In *Confessions of a Knife*. East Lansing: Michigan State University Press.

Senate Committee on the Judiciary. 1955. *Comic Books and Juvenile Delinquency: Interim Report, 1955* [Comic Book Code of 1954]. Washington, DC: U.S. Government Printing Office. (Text at Wikisource, http://en.wikisource.org/wiki/Comic_book_code_of_1954.)

Sequist, Thomas D., Garrett M. Fitzmaurice, and Richard Marshall. 2008. "Physician Performance and Racial Disparities in Diabetes Mellitus Care." *Archives of Internal Medicine* 168 (11): 1145–1151.

Serota, Nicholas. 2011, May 18. *The Times*.

Shahn, Ben. 1996. *It's No Use to Do Any More*. Tempera on board, 64.8 × 99.1 cm. Maier Museum of Art, Randolph-Macon Woman's College, Lynchburg, VA; Louise Jordan Smith Fund. Cover. *Journal of the American Medical Association* 275(3).

Shakespeare, Tom. 2010. "The Social Model of Disability. In *The Disability Studies Reader*, 3rd ed., edited by Lennard J. David, 266–273. New York: Routledge.

Shankman, Adam, dir. 2002. *A Walk to Remember*. Burbank, CA: Warner Bros.

Shannon, Jeff. 2003, May. "Access Hollywood: Disability in Recent Film and Television." *New Mobility*. www.newmobility.com/articleView.cfm?id=690&action=browse.

Sharf, Barbara F. 1990. "Physician-Patient Communication as Interpersonal Rhetoric: A Narrative Approach." *Health Communication* 2:217–231.

Shattuck, Roger. 1963. *Proust's Binoculars: A Study of Memory, Time, and Recognition in "A La Recherche du Temps Perdu."* New York: Random House.

Sheehan, Elizabeth. 1981. "Victorian Clitoridectomy: Isaac Baker Brown and His Harmless Operative Procedure." *Medical Anthropology Newsletter* 12 (4): 9–15.

Shelley, Mary. (1818) 1994. *Frankenstein; or, The Modern Prometheus*, edited by Marilyn Butler. Oxford: Oxford University Press.

———. (1818) 1999. *Frankenstein; or, The Modern Prometheus*. 2nd ed., edited by D. L. Macdonald and Kathleen Scherf. Peterborough, ON: Broadview Press.

———. (1818) 2011. *Frankenstein* (Planet eBook). Accessed February 14, 2012. www.planetebook.com/Frankenstein.asp.

Shenk, Joshua Wolf. 2002. "A Melancholia of My Own." In *Unholy Ghost: Writers on Depression*, edited by Nell Casey, 242–256. New York: HarperPerennial.

Shirley, Jamie Lynn. 2012, October 31. American Society for Bioethics and Humanities Literature and Medicine Listserv. litmed@listserv.com.

Shorter, Edward. 1985. *Bedside Manners: The Troubled History of Doctors and Patients.* New York: Simon & Schuster.

Showalter, Elaine. 1985. *The Female Malady: Women, Madness, and English Culture, 1890–1980.* New York: Penguin.

———. 1997. *Hystories: Hysterical Epidemics and Modern Media.* New York: Columbia University Press.

Shute, Nancy. 2011, September 19. "Teens and Tweens Find They Too Need Vaccinations to Attend." *Morning Edition.* National Public Radio. www.npr.org/blogs/health/2011/09/19/140544546/teens-and-tweens-find-they-too-need-vaccines-to-attend-school.

Shyamalan, M. Night, dir. 2000. *Unbreakable.* Burbank, CA: Buena Vista Pictures.

"Shyness Is Blamed in Mental Illness." 1929, December 29. *New York Times,* 9.

Sia, Calvin, Thomas F. Tonniges, Elizabeth Osterhus, and Sharon Taba. 2004. "History of the Medical Home Concept." *Pediatrics* 113:1473–1478.

Siebers, Tobin. 2006. "Disability in Theory: From Social Constructionism to the New Realism of the Body." In *The Disability Studies Reader,* 2nd ed., edited by Lennard Davis, 173–183. New York: Routledge.

———. 2008. *Disability Theory.* Ann Arbor: University of Michigan Press.

———. 2010. *Disability Aesthetics.* Ann Arbor: University of Michigan Press.

Simon, Jonathan. 1998. "Refugees in a Carceral Age: The Rebirth of Immigration Prisons in the United States." *Public Culture* 10:577–607.

Singer, Tania, Ben Seymour, John O'Doherty, Holger Kaube, Raymond J. Dolan, and Chris D. Frith. 2004, February 20. "Empathy for Pain Involves the Affective but Not Sensory Components of Pain." *Science* 303:1157–1162.

Sinha, Indrani, and Shamita Das DasGupta. 2009. *Mothers for Sale: Women in Kolkata's Sex Trade.* Kolkata: Global Books.

Sirohi, Seema. 2005, March 14. "Zana's Shutters." *Outlookindia.com.* www.outlookindia.com/article.aspx?226761.

Sismondo, Sergio. 2007. "Ghost Management: How Much of the Medical Literature Is Shaped behind the Scenes by the Pharmaceutical Industry?" *PLOS Medicine* 4 (9): 1429–1433.

———. 2008. "How Pharmaceutical Industry Funding Affects Trial Outcomes: Causal Structures and Responses." *Social Science and Medicine* 66:1909–1914.

Skvorecky, Josef. 1994. *The Bass Saxophone.* London: Vintage.

Slack, Paul. 1988. "Responses to Plague in Early Modern Europe: The Implications of Public Health." *Social Research* 55:433–453.

Sloboda, John. 2005. *Exploring the Musical Mind: Cognition, Emotion, Ability, Function.* Oxford: Oxford University Press.

Slobodin, Richard. 1997. *Rivers.* Phoenix Mill, Gloucestershire: Sutton Publishing.

Small, Helen. 2007. *The Long Life.* Oxford: Oxford University Press.

Smalley, Logan, dir. 2007. *Darius Goes West.* Athens, GA: Roll with Me Productions.

Smedley, Brian D., Adrienne Y. Stith, and Alan R. Nelson, eds. 2003. *Unequal Treatment: Confronting Racial and Ethnic Disparities in Health Care.* Washington, DC: National Academies Press.

Smith, Daniel W. 2005. "Critical, Clinical." In *Gilles Deleuze: Key Concepts,* edited by Charles J. Stivale, 182–193. Stocksfield: Acumen.

Smith, Jan. 2011. "Morgellons Exposed: Telling the Truth You Were Never Supposed to Know." www.morgellonsexposed.com.

Smith, Jonathan Z. 1986. "The Bare Facts of Ritual." In *Readings in Ritual Studies,* edited by Ronald L. Grimes, 473–482. Upper Saddle River, NJ: Prentice Hall.

Smith-Rosenberg, Carroll. 1986. New York: Oxford University Press.

Snow, C. P. (1959) 1993. *The Two Cultures.* Cambridge: Cambridge University Press.

Snyder, Sharon L., and David T. Mitchell. 2010. "Body Genres: An Anatomy of Disability in Film." In *The Problem Body: Projecting Disability on Film,* edited by Sally Chivers and Nicole Markotic, 179–204. Columbus: Ohio State University Press.

Sokel, Walter H. 1988. "From Marx to Myth: The Structure and Function of Self-Alienation in Kafka's *Metamorphosis.*" In *Franz Kafka's "The Metamorphosis,"* edited by Harold Bloom, 216–224. New York: Chelsea House Publishers.

Solomon, Andrew. 2001. *The Noonday Demon: An Atlas of Depression.* New York: Scribner.

Solomon, Martha. 1985. "The Rhetoric of Dehumanization: An Analysis of Medical Reports of the Tuskegee Syphilis Project." *Western Journal of Speech Communication* 49:233–247.

Solondz, Todd, dir. 2004. *Palindromes.* Santa Monica, CA: Genius Entertainment.

Solzhenitsyn, Alexander. (1967) 1983. *Cancer Ward.* Translated by Nicholas Bethell and David Burg. New York: Modern Library.

———. 1974. *The Cancer Ward.* Translated by Nicholas Bethell and David Burg. New York: Farrar, Straus & Giroux.

Sonfield, Nik M., and Jessica Ryan. 2008. "The Appointment." *Not Your Mother's Meatloaf,* issue no. 1. http://sexedcomicproject.blogspot.com. Accessed September 23, 2011.

Sonnenfeld, Barry, dir. 1999. *Wild Wild West.* Burbank, CA: Warner Bros.

Sontag, Susan. 1978. *Illness as Metaphor.* New York: Farrar, Straus & Giroux.

———. 1986, November 24. "The Way We Live Now." *New Yorker,* 42–51.

———. 1989. *AIDS and Its Metaphors.* New York: Farrar, Straus & Giroux.

The Sopranos. 1999–2007. Television series. New York: HBO.

Sourkes, Barbara. 1982. *The Deepening Shade: Psychological Aspects of Life-Threatening Illness.* Pittsburgh: University of Pittsburgh Press.

South Park. 1997–. Television series. New York: Comedy Central.

Sox, Harold C., and Steven Woloshin. 2000. "How Many Deaths Are Due to Medical Error? Getting the Number Right." *Effective Clinical Practice* 3:277–283.

Special Correspondent. 1971. "Unheard Voices: The Clinical Scientist." *British Medical Journal* 1:225.

Spielberg, Steven, dir. 1991. *Hook.* Culver City, CA: TriStar Pictures.

Spivak, Gayatri. 1988. "Can the Subaltern Speak?" In *Marxism and the Interpretation of Culture,* edited by Cary Nelson and Lawrence Grossberg, 271–312. Champaign: University of Illinois Press.

Spottiswoode, Roger, dir. 1993. *And the Band Played On.* New York: HBO.

Squier, Susan M. 2007. "Beyond Nescience: The Intersectional Insights of Health Humanities." *Perspectives in Biology and Medicine* 50:334–347.

———. 2011a. E-mail interview with Saiya Miller and Liza Bley, May 20, 2011. http://sexedcomicproject.blogspot.com. Accessed September 23, 2011.

———. 2011b. Presentation. "Comics and Medicine: The Sequential Art of Illness" conference. Chicago: Northwestern University, Feinberg School of Medicine, June 9–11. www.graphicmedicine.org/comics-and-medicine-conferences/2011-chicago-comics-and-medicine-conference.

Stabile, Carol. 1992. "Shooting the Mother: Fetal Photography and the Politics of Disappearance." *Camera Obscura* 28:179–205.

Starfield, Barbara. 1992. *Primary Care: Concept, Education, and Policy.* New York: Oxford University Press.

Starr, C. J., T. T. Houle, and R. C. Coghill. 2010. "Psychological and Sensory Predictors of Experimental Thermal Pain: A Multifactorial Model." *Journal of Pain* 11:1394–1402.

Starr, Paul. 1983. *The Social Transformation of American Medicine.* New York: Basic Books.

Star Trek. 1966–1969. Television series. New York: CBS Television Distribution.

Star Trek: The Next Generation. 1987–1994. Television series. New York: CBS Television Distribution.

Steinbach, Susie. 2004. *Women in England, 1760–1914: A Social History.* London: Weidenfeld & Nicholson.

Stone, Oliver, dir. 1989. *Born on the Fourth of July.* Ixtlan. Orlando, FL: Universal Pictures.

Stras, Laurie. 2006. "The Organ of the Soul: Voice, Damage, and Affect." In *Sounding Off: Theorizing Disability in Music,* edited by Neil Lerner and Joseph N. Straus, 173–184. New York: Routledge.

Straus, Joseph N. 2010. "Autism as Culture." In *The Disability Studies Reader,* 3rd ed., edited by Lennard Davis, 535–562. New York: Routledge.

Strauss, John S., Hisam Hafez, Paul Lieberman, and Courtenay Harding. 1985. "The Course of Psychiatric Disorder: III. Longitudinal Principles." *American Journal of Psychiatry* 142 (3): 289–296.

Studd, John. 2007. "A Comparison of 19th Century and Current Attitudes to Female Sexuality." *Gynecological Endocrinology* 23:673–681.

Styron, William. 1990. *Darkness Visible: A Memoir of Madness.* New York: Random House.

———. 2002. "From *Darkness Visible.*" In *Unholy Ghost: Writers on Depression,* edited by Nell Casey, 114–126. New York: Harper Perennial.

Sulmasy, Daniel P. 2002. "A Biopsychosocial-Spiritual Model for the Care of Patients at the End of Life." *Gerontologist* 42 (3): 24–33.

Sutherland, John. 2007. *Bestsellers: A Very Short Introduction.* Oxford: Oxford University Press.

Svenaeus, Fredrik. 1999. *The Hermeneutics of Medicine and the Phenomenology of Health— Steps towards a Philosophy of Medical Practice.* Linköping, Sweden: Linköping University Press.

———. 2000a. "Das Unheimliche: Towards a Phenomenology of Illness." *Medicine, Health Care and Philosophy* 3 (1): 3–16.

———. 2000b. "The Body Uncanny—Further Steps towards a Phenomenology of Illness." *Medicine, Health Care and Philosophy* 3 (2): 125–137.

———. 2010. *The Hermeneutics of Medicine and the Phenomenology of Health: Steps towards a Philosophy of Medical Practice.* Dordrecht: Kluwer.

Talbott, John. 1979. "Deinstitutionalization: Avoiding the Disasters of the Past." *Hospital and Community Psychiatry* 30 (55): 621–624.

Tanner, Jennifer Lynn, and Jeffrey Jensen Arnett. 2009. "The Emergence of 'Emerging Adulthood': The New Life Stage between Adolescence and Young Adulthood." In *Handbook of Youth and Young Adulthood,* edited by Andy Furlong, 39–45. London: Routledge.

Tanner, Murray Scot. 2005, April 14. "Chinese Government Responses to Rising Social Unrest." Testimony presented to the U.S.-China Economic and Security Review Commission. Santa Monica, CA: RAND Corp. http://www.rand.org/content/dam/rand/pubs/testimonies/2005/RAND_CT240.pdf.

Tatum, Karen E. 2010. "Drawing the Eczema Aesthetic: The Psychological Effects of Chronic Skin Disease as Depicted in the Works of John Updike, Elizabeth Bishop, and Zelda Fitzgerald." *Journal of Medical Humanities* 31:127–153.

Taylor, Carol, and Roberto Dell'Oro. 2006. *Health and Human Flourishing: Religion, Medicine, and Moral Anthropology.* Washington, DC: Georgetown University Press.

Taylor, Janelle. 2003. "The Story Catches You and You Fall Down: Tragedy, Ethnography, and 'Cultural Competence.'" *Medical Anthropology Quarterly* 17 (2): 159–181.

Taylor, Sparky. 2010. "My Body, Myself." *Not Your Mother's Meatloaf,* issue no. 3. http://sexedcomicproject.blogspot.com. Accessed September 23, 2011.

Teal, Cayla R., and Richard L. Street. 2009. "Critical Elements of Culturally Competent Communication in the Medical Encounter: A Review and Model." *Social Science and Medicine* 68:533–543.

Terdiman, Richard. 1993. *Present Past: Modernity and the Memory Crisis.* Ithaca, NY: Cornell University Press.

Terry, Jennifer. 1999. *An American Obsession: Science, Medicine, and Homosexuality in Modern Society.* Chicago: University of Chicago Press.

Tervalon, Melanie, and Jann Murray-García. 1998. "Cultural Humility versus Cultural

Competence: A Critical Distinction in Defining Physician Training Outcomes in Multi-cultural Education." *Journal of Health Care for the Poor and Underserved* 9 (2): 117–125.

Thelwall, Mike, and Liz Price. 2006. "Language Evolution and the Spread of Ideas on the Web: A Procedure for Identifying Emergent Hybrid Word Family Members." *Journal of the American Society for Information Science and Technology* 57:1326–1337.

Thernstrom, Melanie. 2010. *The Pain Chronicles: Cures, Myths, Mysteries, Prayers, Diaries, Brain Scans, Healing, and the Science of Suffering.* New York: Farrar, Straus & Giroux.

Thomas, E. G. 1980. "The Old Poor Law and Medicine." *Medical History* 24:1–19.

Thompson, Kenneth S., and Michael Rowe. 2010. "Social Inclusion." *Psychiatric Services* 61 (8): 735.

Thompson, Teresa L. 1982a. "Gaze Toward and Avoidance of the Handicapped: A Field Experiment." *Journal of Nonverbal Behavior* 6 (3): 188–196.

———. 1982b, Spring. " 'You Can't Play Marbles—You Have a Wooden Hand': Communication with the Handicapped." *Communication Quarterly* 30 (2): 108–115.

Thornicroft, Graham, and Michele Tansella. 2004. "Components of a Modern Mental Health Service: A Pragmatic Balance of Community and Hospital Care." *British Journal of Psychiatry* 185:283–290.

Tishler, Peter V. 1992. " 'The Care of the Patient': A Living Testimony to Francis Weld Peabody." *Pharos of Alpha Omega Alpha* 55 (3): 32–36.

Tollifson, Joan. 1997. "Imperfection Is a Beautiful Thing: On Disability and Meditation." In *Staring Back: The Disability Experience from the Inside Out,* edited by Kenny Fries. New York: Plume.

Tolstoy, Leo. (1886) 1981. *The Death of Ivan Ilyich.* Translated by Lynn Solotaroff. New York: Bantam.

———. 1960. "The Death of Ivan Ilych." Translated by Alymer Maude. In *The Death of Ivan Ilych and Other Stories.* New York: Signet.

———. 2001. *The Death of Ivan Ilyich.* Posted at *Classic Reader.* www.classicreader.com/book/295.

———. 2004. *The Death of Ivan Ilyich and Other Stories.* Translated by Constance Garnett. New York: Barnes & Noble.

———. 2011. *The Death of Ivan Ilych.* Translated by Ian Dreiblatt. Brooklyn: Melville House.

———. n.d. "Last Words of Real People: Thurber to Villa." http://mysite.verizon.net/sanftleben/Last%20Words/lastwords-r-t.html.

Tomes, Nancy. 1998. *The Gospel of Germs: Men, Women, and the Microbe in American Life.* Cambridge, MA: Harvard University Press.

Tomlinson, Tom. 1997. "Perplexed about Narrative Ethics." In *Stories and Their Limits: Narrative Approaches to Bioethics,* edited by Hilde Lindemann Nelson, 123–133. New York: Routledge.

Tompkins, Sandra M. 1992. "The Influenza Epidemic in Western Samoa." *Journal of Pacific History* 27 (2): 181–197.

Tong, Rosemarie. 2007. *New Perspectives in Healthcare Ethics.* Upper Saddle River, NJ: Prentice Hall.

The Tonight Show Starring Johnny Carson. 1962–1992. Television talk show. New York: NBC.

Torres, Jennifer M., and Ronald G. DeVries. 2009. "Birthing Ethics: What Mothers, Families, Childbirth Educators, Nurses, and Physicians Should Know about the Ethics of Childbirth." *Journal of Perinatal Education* 18:12–24.

Torrey, E. Fuller. 2001. *Surviving Schizophrenia: A Manual for Families, Consumers, and Providers,* 4th ed. New York: Quill.

Tournon, Andre. 2005. "Justice and the Law: On the Reverse Side of the Essays." In *The Cambridge Companion to Montaigne,* edited by Ullrich Langer, 96–117. New York: Cambridge University Press.

Trautmann (Banks), Joanne. 1982. "The Wonders of Literature in Medical Education." *Mobius* 2 (3): 22–31.

Treffert, Darold A. 1988. "The Idiot Savant: A Review of the Syndrome." *American Journal of Psychiatry* 145:563–572.

Treichler, Paula. 1999. *How to Have Theory in an Epidemic: Cultural Chronicles of AIDS.* Durham, NC: Duke University Press.

Tresolini, Carol P., and the Pew-Fetzer Task Force. 1994. *Health Professions Education and Relationship-Centered Care.* San Francisco: Pew Health Professions Commission.

Trousdale, Gary, and Kirk Wise, dirs. 1996. *The Hunchback of Notre Dame.* Burbank, CA: Buena Vista Pictures.

True, G., E. J. Phipps, L. E. Braitman, T. Harralson, D. Harris, and W. Tester. 2005. "Treatment Preferences and Advance Care Planning at End of Life: The Role of Ethnicity and Spiritual Coping in Cancer Patients." *Annals of Behavioral Medicine* 30 (2): 174–179.

Tuana, Nancy. 2006. "The Speculum of Ignorance: The Women's Health Movement and Epistemologies of Ignorance." *Hypatia* 21:1–19.

Turk, Dennis C., and Akiko Okifuji. 1999. "Assessment of Patients' Reporting of Pain: An Integrated Perspective." *Lancet* 353:1784–1788.

Turner, Victor Witter. (1967) 1981. *The Forest of Symbols: Aspects of Ndembu Ritual.* Ithaca, NY: Cornell University Press.

———. 1982. *From Ritual to Theatre: The Human Seriousness of Play.* Performance Studies Series, vol. 1. New York City: Performing Arts Journal Publications.

24. 2001–2010. Television series. Joel Surnow et al., producers. Beverly Hills, CA: 20th Century Fox Television and Imagine Entertainment.

Twitchell, Chase. 2002. "An Ars Poetica under the Influence." In *Unholy Ghost: Writers on Depression.* Edited by Nell Casey, 2–29. New York: Harper Perennial.

"Two with Legionnaire's Disease Die at the Downstate Medical Center." 1984, September 9. *New York Times,* sec.1, part 1, 45.

Tyler, Edward A. 1970. "Introducing a Sex Education Course into the Medical Curriculum." *Journal of Medical Education* 45:1025–1031.

Ubell, Earl. 1972, February 6. "Are We Breeding an 'Andromeda Strain'?" *New York Times,* E7.

Updike, John. 1976, July 19. "From the Journal of a Leper." *New Yorker,* 28–33.

U.S. Conference of Catholic Bishops. 2005, July 11. "Commentary on Nutrition and Hydration." http://old.usccb.org/prolife/tdocs/anhcommentary.shtml.

U.S. Department of Health and Human Services. 2010. *National Healthcare Quality Report, 2009.* Rockville, MD: Agency for Healthcare Research and Quality.

U.S. Government Accountability Office. 1977. *Returning the Mentally Disabled to the Community: Government Needs to Do More.* GAO Publication No. HRD-76–152 235. Washington, DC: U.S. Government Accountability Office.

Van der Molen, Beverley. 2000. "Relating Information Needs to the Cancer Experience: 2. Themes from Six Cancer Narratives." *European Journal of Cancer Care* 9 (1): 48–54.

Van Dijkhuizen, Jan Frans, and Karl A. E. Enenkel, eds. 2009. *The Sense of Suffering: Constructions of Physical Pain in Early Modern Culture.* Boston: Brill.

Veatch, Robert. 1981. *A Theory of Medical Ethics.* New York: Basic Books.

Vedantam, Shankar. 2005, June 28. "Racial Disparities Found in Pinpointing Mental Illness." *Washington Post,* A1. www.washingtonpost.com/wp-dyn/content/article/2005/06/27/AR2005062701496.html.

Verhey, Allen. 1987. "The Doctor's Oath—and a Christian Swearing It." In *On Moral Medicine: Theological Perspectives in Medical Ethics,* edited by Stephen E. Lammers and Allen Verhey, 72–82. Grand Rapids, MI: Eerdmans Publishing Co.

Vidor, King. 1925. *The Big Parade.* Beverly Hills, CA: Metro-Goldwyn-Mayer.

Vila-Rodriguez, Fidel, and Bill Macewan. 2008. "Delusional Parasitosis Facilitated by Web-Based Dissemination." *American Journal of Psychiatry* 165 (12): 1612.

Vincent, Charles. 2010. *Patient Safety,* 2nd ed. Oxford: Wiley-Blackwell.

Vonnegut, Mark. 1975. *The Eden Express: A Memoir of Insanity.* New York: Praeger.

Vonnegut, Mark. 2010. *Just Like Someone without Mental Illness Only More So: A Memoir.* New York: Delacorte.

Wailoo, Keith. 2001. *Dying in the City of the Blues: Sickle Cell Anemia and the Politics of Race and Health.* Chapel Hill: University of North Carolina Press.

Waitzkin, Howard. 2006. "One and a Half Centuries of Forgetting and Rediscovering: Virchow's Lasting Contributions to Social Medicine." *Social Medicine* 1:5–10.

Wakefield, A. J., S. H. Murch, A. Anthony, J. Linnell, D. M. Casson, M. Malik, et al. 1998. "Ileal-Lymphoid-Nodular Hyperplasia, Non-specific Colitis, and Pervasive Developmental Disorder in Children" [retracted]. Lancet 351:637–641.

Wald, Hedy S., and Shmuel P. Reis. 2010. "Beyond the Margins: Reflective Writing and Development of Reflective Capacity in Medical Education." *Journal of General Internal Medicine* 25:746–749.

Walker, Laura M., et al. 2011, August 17. "Broad Neutralization Coverage of HIV by Multiple Highly Potent Antibodies." *Nature.* www.nature.com/nature/journal/v477/n7365/abs/nature10373.html.

Walker, Margaret Urban. 2008. "Introduction: Groningen Naturalism in Bioethics." In *Naturalized Bioethics: Toward Responsible Knowing and Practice,* edited by Hilde Lindemann, Marian Verkerk, and Margaret Urban Walker, 1–20. New York: Cambridge University Press.

Wallace, Robin. 1986. *Beethoven's Critics: Aesthetic Dilemmas and Resolutions during the Composer's Lifetime.* Cambridge: Cambridge University Press.

Waller, John. 2008. "Lessons from the History of Medicine." *Journal of Investigative Surgery* 21:53–56.

Walling, H. W., and B. L. Swick. 2007. Psychocutaneous Syndromes: A Call for Revised Nomenclature. *Clinical and Experimental Dermatology* 32 (3): 317–319.

Walsham, Alexandra. 1999. *Providence in Early Modern England.* Oxford: Oxford University Press.

Ward, Mary Jane. 1946. *The Snake Pit.* New York: New American Library.

Ward, W. Dixon. 1999. "Absolute Pitch." In *The Psychology of Music,* 2nd ed., edited by Diana Deutsch, 265–98. San Diego: Academic Press.

Ware, Chris. 1998. *Jimmy Corrigan: The Smartest Kid on Earth.* New York: Fantagraphics.

Ware, Norma, Kim Hopper, Toni Tugenberg, Barbara Dickey, and Daniel Fisher. 2007. "Connectedness and Citizenship: Redefining Social Integration." *Psychiatric Services* 58: 469–474.

Warner, Margaret Humphreys. 1981. "Vindicating the Minister's Medical Role: Cotton Mather's Concept of the Nishmath-Chajim and the Spiritualization of Medicine." *Journal of the History of Medicine and Allied Sciences* 36 (3): 278–295.

Washington, Harriet A. 2006. *Medical Apartheid: The Dark History of Medical Experimentation on Black Americans from Colonial Times to the Present.* New York: Harlem Moon.

Watson, Katie. 2011. "Perspective: Serious Play: Teaching Medical Skills with Improvisational Theater Techniques." *Academic Medicine: Journal of the Association of American Medical Colleges* 86:1260–1265. doi: 10.1097/ACM.0b013e31822cf858.

Waugh, Evelyn. 1948. *The Loved One: An Anglo-American Tragedy.* New York: Little, Brown.

Wear, Andrew, ed. 1992. *Medicine in Society: Historical Essays.* New York: Cambridge University Press.

Wear, Delese. 1992. "The Colonization of the Medical Humanities: A Confessional Critique." *Journal of Medical Humanities* 13 (4): 199–209.

———. 1998. "On White Coats and Professional Development: The Formal and the Hidden Curricula." *Annals of Internal Medicine* 129 (9): 734–737.

———. 2002. "'Face-to-Face with It': Medical Students' Narratives about Their End-of-Life Education." *Academic Medicine* 77 (4): 271–277.

———. 2003. "Insurgent Multiculturalism: Rethinking How and Why We Teach Culture in Medical Education." *Academic Medicine* 78:549–554.

———. 2009. "The Medical Humanities: Toward a Renewed Praxis." *Journal of Medical Humanities* 30 (4): 209–220.

———. 2007. "Creating Difficulties Everywhere." *Perspectives in Biology and Medicine* 50 (3): 348–362.

Weathers, Helen. 2010, November 14. "Broody again at 72: She Became the World's Oldest Mother at 66. Now Her Little Girl's Five—and She Wants ANOTHER." *Daily Mail*. www.dailymail.co.uk/femail/article-1329255/Worlds-oldest-mother-Adriana-Illiescu-broody-72.html.

Weaver, Richard M. 1953. *The Ethics of Rhetoric*. South Bend, IN: Regenery/Gateway.

Webb, Millard. 1926. *The Sea Beast*. Burbank, CA: Warner Bros.

Weber, Max. 1958. *From Max Weber: Essays in Sociology*, edited by C. W. Mills and H. Gerth. New York: Oxford University Press.

WebMD. 2011. "Picture of the Vagina." http://women.webmd.com/picture-of-the-vagina.

Weil, Elizabeth. 2006a, September 24. "What If It's (Sort of) a Boy and (Sort of) a Girl?" *New York Times Magazine*. www.nytimes.com/2006/09/24/magazine/24intersexkids.html.

———. 2006b, March 12. "A Wrongful Birth?" *New York Times*. www.nytimes.com/2006/03/12/magazine/312wrongful.1.html?pagewanted=all.

Weiss, Peter. 2005. *The Aesthetics of Resistance*. Durham, NC: Duke University Press.

Welch, W. Pete, Mark E. Miller, H. Gilbert Welch, Elliott S. Fisher, and John E. Wennberg. 1993. "Geographic Variation in Expenditures for Physicians' Services in the United States." *New England Journal of Medicine* 328 (9): 621–627.

Wendell, Susan. 1996. *The Rejected Body: Feminist Philosophical Reflections on Disability*. New York: Routledge.

Wennberg, John, Elliot S. Fisher, David C. Goodman, and Jonathan S. Skinner. 2008. *Tracking the Care of Patients with Severe Chronic Illness: The Dartmouth Atlas of Health Care, 2008*. Lebanon, NH: Dartmouth Institute for Health Policy and Clinical Practice. www.dartmouthatlas.org/downloads/atlases/2008_Chronic_Care_Atlas.pdf.

Wertham, Fredric. 1954. *The Seduction of the Innocent: The Influence of Comic Books on Today's Youth*. New York: Rinehart.

West, Michael A., and Carol S. Borrill. 2002. *Effective Human Resource Management and Lower Patient Mortality*. Birmingham: University of Aston.

Whale, James, dir. 1931. *Frankenstein*. Orlando, FL: Universal Pictures.

Wharton, Edith. 1911. *Ethan Frome*. New York: Scribner's.

Wharton, Leopold, and Theodore Wharton, dirs. 1917. *The Black Stork*. New York: Sheriott Pictures Corp.

White, Michael. 2007. *Maps of Narrative Practice*. New York: W. W. Norton.

———. 2011. *Narrative Practice: Continuing the Conversations*. New York: W. W. Norton.

White, Michael, and David Epston. 1990. *Narrative Means to Therapeutic Ends*. New York: W. W. Norton.

Whitman, Walt. 1855. "Song of Myself." In *Leaves of Grass*. www.poets.org/viewmedia.php/prmMID/15755.

Wilkerson, Abby. 2002. "Disability, Sex Radicalism, and Political Agency." *NWSA Journal* 14 (3): 33–57.

Wilkin, David, Lesley Hallam, and Marie-Anne Doggett. 1992. *Measures of Need and Outcome for Primary Health Care*. Oxford: Oxford University Press.

Williams, David R. 1999. "Race, Socioeconomic Status and Health: The Added Effects of Racism and Discrimination." *Annals of the New York Academy of Sciences* 896 (1): 173–188.

Williams, Gareth. 1984. "The Genesis of Chronic Illness: Narrative Re-construction." *Sociology of Health and Illness* 6 (2): 175–200.

Williams, Terry Tempest. 2001. *Refuge: An Unnatural History of Place*, 2nd ed. New York: Vintage.

Wilson, Eric G. 2008. *Against Happiness: In Praise of Melancholy.* New York: Farrar, Straus, & Giroux.

Wilson, Keith G., Harvey Max Chochinov, Christine J. McPherson, Katerine LeMay, Pierre Allard, Srini Chary, Pierre R. Gagnon, Karen Macmillan, Marina De Luca, Fiona O'Shea, David Kuhl, and Robin L. Fainsinger. 2007. "Suffering with Advanced Cancer." *Journal of Clinical Oncology* 25 (13): 1.

Wilson, Robert. 2011. "St Louis and the 1918 Influenza: The Impact of Non-pharmaceutical Interventions." *Missouri Historical Review* 105 (2): 94–108.

Winn, Peter A. 1996. "Legal Ritual." In *Readings in Ritual Studies,* edited by Ronald L. Grimes, 552–565. Upper Saddle River, NJ: Prentice Hall.

Winnicott, Donald W. 1971. *Playing and Reality.* London: Tavistock.

Wise, Robert, dir. 1971. *The Andromeda Strain.* Universal City, CA: Universal Pictures.

Wolff, Jonathan. 2009. "Disadvantage, Risk, and the Social Determinants of Health." *Public Health Ethics* 2:214–223.

Woloshin, Steven, Nina A Bickell, Lisa M. Schwartz, Francesca Gany, and H. Gilbert Welch. 1995. "Language Barriers in Medicine in the United States." *Journal of the American Medical Association* 273:724–728.

Wolpe, Paul R. 1998. "The Triumph of Autonomy in American Bioethics: A Sociological View." In *Bioethics and Society,* edited by Raymond DeVries and Janardan Subedi, 1–15. Upper Saddle River, NJ: Prentice Hall.

Woo, Judy. 2010. "Focal Dystonia in Pianists: The Role of the Educational Institution." Ph.D. dissertation, City University of New York.

Wood, Sam, dir. 1949. *The Stratton Story.* Beverly Hills, CA: Metro-Goldwyn-Mayer.

Woolf, Steven, Robert E. Johnson, Robert L. Phillips, Jr., and Maike Philipsen. 2007. "Giving Everyone the Health of the Educated: An Examination of Whether Social Change Would Save More Lives than Medical Advances." *American Journal of Public Health* 97:679–683.

World Health Organization. 2010. Preamble to the Constitution of the World Health Organization. Adopted by the International Health Conference. New York, 19–22 June 1946; signed on 22 July 1946 by the representatives of 61 States and entered into force on 7 April 1948. Official Records of the World Health Organization, no. 2.

———. 2011. "Depression." www.who.int/topics/depression/en. Accessed July 8, 2011.

Worldwide HIV and AIDS Statistics. www.avert.org/worldstats.htm. Accessed July 15, 2011.

Worsley, Wallace, dir. 1920. *The Penalty.* Fort Lee, NJ: Goldwyn Pictures.

———, dir. 1923. *The Hunchback of Notre Dame.* Universal City, CA: Universal Pictures.

"Writes in Defense of Lincoln's Wife." 1935, March 2. *New York Times,* 17.

Wyler, William, dir. 1946. *The Best Years of Our Lives.* New York: RKO Radio Pictures; Beverly Hills, CA: Metro-Goldwyn-Mayer.

The X Files. 1994–2002. Television series. Chris Carter, director. Beverly Hills, CA: 20th Century Fox Television.

Xyrichis, Andreas, and Emma Ream. 2008. "Teamwork: A Concept Analysis." *Journal of Advanced Nursing* 61:232–241.

Yamamoto, Kaoru. 1971, March. "To Be Different." *Rehabilitation Counseling Bulletin* 14 (3): 180–189.

Yancey, Kitty Bean. 2011, February 10. "British Woman Dies after Botched Butt 'Enhancement' in a Hotel." *USA Today.* http://travel.usatoday.com/destinations/dispatches/post/2011/02/british-woman-dies-after-botched-butt-implant-in-a-hotel/142353/1.

Yoder v. Wisconsin. 1972. 406 US 205 (Supreme Court of the United States).

Young, Hugh Hampton. 1937. *Genital Abnormalities, Hermaphroditism, and Related Adrenal Diseases.* Baltimore: Williams & Wilkins.

Zaki, Jamil. 2011, January 19. "What, Me Care? Young Are Less Empathetic: A Recent Study Finds a Decline in Empathy among Young People in the U.S." *Scientific American Mind.* www.scientificamerican.com/article.cfm?id=what-me-care.

Zemeckis, Robert, dir. 1994. *Forrest Gump.* Hollywood, CA: Paramount Pictures.

Zhan, Chunliu, and Marlene R. Miller. 2003. "Excess Length of Stay, Charges, and Mortality Attributable to Medical Injuries during Hospitalization." *Journal of the American Medical Association* 290:1868–1874.

Ziegler, Philip. 1971. *The Black Death.* New York: Harper Perennial.

Zinnemann, Fred, dir. 1950. *The Men.* Beverly Hills, CA: United Artists.

Zussman, Robert. 1992. *Intensive Care: Medical Ethics and the Medical Profession.* Chicago: University of Chicago Press.

NOTES ON CONTRIBUTORS

JULIE M. AULTMAN, Ph.D., is an associate professor of family and community medicine at Northeast Ohio Medical University in Rootstown.

RAYMOND C. BARFIELD, M.D., Ph.D., is an associate professor of pediatrics and Christian philosophy at Duke University in Durham, North Carolina.

JAY BARUCH, M.D., is an associate professor of emergency medicine, director of the Program in Clinical Arts and Humanities, co-director of Medical Humanities and Bioethics Scholarly Concentration, Alpert Medical School at Brown University in Providence, Rhode Island.

CATHERINE BELLING, Ph.D., is an associate professor of medical humanities and bioethics at Feinberg School of Medicine, Northwestern University in Chicago, Illinois.

JEFFREY P. BISHOP, M.D., Ph.D., is a professor of philosophy and health care ethics, Tenet Endowed Chair in Health Care Ethics, and director, Albert Gnaegi Center for Health Care Ethics at St. Louis University in Missouri.

MICHAEL BLACKIE, Ph.D., is an associate professor of family and community medicine at Northeast Ohio Medical University in Rootstown.

ALAN BLEAKLEY, D.Phil., PGDip, PGCert, DipIDHP, BSc (Hons), FAcadMedEd, is a professor of medical education and medical humanities, Collaboration for the Advancement of Medical Education Research and Assessment (CAMERA) at University of Plymouth Peninsula Medical School in Cornwall, United Kingdom.

HOWARD BRODY, M.D., Ph.D., is the John P. McGovern Centennial Chair in Family Medicine and director, Institute for the Medical Humanities, at the University of Texas Medical Branch in Galveston.

RAFAEL CAMPO, M.A., M.D., D.Litt. (Hon.), is an associate professor of medicine, Harvard Medical School; director, Office of Multicultural Affairs; and director, Katherine Swan Ginsburg Humanism in Medicine Program at Beth Israel Deaconess Medical Center in Boston, Massachusetts.

GRETCHEN A. CASE, Ph.D., is an assistant professor, Division of Medical Ethics and Humanities, Departments of Internal Medicine and Pediatrics, at University of Utah School of Medicine in Salt Lake City.

TOD CHAMBERS, Ph.D., is an associate professor of medical humanities and bioethics and director, Medical Humanities and Bioethics Program, Feinberg School of Medicine at Northwestern University in Chicago, Illinois.

MARK CLARK, Ph.D., is an assistant professor and director of the Graduate Program, Institute for the Medical Humanities at the University of Texas Medical Branch in Galveston.

FELICIA COHN, Ph.D., is bioethics director at Kaiser Permanente Orange County in Orange County, California, and a clinical professor at the School of Medicine at University of California, Irvine.

THOMAS R. COLE, Ph.D., is a professor at the School of Medicine, the McGovern Chair in Medical Humanities, and founding director of the McGovern Center for Humanities and Ethics at University of Texas Medical School in Houston.

JACK COULEHAN, M.D., is an emeritus professor of medicine and senior fellow, Center for Medical Humanities, Compassionate Care, and Bioethics at Stony Brook University in New York.

SAYANTANI DASGUPTA, M.D., M.P.H., is an assistant clinical professor of pediatrics; faculty, Master's Program in Narrative Medicine; and co-chair, University Seminar in Narrative, Health, and Social Justice at Columbia University in New York, New York.

ALICE DREGER, Ph.D., is a professor of clinical medical humanities and bioethics, Medical Humanities and Bioethics Program, Feinberg School of Medicine at Northwestern University in Chicago, Illinois.

DAVID H. FLOOD, Ph.D., is a professor, College of Nursing and Health Professions, and ombudsman at Drexel University in Philadelphia, Pennsylvania.

ARTHUR W. FRANK, Ph.D., is professor emeritus in the Department of Sociology at University of Calgary in Alberta, Canada.

LESTER D. FRIEDMAN, Ph.D., is a professor and chair of the Media and Society Program at Hobart and William Smith Colleges in Geneva, New York.

REBECCA GARDEN, Ph.D., is an associate professor of bioethics and humanities at Upstate Medical University in Syracuse, New York.

SANDER L. GILMAN, Ph.D., is Distinguished Professor of the Liberal Arts and Sciences and professor of psychiatry at Emory University in Atlanta, Georgia.

DANIEL GOLDBERG, J.D., Ph.D., is an assistant professor, Department of Bioethics and Interdisciplinary Studies, Brody School of Medicine at East Carolina University in Greenville, North Carolina.

MAREN GRAINGER-MONSEN, MD, is director, Program in Bioethics and Film, and filmmaker-in-residence, Stanford University Center for Biomedical Ethics, School of Medicine at Stanford University in California.

AMY HADDAD, Ph.D., is a professor and the Dr. C. C. and Mabel L. Criss Endowed Chair in the Health Sciences, and director, Center for Health Policy and Ethics, at Creighton University in Omaha, Nebraska.

BERNICE L. HAUSMAN, Ph.D., is the Edward S. Diggs Professor of Humanities in the department of English at Virginia Tech, in Blacksburg, Virginia, and professor at Virginia Tech Carillon School of Medicine in Roanoke.

REBECCA HESTER, M.A., Ph.D., is an assistant professor of social medicine in the Institute for the Medical Humanities, Department of Preventive Medicine and Community Health, the University of Texas Medical Branch in Galveston.

MARTHA STODDARD HOLMES, Ph.D., is a professor of literature and writing studies at California State University in San Marcos.

LISA I. IEZZONI, M.D., M.Sc., is a professor of medicine, Harvard Medical School, and director, Mongan Institute for Health Policy at Massachusetts General Hospital in Boston.

ANNE HUDSON JONES, Ph.D., is a professor and Harris L. Kempner Chair in the Humanities in Medicine, Institute for the Medical Humanities at the University of Texas Medical Branch in Galveston.

THERESE JONES, Ph.D., is an associate professor, Department of Medicine, and director, Arts and Humanities in Healthcare Program, Center for Bioethics and Humanities at University of Colorado Anschutz Medical Campus in Aurora.

E. ANN KAPLAN, Ph.D., is Distinguished Professor of English and Cultural Analysis and Theory and director, The Humanities Institute at Stony Brook University, New York.

ALLISON B. KAVEY, Ph.D., is an associate professor in the History Department at John Jay College of Criminal Justice and CUNY Graduate Center, at City University of New York in New York.

LISA KERÄNEN, Ph.D., is an associate professor and director of Graduate Studies, Department of Communication, at University of Colorado in Denver.

ERIN GENTRY LAMB, Ph.D., is director of the Center for Literature and Medicine and an assistant professor of biomedical humanities at Hiram College in Ohio.

JOHN LANTOS, M.D., is a professor of pediatrics at the University of Missouri–Kansas City, and director of the Children's Mercy Bioethics Center at Children's Mercy Hospitals and Clinics in Kansas City, Missouri.

MARJORIE LEVINE-CLARK, Ph.D., is an associate professor of history and associate dean for planning and initiatives in the College of Liberal Arts and Sciences at University of Colorado in Denver.

BRAD LEWIS, M.D., Ph.D., is an associate professor, Gallatin School of Individualized Study at New York University in New York.

JONATHAN M. METZL, M.D., Ph.D., is the Frederick B. Rentschler II Professor of Sociology, Psychiatry, and Medicine and director, Program in Medicine, Health, and Society at Vanderbilt University in Nashville, Tennessee.

MARTHA MONTELLO, Ph.D., is an associate professor, School of Medicine, at University of Kansas in Kansas City.

JEFF NISKER, M.D., Ph.D., FRCSC, FCAHS, is a professor in the Department of Obstetrics and Gynaecology and past coordinator of Health Ethics and Humanities, Schulich School of Medicine & Dentistry at Western University in London, Ontario, Canada.

MARTIN F. NORDEN, Ph.D., is a professor and associate chair of the Department of Communication at University of Massachusetts in Amherst.

ALLAN PETERKIN, M.D., FRCP, is an associate professor of psychiatry and family medicine and head, Health, Arts, and Humanities Program at University of Toronto in Ontario, Canada.

MICHAEL ROWE, Ph.D., is associate professor of psychiatry, School of Medicine at Yale University in New Haven, Connecticut.

MICHAEL SAPPOL, Ph.D., is historian, History of Medicine Division at National Library of Medicine in Bethesda, Maryland.

BENJAMIN SAXTON is a postdoctoral research fellow, McGovern Center for Humanities and Ethics at University of Texas Health Science Center in Houston.

LUCY SELMAN, B.A., M.Phil., Ph.D., is a Cicely Saunders International Faculty Scholar at King's College London, Cicely Saunders Institute, the Department of Palliative Care, Policy, and Rehabilitation, United Kingdom.

AUDREY SHAFER, M.D., is a professor of anesthesiology, School of Medicine, Stanford University, and Veteran Affairs Palo Alto Health Care System, and director of the Arts, Humanities and Medicine Program, Stanford Center for Biomedical Ethics at Stanford University in Palo Alto, California.

RHONDA L. SORICELLI, M.D., is an adjunct assistant professor, Department of Family, Community, and Preventive Medicine, Division of Medical Humanities, College of Medicine at Drexel University in Philadelphia, Pennsylvania.

SUSAN M. SQUIER, Ph.D., is the Brill Professor of Women's Studies and English at Penn State University in University Park, Pennsylvania.

JOSEPH N. STRAUS, Ph.D., is Distinguished Professor of Music, Graduate Center at the City University of New York in New York.

ROSEMARIE TONG, Ph.D., is Distinguished Professor of Healthcare Ethics at University of North Carolina in Charlotte.

MARK VONNEGUT, MD, is a pediatrician in Quincy, Massachusetts.

SHELLEY WALL, AOCAD, MScBMC, Ph.D., is an assistant professor, Biomedical Communications at University of Toronto in Ontario, Canada.

DELESE WEAR, Ph.D., is a professor of family and community medicine at Northeast Ohio Medical University in Rootstown.

IAN WILLIAMS, MA, MB, BCh, MRCGP, DA, is a comics artist, physician, and Honorary Clinical Lecturer at University of Manchester School of Medicine, United Kingdom.

JERALD WINAKUR, M.D., M.A.C.P., is a clinical professor of medicine, Center for Medical Humanities and Ethics at University of Texas Health Science Center in San Antonio, Texas.

PAUL ROOT WOLPE, Ph.D., is the Asa Griggs Candler Professor of Bioethics; Raymond F. Schinazi Distinguished Research Chair in Jewish Bioethics; and director, Center for Ethics at Emory University in Atlanta, Georgia.

INDEX

References to illustrations are in italics.

A1896 stop mutation, hepatitis B, 414
Aarons, Victoria, 294n.11
Abiomed Corporation, 116
able-bodied people: fearful of death and damage, 87; playing disabled characters, 94–95
ableism, assumptions and prejudices of, 93, 135
abortion: American debate over, 186; and Down syndrome, 496; of fetuses tested positive for genetic diseases, 163; first-trimester, 165; and pregnant women, popular hostility toward, 187
absolute pitch, 79, 80, 86n.3, 163
access, by the disabled, 93; bias influencing built environment, 129
accompaniment, and mutuality, 259
Accordino, Robert, 39, 46
achondroplasia, genetic screening for predisposition to, 492
"active listening," 22
active seeing, 506
activism, social, 66, 252–253
Actors' Equity Association, 95
"adapted" *vs.* "core" self, 297, 301
Adoche, Chimamanda, 253
Adorno, Theodor, 510
adulthood, emerging, 499, 500n.4
advance directives (ADs), 107, 108, 110, 365
Aesculapius, 244
aesthetic approach, to teaching literature and medicine, 3
aesthetic labor, 505
aesthetics: and the male gaze, 167; medical, 505; of resistance, 505, 508
affect, *vs.* emotion, 298
African Americans: and devaluation of blackness, 158; likely to be undertreated for pain, 146; and schizophrenia (*see* schizophrenia); susceptibility to diseases, 271; and white physicians, 145
ageism, 285; internalized by the aging, 292

agency: of children, 129; sexual and political, of the disabled, 67, 70, 73
age studies, 66
aging: in Christian writers of antiquity, 287, 288; and modernity, 289; pagan philosophers on, 287–288
Ai Weiwei, 501
alchemy, 420
Alcoff, Linda, 255
alcohol contamination, and the fetus, 195n.1
alienation, 34; of the chronically ill, 28, 29–31; imposed by caregivers, 35n.4
"aliveness," *vs.* "life," 189
alpha-antitrypis deficiency, 155
Altavilla, Gina M. LeVasseur, 72, 75n.10
alterity, 135; of the fetus, 193; of pain, 291; of pregnancy, 194. *See also* the Other
Alvarez, Walter C., 321
Alzheimer's disease, 8, 295–296, 498; genetic screening for predisposition to, 492; increase in death rate from, 296; persistence of the self in, 303n.1; short- *vs.* long-term memory, 298
"Alzheimer's narrative," 301
ambiguity: created by arts and humanities, 505; in ethical challenges, 493, 494; of inhabiting opposite point of view, 498
American Federation of Television & Radio Artists, 95
American Music Therapy Association, 77
American Pastoral (Roth), 294n.2
Americans with Disabilities Act (ADA), 97–99, 257
amniocentesis, 189
Andrews, Kari, 163
Andrews, Lori B., 163–164
androgens, 208
Andromeda, mythological princess, 413, 417
"Andromeda Strain" as trope, 414–416
The Andromeda Strain (Crichton novel), 410–411, 412, 413–414, 416

Marshall, David, 425

Martin, Emily, 233

Mass Hysteria: Medicine, Culture, and Mothers' Bodies (Kukla), 190, 191–193

Massumi, Brian, 298

mastery, lack of, 509

masturbation, 217, 218, 221, 223, 228

material possessions, end-of-life distribution of, 21

maternity: alternative norm of, 188; and subjectivity, 191

Mather, Cotton, 439

Maudsley, Henry, 217

Maugham, William Somerset, 243

May, William F., 139

Mayflower gene pool, 160

McCloud, Scott, 230

McHugh, Heather, 33

McInnerny, Tim, 93–94

McKenny, Gerald, 377

McRuer, Robert, 72

Me, Myself, and Irene (film), 95

meaning: against backdrop of mortality and lack of control, 385; of life, 479; multiple, ritual symbols' capacity to express, 372; private, in autism, 80 (*see also* private associations); search for, 404; spiritual sources of, 390

meaning-centered therapy, 381, 391

meaninglessness, 390

measurable outcomes, 6

mécanique céleste and *mécanique sociale*, 392

Les Médecins sans Frontières, 440

media: engagement of medical themes by, 38; filtering of reality through, 87; and "medical mystery," 42–43; and Morgellons disease, 40

medical aesthetics, 505

Medical Apartheid (Washington), 262

medical care, delivery of, *vs.* pursuit of health, 7. *See also* care

medical education, 514; aesthetic and moral-reflection approaches to, 3; and empathy, 3; and fault line in medical culture, 508; "intellectually underemployed" scholars drawn to, 2; undergraduate, and patient safety agenda, 502–503

medical errors, 501–502, 507; in medication, 508

medical gaze, 505; democratization of, 506–507, 508

medical history, *see* history, medical

The Medical History (Roth), *see Everyman* (Roth novel)

medical home, 138–139; humanities perspective, 146–148

medical humanities, 136n.3; as aesthetic resistance movement, 508; Clouser's 1980 keynote address, 1, 2–3; and community psychiatry, 337–340; and ethics, 338–339, 479, 483–484; as field within "body studies," 66; *vs.* "health humanities," 504; terminological shift to *health humanities*, 6. *See also* health humanities

medical imaging, 171–172

medical imperialism, 507. *See also* autocracy

medicalization: of deafness, 135; of disability, 135; of female life stages, 135

medical model of disability, 88; *vs.* disability studies, 64–66; dominates TV doctor shows, 71; and music, 77–78

"medical mystery," 41, 42–43, 48

medical publications, Morgellons *vs.* delusional parasitosis in, 44–46

medical soap operas, 507

medication: antidepressant, 316–317; antipsychotic, 46, 265; clinical trials, 279–280; errors in, 508; lithium, and the visualization of color, 313–314; psychotropic, 327. *See also* clinical trials

medicine: autocratic, 501–502; biomedical model, 127, 128; biopsychosocial model, 140; biopsychosociospiritual, 394; culturally embedded, 225; democratic, and the humanities, 508–510; "evidence-based modern," 48; feminist histories of, 215–216, 222–225; gay men "passing" in, 247; and health, rhetoric of, 37; instrumental view of, 165–168; medical-school history of, and omission of women's contributions, 244; narrative, 490; occupational, on-the-job "expertise" in, 149–152; perceived as arrogant and without accountability, 507; psychosomatic, 140; role of, in mediating divine will, 439; systems informing ideologies of sexuality and gender, 216; as theoretical system, effect of disease on, 431. *See also* biomedicine

"Meditations of an Anesthesiologist" (Shafer), 403–404

meekness, of people with disabilities, 89

Meeting the Universe Halfway (Barad), 184–185

Mehlman, Maxwell, 169–170

Meisel, Alan, 367

melancholy, 317. *See also* depression